AF823185

Science in Nursing and Health Care

Visit the *Science in Nursing and Health* Companion Website at **www.routledge.com/9780131869028** to find valuable **student** learning material including:

- Multiple choice questions on each chapter to help test your learning
- Annotated links to relevant sites on the web
- An Online glossary to explain key terms
- Practical Scenarios with reflective questions to help apply your knowledge to your everyday clinical practice.

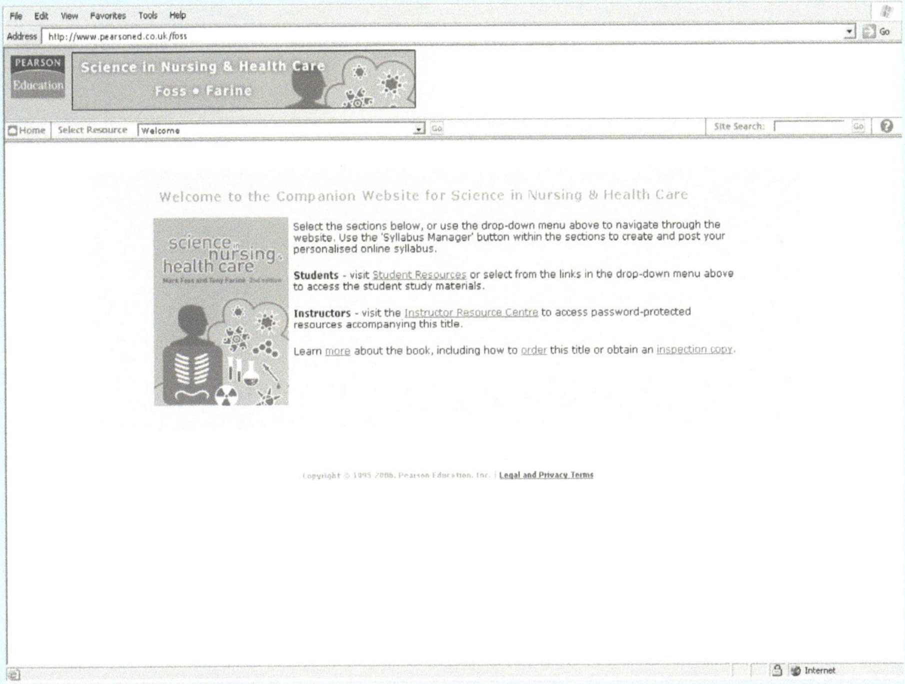

Related titles

Galbraith et al., *Fundamentals of Pharmacology: An Applied Approach for Nursing and Health*

Maltby, Day & Williams, *An Introduction to Statistics for Nurses*

Hawley (editor), *Ethics in Clinical Practice: An Inter-Professional Approach*

Kozier et al., *Fundamentals of Nursing*

Second Edition

Science in Nursing and Health Care

Mark Foss and Tony Farine

Routledge
Taylor & Francis Group
LONDON AND NEW YORK

First published 2000 by Pearson Education Limited
Second edition published 2007

Published 2013 by Routledge
2 Park Square, Milton Park, Abingdon, Oxfordshire OX14 4RN
711 Third Avenue, New York, NY 10017, USA

First issued in hardback 2014

Routledge is an imprint of the Taylor & Francis Group, an informa business

Copyright © 2007, Taylor & Francis.

The rights of Mark Foss and Tony Farine to be identified as authors of this work have been asserted by them in accordance with the Copyright, Designs and Patents Act 1988.

All rights reserved. No part of this book may be reprinted or reproduced or utilised in any form or by any electronic, mechanical, or other means, now known or hereafter invented, including photocopying and recording, or in any information storage or retrieval system, without permission in writing from the publishers.

Notices
Knowledge and best practice in this field are constantly changing. As new research and experience broaden our understanding, changes in research methods, professional practices, or medical treatment may become necessary.

Practitioners and researchers must always rely on their own experience and knowledge in evaluating and using any information, methods, compounds, or experiments described herein. In using such information or methods they should be mindful of their own safety and the safety of others, including parties for whom they have a professional responsibility.

To the fullest extent of the law, neither the Publisher nor the authors, contributors, or editors, assume any liability for any injury and/or damage to persons or property as a matter of products liability, negligence or otherwise, or from any use or operation of any methods, products, instructions, or ideas contained in the material herein.

ISBN 13: 978-1-138-83686-0 (hbk)
ISBN 13: 978-0-13-186902-8 (pbk)

British Library Cataloguing-in-Publication Data
A catalogue record for this book is available from the British Library

Library of Congress Cataloging-in-Publication Data
A catalog record for this book is available from the Library of Congress

Typeset in 9/13 Interstate Light by 35

Contents

Preface ix
Guided tour xii
Publisher's acknowledgements xv

1 Expressing numbers and SI units **1**

Learning outcomes 1
Introduction 2
Expressing numbers 2
Scientific notation 2
Numerical prefixes 3
SI units 4
Summary 6

2 Homeostasis: keeping the body in balance **7**

Learning outcomes 7
Introduction 8
The internal environment 8
Homeostasis 10
Homeostatic control mechanisms 10
Nursing care and homeostasis 12
Summary 13

3 The physical world and basic chemistry **15**

Learning outcomes 15
Introduction 16
States of matter 16
Atoms and elements 16
The Periodic Table 18
Compounds 19
The structure of the atom 20
Chemical bonds 25
Structural formulae 32
Molecular mass 33
The mole 33
Chemical reactions 35
The carbon atom and organic chemistry 44
Summary 51
Self-test questions 52

4 Water, electrolytes and body fluids **55**

Learning outcomes 55
Introduction 56
Water 58
Cohesion and adhesion 61
Aqueous mixtures 65
Electrolytes and non-electrolytes 70
The concept of concentration 72
Diffusion and osmosis 75
Filtration 85
The distribution of water within the body 86
Specialised body fluids 89
The regulation of fluid balance within the body 90
Specific gravity 92
Dialysis 93
Summary 95
Self-test questions 96
Further study/exercises 98

5 Acids, bases and pH balance **99**

Learning outcomes 99
Introduction 100
Acids 101
Bases 102
Properties of acids and bases 103

Measuring acidity 104
Salts as acids and bases 106
Acid-base balance 106
Acid-base imbalance 112
Summary 118
Self-test questions 118
Further study/exercises 120

6 Pressure, fluids, gases and breathing 121

Learning outcomes 121
Introduction 122
Atmospheric pressure 124
Pressure in static liquids 130
Blood flow 133
Gases and breathing 138
Gases in solution and their movement 143
Oxygen therapy 146
Summary 150
Self-test questions 151
Further study/exercises 153

7 Biological molecules and food 155

Learning outcomes 155
Introduction 156
Diet and food 156
Carbohydrates 156
Proteins 161
Lipids 166
Vitamins 172
Minerals 177
Fibre (roughage/non-starch polysaccharide) 180
Summary 181
Self-test questions 182
Further study/exercises 184

8 Energy in the body 185

Learning outcomes 185
Introduction 186
The conservation of energy 188
Units of energy 189
The ATP molecule 192
The energy-liberating reactions of cells 194
Overview of carbohydrate catabolism 195
Fat catabolism 197
Protein catabolism 198
Basal metabolic rate 198
Summary 199
Self-test questions 200
Further study/exercises 202

9 Heat and body temperature 203

Learning outcomes 203
Introduction 204
Heat and temperature 204
Latent heat and changes in state 205
Temperature scales 206
Temperature-measurement devices 207
Body temperature 209
Cyclical variations in body temperature 214
The transmission of heat 214
Temperature homeostasis 220
Thermoregulation abnormalities 221
Other uses of heat and cold 226
Summary 226
Self-test questions 227
Further study/exercises 229

10 Force, mechanics and biomechanics 231

Learning outcomes 231
Introduction 232
Speed and velocity 232
Acceleration 233
Mass and weight 233
Momentum 234
Force 234
Newton's laws of motion 236
The force of gravity 239
Stability 244

Levers 245
Pulleys 249
Vectors 249
Summary 251
Self-test questions 252
Further study/exercises 254

11 Electricity, magnetism and medical equipment **255**

Learning outcomes 255
Introduction 256
Magnetism 256
Electricity 259
Current flow 262
Electrocution 263
Electricity in the body 267
Important items of medical equipment 274
Summary 280
Self-test questions 280
Further study/exercises 282

12 Light and vision **283**

Learning outcomes 283
Introduction 284
Transverse waves 284
The electromagnetic spectrum 285
The properties of light 287
Lenses 290
How do we see? 296
Optical instruments 298
Ultraviolet radiation 303
Summary 307
Self-test questions 308
Further study/exercises 309

13 Sound and hearing **311**

Learning outcomes 311
Introduction 312
Sound 312
Ultrasound and the piezoelectric effect 322
The Doppler effect 323
Summary 325
Self-test questions 325
Further study/exercises 327

14 Radiation in diagnosis and treatment **329**

Learning outcomes 329
Introduction 330
The nature of ionising radiation 330
Radioactivity and radioactive decay 331
The concept of half-life 333
The effects of ionising radiation 336
The measurement of radiation 338
Summary 342
Self-test questions 343
Further study/exercises 345

15 Genetics in health and illness **347**

Learning outcomes 347
Introduction 348
The nucleus of the cell 348
DNA: the genetic code 350
DNA replication 352
Mitosis and the cell cycle 353
Meiosis 355
Protein synthesis 357
Genetic inheritance 360
Genetic disease 364
Summary 369
Self-test questions 370
Further study/exercises 372

16 Microbiology **373**

Learning outcomes 373
Introduction 374
Naming microorganisms 374
Bacteria 375
Viruses 378
Fungi 380
Protozoa 380
Host-microorganism relationships 384
The response to infection 387

Virulence 392
Sources of infection 394
Microbiology samples 403
Microbiological tests 407
The microbiology laboratory 408
Cleaning, disinfection and sterilisation 411
Treating infections 414
Summary 418
Self-test questions 419
Further study/exercises 421

Answers to self-test questions 423
Appendix: The Periodic Table 425
Glossary 426
Index 465

Supporting resources

Visit **www.routledge.com/9780131869028** to find valuable online resources

Companion Website for students

- Multiple choice questions on each chapter to help test your learning
- Annotated links to relevant sites on the web
- An Online glossary to explain key terms
- Practical Scenarios with reflective questions to help apply your knowledge to your everyday clinical practice.

For instructors

- Downloadable PowerPoint slides of section summaries and figures in the book
- Practical Scenario suggestions for class discussions

Also: The Companion Website provides the following features:

- Search tool to help locate specific items of content
- E-mail results and profile tools to send results of quizzes to instructors
- Online help and support to assist with website usage and troubleshooting

Preface

This second edition of *Science in Nursing and Health Care* has been written with the aim of introducing readers to aspects of basic science that inform a number of health-care disciplines. The authors are involved in the teaching of science to nursing students at a British university and the text is primarily intended for use by those studying nursing at diploma and undergraduate levels. However, the general nature of the material means that other health-care students may find the text of use, including those studying midwifery, physiotherapy, occupational therapy and dietetics. The expanding number of professionals involved in health care means that this book may also find its way on to the shelves of operating-department assistants, perfusionists and paramedics.

How topics are approached

Topics covered in this text are also dealt with in a variety of other sources. For example, the concept of homeostasis is described widely in physiology texts, acids and bases in science texts and mechanical force in physics texts. The particular contribution this book makes is to bring together in one text diverse topic areas. Furthermore, the content of each chapter is also given a context. For example, acids and bases are not described in isolation but are discussed in the context of the acid-base balance of the body and electromagnetic radiation is placed in the context of diagnosis and treatment.

The aim of the authors is to produce a text that is accurate and thorough, while at the same time integrating science with the nursing context. The assumption made is that as far as the physical care of individuals is concerned, the prescription of appropriate nursing interventions depends upon a thorough understanding of physical problems. This means that nurses caring for physically ill patients must make reference to anatomy, physiology and pathology. A problem arises when students lack knowledge of basic science, and this prevents them from developing a better understanding of the function of the body in health and illness and thus of nursing care too. It is intended that this text will help students to deal with this problem. In the completion of this second edition, the text was reviewed widely by teachers of science to nurses. This led to revisions of each of the chapters in an attempt to relate the material even more closely to the needs of student nurses. Some chapters have been expanded and others reduced. For example, more information about the nervous system has been included in Chapter 11, Electricity and magnetism, while the material contained in Chapter 8, Energy in the body, has been simplified. There are two additional chapters - Expressing numbers and SI units has been removed from the appendix and now forms Chapter 1, while a chapter on Microbiology has been added as Chapter 16.

How this book is organised

The text is divided into 16 chapters. Although it is possible to read this book from cover to cover, it is expected that students will usually dip into chapters as particular questions arise in their studies. Consequently, as far as possible, each chapter stands alone. However, information covered in one chapter is not repeated in another. For this reason, it makes sense to read Chapter 3, The physical world and basic chemistry, before Chapter 5, Acids, bases and pH balance.

Each chapter begins with a list of learning outcomes, and you may wish to think about these both before and after reading a chapter. Throughout, text questions appear in *italics*. These are intended to provoke thought as you read. When you come across such a question, pause for a moment and think about the answer. If you are unsure about the correct response, do not worry: the answer is given immediately below the question. However, do get into the habit of attempting to answer these questions before moving on. Periodically, and especially in the longer chapters, the content is reviewed in boxed sections called in-text reviews. When you reach one such feature, ponder each point in turn. Make sure that you understand it before moving on. If you do not, it may be helpful to go back and read the relevant section again. You will find that the text is a practical one in which science and health care are linked closely. Some aspects, however, are of a particularly practical nature and appear in boxed sections called practice points. In addition, chapter summaries help you to reflect on the information covered, and these are followed by a number of self-test questions. The correct answers are also given, but it is clearly a good idea to attempt the questions before looking at the correct responses. Three types of question are used:

Simple multiple choice questions

Simply choose the correct response from a short list of possible answers. For example:

1 Which one of the following is considered to be a normal systolic blood pressure in mmHg?
  (a) 12.
  (b) 120.
  (c) 8.
  (d) 80.

The correct answer is b.

True/false questions

Identify which of a list of statements are true. There is no fixed number of true statements, but at least one statement will be true. For example:

1 Which of the following statements are true?
  (a) Light is a transverse wave.
  (b) Sound is a transverse wave.
  (c) Sound is a mechanical wave.
  (d) Light is an electromagnetic wave.

In this case, a, c and d are true.

Matching-pairs questions

These questions consist of two short lists. The items in each list have to be matched. For example:

1 Match the substances on the left with the appropriate descriptions on the right.

(a) Na	(i) An ion
(b) CO_2	(ii) An atom
(c) NaCl	(iii) A covalent compound
(d) HCO_3^-	(iv) An ionic compound

The above match in the following way:

(a) (ii)

(b) (iii)

(c) (iv)

(d) (i)

At the end of each chapter there are also further study questions/exercises with references. You may not always have the time to complete these at once, but keep it in mind to return to them when time allows. You will find that the questions asked are often of a practical nature, and the references make interesting reading.

Summary of key features

- A practical text that integrates science and health care.
- Learning outcomes for each chapter.
- Key terms are highlighted.
- Friendly style with thought-provoking questions included in the text.
- Boxed in-text reviews and practice points illustrate important practical applications.
- Chapter summaries.
- Self-test questions at the end of each chapter.
- Further study questions/exercises.

All that now remains is for me to wish you well with your studies.

Mark Foss
Tony Farine
Nottingham, August 2006

Guided tour

Setting the scene

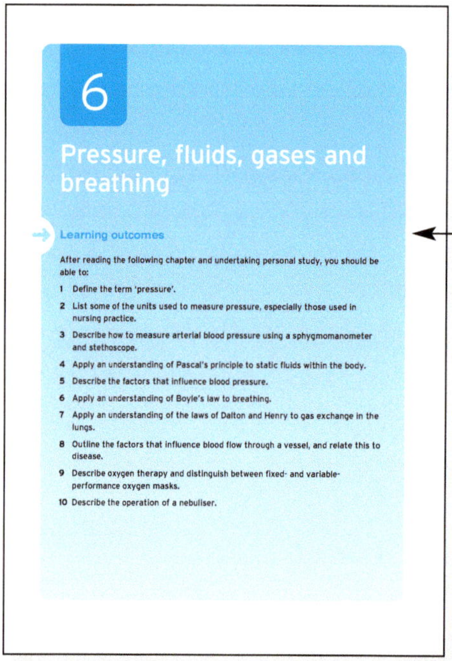

6

Pressure, fluids, gases and breathing

Learning outcomes

After reading the following chapter and undertaking personal study, you should be able to:

1 Define the term 'pressure'.
2 List some of the units used to measure pressure, especially those used in nursing practice.
3 Describe how to measure arterial blood pressure using a sphygmomanometer and stethoscope.
4 Apply an understanding of Pascal's principle to static fluids within the body.
5 Describe the factors that influence blood pressure.
6 Apply an understanding of Boyle's law to breathing.
7 Apply an understanding of the laws of Dalton and Henry to gas exchange in the lungs.
8 Outline the factors that influence blood flow through a vessel, and relate this to disease.
9 Describe oxygen therapy and distinguish between fixed- and variable-performance oxygen masks.
10 Describe the operation of a nebuliser.

Learning outcomes - introduce topics covered and summarises what you should have learnt by the end of the chapter

Chapter introductions - give you an overview of the topics covered in the chapter by drawing on interesting real-life examples to show you how they relate to you everyday practice

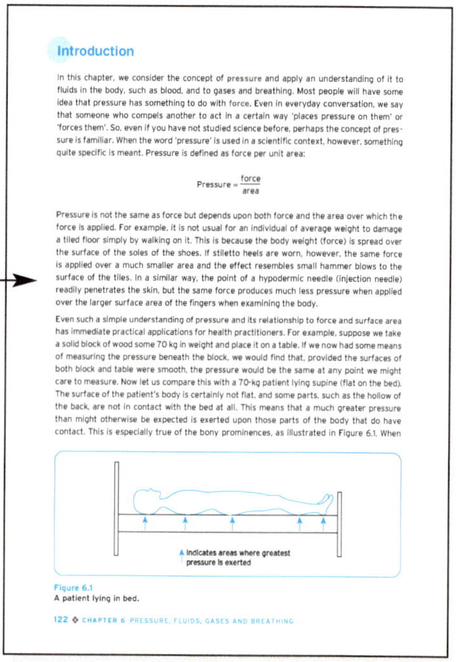

Introduction

In this chapter, we consider the concept of pressure and apply an understanding of it to fluids in the body, such as blood, and to gases and breathing. Most people will have some idea that pressure has something to do with force. Even in everyday conversation, we say that someone who compels another to act in a certain way 'places pressure on them' or 'forces them'. So, even if you have not studied science before, perhaps the concept of pressure is familiar. When the word 'pressure' is used in a scientific context, however, something quite specific is meant. Pressure is defined as force per unit area:

$$\text{Pressure} = \frac{\text{force}}{\text{area}}$$

Pressure is not the same as force but depends upon both force and the area over which the force is applied. For example, it is not usual for an individual of average weight to damage a tiled floor simply by walking on it. This is because the body weight (force) is spread over the surface of the soles of the shoes. If stiletto heels are worn, however, the same force is applied over a much smaller area and the effect resembles small hammer blows to the surface of the tiles. In a similar way, the point of a hypodermic needle (injection needle) readily penetrates the skin, but the same force produces much less pressure when applied over the larger surface area of the fingers when examining the body.

Even such a simple understanding of pressure and its relationship to force and surface area has immediate practical applications for health practitioners. For example, suppose we take a solid block of wood some 70 kg in weight and place it on a table. If we now had some means of measuring the pressure beneath the block, we would find that, provided the surfaces of both block and table were smooth, the pressure would be the same at any point we might care to measure. Now let us compare this with a 70-kg patient lying supine (flat on the bed). The surface of the patient's body is certainly not flat, and some parts, such as the hollow of the back, are not in contact with the bed at all. This means that a much greater pressure than might otherwise be expected is exerted upon those parts of the body that do have contact. This is especially true of the bony prominences, as illustrated in Figure 6.1. When

Indicates areas where greatest pressure is exerted

Figure 6.1
A patient lying in bed.

122 CHAPTER 6 PRESSURE, FLUIDS, GASES AND BREATHING

Helping your understanding and applying your knowledge

In-text reviews – remind you of the key concepts to take away with you from the areas you have just read about

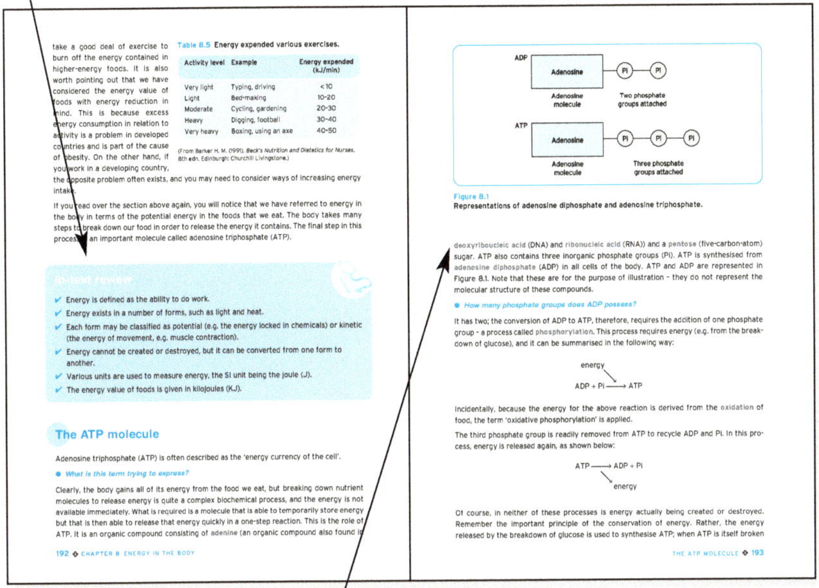

take a good deal of exercise to burn off the energy contained in higher-energy foods. It is also worth pointing out that we have considered the energy value of foods with energy reduction in mind. This is because excess energy consumption in relation to activity is a problem in developed countries and is part of the cause of obesity. On the other hand, if you work in a developing country, the opposite problem often exists, and you may need to consider ways of increasing energy intake.

Table 8.5 Energy expended various exercises.

Activity level	Example	Energy expended (kJ/min)
Very light	Typing, driving	<10
Light	Bed-making	10–20
Moderate	Cycling, gardening	20–30
Heavy	Digging, football	30–40
Very heavy	Boxing, using an axe	40–50

(From Barker H. M. (1991). *Beck's Nutrition and Dietetics for Nurses*, 8th edn. Edinburgh: Churchill Livingstone.)

If you read over the section above again, you will notice that we have referred to energy in the body in terms of the potential energy in the foods that we eat. The body takes many steps to break down our food in order to release the energy it contains. The final step in this process uses an important molecule called adenosine triphosphate (ATP).

In-text review

- Energy is defined as the ability to do work.
- Energy exists in a number of forms, such as light and heat.
- Each form may be classified as potential (e.g. the energy locked in chemicals) or kinetic (the energy of movement, e.g. muscle contraction).
- Energy cannot be created or destroyed, but it can be converted from one form to another.
- Various units are used to measure energy, the SI unit being the joule (J).
- The energy value of foods is given in kilojoules (kJ).

The ATP molecule

Adenosine triphosphate (ATP) is often described as the 'energy currency of the cell'.

- *What is this term trying to express?*

Clearly, the body gains all of its energy from the food we eat, but breaking down nutrient molecules to release energy is quite a complex biochemical process, and the energy is not available immediately. What is required is a molecule that is able to temporarily store energy but that is then able to release that energy quickly in a one-step reaction. This is the role of ATP. It is an organic compound consisting of adenine (an organic compound also found in

192 ◆ CHAPTER 8 ENERGY IN THE BODY

Figure 8.1
Representations of adenosine diphosphate and adenosine triphosphate.

deoxyribonucleic acid (DNA) and ribonucleic acid (RNA)) and a pentose (five-carbon-atom) sugar. ATP also contains three inorganic phosphate groups (Pi). ATP is synthesised from adenosine diphosphate (ADP) in all cells of the body. ATP and ADP are represented in Figure 8.1. Note that these are for the purpose of illustration – they do not represent the molecular structure of these compounds.

- *How many phosphate groups does ADP possess?*

It has two; the conversion of ADP to ATP, therefore, requires the addition of one phosphate group – a process called phosphorylation. This process requires energy (e.g. from the breakdown of glucose), and it can be summarised in the following way:

$$\text{ADP} + \text{Pi} \xrightarrow{\text{energy}} \text{ATP}$$

Incidentally, because the energy for the above reaction is derived from the oxidation of food, the term 'oxidative phosphorylation' is applied.

The third phosphate group is readily removed from ATP to recycle ADP and Pi. In this process, energy is released again, as shown below:

$$\text{ATP} \longrightarrow \text{ADP} + \text{Pi} + \text{energy}$$

Of course, in neither of these processes is energy actually being created or destroyed. Remember the important principle of the conservation of energy. Rather, the energy released by the breakdown of glucose is used to synthesise ATP; when ATP is itself broken

THE ATP MOLECULE ◆ 193

Key terms – are highlighted in the text when they first appear, followed by a brief explanation of their meaning. These are also included in the Glossary section at the back of the book

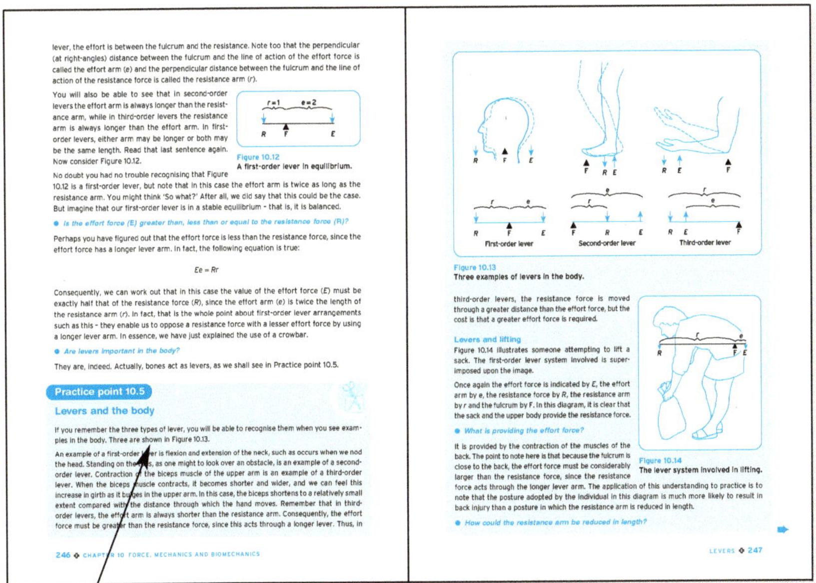

lever, the effort is between the fulcrum and the resistance. Note too that the perpendicular (at right-angles) distance between the fulcrum and the line of action of the effort force is called the effort arm (*e*) and the perpendicular distance between the fulcrum and the line of action of the resistance force is called the resistance arm (*r*).

You will also be able to see that in second-order levers the effort arm is always longer than the resistance arm, while in third-order levers the resistance arm is always longer than the effort arm. In first-order levers, either arm may be longer or both may be the same length. Read that last sentence again. Now consider Figure 10.12.

Figure 10.12
A first-order lever in equilibrium.

No doubt you had no trouble recognising that Figure 10.12 is a first-order lever, but note that in this case the effort arm is twice as long as the resistance arm. You might think 'So what?' After all, we did say that this could be the case. But imagine that our first-order lever is in a stable equilibrium – that is, it is balanced.

- *Is the effort force (E) greater than, less than or equal to the resistance force (R)?*

Perhaps you have figured out that the effort force is less than the resistance force, since the effort force has a longer lever arm. In fact, the following equation is true:

$$Ee = Rr$$

Consequently, we can work out that in this case the value of the effort force (*E*) must be exactly half that of the resistance force (*R*), since the effort arm (*e*) is twice the length of the resistance arm (*r*). In fact, that is the whole point about first-order lever arrangements such as this – they enable us to oppose a resistance force with a lesser effort force by using a longer lever arm. In essence, we have just explained the use of a crowbar.

- *Are levers important in the body?*

They are, indeed. Actually, bones act as levers, as we shall see in Practice point 10.5.

Practice point 10.5
Levers and the body

If you remember the three types of lever, you will be able to recognise them when you see examples in the body. Three are shown in Figure 10.13.

An example of a first-order lever is flexion and extension of the neck, such as occurs when we nod the head. Standing on the toes, as one might to look over an obstacle, is an example of a second-order lever. Contraction of the biceps muscle of the upper arm is an example of a third-order lever. When the biceps muscle contracts, it becomes shorter and wider, and we can feel this increase in girth as it bulges in the upper arm. In this case, the biceps shortens to a relatively small extent compared with the distance through which the hand moves. Remember that in third-order levers, the effort arm is always shorter than the resistance arm. Consequently, the effort force must be greater than the resistance force, since this acts through a longer lever. Thus, in

246 ◆ CHAPTER 10 FORCE, MECHANICS AND BIOMECHANICS

Figure 10.13
Three examples of levers in the body.

third-order levers, the resistance force is moved through a greater distance than the effort force, but the cost is that a greater effort force is required.

Levers and lifting

Figure 10.14 illustrates someone attempting to lift a sack. The first-order lever system involved is superimposed upon the image.

Once again the effort force is indicated by *E*, the effort arm by *e*, the resistance force by *R*, the resistance arm by *r* and the fulcrum by F. In this diagram, it is clear that the sack and the upper body provide the resistance force.

- *What is providing the effort force?*

It is provided by the contraction of the muscles of the back. The point to note here is that because the fulcrum is close to the back, the effort force must be considerably larger than the resistance force, since the resistance force acts through the longer lever arm. The application of this understanding to practice is to note that the posture adopted by the individual in this diagram is much more likely to result in back injury than a posture in which the resistance arm is reduced in length.

Figure 10.14
The lever system involved in lifting.

- *How could the resistance arm be reduced in length?*

LEVERS ◆ 247

Practice points – show how science is applicable to your everyday clinical practice

Helping your understanding and applying your knowledge – continued

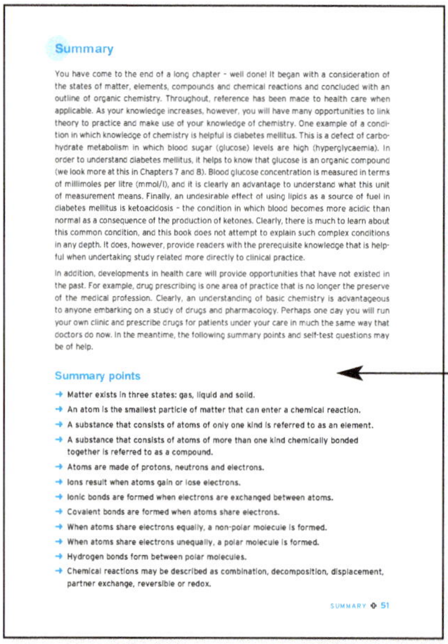

Summary

You have come to the end of a long chapter - well done! It began with a consideration of the states of matter, elements, compounds and chemical reactions and concluded with an outline of organic chemistry. Throughout, reference has been made to health care when applicable. As your knowledge increases, however, you will have many opportunities to link theory to practice and make use of your knowledge of chemistry. One example of a condition in which knowledge of chemistry is helpful is diabetes mellitus. This is a defect of carbohydrate metabolism in which blood sugar (glucose) levels are high (hyperglycaemia). In order to understand diabetes mellitus, it helps to know that glucose is an organic compound (we look more at this in Chapters 7 and 8). Blood glucose concentration is measured in terms of millimoles per litre (mmol/l), and it is clearly an advantage to understand what this unit of measurement means. Finally, an undesirable effect of using lipids as a source of fuel in diabetes mellitus is ketoacidosis - the condition in which blood becomes more acidic than normal as a consequence of the production of ketones. Clearly, there is much to learn about this common condition, and this book does not attempt to explain such complex conditions in any depth. It does, however, provide readers with the prerequisite knowledge that is helpful when undertaking study related more directly to clinical practice.

In addition, developments in health care will provide opportunities that have not existed in the past. For example, drug prescribing is one area of practice that is no longer the preserve of the medical profession. Clearly, an understanding of basic chemistry is advantageous to anyone embarking on a study of drugs and pharmacology. Perhaps one day you will run your own clinic and prescribe drugs for patients under your care in much the same way that doctors do now. In the meantime, the following summary points and self-test questions may be of help.

Summary points

- Matter exists in three states: gas, liquid and solid.
- An atom is the smallest particle of matter that can enter a chemical reaction.
- A substance that consists of atoms of only one kind is referred to as an element.
- A substance that consists of atoms of more than one kind chemically bonded together is referred to as a compound.
- Atoms are made of protons, neutrons and electrons.
- Ions result when atoms gain or lose electrons.
- Ionic bonds are formed when electrons are exchanged between atoms.
- Covalent bonds are formed when atoms share electrons.
- When atoms share electrons equally, a non-polar molecule is formed.
- When atoms share electrons unequally, a polar molecule is formed.
- Hydrogen bonds form between polar molecules.
- Chemical reactions may be described as combination, decomposition, displacement, partner exchange, reversible or redox.

SUMMARY ◆ 51

Chapter summary points - quickly recap and reinforce the key points to take away from the chapter

Self test questions - provide a chance to check your knowledge and understanding of the topics covered in the chapter with answers provided at the back of the book

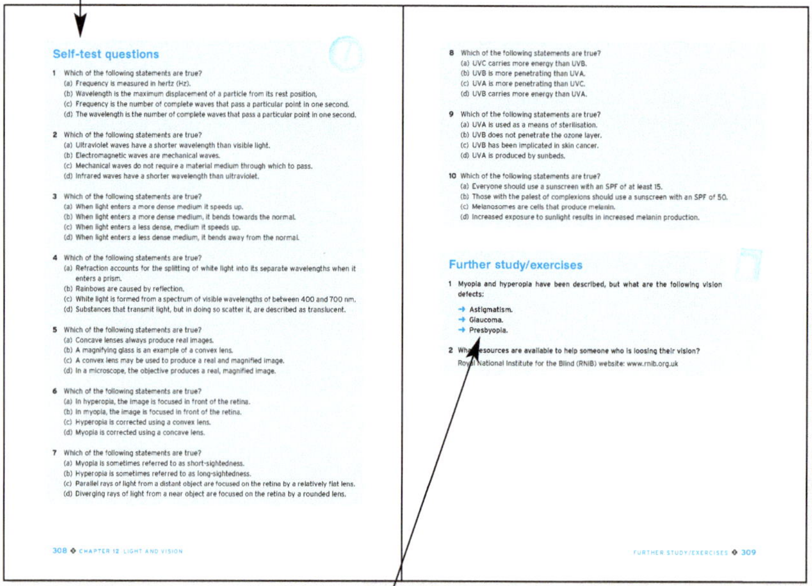

Self-test questions

1 Which of the following statements are true?
(a) Frequency is measured in hertz (Hz).
(b) Wavelength is the maximum displacement of a particle from its rest position,
(c) Frequency is the number of complete waves that pass a particular point in one second.
(d) The wavelength is the number of complete waves that pass a particular point in one second.

2 Which of the following statements are true?
(a) Ultraviolet waves have a shorter wavelength than visible light.
(b) Electromagnetic waves are mechanical waves.
(c) Mechanical waves do not require a material medium through which to pass.
(d) Infrared waves have a shorter wavelength than ultraviolet.

3 Which of the following statements are true?
(a) When light enters a more dense medium it speeds up.
(b) When light enters a more dense medium, it bends towards the normal.
(c) When light enters a less dense, medium it speeds up.
(d) When light enters a less dense medium, it bends away from the normal.

4 Which of the following statements are true?
(a) Refraction accounts for the splitting of white light into its separate wavelengths when it enters a prism.
(b) Rainbows are caused by reflection.
(c) White light is formed from a spectrum of visible wavelengths of between 400 and 700 nm.
(d) Substances that transmit light, but in doing so scatter it, are described as translucent.

5 Which of the following statements are true?
(a) Concave lenses always produce real images.
(b) A magnifying glass is an example of a convex lens.
(c) A convex lens may be used to produce a real and magnified image.
(d) In a microscope, the objective produces a real, magnified image.

6 Which of the following statements are true?
(a) In hyperopia, the image is focused in front of the retina.
(b) In myopia, the image is focused in front of the retina.
(c) Hyperopia is corrected using a convex lens.
(d) Myopia is corrected using a concave lens.

7 Which of the following statements are true?
(a) Myopia is sometimes referred to as short-sightedness.
(b) Hyperopia is sometimes referred to as long-sightedness.
(c) Parallel rays of light from a distant object are focused on the retina by a relatively flat lens.
(d) Diverging rays of light from a near object are focused on the retina by a rounded lens.

308 ◆ CHAPTER 12 LIGHT AND VISION

8 Which of the following statements are true?
(a) UVC carries more energy than UVB.
(b) UVB is more penetrating than UVA.
(c) UVA is more penetrating than UVC.
(d) UVB carries more energy than UVA.

9 Which of the following statements are true?
(a) UVA is used as a means of sterilisation.
(b) UVB does not penetrate the ozone layer.
(c) UVB has been implicated in skin cancer.
(d) UVA is produced by sunbeds.

10 Which of the following statements are true?
(a) Everyone should use a sunscreen with an SPF of at least 15.
(b) Those with the palest of complexions should use a sunscreen with an SPF of 50.
(c) Melanosomes are cells that produce melanin.
(d) Increased exposure to sunlight results in increased melanin production.

Further study/exercises

1 Myopia and hyperopia have been described, but what are the following vision defects:
- Astigmatism.
- Glaucoma.
- Presbyopia.

2 What resources are available to help someone who is loosing their vision?
Royal National Institute for the Blind (RNIB) website: www.rnib.org.uk

FURTHER STUDY/EXERCISES ◆ 309

Further study exercises - provide practical clinical problems that are designed to stimulate further individual investigation

Publisher's acknowledgements

The publisher would like to thank all the reviewers who contributed to the development of this text:

Tony Blacket at the University of Sheffield

Alistair Farley at the University of Dundee

Chris Johnson at Queen's University Belfast

John Knight at Swansea University

Lorraine Carline at Staffordshire University

Patricia Pass at the University of Greenwich

Morag Prowse at the University of Plymouth

We are also grateful to the following for permission to reproduce copyright material:

Figure 7.2 from *The Addison-Wesley Science Handbook for Students, Writers and Science Buffs,* Addison Wesley, Pearson Canada (Coleman & Dewar, 1997); Figure 15.1 from *Longman Study Guides: A-level and AS-level Biology*, Longman, Harlow (Cornwell & Miller, 1997); Figure 15.7 from *Essentials of Human Physiology*, William C. Brown (Sheeler, P. et al., 1996), reproduced with permission of The McGraw-Hill Companies.

In some instances we have been unable to trace the owners of copyright material, and we would appreciate any information that would enable us to do so.

1

Expressing numbers and SI units

Learning outcomes

After reading the following chapter and undertaking personal study, you should be able to:

1 Identify situations in clinical practice in which numerical values are important.

2 Identify the following as two different ways in which numerical values are expressed:
  (a) Scientific notation
  (b) Numerical prefixes.

3 State what is mean by Système Internationale (SI) units.

4 Identify the units of measurement of the following:
  (a) Length
  (b) Mass
  (c) Volume.

5 List situations in clinical practice in which the above units of measurement are used.

Introduction

Most students who chose nursing as a career do so because they are interested in people. They do not necessarily get enthusiastic about mathematics! Nonetheless, being interested in people and being concerned to use numbers correctly certainly do go together. For example, think about the issue of unplanned teenage pregnancy in the UK. Why is it important? Apart from concern for individuals involved, teenage pregnancy in the UK is important because the numbers involved are high compared with those in other European countries. We might now start to think about why this is so, but it is numbers that have triggered our concern. Similarly, we might try to develop a programme to deal with teenage pregnancy, but how would we know whether it was successful? Once again, we come back to numbers. Even the most human, people-centred issues with significant ethical aspects involve numbers at some point. Numbers are also involved in a number of the important day-to-day tasks that nurses undertake. For example, nurses dispense drugs in specific doses, and some nurses prescribe drugs. We adjust the rate at which fluid is flowing in an intravenous infusion (drip) or the energy of the electric shock delivered by a defibrillator used to restart a heart that has stopped beating. In each of these cases, it is of the utmost importance that we get the numbers right. Clearly we do not want to endanger a patient by giving too much of a drug, by overloading the circulation with fluid or by administering a shock of too great an energy. At times, we have to deal with very small numbers such as the dose of some drugs, while at other times the numbers are quite large - energy values of food, for example.

Expressing numbers

When, as nurses, we have a problem with numbers, to whom do we look for help? Perhaps we should turn to people whose main business is numbers. Scientists understand the problems that numbers present, since they have to deal with a very wide range of numerical values. Consider the following two extremes: the earth, which is very large, and the hydrogen atom, which is very small. The mass of each is as follows:

- The earth = 5 980 000 000 000 000 000 000 000 kg.
- The hydrogen atom = 0.000 000 000 000 000 000 000 000 001 674 kg.[1]

The range of values that health-care professionals meet is not quite so wide, but sometimes we do find ourselves writing out a great many zeros. We could write very large or very small numbers in a more convenient way by doing what scientists do - using **scientific notation.**

Scientific notation

Have you ever wondered why we write numbers as we do? In human history, numbers have been written in different ways. For example, the Romans expressed numbers as letters, e.g. I, II, III, IV, V. Fortunately for them, they did not have to deal with something as big as the

[1] Coleman G. J. and Dewar D. (1997). *The Addison-Wesley Science Handbook for Students, Writers and Science Buffs*. Don Mills, Ontario: Addison-Wesley.

earth or as small as an atom. Still today, we sometimes use simple tally systems for counting – for example, making a mark each time a count is made, e.g. I, II, III, IIII. At the count of five, we usually score through a group of four and start again, thus ~~IIII~~; we can then readily add up groups of five. The point is to note that there is more than one way to write numbers, and scientific notation is simply one way to make very large or small numbers easier to record. To change a large number to scientific notation, move the decimal point to the left and place it between the first and second digits. Next, count the number of spaces moved and write this figure as a power of 10.

- ***What does power of 10 mean?***

It is simply a way of showing how many times you moved the decimal point. For example:

→ $100 = 10 \times 10$ or as a power of ten $= 1 \times 10^2$ (or simply 10^2)

→ $1000 = 10 \times 10 \times 10$ or as a power of ten $= 1 \times 10^3$ (or simply 10^3)

Using scientific notation, the mass of the earth becomes 5.98×10^{24} kg.

- ***What about very small numbers?***

To change a small number to scientific notation, move the decimal point to the right and stop immediately after the first digit that is not a zero. To show that you have moved the decimal point to the right, express the power of 10 as a negative value. In this way, the mass of a hydrogen atom becomes 1.674×10^{-27} kg.

- ***Is there not an even more convenient method of expressing very large and very small numbers?***

Indeed there is – we could use **numerical prefixes**.

Numerical prefixes

A prefix is a word that is added before another in order to change its size. Let us take an everyday example. A 'store' is a shop – right? So what, then, is a 'megastore'? Yes – it is a big shop. We can tell it is a big shop from the prefix 'mega', which means big. Actually, 'mega' is a numerical prefix with a precise meaning – it means one million. So, then, numerical prefixes are used to replace powers of 10. We use numerical prefixes all the time; for example, we do not usually say 'two thousand metres' but 'two kilometres'. 'Kilo' is a numerical prefix that means one thousand. We also use prefixes to deal with very small numbers (sub-powers of ten). Let us use an example from our bodies. Instead of writing the diameter of an erythrocyte (red blood cell) as 0.000 008 m (or 8×10^{-6} m), we could use the numerical prefix 'micro', which means one-millionth. Now we say that the erythrocyte has a diameter of eight micrometres (8 μm). Actually, we even simplify that and contract the word micrometres to microns, which is easier to say. Some important prefixes are given in Table 1.1.

Table 1.1 Numerical prefixes.

Powers of ten		
Power	**Prefix**	**Symbol**
10^3	Kilo	k
10^6	Mega	M
Sub-powers of ten		
Power	**Prefix**	**Symbol**
10^{-1}	Deci	d
10^{-2}	Centi	c
10^{-3}	Milli	m
10^{-6}	Micro	μ
10^{-9}	Nano	n

SI units

Let me ask you an unexpected question: 'How are you getting on with euros?' This is not a political question about monetary union. I am simply pointing out that having the same currency in many countries certainly makes things more convenient for the traveller. Of course, it is still quite difficult to change from miles per hour to kilometres per hour, but one day that too may change. Scientists do not have a problem here – they mostly use an agreed system of standard units called the Système Internationale (SI). This is also the system normally used in health care, although, for convenience, hospitals sometimes use non-SI units too. The system is comprised of a number of base units (Table 1.2) and a much larger number of derived units (Table 1.3), which, as their name implies, are derived from the base units.

Length

The SI unit of length is the **metre**, and this unit is certainly used by health-care professionals. For example, the height of adults is recorded in metres. It may be more convenient

Table 1.2 Selected SI base units.

Quantity	Symbol	Name	Abbreviation
Amount of a substance	N	Mole	mol
Electrical current	I	Ampere	A
Length	L	Metre	m
Mass	m	Kilogram	kg
Temperature	T	Kelvin	K
Time	t	Second	s

Table 1.3 Selected SI derived units.

Quantity	Symbol	Unit	Quantity	Symbol	Unit
Acceleration	a	m/s^2 or ms^{-2}	Power	P	Watt (W)
Area	A	m^2	Pressure	P	Pascal (Pa)
Electrical potential	V	Volt (V)	Radiation absorbed dose	D	Gray (Gy) (J/kg)
Electrical resistance	R	Ohm (Ω)	Radioactivity	A	Becquerel (Bq)
Energy	E	Joule (J)	Solubility	s	g/l
Force	F	Newton (N)	Speed	s	m/s or ms^{-1}
Frequency	F	Hertz (Hz)	Volume	V	m^3
Molality	m	mol/kg	Wavelength	λ	m
Molarity	M	mol/l	Weight	W	Newton (N)
Period	T	s	Work	W	Joule (J)

to use centimetres to measure the height of infants and children. As the prefix 'centi' implies, there are 100 centimetres in each metre:

$$1\ \text{cm} = 1 / 10 \times 10\ \text{m or } 10^{-2}\ \text{m}.$$

You will also see millimetres used - for example, in expressing the length of a suture needle used to sew together the edges of a wound. There are 1000 millimetres in each metre:

$$1\ \text{mm} = 1 / 10 \times 10 \times 10\ \text{m or } 10^{-3}\ \text{m}.$$

Of course, much smaller units are also used. For example, the bacterium that causes anthrax (*Bacillus anthracis*) is about 6 μm (microns) in diameter. There are one million (1 000 000) microns in one metre:

$$1\ \mu\text{m} = 1 / 10 \times 10 \times 10 \times 10 \times 10 \times 10 \text{ or } 10^{-6}\ \text{m}.$$

The smallpox virus is even smaller - only about 300 nm in diameter. There are one thousand million nanometres (1 000 000 000) in each metre:

$$1\ \text{nm} = 1 / 10 \times 10 \times 10 \times 10 \times 10 \times 10 \times 10 \times 10 \times 10 \text{ or } 10^{-9}\ \text{m}.$$

Mass

The SI unit of mass is the **kilogram**. Adult body weight is normally expressed in kilograms. A kilogram is 1000 grams:

$$1\ \text{kg} = 10 \times 10 \times 10\ \text{g or } 10^{3}\ \text{g}.$$

In contrast, the gram is used to express some drug doses. For example, a normal adult dose of aspirin is 0.6 g. Many other drugs, however, are given in smaller doses, expressed in milligrams. Just as there are 1000 millimetres in a metre, there are 1000 milligrams in a gram:

$$1\ \text{mg} = 1 / 10 \times 10 \times 10 \text{ or } 10^{-3}\ \text{g}.$$

For example, the initial adult dose of the drug propranolol, which is used to treat hypertension (high blood pressure), is 80 mg. Occasionally, drug doses are expressed in micrograms. There are one million micrograms in a gram:

$$1\ \text{mcg} = 1 / 10 \times 10 \times 10 \times 10 \times 10 \times 10\ \text{g or } 10^{-6}\ \text{g}.$$

For example, the adult daily maintenance dose of the heart drug digoxin may be as low as 125 mcg.

- ***What's that again – mcg?***

Yes, that's right. Although the normal numerical prefix for micro is the Greek letter μ, when μg is written by hand it may be mistaken for mg. This would clearly be unhelpful, since it would appear that 1000 times the required dose should be given. Consequently, in health care we use mcg as the abbreviation for micrograms.

Volume

The SI unit of volume is the cubic metre (m^3), but this is a rather large unit. Consequently, in both health care and everyday life it is more convenient to use a smaller unit - the **litre**. There are 1000 litres in a cubic metre. This unit is used widely to measure the volume of commodities such as soft drinks and petrol; in health care, bags of intravenous fluid commonly have a volume of 1 l. In health care, however, the millilitre (ml) is an even more commonly used unit. There are 1000 millilitres in a litre. For example, the volume of drug solution for injection is usually measured in millilitres. Incidentally, 1 ml is equal to 1 cm^3.

Summary

We began this short chapter by considering a highly person-centred issue - teenage pregnancy. We noted that numbers are important even when considering such human issues because we want to know how many people are affected and because we want to be able to measure the effect of any interventions we make. We then moved on to consideration of the wide range of numerical values that health-care workers have to deal with on a daily basis. We considered how we make using such numbers easier, including scientific notation and numerical prefixes. Finally, SI units and other units used in clinical practice were described.

Summary points

- Scientific notation is a way of getting rid of zeros in very large or very small numbers.
- To change a large number to scientific notation, move the decimal point to the left and place it between the first and second digits. Count the number of spaces moved and express this figure as a power of 10.
- To change a small number to scientific notation, move the decimal point to the right and stop immediately after the first digit that is not a zero. To show that you have moved the decimal point to the right, express the power of 10 as a negative value.
- Numerical prefixes can be used to replace powers of 10. For example, kilo refers to 10^3 and milli to 10^{-3}.
- The Système Internationale (SI) is an agreed system of standard units that is used throughout the world. The SI unit of length is the metre (m), of weight it is the kilogram (kg) and of volume it is the cubic metre (m^3).
- In health care, we use SI units to measure length (m) and mass (kg), but the SI unit of volume (m^3) is large and so we use litre (l) instead. There are 1000 litres (l) in a cubic metre (m^3).

2

Homeostasis: keeping the body in balance

Learning outcomes

After reading the following chapter and undertaking personal study, you should be able to:

1. Explain what is meant by the term ‘internal environment’.
2. Explain what is meant by the term ‘controlled condition’ and give examples.
3. Define the term ‘homeostasis’.
4. Identify the components of homeostatic control mechanisms and explain the principle of feedback.
5. Distinguish between negative feedback mechanisms and positive feedback mechanisms and give examples of each.
6. Identify conditions that are characterised by imbalance of homeostatic control.
7. Discuss how certain nursing interventions attempt to restore homeostatic control.

Introduction

Imagine that you are ill and the doctor has just told you that he wants to send you for some tests.

- ***What would you feel like?***

You might have a mixture of emotions: fear that your illness might be serious or encouragement that the doctor is taking it seriously. You are unlikely to think that tests are a waste of time. We assume that if something is wrong with our body, it will show up on tests.

- ***But what do tests do?***

Of course, there are many different kinds of test, but each one measures a specific property of the body. For example, in the condition **diabetes mellitus**, there is an abnormality of carbohydrate metabolism that affects blood sugar levels. Not surprisingly, the doctor or nurse may wish to find out the level of sugar in the blood. This condition is mentioned again later in this book. However, for now let us note that the conditions that exist within our bodies are referred to as the **internal environment**.

The internal environment

Before thinking further about the internal environment, consider the smallest units of life, which are referred to as **cells**. The word 'cell' refers to a small cavity or compartment, like a room in a monastery. When an early scientist first used a primitive microscope, he thought that the small living units he observed resembled in appearance rows of monks' cells. Consequently, the term 'cell' took on a new meaning. Some organisms consist of just a single cell, whereas the body of an adult man or woman is comprised of billions of cells. Whether the entire body of an organism consists of a single cell or billions of cells, each cell has chemical reactions taking place within it. We often use the word **metabolism** to describe this activity. The prefix 'meta' refers to 'all' and the suffix 'anabolism' refers to 'manufacture', although the latter actually comes from a Greek word meaning 'to pile up'. Consequently, metabolism is all the manufacturing reactions of the cell. Metabolism depends upon a continuous supply of raw materials and it produces a number of waste products. Consequently, a cell must have access to the nutrients required for its metabolism and must be able to eliminate its waste products. The similarity between single-celled organisms and the cells of the human body probably ends here, as the following question demonstrates.

- ***From where do cells acquire nutrients, and where are waste products eliminated?***

The answer to this question is the environment in which the cell lives. However, the environment of a single-celled organism and that of one of the cells of the human body are very different. Let us consider the single-celled drifting organism of the ocean, plankton. Its body is so small that it can be seen only with the aid of a microscope; in comparison, its environment (the ocean) is enormous. This means that the metabolic activity (the consumption of nutrients and the production of waste products) of a single plankton has an extremely small impact on the environment in which it lives. Compare this condition with that of a cell found within the human body. Very few of the cells of a multicellular (many-celled) organism are actually in contact with the environment in which the organism lives.

- ***What then is the environment of the cells of a multicellular organism?***

The environment of a cell within the human body is best thought of as the conditions that exist around it. Cells are bathed in a fluid called **interstitial fluid**; it is from this fluid that cells obtain nutrients and into this fluid that they eliminate waste products. Therefore, the environment of the cells of our bodies is not the conditions that exist outside the body (external environment) but rather those that exist within it - the **internal environment**. Interstitial fluid forms what might be regarded as a kind of 'internal ocean'. However, there is a great difference between interstitial fluid and a real ocean, and that is its size. Even though interstitial fluid forms about 16% of the adult body weight, if it were stagnant it would quickly become depleted of nutrients and contaminated by waste products. Clearly, there must be a turnover of interstitial fluid, so that fresh nutrients replace those that are consumed by cells and so that waste products are eliminated. A number of organ systems contribute to maintaining the constancy of the interstitial fluid, although the cardiovascular system plays the principal role. The circulation of blood provides the means by which fresh materials are brought to cells and waste products are removed from cells. Indeed, interstitial fluid is formed from the blood and is resorbed into it. Other systems also play a part by interacting with the environment outside the body. For example, the respiratory system replenishes the blood with oxygen and removes the waste gas carbon dioxide. The digestive system replenishes the blood with nutrients such as glucose, and the urinary system removes waste products (other than carbon dioxide) from the blood and eliminates them to the external environment. These relationships are illustrated in Figure 2.1.

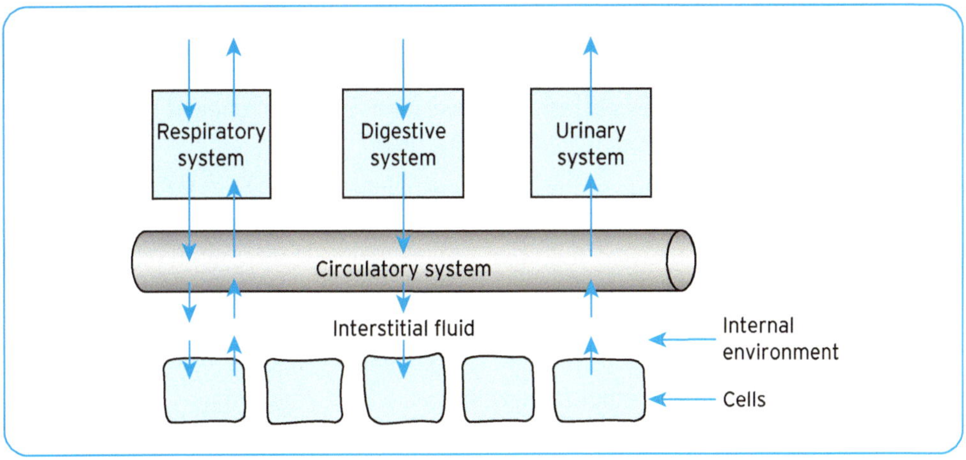

Figure 2.1
The relationship between the body's systems and the internal and external environments.

Homeostasis

Walter B. Cannon, an American physiologist of the early twentieth century, noted that if the heat produced by exercising muscles was not dissipated, then the ensuing rise in temperature would inactivate the body's regulatory proteins. In 1932, Cannon introduced the concept of **homeostasis** in order to explain the way in which our bodies strive to maintain the constancy of the internal environment. Remember that the term 'internal environment' refers primarily to the composition of the interstitial fluid. However, this is regulated not directly but indirectly, as a consequence of the regulation of the composition of blood. Any variable that the body regulates is referred to as a 'controlled condition'. Examples of controlled conditions are given in Table 2.1. Any occurrence that provokes a change in controlled condition is referred to as a 'stimulus'. How the body responds to stimuli is explained in the next section.

Table 2.1 Some controlled conditions.

Temperature
Water balance
Electrolyte balance
Blood pH (level of acidity)
Blood glucose level
Blood pressure

Homeostatic control mechanisms

Regardless of the variable that is regulated, all homeostatic mechanisms possess the same three basic components - **receptors**, a **control centre** and **effectors**. Receptors are sensors that respond to a stimulus that brings about a change in a controlled condition. For example, **thermoreceptors** respond to changes in temperature and **osmoreceptors** to changes in blood osmolarity (concentration of dissolved substances). Information about the controlled condition (input) is conveyed to the control centre, which then determines the set point or range at which a controlled condition is to be maintained. It analyses the input from receptors and determines the appropriate response (output). Effectors are the means by which the control centre regulates the controlled condition. Effectors may be muscles or glands. For example, when we are cold, uncontrollable contraction and relaxation of our muscles (shivering) generates heat. In contrast, when we are hot, the secretion of sweat, by sweat glands, cools down our bodies.

Receptors continuously provide control centres with information about the effectiveness of the responses that they initiate. We might say that receptors provide control centres with feedback. Indeed, this is the very term that is used. Homeostatic control mechanisms are described as **feedback mechanisms** or **feedback loops**. The principle of feedback is illustrated in Figure 2.2. As you consider this diagram, remember that feedback loops operate not intermittently but continuously. There is a continuous input to control centres from receptors, and a continuous output from control centres to effectors.

Even the briefest description of homeostasis demonstrates that a key feature of control mechanisms is communication within the body (internal communication). The nervous system and the endocrine system accomplish internal communication. In the nervous system, information is conveyed in the form of electrical impulses in nerves; in the endocrine system, ductless glands secrete chemicals called **hormones** directly into the bloodstream. Take

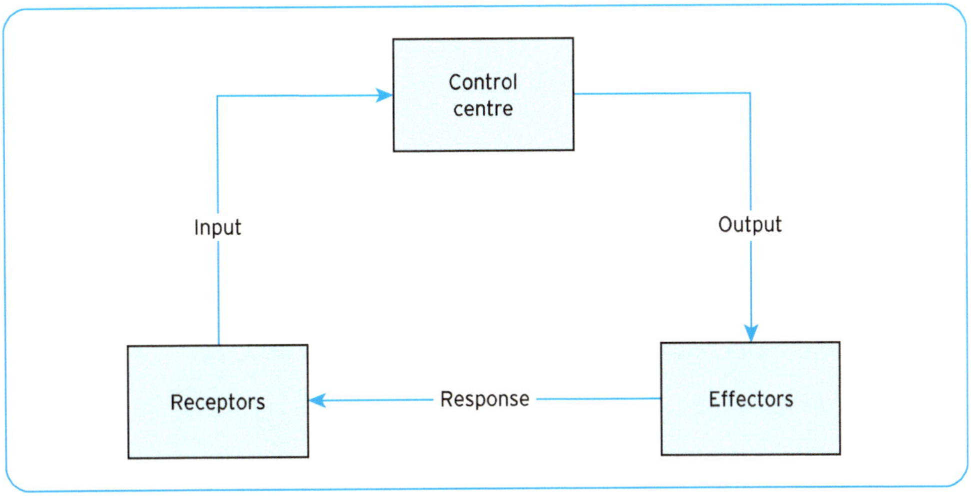

Figure 2.2
The principle of feedback.

temperature regulation as an example. The control centre for temperature is located in the part of the brain called the **hypothalamus**. This receives input from thermoreceptors in the form of nervous impulses, and subsequently nervous impulses form the output to muscles and sweat glands. In a somewhat more complicated example, the cardiac control centres of the **brain stem** (the lower part of the brain) receive nervous inputs from a number of sources and produce nervous outputs to several structures, including the heart and the **adrenal medulla** (the inner part of the adrenal glands). Consider the condition of a heart rate that is too slow. In this case, the nervous output of the cardiac centres serves to raise the heart rate. The heart rate is also increased, however, because of the effects of two hormones of the adrenal medulla - **epinephrine** (adrenaline) and **norepinephrine** (noradrenaline). This is an example of internal communication by both the nervous and endocrine systems.

Negative feedback mechanisms and positive feedback mechanisms

Suppose you step outside on a cold day. After some time, your body temperature starts to fall.

- ***Is the response of the body to initiate heat-generating mechanisms or cooling mechanisms?***

This is perhaps an obvious question - heat-generating mechanisms are indeed initiated. Now let us take an example with which you might not be so familiar. Suppose it is some time since you ate and your blood glucose level has started to fall.

- ***Is the response of your body to raise blood glucose or to lower it further still?***

The body attempts to raise the blood glucose once again. The purpose of these questions is to illustrate a characteristic of most homeostatic control mechanisms - they operate in such a way that the response of the control centre is to reverse the change in the controlled condition. Such mechanisms are described as **negative feedback mechanisms**. You might say that this kind of mechanism is designed to keep the body in balance – that is, to keep controlled conditions within a specific range of values.

- ***What, then, are positive feedback mechanisms?***

Positive feedback mechanisms are those in which a change in a controlled condition is intensified rather than reversed. There are fewer examples of positive feedback mechanisms than negative feedback mechanisms because they do not result in the stability and control that are the essence of homeostasis. In contrast, positive feedback mechanisms are self-perpetuating and appear to be out of control.

- ***What is their purpose?***

Positive feedback mechanisms reinforce a stimulus until a key event is reached that terminates the feedback loop. The birth of a baby is a good example. As the mother's uterus contracts during labour, the baby is pushed against the cervix (the muscular neck of the uterus). The stretching of the cervix is detected by pressure receptors, which convey impulses (input) to the brain (control centre), which responds by causing the release of the hormone **oxytocin** (output) from the posterior lobe of the pituitary gland located beneath the brain.

- ***What is the effect of oxytocin on the uterus?***

Perhaps you have already been able to predict that the effect of oxytocin is to cause more vigorous uterine contractions, which push the baby further towards the cervix, stretching the cervix still further and leading to the release of more oxytocin. This sequence of events is terminated only when the baby is finally expelled from the uterus and is born. Incidentally, this example illustrates the joint role played in internal communication by the nervous and endocrine systems. Nervous impulses from pressure receptors form the input to the control centre, while the output is in the form of the hormone oxytocin.

Nursing care and homeostasis

We revisit homeostasis in a number of chapters later on in this book. For now, let us consider how, when giving physical care to patients, as nurses we are often trying to assist homeostatic control mechanisms. You might say that we work along with patients' own bodies to restore control. An obvious example is temperature imbalance. When an elderly person develops **hypothermia** (low temperature), we undertake actions to try to raise body temperature. When a marathon runner has heat exhaustion caused by too high a body temperature and fluid loss, we use gentle cooling and fluid replacement with special drinks or an intravenous infusion/drip.

The purpose of this chapter has been to introduce the concept of homeostasis and to distinguish between negative and positive feedback mechanisms. As you work through this book, you will encounter a number of controlled conditions, including water balance (Chapter 4), acid-base balance (Chapter 5), blood pressure (Chapter 6), blood glucose level (Chapter 7) and body temperature (Chapter 9). A detailed discussion of the homeostatic mechanisms involved in each case is beyond the scope of this book. You will look at these in more detail, however, as you move on from basic science to studying physiology as part of your course.

Summary

We began this chapter by thinking about what medical tests measure as a way of introducing the concept of the internal environment before moving on to consider how the internal environment is regulated - a phenomenon called homeostasis. Three elements of homeostatic mechanisms were described - receptors, a control centre and effectors - and a distinction was made between positive and negative feedback. The purpose of the chapter has been to suggest that nursing care often involves working with patients' bodies to assist the restoration of normal homeostatic control.

Summary points

- Interstitial fluid forms the internal environment.
- Homeostasis refers to the regulation of the internal environment.
- Any variable of the internal environment that is controlled is referred to as a controlled condition.
- Any event that provokes a change in a controlled condition is referred to as a stimulus.
- The basic components of all homeostatic control mechanisms are receptors, a control centre and effectors.
- Control mechanisms are described as either negative feedback mechanisms or positive feedback mechanisms.
- Negative feedback mechanisms operate in such a way that the response of the control centre is to reverse the change in the controlled condition.
- Positive feedback mechanisms operate in such a way that the response of the control centre is to reinforce the change in the controlled condition.
- Nursing care often involves working with patients' bodies to assist the restoration of normal homeostatic control.

3

The physical world and basic chemistry

Learning outcomes

After reading the following chapter and undertaking personal study, you should be able to:

1 Identify three states of matter.
2 Describe the structure of the atom and differentiate between atoms and ions.
3 Define the terms 'atomic number', 'mass number' and 'relative atomic mass'.
4 Define the term 'compound' and differentiate between ionic and covalent compounds.
5 Differentiate between polar and non-polar molecules and describe hydrogen bonds.
6 Define the terms 'molecular mass' and 'mole'.
7 Briefly explain the following types of chemical reaction: combination, decomposition, displacement, partner exchange, reversible and redox.
8 Explain the action of enzymes.
9 Differentiate between organic and inorganic chemistry.
10 Differentiate between aliphatic and aromatic compounds.
11 Outline the structure of the following groups of organic compounds: alkanes, alkenes, alkynes, alcohols, aldehydes, ketones, carboxylic acids and amines.
12 Identify physical conditions affecting a patient in which knowledge of chemistry helps in understanding the processes taking place.
13 Identify aspects of nursing care of which the understanding is helped by knowledge of chemistry.

Introduction

To some students, the prospect of studying chemistry is a daunting one. Nonetheless, a brief examination of the world around us reveals how important this subject is to both nurses and other health-care workers. Our bodies are made up of chemicals, the foods we eat and drink are chemicals, and we use some chemicals as drugs. Consequently, knowledge of chemistry becomes important when we study health and illness, give dietary advice and administer medicines. Therefore, this chapter may be more important than you initially imagine. Despite its daunting appearance, the study of chemistry does not have to be difficult. Let us begin with a simple but important point about matter.

Think about the universe for a moment.

- ***What is it made up of?***

At the simplest level, we might say that the entire universe consists of matter and energy. The nature of energy is dealt with in Chapter 8, while in this chapter we shall think more about matter. Matter is anything that occupies space; it can exist in one of three states.

States of matter

Matter may exist in the **solid**, **liquid** or **gaseous** state. When we think of a substance, we tend to think of it in the state in which we commonly encounter it. For example, we think of solid iron but gaseous oxygen. On the other hand, if we worked in an iron-smelting works we would be familiar with molten (liquid) iron and oxygen is delivered to hospitals under high pressure as liquid oxygen. In other cases, we are familiar with a substance in all three states. Water is a case in point, since its melting point (0 °C) and its boiling point (100 °C) are within the range of our everyday experience of temperature. Our kitchen refrigerators are capable of creating temperatures below the freezing point of water and we can certainly boil water on a kitchen cooker. We are familiar with this important substance in its solid state (ice), in its liquid state (water) and as a gas (water vapour or steam). We also have some idea, from everyday experience, about the behaviour of matter in each of these states. For example, we know that solids have a shape and do not adapt to the shape of the container into which they are placed. If we take a rubber ball and place it in a square box, it remains round and does not become square like the box. In contrast, liquids have a much less rigid structure and conform to the shape of the container into which they are poured. Nonetheless, their structure is still more rigid than that of a gas. It is possible, for example, to have a container half-filled with a liquid, but gases not only conform to the shape of the container into which they are placed but actually occupy the whole space of the container.

All matter, then, exists in these three states, but what does matter actually consist of? All matter is made up of particles called **atoms**.

Atoms and elements

Some time ago, an elderly woman was stopped in the street by a television interviewer and asked about which political party she hoped would win the next general election. In response she said, 'I don't give an atom!' Her reply indicated that she knew that an atom was something very small, and that was how much she cared about politics. The word 'atom' is derived from a Greek word meaning 'indivisible', and it was coined at a time when it was believed that the atom was the smallest particle of matter. We now know that atoms can be split into smaller particles called subatomic particles, but the atom remains the smallest unit of matter that can enter a chemical reaction. Atoms differ according to the number of different subatomic particles that they contain. This is explained more fully later in this chapter. For the time being, it is important simply to note that matter that consists of atoms of only one type is referred to as an **element**. There are 92 naturally occurring elements and other elements that are created artificially as a part of nuclear reactions. Some of the common naturally occurring elements are hydrogen, oxygen, carbon and nitrogen. In fact, over 95% of a living organism is made up of these four elements alone, so they will often feature in your studies. Table 3.1 lists some of the elements that are important in the body.

Writing the names of elements is often a laborious process, so each is given a symbol (abbreviation) that usually consists of the first letter, or first and second letters, of its English or Latin name. If only one letter is used, it is given as a capital. For example, the chemical symbol for oxygen is O. If two letters are used, then the first is given as a capital and the second as a lower-case letter. Consequently, the symbol for calcium is Ca. The symbol Na for sodium looks confusing at first, but if you know that the Latin name for this element is *natrium* you will see that the same rules apply. When elements have similar names, the first letter and another instead of the first and second letters are used. For example, the symbol for chlorine is Cl and for chromium it is Cr. Similarly, Mg is the symbol for magnesium and Mn is the symbol for manganese.

For convenience, the elements are grouped in a table referred to as the **Periodic Table**, an example of which is given in the appendix. Examine this table for a moment. You will see that in addition to the symbol, the table gives a number of items of numerical data, including the **atomic number** and the **atomic mass**, which we shall use later.

Table 3.1 Important elements in the body.

Element	Importance
Calcium	Muscle contraction, nervous impulses, blood coagulation, structure of bones and teeth
Carbon	Principal element in organic compounds
Chlorine	Principal extracellular anion
Hydrogen	Component of all organic compounds
Iodine	Component of thyroxine
Iron	Component of haemoglobin
Nitrogen	Component of amines, amino acids and nucleic acids
Oxygen	Necessary for cellular respiration
Phosphorus	Component of adenosine triphosphate (ATP) - the body's chemical form of energy
Potassium	Nervous impulses, main intracellular cation
Sodium	Fluid balance, nervous impulses, main extracellular cation

- ***Now that you have seen the Periodic Table, you are in a position to check the symbols of the elements in Table 3.1. Take a moment to do this now.***

In-text review

- ✔ The entire universe consists of matter and energy.
- ✔ Matter is anything that occupies space.
- ✔ Matter exists in one of three states - solid, liquid or gas.
- ✔ In both everyday life and clinical practice, we encounter substances in one or more of these states.
- ✔ The atom is the smallest unit of matter that can enter a chemical reaction.
- ✔ Matter that consists of atoms of only one type is referred to as an element.
- ✔ Some of the most important elements in the body are hydrogen, oxygen, carbon and nitrogen.
- ✔ Elements are given symbols usually consisting of the first, or first and second, letters of the English or Latin name, e.g. calcium (Ca) and sodium (Na).

The Periodic Table

Having begun to use the Periodic Table, we ought to consider it in a little more detail. Perhaps you have already begun to wonder why the elements are arranged in the way that they are and why the table of elements was given the name 'periodic' in the first place. Early scientists performed experiments that led them to conclude that atoms of different elements had different weights. The absolute weight of atoms was not being measured, but rather their **relative weights** were considered. At this early time, scientists had no agreed unit against which to measure the weight of atoms. Consequently, they did what people have done for centuries and measured one thing against another - how much heavier one atom was compared with another. For example, it was shown that in the reaction between hydrogen and chlorine, the weight of chlorine consumed was approximately 36 times that of hydrogen. It was then concluded that a chlorine atom weighs 36 times as much as a hydrogen atom. Such conclusions were based upon a number of assumptions, not all of which proved to be true (e.g. that all elements reacted in equal ratios). Despite such false assumptions, early scientists were able to ascribe a number, referred to as the **atomic mass**, which indicated the relative masses of different atoms.

A Russian chemist Dmitri Mendeleyev noticed that when the known elements were listed in order of ascending atomic mass, the properties of the elements, such as physical state and ability to conduct heat and electricity, varied in a regular, or periodic, manner. This led to the construction of a table in which elements with similar properties fell into the same vertical columns, and to this table the name 'periodic' was then applied. Incidentally, when using the Periodic Table, it might be helpful to know that the vertical columns are referred to as **groups** and the horizontal rows as **periods**.

Elements on the left-hand side of the Periodic Table are nearly all solids, and they more readily conduct heat and electricity than elements on the right of the table.

- ***What name is given to these elements on the left?***

Perhaps you know that they are metals. In contrast, non-metals are generally poor conductors of heat and electricity. They may be solids, but many are gases. Of the elements on the right-hand side, only bromine is liquid at room temperature.

- ***So where is the dividing line between metals and non-metals in the Periodic Table?***

Unfortunately, a rigid dividing line between metals and non-metals cannot be drawn. However, if you look at the Periodic Table once again, you will see a step-like line drawn between the elements boron and aluminium, silicon and germanium, and so on. Elements on either side of this line may have characteristics of both metals and non-metals. For example, carbon is a non-metal that exists in a number of forms, some of which do conduct electricity.

In-text review

- ✔ Elements are arranged in the Periodic Table, which is so called because of the manner in which physical properties, such as the ability to conduct heat, recur in a periodic matter.
- ✔ In the Periodic Table, columns are called groups and rows are called periods.
- ✔ Elements on the left-hand side of the table (metals) conduct heat and electricity more readily than those to the right (non-metals).

Compounds

Thus far, we have considered only matter that consists of atoms of only one type. Some substances, however, consist of atoms of more than one type that are joined together by chemical bonds. Such substances are referred to as **compounds** and we consider some of these in this section.

Compounds are named after the elements that comprise them. For example, sodium chloride is a compound formed from sodium and chlorine. In order to avoid the labour of writing the name of compounds, the chemical formula is often used. This is made up of the symbols of the elements that are contained in the compound. For example, since sodium is designated by the symbol Na and chlorine by the symbol Cl, the chemical formula of sodium chloride is NaCl. Sometimes, compounds have common names.

● ***What is the common name for NaCl?***

NaCl is common (table) salt. It is generally better to avoid the use of common names, since they can be confusing. For example, there is a great deal of difference between bicarbonate of soda ($NaHCO_3$), caustic soda (NaOH) and washing soda ($NaCO_3$). Bicarbonate of soda is added to cakes to make them rise, caustic soda can cause burns but is very useful for unblocking drains, and washing soda is so called because it is used to create a better lather when soap, rather than laundry detergent, is used to wash clothes. Despite their very different properties, each of these substances is called 'soda'. In nursing, it is always better to refer to the chemical name of a substance, or some other form of agreed name, such as the generic name of a drug, e.g. paracetamol. The likelihood of an error is much less if we stick to using agreed names. Some common names in health care are dealt with in Practice point 3.1.

Practice point 3.1

Common names in health care

Although a word of caution has been given about using common names, some expressions are used regularly in clinical practice. It is worth noting that a 0.9% solution of NaCl for intravenous infusion (drip) is usually referred to as 'normal saline'. This expression refers to the concentration of salt solution that is normally used (0.9%). If you are asked to collect a bag of normal saline, it will be identified by the chemical formula (NaCl) and the numerical expression of concentration (0.9%). Expressions of concentration are explained more fully in Chapter 4.

When different elements combine to form compounds, they do not always do so in equal proportions. In the chemical formula, this is taken into account by the use of numerical subscripts. For example, one atom of carbon combines with two atoms of oxygen to form carbon dioxide (CO_2). You are probably familiar with this compound as the main greenhouse gas responsible for rising global temperatures. This compound is also a respiratory stimulant found on anaesthetic machines and the waste product of living cells excreted by the respiratory system in exhaled breath.

The structure of the atom

An atom is the smallest particle of an element that retains the characteristics of that element. Although atoms are very small, they are made up of even smaller particles referred to as subatomic particles or elementary particles. These have been given the names **protons** (p), **neutrons** (n) and **electrons** (e^-). These particles have different characteristics. For example, although protons and neutrons have equal mass, that of an electron is negligible. In fact, it is only 1/1837 of the mass of a proton or neutron. In addition, although the neutron carries no charge, the proton has a single positive charge and the electron a single negative charge. (Charge is explained more fully in Chapter 11.)

● ***But how are these particles distributed within the atom?***

The atom contains a dense core, or **nucleus**, in which the protons and neutrons are located.

- ***Does the nucleus have an overall charge?***

Since the nucleus contains neutral neutrons and positively charged protons, it has an overall positive charge.

- ***Where are the electrons located?***

Electrons rapidly orbit the central nucleus in what may be referred to as the **electron cloud**. This is illustrated in Figure 3.1. The numbers of subatomic particles that an atom contains is given by two items of data – the atomic number and the mass number.

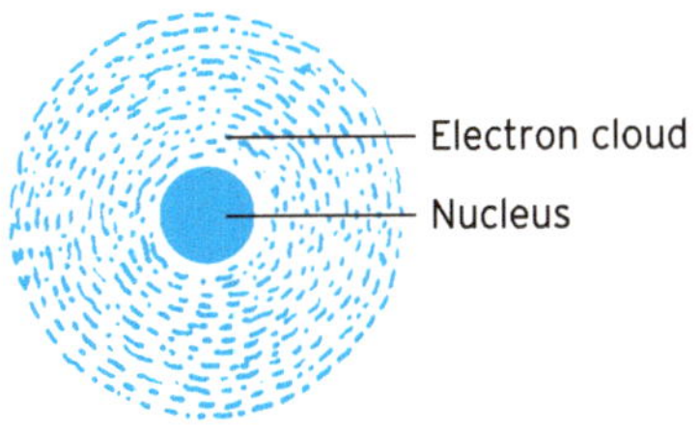

Figure 3.1
The nucleus and electron cloud of an atom.

Atomic number and mass number

The **atomic number** is simply the number of protons that an atom contains. All the atoms of a particular element have the same atomic number. For example, the atomic number of sodium is 11 and all atoms of sodium have 11 protons in the nucleus. The atomic number is usually written as a subscript before or after the symbol for the element concerned. In the case of sodium, it is $_{11}Na$.

- ***Go back to the Periodic Table in the appendix and find out the atomic numbers of the elements in Table 3.1.***

At this point, it is also worth pointing out that atoms are electrically neutral.

- ***This being so, what can you say about the number of electrons in an atom?***

The number of electrons equals the number of protons. For the sake of definition, however, and for reasons that you will understand later, the atomic number is defined as the number of protons that an atom contains.

Atoms are also given a **mass number**, which is simply the sum of the number of protons and neutrons in the nucleus. The mass number is usually given as a superscript before or after the symbol for the element concerned. In the case of sodium, it is written as ^{23}Na.

- ***Why is the number of electrons not included in the mass number?***

To answer this question, remember that the mass of an electron is only 1/1837 of that of a proton or a neutron. Consequently, electrons make a negligible contribution to the mass of an atom. Furthermore, if both the mass number and the atomic number of an element are known, then the number of neutrons can be calculated easily.

- ***How many neutrons are there in $^{23}_{11}Na$?***

If you have written 12, then you have the right answer (that is, 23 – 11).

Isotopes

At this point, it is worth introducing the term **isotope**, which is sometimes encountered in clinical practice and in the study of chemistry. Isotopes are atoms that have the same atomic numbers but different mass numbers. Isotopes are, therefore, atoms of the same element but with different numbers of neutrons. This is probably best illustrated by the case of hydrogen. All atoms of hydrogen have an atomic number of 1. The most common isotope of hydrogen also has a mass number of 1 ($^{1}_{1}H$), but there is an isotope of hydrogen with a mass number of 2 ($^{2}_{1}H$) and another with a mass number of 3 ($^{3}_{1}H$).

- ***How many neutrons are there in $^{1}_{1}H$, $^{2}_{1}H$ and $^{3}_{1}H$?***

→ In $^{1}_{1}H$ there are no neutrons (1 – 1).

→ In $^{2}_{1}H$ there is one neutron (2 – 1).

→ In $^{3}_{1}H$ there are two neutrons (3 – 1).

Isotopes in clinical practice are dealt with in Practice point 3.2.

Practice point 3.2

Isotopes in clinical practice

The atoms of certain isotopes are unstable and decay, with the emission of **radiation**. Isotopes that decay in this fashion are described as **radioisotopes**. You will encounter radioisotopes in a number of diagnostic investigations and in some treatments for cancer. For example, in creating an image (scan) of the thyroid gland of the neck, the radioisotope iodine-131 (^{131}I) is used. Once this isotope has been administered to a patient, it concentrates in the thyroid gland. The radiation given off by the gland can then be detected and used to produce an image of the gland that is used by medical staff in making diagnosis. This is explained more fully in Chapter 14.

Relative atomic mass

Relative atomic mass is a concept that is easier to understand than to define. For this reason, we will consider an example before moving on to give a definition. There are two isotopes of the element chlorine, and they have the mass numbers 35 and 37. Both of the isotopes have the atomic number 17.

- ***So how many neutrons are there in the atoms of each of these isotopes of chlorine?***

The lighter isotope (^{35}Cl) has 18 (35 – 17) neutrons and the heavier isotope (^{35}Cl) has 20 (37 – 17) neutrons. In a sample of chlorine gas, both isotopes are present, but not in equal proportions. The lighter isotope is more abundant, comprising 77.5% of the sample compared with the heavier isotope's 22.5%.

- ***How is the existence of two isotopes taken into account when we want to express the relative weight of chlorine atoms?***

We clearly need to calculate an average of the mass numbers that takes into account the relative proportions of the two isotopes, as shown below:

$$(35 \times 77.5\%) + (37 \times 22.5\%) = 27.125 + 8.325$$
$$= 35.45$$

It is this value that is referred to as the relative atomic mass, and we are now in a position to define relative atomic mass as the average mass of a single atom of an element that takes into account the relative proportions of the different isotopes of that element.

The units in which relative atomic mass is measured are referred to as **atomic mass units** (amu or u). All units of measurement are based upon a standard - for example, length in terms of metres.

- ***But what is the standard in this case? What has a mass of 1 amu?***

From the discussion on isotopes, you may recall that there is an isotope of hydrogen that has a mass number of 1 (^{1}H). This is not used as the standard unit, however. The standard amu is defined in terms of the most abundant isotope on earth - that is, the carbon-12 isotope (^{12}C).

- ***But surely ^{12}C has a mass of 12 amu?***

Indeed it does, and consequently the amu is defined so that 12 amu equals the mass of the most abundant isotope of carbon (^{12}C).

The orbital model of the atom

Electrons are not distributed randomly within the atom but circle the nucleus in orbits of varying distance from the nucleus. This model of atomic structure may be described as an orbital model - an electron orbiting the nucleus of an atom may be likened to a satellite orbiting a planet. It often helps to think about atoms in this way, but orbits are more usually referred to as **energy levels** or **energy shells**. There is a good reason for this. Let's think about the satellite illustration further.

- ***What would happen to the satellite as it lost energy and started to slow down?***

Its orbit would decay - that is, it would be pulled closer to the earth by gravity. In a similar way, electrons with the least amount of energy are found nearer the nucleus and those with the greatest amount of energy are furthest away. At this point, the satellite model is beginning to show its weakness. Electrons do not orbit the nucleus in infinitely variable orbits. Instead, a specific amount of energy is required to promote an electron from a low energy level (orbit) near the nucleus to the next energy level further away from the nucleus. An electron may move to a higher or lower energy level, but it cannot exist in between.

A letter designates each energy level. Strangely, the first energy level (the one nearest the nucleus) is designated the K shell; next comes the L shell, and then the M shell, and so on. Each energy level holds a specific number of electrons, and this can be calculated using the formula $X = 2n^2$, where X is the maximum number of electrons in the energy level n. For the K, L and M energy levels, n equals 1, 2 and 3, respectively.

- ***So how many electrons does the first energy level hold?***

Let us work through this using our formula:

Formula	$X = 2n^2$
First energy shell	$n = 1$
Calculation	2×1^2
	2×1
Answer	2

- ***And what about the second energy level?***

Formula	$X = 2n^2$
Second energy shell	$n = 2$
Calculation	2×2^2
	2×4
Answer	8

Have a go yourself at the calculation for the third energy level. You will find it holds 18 electrons (2×3^2). Also, note that the energy levels are filled in order, beginning with the lowest. Therefore, K is filled before L, and L is filled before M. Let us now consider how the electrons are arranged in the atoms of some familiar elements, beginning with sodium. Perhaps you remember that sodium has an atomic number of 11.

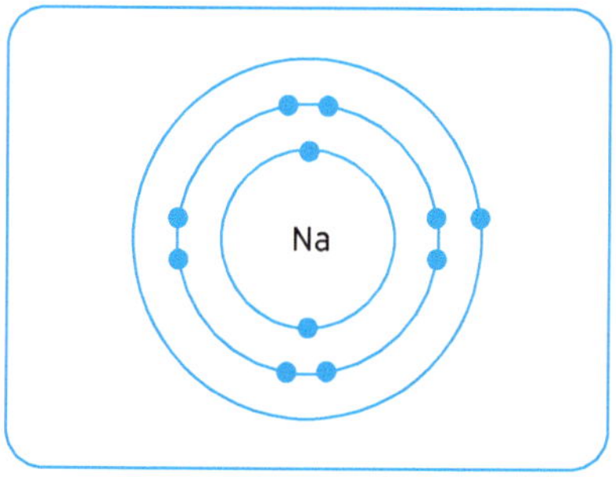

Figure 3.2
The arrangement of electrons in an atom of sodium.

- ***How are the 11 electrons of sodium arranged?***

The K level is filled with two electrons and the L level with eight; this leaves one electron left over in the M level. This electron configuration is usually written as 2.8.1, although it may also be given in diagrammatic form, as Figure 3.2 shows.

We can consider chlorine in a similar manner. Chlorine has an atomic number of 17.

- ***What is the electron configuration of chlorine?***

It is 2.8.7, and once again this arrangement can be given in diagrammatic form (Figure 3.3).

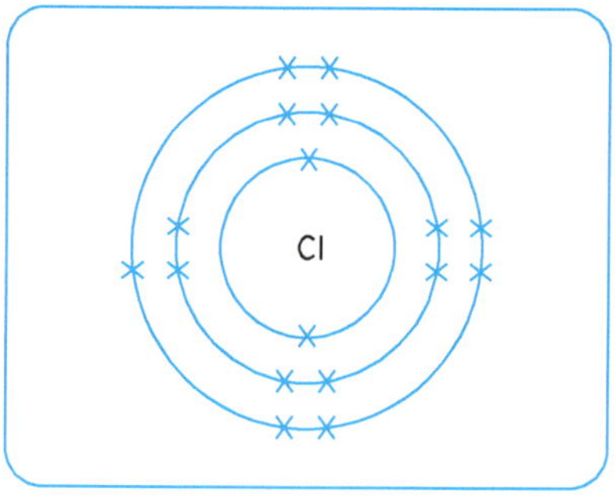

Figure 3.3
The arrangement of electrons in an atom of chlorine.

● *Take time to work out the electron configurations of the other elements listed in Table 3.1.*

Two observations about atomic structure and the position of elements within the Periodic Table are worth noting:

- Elements that have the same number of electrons in the outer energy level fall into the same group, e.g. sodium and potassium are both found in group 1.
- Elements that have the same number of energy levels occupied by electrons fall into the same period, e.g. potassium and calcium.

In-text review

- ✔ Atoms consist of subatomic particles such as protons, neutrons and electrons. Protons and neutrons have equal mass, but the mass of electrons is negligible. Protons carry a positive charge and electrons a negative charge. Neutrons are neutral.
- ✔ Atoms consist of a dense core of protons and neutrons.
- ✔ The atomic number is the number of protons an atom contains. It is given as a subscript before the element symbol. The mass number is the sum of the number of protons and neutrons and is given as a numerical superscript before the element symbol. For example, the atomic number and mass number for sodium are $^{23}_{11}Na$.
- ✔ Isotopes are atoms that have the same atomic number but different mass numbers. Consequently, they are atoms of the same element, but with different numbers of neutrons. For example, three isotopes of hydrogen are $^{1}_{1}H$, $^{2}_{1}H$ and $^{3}_{1}H$.
- ✔ The relative atomic mass is the average mass of a single atom of an element that takes into account the relative proportions of the different isotopes of that element.
- ✔ Electrons orbit the nucleus in orbits called energy levels (energy shells). A letter designates each energy level. The first energy level (the one nearest the nucleus) is designated the K shell; next comes the L shell and then the M shell.
- ✔ Each energy level holds a specific number of electrons, and this can be calculated using the formula $X = 2n^2$, where X is the maximum number of electrons in the energy level n. For the K, L and M energy levels, n equals 1, 2 and 3, respectively.

Chemical bonds

It has been noted that compounds, such as sodium chloride (NaCl), are substances that consist of atoms of more than one kind joined by chemical bonds. We now study compounds in a little more detail and examine the different kinds of chemical bond that are formed. Before we do this, it is helpful to look at a group of elements called inert gases (or noble gases). They can be found in Group VIII of the Periodic Table.

- ***Take a moment to find these elements.***

The first three members of this group are helium, neon and argon. Perhaps you are already familiar with the inert gases. Helium is lighter than air and is sometimes used to fill party balloons, while neon is used in street lights and illuminated advertisements.

- ***Using the Periodic Table in the appendix, identify the atomic numbers of helium, neon and argon.***

They are 2, 10 and 18, respectively.

- ***How are the electrons of helium, neon and argon arranged?***

Helium	2
Neon	2.8
Argon	2.8.8

- ***Do you notice anything about the number of electrons in the outer energy levels of these elements?***

In each case, the outer energy level either is full or contains eight electrons. This observation has an important significance. The description of members of Group VIII as inert gases is made in reference to the fact that they do not react with other elements to form compounds. In contrast to the inert gases, some elements are highly reactive - that is, they readily form compounds with other elements. Sodium is one example of a reactive metal and chlorine is an example of a reactive non-metal. Examine the outer energy levels of sodium and chlorine for a moment. Remember that the atomic numbers of sodium and chlorine are 11 and 17, respectively.

- ***How many electrons are there in the outer energy levels of sodium and chlorine?***

The outer energy level of sodium contains only one electron (configuration 2.8.1), while the outer energy level of chlorine possesses seven electrons (configuration 2.8.7).

So, then, the outer energy levels of highly reactive metals such as sodium are nearly empty, and the outer energy levels of non-metals such as chlorine are nearly full. In contrast, the inert gases are not reactive, and each has a full outer energy level. The importance of this observation becomes obvious when we examine chemical bonds such as **ionic bonds**.

Ions and ionic bonding

Remember that compounds are substances that consist of atoms of more than one element joined by chemical bonds. In this section, one form of bonding - ionic bonding - is described. Remember that atoms contain equal numbers of protons and electrons, so they are electrically neutral.

- ***But what would happen if an atom either lost or gained electrons?***

It would no longer be electrically neutral but would possess a net charge. This charged structure is no longer called an atom but instead is referred to as an **ion**. An ion is an electrically charged particle that results when an atom loses or gains electrons. Let us think about the atomic structure of sodium and chlorine again.

- ***How could sodium (configuration 2.8.1) achieve the stability of the noble gas neon (configuration 2.8)?***

It could do so by losing the single electron from its outer energy level.

- ***What would be the effect of this on the sodium atom?***

It would become a sodium ion with a single positive charge (Na^+).

- ***What about chlorine? How could a chlorine atom (configuration 2.8.7) attain the stability of the inert gas argon (configuration 2.8.8)?***

Chlorine achieves stability by gaining an additional electron in its outer energy level and thus becoming a chloride ion with a single negative charge (Cl^-). Incidentally, positively charged ions are referred to as **cations** and negatively charged ions are referred to as **anions**.

You might now wonder whether all atoms produce ions. The answer is no. Generally, atoms with up to three electrons in the outer energy level achieve stability by losing electrons to form cations. Examples include potassium (configuration 2.8.8.1) and magnesium (configuration 2.8.2). In contrast, atoms with six or seven electrons in the outer energy level achieve stability by gaining electrons to form anions. Examples include fluorine (configuration 2.7) and sulphur (configuration 2.8.6). Atoms with four or five electrons in the outer energy level do not form ions, although it is worth pointing out that there are exceptions to these general rules.

We are now in a position to explain the chemical reaction between sodium and chlorine that leads to the formation of the compound sodium chloride. Both atoms achieve their most stable state when sodium donates an electron to chlorine. This is represented in the form of an equation:

$$Na + Cl \rightarrow Na^+ + Cl^-$$

Note that the sodium ion and the chloride ion carry opposite charges, and, as a consequence, they are attracted strongly to each other. We say that there is an ionic bond between them, and this results in a new substance - the compound sodium chloride (NaCl). Note that it is not usual to include the charges when writing the formula of ionic compounds. Ionic bonding can also be represented diagrammatically, as shown in Figure 3.4.

Before we leave ionic bonding, let us consider a further example - calcium chloride. We have already seen how chlorine (Cl) gains an electron to become a chloride ion (Cl^-). We now examine how calcium ions are formed.

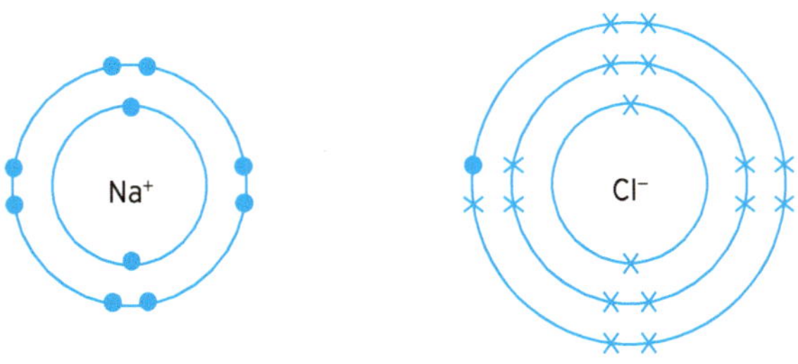

Figure 3.4
The ionic bonding of sodium and chlorine to form sodium chloride.

Element	Calcium (Ca)
Atomic number	20
Electron configuration	2.8.8.2
Nearest (most similar) inert gas	Argon (Ar)
Atomic number	18
Electron configuration	2.8.8
How could Ca achieve the configuration of Ar?	By losing two electrons from its outer energy level to form a calcium ion
What charge does a calcium ion carry?	Since two electrons have been lost, the calcium ion carries a double positive charge (Ca^{2+})

- ***Suppose calcium reacted with chlorine. How many atoms of chlorine would react with each atom of calcium?***

Two atoms of chlorine would react with each atom of calcium to produce calcium chloride ($CaCl_2$), as illustrated in Figure 3.5. This is because each atom of calcium has two electrons to donate, and atoms of chlorine are able to accept only a single electron each. An important point to note here is that not all atoms have the same combining power - a concept referred to as **valency**. Valency is the ability of an atom to combine with other atoms measured by the number of its electrons that are involved in the formation of a chemical bond. Sodium and chlorine both have valencies of 1, since in both cases a single electron is involved in the formation of a chemical bond. In contrast, calcium has a valency of 2, since two of its electrons are involved in the formation of a chemical bond. Since it is only the electrons in the outermost energy level that are involved in chemical bonding, this energy level is referred to as the valence shell.

Polyatomic ions

Thus far, we have considered ions that result when an atom loses or gains electrons. Some ions, however, such as the hydrogen carbonate ion, are actually made up of atoms of more than one element - in this case, hydrogen, carbon and oxygen (HCO_3^-). Such ions are referred to as **polyatomic ions**. Although their structures appear complex, they behave in the way as

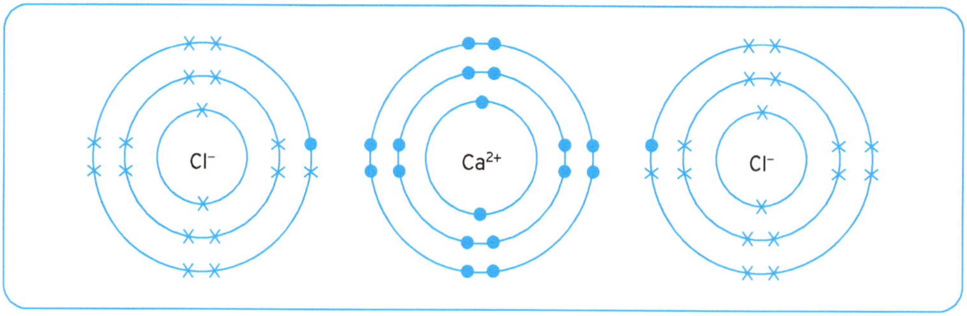

Figure 3.5
The formation of calcium chloride.

the more simple ions considered earlier. For example, the hydrogen carbonate ion possesses a single negative charge, and consequently it forms an ionic bond with a sodium ion to form sodium hydrogen carbonate ($NaHCO_3$). Polyatomic ions are considered in Practice point 3.3.

Practice point 3.3

Polyatomic ions in the body

The hydrogen carbonate ion is important in the regulation of blood acidity. Intravenous infusions (drips) of a solution of sodium hydrogen carbonate are used to control excessive blood acidity. You can recognise a bag containing sodium hydrogen carbonate from the structural formula $NaHCO_3$. The old-fashioned name for this compound, sodium bicarbonate, is still in common use too. Table 3.2 lists some polyatomic radicals that are important within the body.

Table 3.2 Important polyatomic ions.

Polyatomic radical	Importance
Ammonium (NH_4^+)	Regulation of urinary pH
Dihydrogen phosphate ($H_2PO_4^-$)	Regulation of urinary pH
Hydrogen carbonate (HCO_3^-)	Regulation of blood pH; transport of CO_2
Hydroxide (OH^-)	Produced by many bases
Monohydrogen phosphate (HPO_4^{2-})	Regulation of urinary pH
Phosphate (PO_4^-)	Component of adenosine triphosphate (ATP), the body's chemical form of energy

In-text review

- ✔ Compounds are substances that consist of atoms of more than one kind, joined by chemical bonds.
- ✔ Atoms are most stable when they have a full outer energy level.
- ✔ Atoms can achieve stability by losing or gaining electrons in order to achieve the electron configuration of the nearest inert gas. For example, sodium (Na, configuration 2.8.1) loses an electron in order to achieve the electron configuration of neon (Ne, configuration 2.8). Chlorine (Cl, configuration 2.8.7) gains an electron to achieve the configuration of argon (Ar, configuration 2.8.8).
- ✔ When atoms lose or gain electrons, they become charged particles called ions. When sodium (Na) loses a single electron, it becomes a sodium ion with a single positive charge (Na^+). When chlorine gains an electron, it becomes a chlorine ion with a single negative charge (Cl^-).
- ✔ A bond formed by the attraction of two oppositely charged ions is referred to as an ionic bond. Sodium chloride (NaCl) is one example of an ionic compound.

Covalent bonding

Earlier we noted that certain atoms, particularly those with four or five electrons in the outer energy level, do not form ions. You might then wonder whether this means that they do not form compounds by bonding with other atoms. In fact, atoms that do not form ions do form compounds with other atoms. They do so not through the exchange of electrons but through a process of electron sharing. The bonds that result from the sharing of electrons are called **covalent bonds**, and the structure that results from the covalent bonding of atoms is referred to as a molecule. Water (H_2O) is one example of a covalent compound. In the water molecule, an atom of oxygen shares two of its electrons with two atoms of hydrogen.

- ***Refer to the Periodic Table in the appendix and make a note of the atomic numbers and electron configurations of oxygen and hydrogen.***

Oxygen has an atomic number of 8 and its electron configuration is 2.6. This means that its valency is 2, since it requires two more electrons to achieve a stable valence shell. In contrast, hydrogen has an atomic number of 1 and possesses a single electron in its only energy level. It therefore has a valency of 1, since it requires one further electron in order to achieve a stable valence shell. In water molecules, the oxygen atom has six of its own electrons in its valence shell plus one shared with each of the two hydrogen atoms, as shown is Figure 3.6. Similarly, the valence shell of each of the two hydrogen atoms has one of its own electrons plus one shared with the oxygen atom.

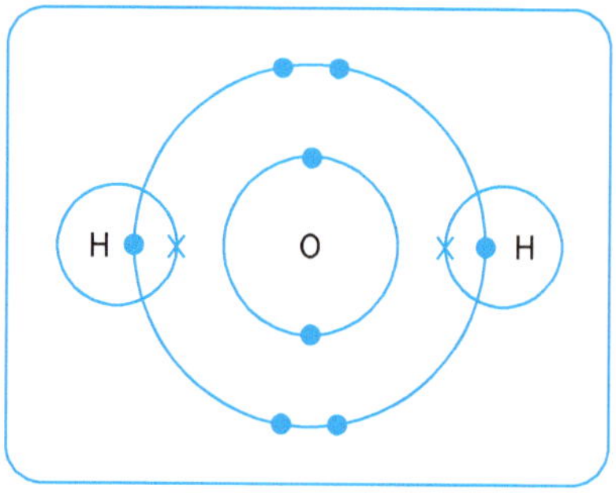

Figure 3.6
The covalent bonding of oxygen and hydrogen to form water.

At this point, it is worth pointing out that covalent bonds can be formed between atoms of the same element. For example, two atoms of hydrogen share electrons to form a molecule of hydrogen (H_2), as shown in Figure 3.7. Similarly, oxygen and nitrogen exist not as individual atoms but as the molecules O_2 and N_2, respectively. Consequently, these elements are referred to as diatomic gases (literally, two-atom gases).

Double and triple covalent bonds

Have a look at Figure 3.7 again.

- ***In the formation of molecules of hydrogen, oxygen and nitrogen, how many electrons are shared in each case?***

You should have noted that in the case of hydrogen, each atom shares one of its electrons with another, and a single covalent bond is formed. In the case of oxygen, each atom achieves a stable (full) outer energy level by sharing two of its electrons with another oxygen atom, and this is referred to as a double covalent bond. Not surprisingly, when nitrogen atoms each share three electrons, a triple covalent bond is formed.

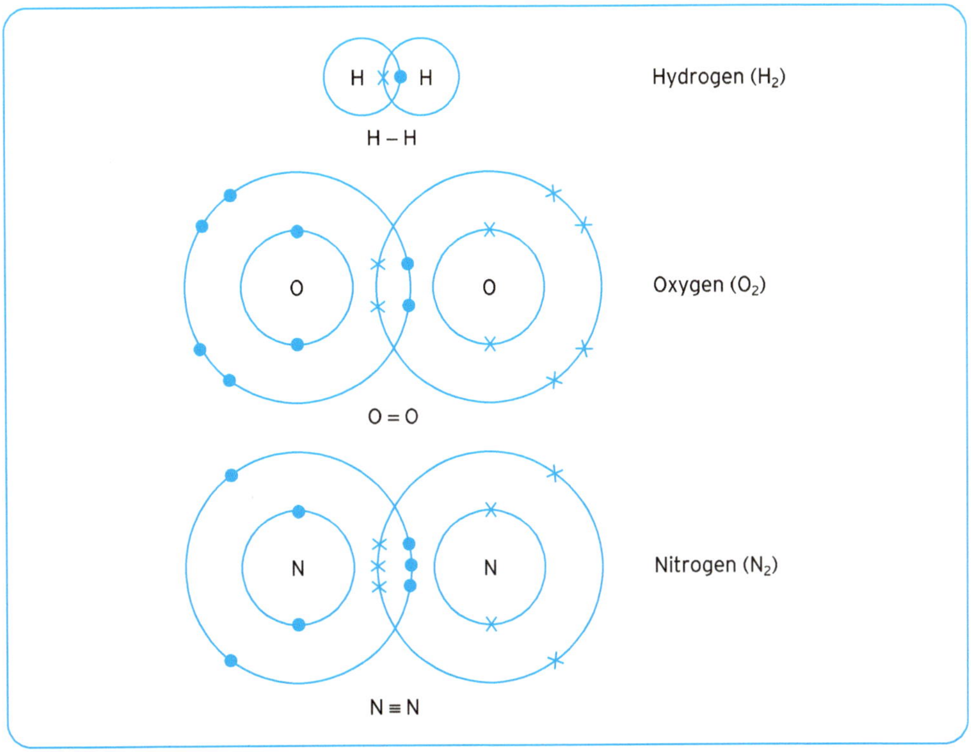

Figure 3.7
Covalent bonding in diatomic gases.

Non-polar and polar molecules

Although electron sharing forms covalent compounds, the atoms that make up a molecule do not necessarily share electrons equally. If the electrons that take part in a covalent bond are not shared equally between the atoms of the molecule, it is described as being **polar**.

- ***Why might the electrons in a covalent bond not be shared equally between the atoms of the molecule?***

An atom with a greater number of protons will exert a greater attraction over shared electrons than will an atom with fewer protons, because of the greater positive charge carried by the larger nucleus. Such is the case in the water molecule, in which each oxygen atom shares electrons with two atoms of hydrogen.

- ***How many protons do the nuclei of oxygen and hydrogen possess?***

Remember that this information is given by the atomic number. The oxygen nucleus is larger than the hydrogen nucleus. The oxygen nucleus possesses eight protons, while hydrogen has only one proton. Consequently, the oxygen atom attracts shared electrons more strongly than do the hydrogen atoms; this leads to the oxygen atom possessing a slight negative charge and the hydrogen atoms possessing a slight positive charge. The polar nature of water is explained more fully in Chapter 4.

Table 3.3 Characteristics of ionic and covalent compounds.

Ionic bonds	Covalent bonds	Ionic compounds	Covalent compounds
Formed by the transfer of electrons	Formed by sharing electrons	Tend to have high melting points	Tend to have low melting points
Involve the formation of oppositely charged ions that attract each other		Soluble in polar solvents such as water	Dissolve in non-polar solvents such as alcohol

In contrast, non-polar molecules are the result of covalent bonding between identical atoms, as is the case in H_2 (two hydrogen atoms bonding), O_2 (two oxygen atoms bonding) and N_2 (two nitrogen atoms bonding).

Thus far, we have discussed two types of bond (ionic bonds and covalent bonds) that are formed in different ways. The types of compound that possess these bonds (ionic compounds and covalent compounds) have different characteristics, and these are compared in Table 3.3.

Hydrogen bonds

When the covalent bonding of a hydrogen atom to an atom of another element results in the formation of a polar molecule, the positive (hydrogen) end of one molecule is attracted to the negative end of a second polar molecule, and the resultant bond is called a **hydrogen bond**. Hydrogen bonds occur between water molecules when the slightly positive hydrogen ends attract the partially negative oxygen ends of other molecules. Hydrogen bonds also occur between hydrogen atoms that are attached to nitrogen atoms and oxygen atoms that are part of a C=O group. Such hydrogen bonds are present in most proteins (see Chapter 7) and in deoxyribonucleic acid (DNA). In fact, hydrogen bonds are important in the unique shape of DNA – the double helix. You can read more about DNA in Chapter 15.

Structural formulae

The type of chemical formula that we have used so far (for example, CO_2) is referred to more correctly as the **molecular formula**. This provides us with information about the atoms present in a compound and the ratios in which they occur. Although this information is useful, a molecular formula does not show how the atoms of a compound are arranged. This information is indicated by the **structural formula**, in which bonds between atoms are shown as solid lines. By way of example, the structural formulae of three compounds are given in Figure 3.8. It is also worth noting here that compounds that share the same molecular formulae but have different arrangements of atoms are referred to as **isomers**.

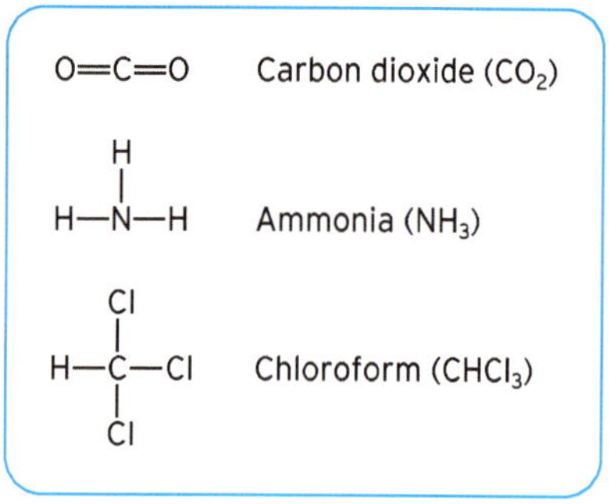

Figure 3.8
Three examples of structural formulae.

Molecular mass

The **molecular mass** of a compound is the sum of the relative atomic masses of the elements that make up the compound. Taking carbon dioxide (CO_2) as an example:

Element	Relative atomic mass	Number of atoms/ions	Total
Carbon (C)	12.01	1	12.01
Oxygen (O)	16	2	32
			44.01

In a similar way, the molecular mass of larger molecules such as glucose ($C_6H_{12}O_6$) is calculated as follows:

Element	Relative atomic mass	Number of atoms/ions	Total
Carbon (C)	12.01	6	72.06
Hydrogen (H)	1.01	12	12.12
Oxygen (O)	16	6	96
			180.18

Understanding molecular mass becomes important when the concept of the **mole** is examined and in clinical practice when dealing with millimoles per litre (mmol/l) as an expression of concentration. This unit is used in a variety of situations, such as in the expression of concentration of glucose in the blood of a **diabetic** patient.

The mole

In everyday, language we sometimes use expressions to designate numbers, for example couple and dozen. Let us now ask two rather obvious questions.

- ***How many apples are a couple? How many apples are a dozen?***

Yes: there are 2 and 12, respectively. If we were then to ask the same questions of a couple of oranges and a dozen oranges, the answers would be the same - a couple is always two and a dozen always refers to 12. In a similar way, a mole is an expression of the amount of a substance that contains a specific number of particles. They could be atoms, ions or molecules.

- ***So what number of particles does a mole of a substance contain?***

Certainly not a couple or a dozen, but a very large number indeed - 6.022×10^{23} in fact. This number is sometimes referred to as **Avogadro's number**, which for the purpose of definition is the number of atoms in 12 g of the ^{12}C isotope.

- ***But what about other elements – what is the weight of one mole of sodium atoms, for example?***

This is actually very easy to work out. The weight of a mole of atoms is equal to the relative atomic mass of an element expressed in grams. Since the relative atomic mass of sodium is 22.99, one mole of sodium atoms weighs 22.99 g.

- ***And what about the weight of one mole of a compound, such as NaCl?***

Once again, this is easy to work out - one mole of a compound is equal to the molecular mass of that compound expressed in grams. Remember that the molecular mass of NaCl is calculated as follows:

Element	Relative atomic mass	Number of atoms/ions	Total
Sodium (Na)	22.99	1	22.99
Chlorine (Cl)	35.45	1	35.45
			58.44

Therefore, one mole of NaCl weighs 58.44 g.

- ***Is there any point in learning about moles?***

Indeed, there is. Moles and millimoles (there are 1000 millimoles in a mole) are used by nurses, other health-care workers and scientists as shown in Practice point 3.4.

Practice point 3.4

Moles in clinical practice

One of the most common uses of the mole is in expressing concentration, whether of substances dissolved in blood, intravenous fluids or solutions of drugs. This is explained more fully in Chapter 4. For the time being, we shall give one example: the normal blood glucose concentration is 3.9–5.6 mmol/l (millimoles per litre), but it becomes elevated in diabetes mellitus. A practice nurse seeing patients in a diabetes clinic would clearly need to understand the units of measurement of blood sugar as well as the condition diabetes mellitus if a patient's condition is to be effectively monitored and treated.

In-text review

- ✔ Certain atoms, particularly those with four or five electrons in the outer energy level, do not form ions. Instead, such atoms form compounds with other atoms through a process of electron sharing. The bonds that result from the sharing of electrons are called covalent bonds.
- ✔ The structure that results from the covalent bonding of atoms is referred to as a molecule. Water (H_2O) is one example of a covalent compound. In the water molecule, an atom of oxygen shares two of its electrons with two atoms of hydrogen.

- ✔ Compounds with the same molecular formula but different structural formulae are called isomers.
- ✔ The molecular mass of a compound is the sum of the masses of the elements that make up that compound.
- ✔ A mole of a substance contains 6.022×10^{23} particles of that substance.
- ✔ The weight of a mole of atoms is equal to the relative atomic mass of an element expressed in grams. Since the relative atomic mass of sodium is 22.99, one mole of sodium atoms weighs 22.99 g.
- ✔ In clinical practice, concentration is often expressed in terms of millimoles per litre (mmol/l).

Chemical reactions

A chemical reaction is an interaction between chemical substances that results in a change of bonding between atoms. The substances that take part in a chemical reaction are referred to as **reactants** and the new substances produced as a consequence of a reaction are referred to as **products**. For example, when the reactants are sodium (Na) and chlorine (Cl), the product is the compound sodium chloride (NaCl). Chemical reactions are described in the form of an equation using chemical symbols. In such equations, reactants and products are separated by a horizontal arrow pointing away from the reactants on the left and towards the products on the right. When there is more than one reactant or more than one product, the substances are separated by a plus (+) sign, in the manner shown below:

$$A + B \rightarrow AB$$

$$\text{Reactants} \rightarrow \text{Products}$$

When using chemical equations, it is important to remember the principle of the conservation of matter, which states that matter cannot be created or destroyed in a chemical reaction. That is, there must be the same number of atoms of each element on the left- and right-hand sides of the equation. When this is the case, the equation is said to be balanced.

There are many different types of chemical reaction, including combination reactions and decomposition reactions, both of which are important in the body. Some of the different types of reaction are described below.

Combination reactions

Combination reactions involve two or more substances combining to form a single substance. Such reactions are sometimes referred to as synthesis reactions, and they conform to the pattern shown below:

$$A + B \rightarrow AB$$

One simple example of a combination reaction is that between sodium and chlorine to form sodium chloride:

$$Na + Cl \rightarrow NaCl$$

Note that this equation is balanced - there is one atom of sodium and one atom of chlorine on the left and one ion of each on the right.

- ***Are there examples of combination reactions in the body?***

There are, as Practice point 3.5 shows.

Practice point 3.5

Combination reactions in the body

The combination of oxygen with the erythrocyte (red blood cell) pigment **haemoglobin** (Hb) to form **oxyhaemoglobin** (HbO) is an example of a combination reaction. Haemoglobin is a rather complex molecule, so no attempt is made here to give its chemical formula. We can, however, illustrate its reaction with oxygen in the following way:

$$Hb + 4O_2 \rightarrow HbO$$

- ***Where does this reaction take place?***

It takes place in the lungs - this will be considered in more detail in Chapter 6.

- ***What kinds of problem relating to this combination might arise?***

It is possible to have insufficient haemoglobin to carry O_2 - a condition referred to as **anaemia**. Alternatively, haemoglobin might be 'blocked' and unable to take up oxygen. This occurs in carbon monoxide (CO) poisoning, for example from engine fumes. CO combines with haemoglobin to form **carboxyhaemoglobin**, which can no longer carry oxygen. Finally, in some forms of lung disease, insufficient O_2 passes through the damaged lungs to be picked up by haemoglobin into the blood.

Decomposition reactions

Decomposition reactions involve the breakdown of one substance to produce two or more products according to the pattern shown below:

$$AB \rightarrow A + B$$

Practice point 3.6 identifies where such reactions occur within the body.

Some compounds decompose (dissociate) into ions when dissolved in water. This form of decomposition is referred to as **ionisation**. It is illustrated below using the examples of

Practice point 3.6

Decomposition reactions in the body

You will no doubt realise that an example of a decomposition reaction in the body is the reverse of that noted in Practice point 3.5:

$$HbO \rightarrow Hb + 4O_2$$

- ***Where does this reaction occur?***

It occurs in the tissues where haemoglobin gives up its O_2 to the body's cells. The digestion of food in the gut is also a form of decomposition reaction, and you can read more about this in Chapter 7. Decomposition reactions in the body are sometimes referred to as catabolic and the sum of these reactions as catabolism. The word metabolism is used to collectively describe **anabolism** and **catabolism**.

hydrochloric acid, sodium hydroxide and sodium chloride. In the examples below, the subscript (aq) refers to water (*aqua*) and means the substance is dissolved in water.

$HCl_{(aq)}$	$\rightarrow$	H^+	+	Cl^-
hydrochloric acid		hydrogen ions		chloride ions
$NaOH_{(aq)}$	$\rightarrow$	Na^+	+	OH^-
sodium hydroxide		sodium ions		hydroxyl ions
$NaCl_{(aq)}$	$\rightarrow$	Na^+	+	Cl^-
sodium chloride		sodium ions		chloride ions

In the case of hydrochloric acid, ionisation produces hydrogen ions and chloride ions. **Acids** are substances that liberate hydrogen ions. In the case of sodium hydroxide, ionisation results in sodium ions and hydroxyl ions. A substance that liberates hydroxyl ions is referred to as a **base**. Acids and bases are discussed in Chapter 5. Finally, in the case of sodium chloride, ionisation produces sodium ions and chloride ions. A substance that ionises to produce ions other than hydrogen ions or hydroxyl ions is referred to as a **salt**.

In-text review

- ✔ A chemical reaction is an interaction between chemical substances that results in a change of bonding between atoms.
- ✔ Substances that take part in a chemical reaction are referred to as reactants, and new substances produced as a consequence of a reaction are referred to as products. For example, when the reactants are sodium (Na) and chlorine (Cl), the product is the compound sodium chloride (NaCl).

- ✔ Combination reactions involve two or more substances combining to form a single substance. Such reactions are sometimes referred to as synthesis reactions. They conform to the pattern shown below:

$$A + B \rightarrow AB$$

  For example, that between sodium and chlorine to form sodium chloride:

$$Na + Cl \rightarrow NaCl$$

- ✔ Decomposition reactions involve the breakdown of one substance to produce two or more products, according to the pattern shown below:

$$AB \rightarrow A + B$$

  For example, when oxyhaemoglobin (HbO) gives up oxygen (O_2) to become haemoglobin (Hb):

$$HbO \rightarrow Hb + 4O_2$$

Displacement reactions

Displacement reactions involve the displacement of a less reactive element by a more reactive element. They conform to the general pattern shown below:

$$AB + C \rightarrow AC + B$$

This type of reaction is sometimes described as a substitution reaction, since one element is substituted for another. An example is given in Practice point 3.7.

Practice point 3.7

Displacement reactions in the body

An abnormally elevated concentration of potassium ions (K^+) in the blood is referred to as **hyperkalaemia**. The prefix 'hyper' refers to high, 'kal' is derived from the Greek word *kallium* (potassium) and 'aemia' refers to the blood. Hyperkalaemia is a potentially dangerous condition that may cause cardiac arrest (the heart stops effective pumping). Since the kidneys play an important role in excreting potassium ions, renal failure (kidney failure) is one possible cause of hyperkalaemia. This is treated using a displacement reaction involving calcium polystyrene sulphonate. Following the oral administration of this medicine, calcium polystyrene sulphonate is absorbed from the gut into the bloodstream. Here, calcium is displaced by potassium in the following way:

$$K^+ + \text{calcium polystyrene sulphonate} \rightarrow Ca^{2+} + \text{potassium polystyrene sulphonate}$$

By this means, free potassium ions are removed from the blood and hyperkalaemia is treated.

Partner exchange

Partner exchange reactions could be regarded as those in which there is a double displacement. That is, the substitution of elements between compounds results in the formation of more than one new compound. Such reactions conform to the pattern noted below:

$$AB + CD \rightarrow AD + CB$$

An example of such a reaction is that between hydrochloric acid (HCl) and sodium hydrogen carbonate ($NaHCO_3$) according to the equation shown below:

$$\underset{\text{hydrochloric acid}}{HCl_{(aq)}} + \underset{\text{sodium hydrogen carbonate}}{NaHCO_3} \rightarrow \underset{\text{carbonic acid}}{H_2CO_3} + \underset{\text{sodium chloride}}{NaCl}$$

The relevance of this reaction to the body is explained in Practice point 3.8.

Practice point 3.8

Partner exchange reactions in the body

The stomach produces hydrochloric acid, which performs the important role of turning a protein called **pepsinogen** into an active protein-digesting enzyme called **pepsin**. Excessive acidity, however, causes pain and can result in damage to the lining of the stomach. Sodium hydrogen carbonate is a component of a number of antacid medicines used to treat excess stomach acidity. When such medicines are swallowed, the above reaction takes place in the stomach.

- ***What does this achieve?***

The result is that a strong acid (HCl) is replaced by a weak acid (H_2CO_3). In addition, H_2CO_3 decomposes into the gas CO_2 and water, according to the following equation:

$$H_2CO_3 \rightarrow CO_2 + H_2O$$

- ***What now happens to this CO_2? Hint: CO_2 is a gas.***

It causes burping!

Reversible reactions

In view of the convention of placing reactants on the left-hand side of an equation arrow and products on the right, we can think of reactions as having a direction. We might say that a reaction proceeds from left to right. In some cases, however, the reverse reaction also takes place - that is, the reactants can be reformed from the products. Consequently, we might say in such cases that the reaction also proceeds from right to left. Such reactions are then said to be **reversible reactions**, and this is indicated by the presence of a double arrow in the equation. An example of such a reaction is shown below:

$$\underset{\text{carbonic acid}}{H_2CO_3} \rightleftharpoons \underset{\text{hydrogen carbonate ion}}{HCO_3^-} + \underset{\text{hydrogen ion}}{H^+}$$

After a period of time, the rate of the decomposition reaction (left to right in the above example) and the combination reaction (right to left) become equal, and we say that a chemical equilibrium has been reached. For this reason, reversible reactions are sometimes called equilibrium reactions.

- ***Does this mean that there is an equal concentration of reactants and products?***

No. When a reversible reaction reaches equilibrium, it simply means that the rate of the two reactions (left to right and right to left) are equal and there is no net increase in the concentration of the reactants and products. In the above reaction, the concentration of hydrogen carbonate ions in blood is 20 times that of carbonic acid molecules.

- ***So could anything occur to change the rate of the reactions?***

Indeed, it could. For example, if the concentration of carbonic acid became elevated, the rate of the decomposition reaction (left to right) would increase until the carbonic acid : hydrogen carbonate ion concentration was restored to 1 : 20 again. We might say that the reaction equilibrium had been displaced to the right. In fact, this is an important principle behind the behaviour of reversible reactions - any change in concentration of reactants or products displaces the equilibrium in order to restore these concentrations.

You will become very familiar with the above reaction, since carbonic acid is formed in the blood when carbon dioxide (CO_2) produced by metabolising cells reacts with water. The complete reaction is given below:

$$\underset{\text{carbon dioxide}}{CO_2} + \underset{\text{water}}{H_2O} \rightleftharpoons \underset{\text{carbonic acid}}{H_2CO_3} \rightleftharpoons \underset{\text{hydrogen ion}}{H^+} + \underset{\text{hydrogen carbonate ion}}{HCO_3^-} \rightleftharpoons \underset{\text{hydrogen ion}}{H^+} + \underset{\text{carbonate ion}}{CO_3^{2-}}$$

You will read more about acids and the body's regulation of acid-base balance in Chapter 5.

Oxidation–reduction reactions

Oxidation reactions are very important in the world around us, for example in the rusting of iron. They are also important within our bodies, for example in breaking down glucose to release energy.

- ***What actually happens in an oxidation reaction?***

The original definition of oxidation was a reaction in which a substance gained an oxygen atom or lost a hydrogen atom. Consider the example of ethanal (acetaldehyde), which gains an oxygen atom to form ethanoic acid (acetic acid). You may be unfamiliar with these compounds, but simply count the number of oxygen atoms that each possesses. Ethanal has one and acetic acid has two.

$$\underset{\text{ethanal}}{CH_3CHO} \rightarrow \underset{\text{ethanoic acid}}{CH_3COOH}$$

Now consider another example that occurs as part of the energy-producing reactions within our bodies. It involves nicotinamide adenine dinucleotide. This is a rather complex molecule, so instead of giving its molecular formula the abbreviation NAD is used. The reaction also involves a compound that NAD forms with hydrogen - NADH.

$$NADH \rightarrow NAD^{+}$$

We say that NADH has been oxidised to NAD^{+} because it has lost hydrogen. Chemical reactions similar to these also occur in the absence of oxygen and hydrogen, and so oxidation is currently defined as a chemical reaction in which a substance loses one or more electrons. In fact, in the above example, NADH actually loses two electrons and a hydrogen ion (H^{+}). Consequently, the product is NAD^{+}, not NAD.

● ***And what about reduction – how is it defined?***

Originally, **reduction** was defined as a reaction in which a substance lost an oxygen atom or gained a hydrogen atom. This definition has also been revised, however, so that reduction is currently defined as a reaction in which a substance gains one or more electrons.

● ***So reduction is in fact the opposite of oxidation?***

Indeed, it is. In fact, oxidation can never occur without reduction, as the electrons lost from one substance will be picked up by another. Consequently, it is more accurate to speak of oxidation-reduction reactions rather than one or the other. Chemists usually abridge this expression to **redox** reactions. You will read more about this in Chapter 8.

In-text review

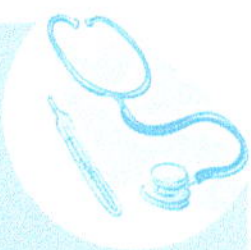

✔ Displacement reactions involve the displacement of a less reactive element by a more reactive element and conform to the general pattern shown below:

$$AB + C \rightarrow AC + B$$

✔ An example of such a reaction is that between hydrochloric acid (HCl) and sodium hydrogen carbonate ($NaHCO_3$), according to the equation shown below:

$HCl_{(aq)}$	+	$NaHCO_3$	$\rightarrow$	H_2CO_3	+	NaCl
hydrochloric acid		sodium hydrogen carbonate		carbonic acid		sodium chloride

✔ When reactants can be reformed from the products, we say that the reaction proceeds from right to left as well as from left to right. Such reactions are said to be reversible reactions, an example of which is:

H_2CO_3	$\rightleftharpoons$	HCO_3^-	+	H^+
carbonic acid		hydrogen carbonate ion		hydrogen ion

✔ Redox reactions are those in which oxidation and reduction take place. Oxidation is a chemical reaction in which a substance loses electrons and reduction is a reaction in which electrons are gained.

Chemical reactions and energy

Chemical reactions invariably involve energy. A certain amount of energy is required to bring about a chemical reaction in the first place, and this is referred to as the **activation energy**. This represents the energy required to break the chemical bonds of the reactants. If the products of a chemical reaction possess less energy than the reactants themselves, then energy will be liberated during the reaction. Such a reaction is then described as **exothermic**. For example, in the body's cells, the substance adenosine triphosphate (ATP) is broken down to adenosine diphosphate (ADP) in order to liberate energy. In contrast, if the products of a chemical reaction possess more energy than the reactants themselves, then energy will have to be supplied in order for the reaction to proceed. Such chemical reactions are described as **endothermic**. The reverse of the above process - the formation of ATP from ADP - is an example of an endothermic reaction. The role of ATP and ADP are described more fully in Chapter 8.

- ***But where does this energy come from in the first place?***

It comes from the breakdown of the food that we eat. It may seem an obvious point, but we have to eat since we cannot make our own nutrients, like plants and some microorganisms can. When we digest food, we break down large compounds to smaller compounds that can be absorbed into the blood and subsequently used by the cells. When the end products of digestion are metabolised in the body, the cells take high-energy compounds such as glucose and convert them into low-energy compounds such as carbon dioxide and water. The energy released by such exothermic reactions can then be used by the cells. The energy may be given off as heat or used in some other chemical process.

Factors that affect the rate of chemical reactions

A number of factors affect the rate of chemical reactions, including the concentration of reactants and the temperature at which the reaction takes place. In order to illustrate how these two factors affect reaction rate, consider the example of a simple combination reaction. Remember that this type of reaction conforms to the following equation:

$$A + B \rightarrow AB$$

$$\text{reactants} \rightarrow \text{products}$$

A reaction will take place only when the reactants (A and B) collide.

- ***How would an increase in the concentration of reactants affect the likelihood of a collision?***

It would increase the likelihood of a collision. In addition, an increase of temperature causes reactants to collide with greater energy, and this makes a reaction following collision more likely too. The rate of reaction can also be affected in other ways - by the presence of a substance called a **catalyst**.

Catalysts

A catalyst is a substance that increases the rate of a chemical reaction without being changed itself by that reaction. Catalysts achieve their effect by lowering the activation energy, which is the amount of energy required to cause a reaction in the first place. They are responsible for considerable improvements in the efficiency of industrial processes. More importantly to us, they are proteins that fulfil the role of catalysts within the body.

- ***What is the name by which biological catalysts are known?***

They are called **enzymes**, one example of which is **carbonic anhydrase**. This enzyme is present in red blood cells and catalyses the reaction between carbon dioxide (CO_2) and water (H_2O) to form carbonic acid (H_2CO_3). When an enzyme is involved in a reaction, placing its name above the equation arrow, as shown below, identifies it:

$$CO_2 + H_2O \xrightarrow{\text{carbonic anhydrase}} H_2CO_3$$

Enzymes are highly effective catalysts, and life would not be possible without them. They are also highly specific - each has an effect on one substance alone or on a number of closely related substances known as **substrates**.

- ***But how do catalysts work?***

The lock-and-key hypothesis is an attempt to explain enzyme action. It is illustrated in Figure 3.9 in the context of a decomposition reaction, but it should be remembered that enzymes also catalyse combination reactions, as the previous example has shown. The first step in enzyme action is the formation of a complex with the substrate. An enzyme-substrate complex forms because the unique three-dimensional structure of an enzyme leads to the existence of an active site. This is a small region that has a reciprocal shape to that of the substrate, into which the substrate fits, rather like a key fitting into a lock. The enzyme is believed to stretch, weaken and finally break chemical bonds within the substrate, and this allows new products to form. These new products then move away from the active site, leaving the enzyme unchanged. Another related model of enzyme action is described as **induced fit**. In this explanation, the active site is regarded as being flexible rather than rigid. It is suggested that the active site undergoes a change in shape during the formation of the enzyme-substrate complex in order to accommodate the substrate.

Although some proteins are capable of functioning as enzymes alone, others need to be joined to other substances. In such cases, the protein part of the enzyme is referred to as the **apoenzyme** and the non-protein part as a **cofactor**. Some cofactors are simple metal ions, while others are complex organic molecules called **coenzymes**. Many vitamins function as coenzymes. Vitamins are described in Chapter 7.

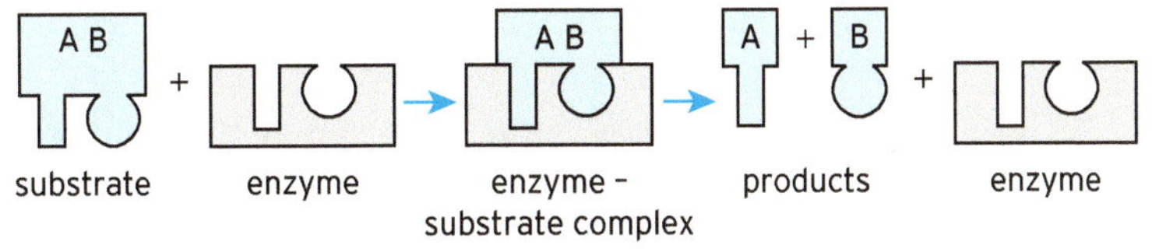

Figure 3.9
The lock-and-key hypothesis of enzyme action.

Sometimes enzymes lose their ability to function, and they are then said to have been **denatured**. Heat, a change in pH and some chemical substances are commonly responsible for denaturing enzymes.

- ***What actually happens when an enzyme is denatured?***

Essentially, denaturation occurs when the active site is lost because of damage to the three-dimensional structure of the enzyme. This occurs because of the disruption of the weak hydrogen bonds responsible for the unique shape of protein molecules.

Finally, you might find it helpful to know that enzymes are usually named by adding the suffix 'ase' to a prefix derived from the name of the substrate.

- ***So what substrate does sucrase act upon?***

It acts on sucrose – the sugar commonly known as table sugar.

In-text review

- ✔ Activation energy is the energy required to break the chemical bonds of reactants.
- ✔ In exothermic reactions, the products have less energy than the reactants and energy is liberated.
- ✔ In endothermic reactions, the products have more energy than the reactants and energy is used.
- ✔ The rate of chemical reactions is affected by the concentration of reactants and the temperature.
- ✔ A catalyst is a substance that increases the rate of a chemical reaction without being changed itself by that reaction.
- ✔ Biological catalysts are known as enzymes.

The carbon atom and organic chemistry

The word **organic** was originally used to refer to compounds found in organisms, but it then came to mean compounds containing carbon. Most compounds within the body contain carbon, and often hydrogen and oxygen too. In current popular usage, the word 'organic' has connotations of naturalness and safety, but many of the products of the petrochemical industry, which certainly do not occur in nature, also contain carbon and are, therefore, organic. In this text, the term 'organic' is used in the way a chemist would use it – meaning a substance containing carbon. In contrast, inorganic chemistry is the study of substances that do not contain carbon.

- ***Using the Periodic Table in the appendix, look up the atomic number of carbon and work out its electron configuration.***

The atomic number of carbon is 6, and therefore its electron configuration is 2.4.

Table 3.4 Carbon-atom chain prefixes.

Prefix	Number of C atoms	Example	Prefix	Number of C atoms	Example
Meth-	1	Methane	Hex-	6	Hexane
Eth-	2	Ethane	Hept-	7	Heptane
Prop-	3	Propane	Oct-	8	Octane
But-	4	Butane	Non-	9	Nonane
Pent-	5	Pentane	Dec-	10	Decane

- ***How many more electrons does carbon require in order to achieve a stable valence shell?***

The correct answer is 4, and these may of course be obtained by sharing. Were someone to attempt to count the number of organic molecules, the figure would run into millions. One of the reasons for this abundance is the ability of carbon atoms to bond covalently with each other and thus form chains of varying lengths. Compounds in which the ends of these chains are not joined together are said to be **aliphatic**, while those in which the chains form a ring are said to be **cyclic**. Since many of these cyclic compounds have a characteristic smell, they are also known as **aromatic**. We shall consider examples of each a little later in this chapter. Some of the most important organic molecules within our bodies are **carbohydrates**, **proteins**, **fats** and **vitamins**. Indeed, they are so important that Chapter 7 has been given over to them along with other substances found in our food. In this section, we concentrate on other important organic molecules, such as alcohols. Let us first clarify how organic molecules are named.

The names of organic molecules usually begin with a prefix that indicates the length of the carbon atom chain. Table 3.4 identifies the first ten carbon atom prefixes. In each case, an example is given from a group of compounds called **alkanes**. You may be unfamiliar with many of these, but if you have ever used a camping stove, you may be familiar with propane and butane as fuels. Petrol is a mixture of organic molecules, including alkanes.

Chemical groups that are attached to a carbon-atom chain are called **substituents**. The simplest organic molecules result when carbon forms compounds with the substituent hydrogen alone. The resultant compounds are collectively referred to as **hydrocarbons**. Alkanes are examples of hydrocarbons, since they consist of hydrogen and carbon alone.

Hydrocarbons

Organic molecules that contain only single bonds between carbon atoms are said to be **saturated**. The group of aliphatic hydrocarbons (compounds containing only hydrogen and carbon in a straight chain) that are saturated are called **alkanes**, and they are named by adding the suffix -ane to the appropriate prefix. The simplest alkane is, therefore, methane.

- ***How many carbon atoms does methane possess?***

Remember those prefixes? If you do, you will have worked out that methane contains only one carbon atom (CH_4). Its structural formula is given in Figure 3.10. Perhaps you are already familiar with methane, since it is the main component of natural gas. You may also have used propane (C_3H_8) and butane (C_4H_{10}) as fuels in portable heaters and cookers.

- ***Take a moment to draw the structures of butane and propane.***

Now check your diagrams against Figure 3.10.

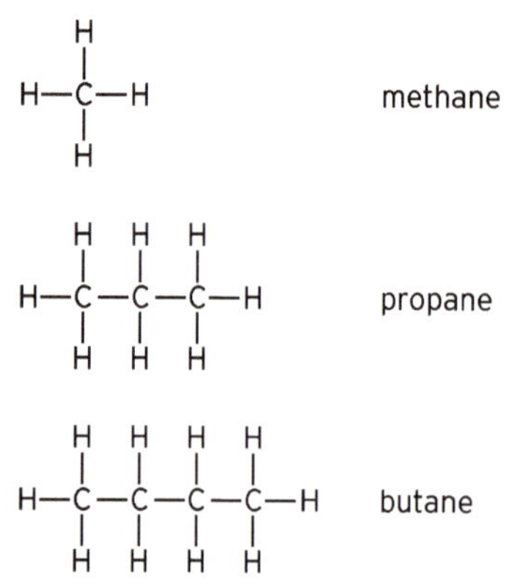

Figure 3.10
The structural formulae of methane, butane and propane.

Hydrocarbons that contain double or triple bonds are said to be **unsaturated**. This is a reference to the fact that the molecule contains less than the maximum number of substituents. The multiple bond could be chemically broken and further hydrogen atoms added, a process called **hydrogenation**. You will find reference is made to it on the back of margarine tubs. In this case, hydrogenation ensures that margarine remains solid at room temperature. **Alkenes** contain a double bond; the simplest member of this family is ethene (C_2H_4), the structure of which is shown in Figure 3.11. Note that alkenes are named using the suffix -ene. **Alkynes** contain a triple bond; the simplest member of this group is ethyne (C_2H_2), the structure of which is also given in Figure 3.11. Once again, note that the family to which this molecule belongs is given by the use of a suffix - in this case, it is -yne. You may be more familiar with ethyne by its alternative name, acetylene - the gas used in welding torches.

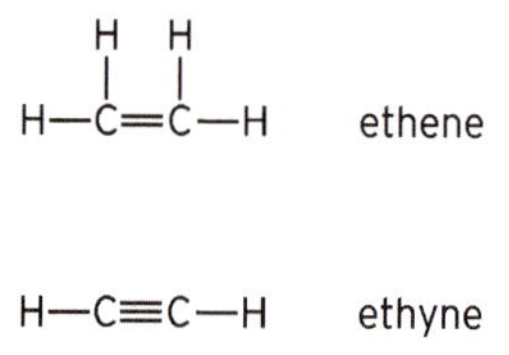

Figure 3.11
The structural formulae of ethene and ethyne.

- ***So are hydrocarbons important in health care?***

The alkanes, alkenes and alkynes are among the simplest organic molecules. In health care, we are interested in the function of the body, which contains some very complex organic molecules. You will no doubt encounter them later in your studies, but it would be too much to introduce them now. Many, such as **saturated fats**, contain chains of carbon atoms such as the alkanes and some, such as **polyunsaturated fats**, contain double bonds such as the alkenes. If you learn about the simpler organic molecules now, you will find it easier later on to understand the structure of more complex molecules found in the body. Some of these large, more complex organic molecules are introduced as nutrients in Chapter 7.

Many different organic compounds share chemical and physical properties. For example, most are flammable. Some properties, however, are characteristic of only certain groups. Consider odour for a moment. Methane has no smell; its use as a fuel, therefore, would be problematic, since gas leaks might go undetected were it not for the fact that gas companies add an odour to it. Other organic molecules have characteristic odours. For example, **ketones** (see later), which smell like pear drops, can be smelled on the breath of poorly controlled diabetic patients who produce ketones in excess. Consequently, smelling ketones on the breath of a patient is an important nursing observation. The distinctive chemical or physical properties of organic compounds exist as a consequence of the possession of certain chemical groups called **functional groups**. These often contain elements such as oxygen and hydrogen, and sometimes nitrogen too. We shall continue our study of organic molecules by thinking about **alcohols**.

Alcohols

Alcohols are compounds that contain one or more **hydroxyl groups** (OH) and conform to the general formula RCH_2OH. In organic chemistry, R stands for either a hydrogen atom or a carbon-atom chain with hydrogen atoms attached. Alcohols are named by adding the suffix -ol to the relevant prefix. Consequently, the simplest alcohol is methanol (CH_3OH). You might buy methanol in the form of methylated spirits in order to fuel a camping stove or for use as a solvent. If ingested, methanol may lead to blindness; therefore, in addition to methanol, methylated spirit contains colouring in order to draw attention to its toxic nature. When the term 'alcohol' is used in everyday language, it is not methanol that we are referring to but ethanol (CH_3CH_2OH). The structural formulae of both of these alcohols are given in Figure 3.12.

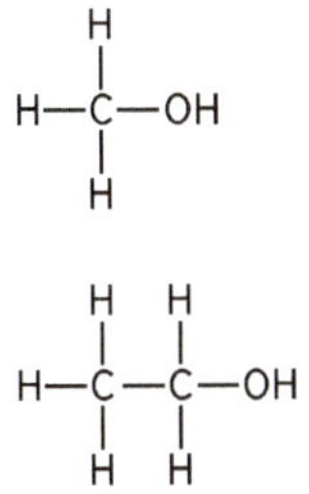

Figure 3.12
The structural formulae of methanol and ethanol.

- ***Now draw the structural formula of propanol.***

Remember that the prefix prop- indicates the presence of three carbon atoms.

- ***Is there a problem in drawing the structural formula of propanol?***

The hydroxyl group could be placed on an end carbon atom or on the middle atom. We clearly need to be told which; adding a number to the name does this. For example, 2-propanol (propan-2-ol) tells us to place the hydroxyl group on the second carbon atom, as shown in Figure 3.13. Incidentally, 2-propanol, sometimes called isopropyl alcohol, is used in injection swabs and some preparations that are used to clean the skin before an invasive procedure (a procedure that produces a wound). Isopropyl alcohol readily evaporates from the skin, producing a cooling effect. It is during this drying process that microorganisms on the skin are killed, and so it is necessary to wait for drying to occur before carrying out the invasive procedure.

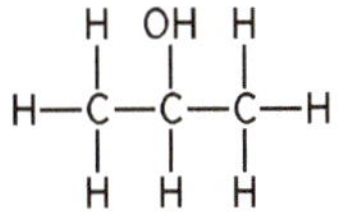

Figure 3.13
The structural formulae of 2-propanol.

Some alcohols possess more than one hydroxyl group. A good example is **glycerol** (glycerine), the structural formula of which is given in Figure 3.14. Glycerol is an important component of **glycerides** (a form of lipid), discussed more fully in Chapter 7. Glycerol is used as an emollient (a substance that softens the skin) and as a component of topical medications, while glycerol suppositories are sometimes used to soften the stool when constipation is present. In addition, since glycerol tastes sweet and has low toxicity, it is also found as a dilutent in liquid oral medications. Note that in the name glycerol, the aforementioned standard nomenclature has not been followed precisely. However, since 'glycerol' is the most commonly used name, it is the one given here.

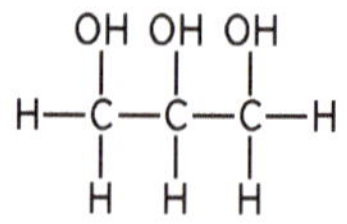

Figure 3.14
The structural formulae of glycerol.

Aldehydes

In this section, we consider the first of three groups of organic compounds that possess a carbonyl group (C=O) - the **aldehydes**. In aldehydes, a hydrogen atom is attached to the carbonyl group so that they conform to the general formula RCHO. They are named using the suffix -al and the simplest aldehyde is therefore methanal, the structural formula of which is shown in Figure 3.15. Although the aldehydes are not of major importance in health care, the carbonyl group is present in more complex molecules that *are* important. One example is the ketones.

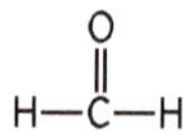

Figure 3.15
The structural formulae of methanal.

Ketones

Like aldehydes, **ketones** are characterised by the possession of a carbonyl group (C=O), but in this case it is located part way along a carbon-atom chain. Ketones conform to the general formula RCOR; the simplest ketone is, therefore, propanone, a compound that is more usually known by the name acetone (Figure 3.16). Nurses sometimes use acetone as a solvent of sticking plaster adhesive, but more importantly it is one of the ketones that is sometimes produced by the body and excreted in the urine. This occurs in fasting and in patients with diabetes mellitus, when lipids, instead of glucose, are used as a source of energy. Some ketones also possess an acidic carboxyl group (see later); the resultant accumulation of these leads to a condition referred to as ketoacidosis. (Acids are explained in Chapter 5.) Ketoacidosis may in turn lead to coma and death. Consequently, ketones will feature in your clinical studies.

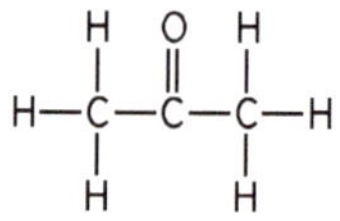

Figure 3.16
The structural formulae of acetone.

Carboxylic acids

In **carboxylic acids**, a hydroxyl group is attached to the carbonyl group to form a carboxyl group (COOH). Carboxylic acids therefore conform to the general formula RCOOH. The simplest member of this group is methanoic acid (formic acid) (HCOOH), but the most familiar is undoubtedly ethanoic acid (CH_3COOH) - sometimes called acetic acid or vinegar. The structural formula of both these compounds is shown in Figure 3.17. Carboxylic acids are sometimes referred to as fatty acids, since they are involved in the formation of **lipids** (fats). Lipids are explained in Chapter 7.

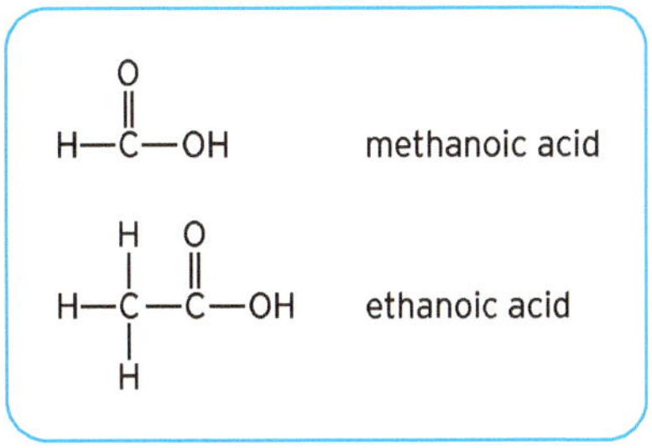

Figure 3.17
The structural formulae of methanoic acid and ethanoic acid.

Esters

Esters conform to the general formula RCOOR. They are formed from a reaction between an alcohol and a carboxylic acid, such as that shown in Figure 3.18.

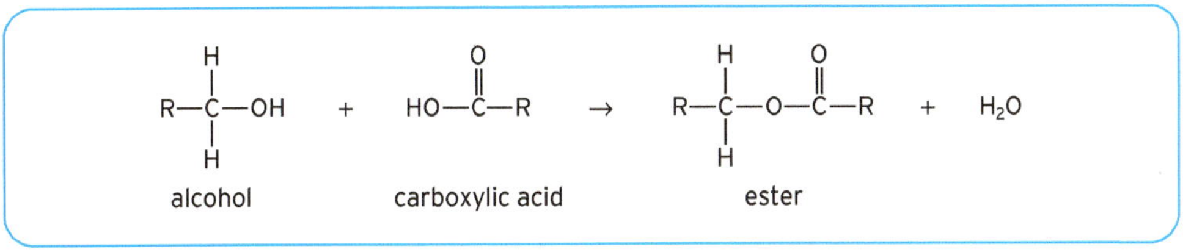

Figure 3.18
The formation of an ester.

- ***What type of reaction is this?***

It is a combination reaction, but since it results in the elimination of water, it is referred to as a **condensation reaction**. Of course, it is possible for an ester to undergo a decomposition reaction in order to reform a carboxylic acid and an alcohol, but in order for this to take place a water molecule would be required. A decomposition reaction of this type is referred to as **hydrolysis** - meaning to break with water. Since lipids (fats) are esters, this group of organic compounds will be encountered frequently during your study of health and illness. Lipids are explained in Chapter 7.

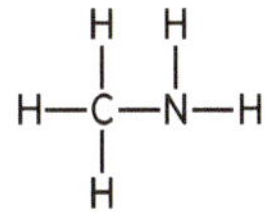

Figure 3.19
The structural formulae of methyl amine.

Amines

Amines are organic compounds that possess an amino group (NH_2) and conform to the general formula RCH_2NH_2. The simplest amine is, therefore, methyl amine, the structural formula of which is given in Figure 3.19. **Amino acids**, the molecules that join together to form proteins, possess both an amino group and a carboxyl group. Proteins are explained in Chapter 7. The structure of the amino acid glycine is shown in Figure 3.20. Other important molecules that occur in the body and that contain an amino group include the catecholamines

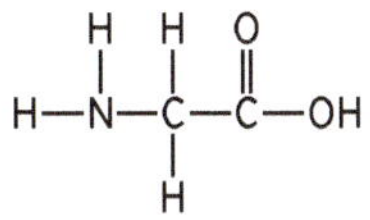

Figure 3.20
The structural formulae of the amino acid glycine.

epinephrine (adrenaline), norepinephrine (noradrenaline) and dopamine. Adrenaline is a hormone and dopamine is a neurotransmitter, while noradrenaline functions in both these roles. The analgesic (pain reliever) morphine and amphetamines are also amines, as their names imply.

Aromatic compounds

Aromatic hydrocarbons consist of unsaturated molecules in which the carbon atom chain is arranged in a ring, as the example of benzene (C_6H_6) shows in Figure 3.21. It is not usual to draw the structural formula of benzene in full, and a simplified version is also shown. You may have heard of benzene, since it is commonly used in industrial processes and is known to be carcinogenic (causes cancer). The benzene ring features in many aromatic compounds, including phenol, in which a hydroxyl group is attached directly to the benzene ring, as Figure 3.22 shows.

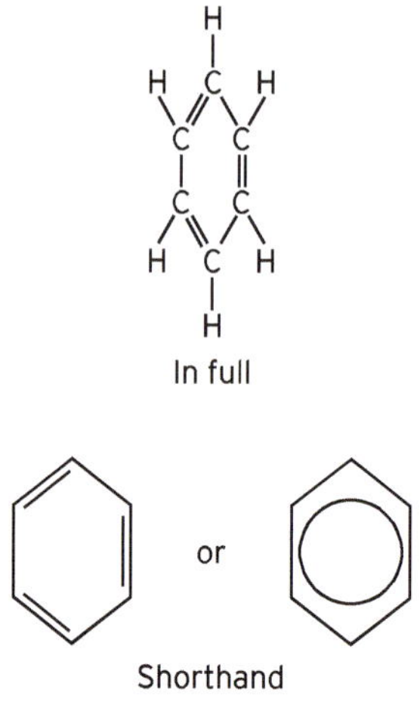

Figure 3.21
The structural formulae of benzene.

- ***What kind of organic compound is phenol?***

It is an alcohol, since it possess a hydroxyl group. Phenol kills bacteria, and Joseph Lister originally used it in 1867 as a surgical antiseptic, which he called carbolic acid. Through the use of phenol, Lister was able to improve the survival of his surgical patients. Bacteria, and the methods used to kill them, are described more fully in Chapter 16.

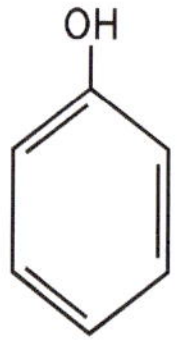

Figure 3.22
The structural formulae of phenol.

In-text review

- ✔ Organic chemistry is the study of compounds that contain carbon.
- ✔ In order to achieve stability, carbon shares four electrons.
- ✔ Organic molecules are either aliphatic (chain structure) or aromatic (ring structure).
- ✔ Hydrocarbons are aliphatic compounds that contain carbon and hydrogen.
- ✔ Important hydrocarbons include alkanes, alkenes and alkynes.
- ✔ Other important aliphatic compounds are alcohols, aldehydes, ketones, carboxylic acids and amines.
- ✔ Phenol is an example of an aromatic alcohol with antiseptic properties.

Summary

You have come to the end of a long chapter - well done! It began with a consideration of the states of matter, elements, compounds and chemical reactions and concluded with an outline of organic chemistry. Throughout, reference has been made to health care when applicable. As your knowledge increases, however, you will have many opportunities to link theory to practice and make use of your knowledge of chemistry. One example of a condition in which knowledge of chemistry is helpful is diabetes mellitus. This is a defect of carbohydrate metabolism in which blood sugar (glucose) levels are high (hyperglycaemia). In order to understand diabetes mellitus, it helps to know that glucose is an organic compound (we look more at this in Chapters 7 and 8). Blood glucose concentration is measured in terms of millimoles per litre (mmol/l), and it is clearly an advantage to understand what this unit of measurement means. Finally, an undesirable effect of using lipids as a source of fuel in diabetes mellitus is ketoacidosis - the condition in which blood becomes more acidic than normal as a consequence of the production of ketones. Clearly, there is much to learn about this common condition, and this book does not attempt to explain such complex conditions in any depth. It does, however, provide readers with the prerequisite knowledge that is helpful when undertaking study related more directly to clinical practice.

In addition, developments in health care will provide opportunities that have not existed in the past. For example, drug prescribing is one area of practice that is no longer the preserve of the medical profession. Clearly, an understanding of basic chemistry is advantageous to anyone embarking on a study of drugs and pharmacology. Perhaps one day you will run your own clinic and prescribe drugs for patients under your care in much the same way that doctors do now. In the meantime, the following summary points and self-test questions may be of help.

Summary points

- **Matter exists in three states: gas, liquid and solid.**
- **An atom is the smallest particle of matter that can enter a chemical reaction.**
- **A substance that consists of atoms of only one kind is referred to as an element.**
- **A substance that consists of atoms of more than one kind chemically bonded together is referred to as a compound.**
- **Atoms are made of protons, neutrons and electrons.**
- **Ions result when atoms gain or lose electrons.**
- **Ionic bonds are formed when electrons are exchanged between atoms.**
- **Covalent bonds are formed when atoms share electrons.**
- **When atoms share electrons equally, a non-polar molecule is formed.**
- **When atoms share electrons unequally, a polar molecule is formed.**
- **Hydrogen bonds form between polar molecules.**
- **Chemical reactions may be described as combination, decomposition, displacement, partner exchange, reversible or redox.**

- Catalysts are substances that increase the rate of chemical reactions.
- Enzymes are protein catalysts.
- Organic chemistry is the study of compounds that contain carbon.
- Organic molecules are either aliphatic or aromatic.
- Important hydrocarbons include alkanes, alkenes and alkynes.
- Other aliphatic compounds are alcohols, aldehydes, ketones, carboxylic acids and amines.
- Phenol is one example of an aromatic alcohol.

Self-test questions

1 Which of the following statements are true?
(a) Matter exists in three states.
(b) Elements consist of atoms of only one type.
(c) Atoms are the smallest particles of matter.
(d) Compounds consist of atoms of more than one type that are chemically bonded together.

2 Which of the following statements are true?
(a) Protons are found in the nucleus.
(b) Electrons carry a negative charge.
(c) Neutrons orbit the nucleus.
(d) Protons and neutrons have identical mass.

3 Which of the following statements are true?
(a) The atomic number is the number of protons.
(b) The mass number is the sum of the number of protons and electrons.
(c) Atoms have no net charge.
(d) In an ion, there are the same number of protons as electrons.

4 Which of the following statements are true?
(a) Ionic bonds result from the sharing of electrons.
(b) Positively charged ions are called cations.
(c) Negatively charged ions are called anions.
(d) Sodium chloride is an example of an ionic compound.

5 Which of the following statements are true?
(a) Covalent bonds result from the sharing of electrons.
(b) Covalent bonds cannot form between identical atoms.
(c) Polar molecules result when electrons are shared equally between atoms.
(d) Hydrogen bonds are weak forces of attraction that exist between polar molecules.

6 Which of the following statements are true?

(a) The second energy level contains a maximum of eight electrons.

(b) The electrons in the outermost energy level are called valence electrons.

(c) The first energy level contains a maximum of eight electrons.

(d) An atom with electrons in the M energy level is most stable when this level contains eight electrons.

7 Match the equations of the left with the descriptions on the right.

(a) $A + B \rightarrow AB$	(i) Decomposition
(b) $A + BC \rightarrow AC + B$	(ii) Partner exchange
(c) $AB + CD \rightarrow AD + CB$	(iii) Displacement
(d) $AB \rightarrow A + B$	(iv) Combination

8 Match the general formulae on the left with the chemical groups on the right.

(a) RCH_2NH_2	(i) Alcohol
(b) RCH_2OH	(ii) Amine
(c) RCOR	(iii) Ketone
(d) RCOOH	(iv) Carboxylic acid

9 Match the substances on the left with the chemical groups on the right.

(a) Methane	(i) Alcohol
(b) Acetone	(ii) Amine
(c) Epinephrine (adrenaline)	(iii) Alkane
(d) Ethanol	(iv) Ketone

10 Match the equations on the left with the descriptions on the right.

(a) $CHOOH + CH_3OH \rightarrow CHOOCH_3 + H_2O$	(i) Oxidation
(b) $CHOOCH_3 + H_2O \rightarrow CHOOH + CH_3OH$	(ii) Condensation
(c) $NADH \rightarrow NAD^+$	(iii) Reduction
(d) $NAD^+ \rightarrow NADH$	(iv) Hydrolysis

4

Water, electrolytes and body fluids

Learning outcomes

After reading the following chapter and undertaking personal study, you should be able to:

1. Identify three states of matter and describe what happens when a substance undergoes a change of state.
2. Describe the structure of the water molecule and distinguish between polar and non-polar molecules.
3. Distinguish between forces of cohesion and adhesion and describe meniscus formation.
4. Describe what is meant by the term 'surface tension' and give practical examples of surface-tension effects, including those encountered in clinical practice.
5. Distinguish between different types of aqueous mixture and give examples of each found in clinical practice.
6. Distinguish between electrolytes and non-electrolytes and give examples of each found in clinical practice.
7. Define the term 'concentration' and explain the different units commonly used to express it in clinical practice, including percentage concentration and molarity.
8. Explain the physical processes diffusion, osmosis and filtration and give examples of each.
9. Define the terms 'osmotic pressure', 'osmolarity', 'osmolality' and 'tonicity' and apply these to clinical practice.
10. Define the term 'oedema' and indicate possible causes in clinical practice.
11. Outline the means by which the body maintains sodium and water balance.
12. Briefly describe dialysis.

Introduction

In this chapter, we consider water - after all, it does form approximately 60% of the body weight of an adult. Water is so important that we can survive only a few days without drinking, and if water is lost from the body in excessive volumes death may occur in only a few hours. In addition to water, we also consider in this chapter important substances dissolved in it, such as **electrolytes**, and body fluids, such as **interstitial fluid**. Of course, we do not do this simply as a theoretical exercise - we also look at fluid balance in the body and some of the different fluids used in **intravenous infusions** (drips).

Before we do this, recall that all matter exists in one of three states - the solid, liquid and gaseous states. Since the melting point of water (0 °C) and its boiling point (100 °C) are within the range of our everyday experience of temperature, we are familiar with this compound in its solid state (ice), in its liquid state (water) and as a gas (water vapour or steam).

- ***But what actually happens when matter undergoes a change of state?***

To answer this question, we shall describe a simple experiment that is illustrated below. In Figure 4.1, ice is taken from a deep freezer and placed in a beaker at room temperature. A

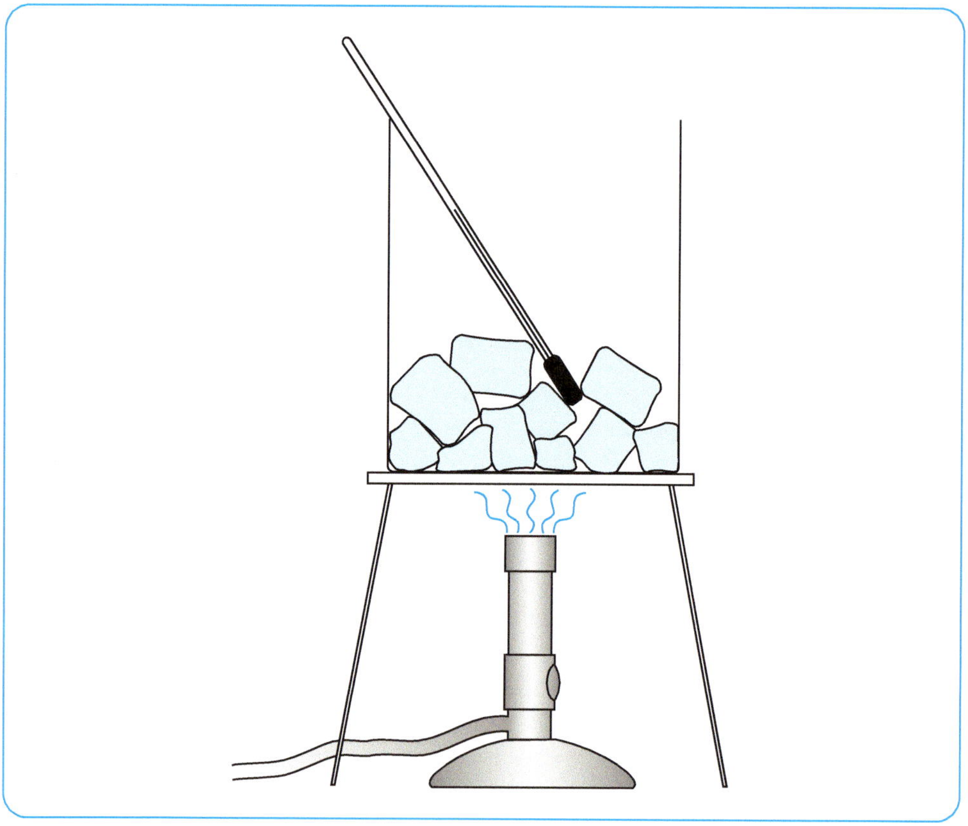

Figure 4.1
A simple experiment to record the temperature of ice as it is heated.

thermometer is also placed in the beaker. As the temperature of the ice rises slowly, it undergoes a change in state from solid to liquid - in ordinary language, we say that it melts.

- ***Remind yourself at what temperature ice melts.***

Ice melts at 0 °C.

- ***But what has actually happened to the ice?***

The first thing to note is that ice and liquid water are both water - no molecules have been broken. The change in state is a result of a change in the arrangement of the molecules. Perhaps we should say a little more about this. Solids consist of particles, atoms, molecules or ions, which are held together in a rigid arrangement by chemical bonds. Even though we regard solids as having a rigid structure, the particles of which they are comprised do have some energy of movement, which we call **kinetic energy**. In the solid state, they are not moving freely, but instead they vibrate about a fixed position. Now let us consider what happens when being allowed to stand at room temperature warms the ice in our experiment. When a solid is heated, the kinetic energy of the particles begins to increase and they vibrate more rapidly. Eventually, the particles have sufficient energy to escape the strong attraction that they have for each other and that is responsible for the rigidity of the solid state. At this point, we observe a change in state (that is, the solid melts), and the temperature at which this occurs is called the melting point. In the liquid state, the particles are not completely free of the attraction that they have for each other, but they are not held together in a rigid arrangement either. If we now light the Bunsen burner (a type of gas burner used in laboratories) beneath the vessel that contains liquid water, the kinetic energy of the water molecules is increased further. Eventually, some of the water molecules are able to break free from the attraction of others and enter the gaseous state.

- ***Have you noticed that when water is heated in this way, bubbles form? Where do they come from?***

The bubbles are bubbles of gaseous water (steam).

- ***Where in the container do they tend to form?***

If you look carefully, they form first at the bottom - that is, at the hottest part of the container. As the temperature of the water rises, more and more of the liquid molecules enter the gaseous phase.

- ***But does the temperature of the water continue to rise indefinitely?***

You will no doubt realise that the temperature of the water continues to rise until the boiling point is reached. Then, no matter how strongly the water is heated, the temperature remains stable.

- ***Remind yourself what the boiling point of water is.***

It is 100 °C.

- ***But why does the temperature remain constant at this point?***

The reason for this is that at the boiling point, all the energy being delivered to the container is being used to convert water molecules from the liquid state to the gaseous state.

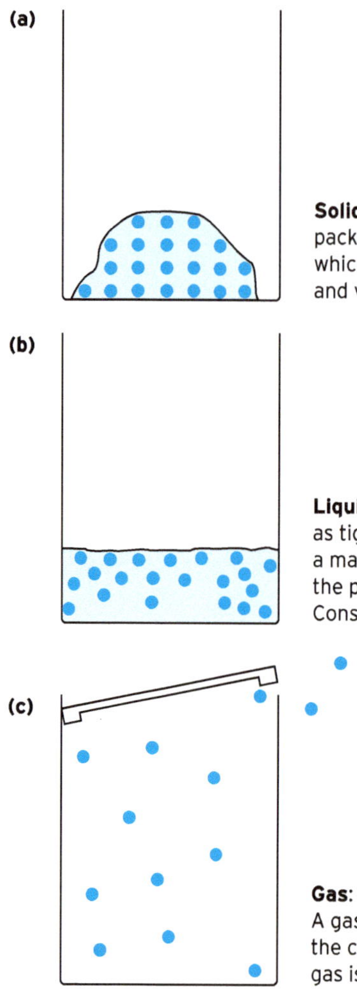

Solid: the arrangement of particles is regular. They are packed together tightly and occupy fixed positions, about which they vibrate. Therefore, solids have fixed shapes and volumes.

Liquid: the particles are packed together tightly, but not as tightly as in a solid. Nonetheless, at a given temperature, a mass of liquid has a fixed volume. In contrast to solids, the particles in a liquid do not occupy a fixed position. Consequently, liquids flow and do not have a fixed shape.

Gas: the particles are spaced widely and move independently. A gas does not have a fixed shape or volume. Here, the lid of the container has not been closed properly and some of the gas is escaping.

Figure 4.2
The states of matter.

Thus, melting and boiling are physical changes - that is, they involve a change in state. There has been no chemical change - no molecules have been broken and no new molecules created. The three states of matter are illustrated in Figure 4.2.

Water

Water is very abundant - two-thirds of the earth's surface are covered by water and water forms 60% of the weight of our bodies.

- ***Do you remember which elements the water molecule consists of?***

Water molecule consists of hydrogen and oxygen.

- ***But how many atoms of these two elements does it take to form one water molecule?***

In each water molecule, there are two atoms of hydrogen and one of oxygen - hence, the molecular formula of water is H_2O. Water is a covalent compound.

- ***Do you remember how covalent bonds are formed?***

If not, it might be a good idea to go back and look at Chapter 3. If you remember that covalent bonds are formed when atoms share electrons, you should have no difficulty in understanding the water molecule. Let us look at the oxygen and hydrogen atoms in turn.

Oxygen has an atomic number of 8, and the arrangement of electrons in its electron shells is 2.6.

- ***How many electrons are required in order to fill the outer shell of oxygen and so achieve stability?***

If you have the answer 8 in mind, then you are quite right. This means that a single oxygen atom can achieve stability by sharing two electrons of another element. Now let us turn to hydrogen, which has an atomic number of only 1 and, as a consequence, has a single electron in its first electron shell.

- ***How many electrons does it take to fill this shell and so achieve stability?***

Two electrons are required in the shell. This means that both elements could achieve stability if one atom of oxygen were to share one electron each with two atoms of hydrogen. This arrangement is illustrated in Figure 4.3.

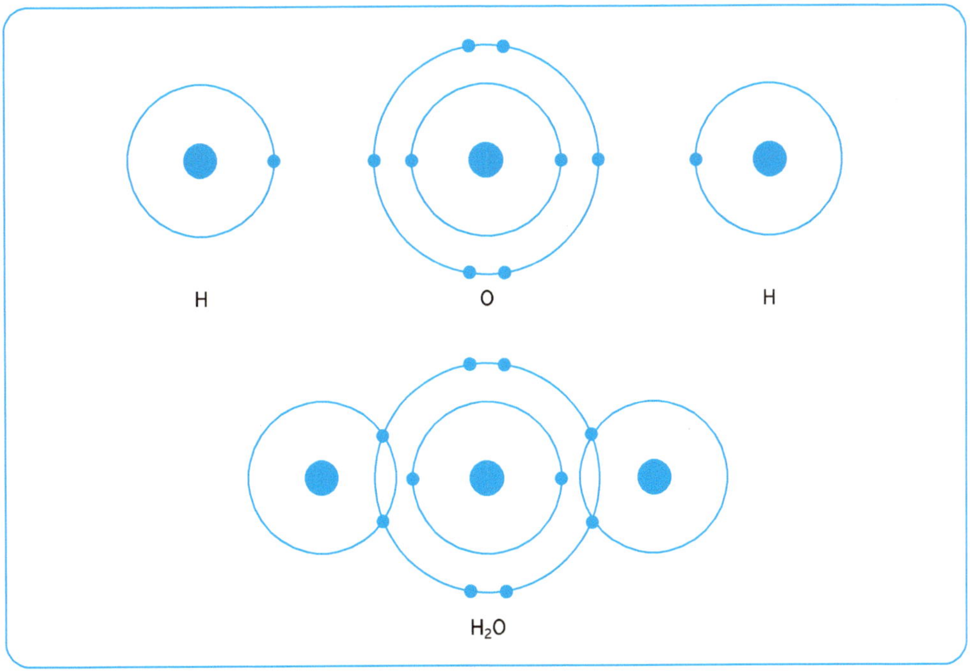

Figure 4.3
The covalent bonding of oxygen and hydrogen to form water.

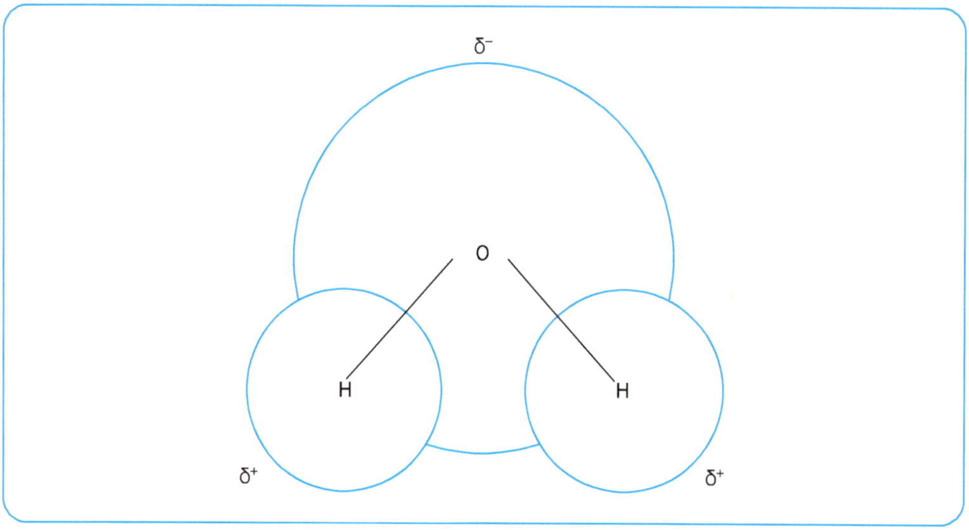

Figure 4.4
The polar nature of the water molecule.

● *Are the electrons shared equally?*

You have probably realised that they are not. The nucleus of oxygen is much larger than that of hydrogen, having eight protons to hydrogen's one. This means that the oxygen nucleus exerts a greater pull on the electrons of the two hydrogen atoms than do the two hydrogen nuclei. This attraction is not sufficient to pull the electrons clean away from hydrogen, but it does result in an unequal sharing.

● *Does this unequal sharing have any important effects?*

Electrons do, of course, carry a negative charge, and so the unequal sharing of them means that the oxygen end of the water molecule has a partial negative charge and the hydrogen end has a partial positive charge. Consequently, we describe water as a **polar** molecule. This is illustrated in Figure 4.4.

It is important to note that covalent molecules have no net charge, as ions do, and the redistribution of charge is small compared with the transfer of electrons in ionic bonding. Consequently, we do not use the symbols + and – to identify this redistribution of charge but use δ^+ (delta +) and δ^- (delta –) instead.

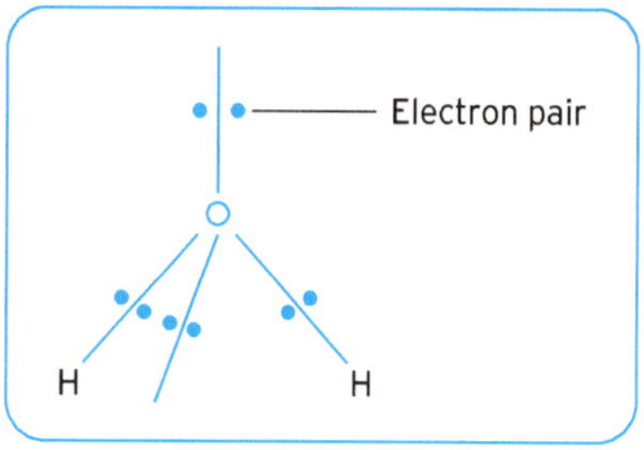

Figure 4.5
Explanation of the non-linear shape of the water molecule.

Incidentally, you may notice from Figure 4.4 that the atoms in a water molecule do not lie in a straight line - the molecule is bent.

● *Why is this?*

This happens because the four separate pairs of electrons in the outer shell repel each other and orient themselves as far from each other as possible. This is illustrated in Figure 4.5. In figuring out this arrangement, you will need to remind yourself that only two electron pairs actually take part in bond formation - these are the bonding electrons. The other two pairs are non-bonding electrons.

- ***What practical relevance does an understanding of the water molecule have?***

It is important for several reasons. First, water is an important solvent, and the polar nature of the water molecule determines which kinds of substance dissolve in it readily.

- ***Can you work out which kinds of substance readily dissolve in water?***

Polar water molecules are able to pull ions out of a solid crystalline lattice, and so ionic compounds, such as sodium chloride, readily dissolve in water. In fact, in our bodies sodium ions are the most abundant extracellular cations (positively charged ions outside cells) and chloride ions are the most abundant extracellular anions (negatively charged ions outside cells). You will see the importance of this when you study aspects of physiology such as nerve and muscle function and when you are nursing patients with intravenous infusions (drips). More information about solutions is given a little later. In contrast, covalent compounds such as lipids (fats) are not readily soluble in water. You might like to ask yourself the question: How does the body transport lipids around the body in the bloodstream? This is clearly important when looking at fats in the diet and their role in disease processes such as **atherosclerosis**. More information about this is given in Chapter 7. In addition, polar water molecules are attracted strongly to each other - that is, there are strong **cohesive forces** within water, and this produces a strong **surface tension** effect. This is explained later. Finally, it is also worth pointing out that a very small number of water molecules dissociate to form ions according to the equation

$$H_2O \rightarrow H^+ + OH^-$$

The importance of this will be explained in Chapter 5. For now, let us return to a consideration of the forces between water molecules and surface tension.

Cohesion and adhesion

We have already noted that the particles of a solid or liquid attract each other and that the strength of these forces of attraction determines the physical state of the substance. The forces of attraction between like particles, such as molecules of water, are referred to as forces of cohesion. The effect of cohesive forces is quite simple to demonstrate. For example, suppose that you were to spill a little water on a flat surface.

- ***Does the water spread out evenly?***

No - instead, it forms into droplets. Perhaps this is such a familiar phenomenon that we don't even think about it. Nonetheless, forces of cohesion do influence the behaviour of water, and one simple application of this can be seen in Practice point 4.1. Before this, however, we should also note that there are forces of attraction between dissimilar molecules - these are called forces of **adhesion**. One example is the attraction between molecules of a liquid and the glass of the container in which they are held.

Practice point 4.1

Meniscus formation and reading manometers

Forces of cohesion and adhesion lead to the formation of a **meniscus** - the bending of the surface of a liquid. Figure 4.6 shows the menisci formed by water and mercury, such as might be seen in the case of the saline manometer and sphygmomanometer, respectively. (Manometers are explained more fully in Chapter 6.)

- ***Note that the shapes of the menisci formed by water and mercury differ.***

In the case of water, the forces of adhesion are greater than the forces of cohesion, and this results in a bowl-shaped meniscus. The opposite is true of mercury, which produces a dome-shaped meniscus. This has practical relevance - ask yourself the following question:

- ***If you had to read the level of fluid in a manometer, would you take your reading from the top or the bottom of the meniscus?***

Clearly, this might be important when you are measuring **blood pressure** with a mercury **sphygmomanometer** or **central venous pressure** with a saline **manometer**. An accurate reading will be obtained if measurements are taken from the bottom of the meniscus in the case of water and the top of the meniscus in the case of mercury.

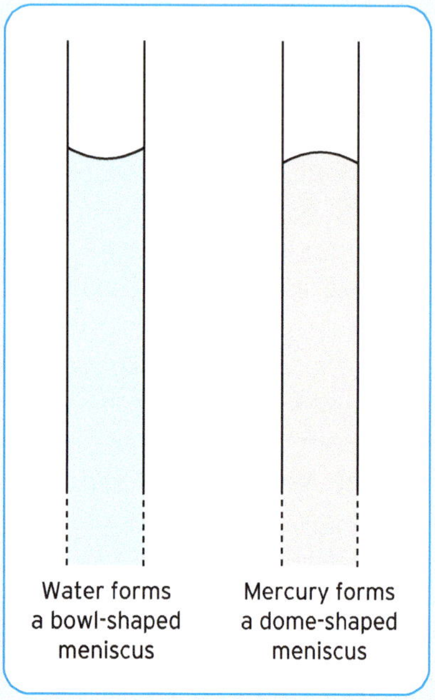

Figure 4.6
The shape of the menisci formed by water and mercury.

(At this point it is probably worth pointing out that, since mercury is toxic, manometers that contain mercury have been replaced in the West with devices that do not contain this substance. Nonetheless, mercury manometers remain in use in many developing countries and for this reason the above explanation is given.)

Surface tension

Have you ever noticed how some insects, such as pond skaters, have the ability to glide across the surface of a pond? The water seems to behave as though it has a kind of skin. In a similar way, it is possible to take a pin, made from a substance denser than water, and with care place it on the water surface. If you can't find a pond with pond skaters, you might like to have a go at this simple experiment instead. Clearly, the water doesn't really have a skin, since if we agitate the surface a little the pin sinks. Perhaps it would be better to say that there appears to be a tension over the surface of the water - in fact, that is exactly the expression that is used - **surface tension**.

- ***What could account for this surface tension?***

In a body of water, all the water molecules except those on the surface of the water are completely surrounded by other water molecules and subject to cohesive forces in all directions. Cohesive forces also pull down surface molecules from below, but there is no corresponding force from above. Consequently, the surface of the water behaves like a skin. We have already noted how some insects put this surface tension effect to good use. On the other hand, you might have noticed what happens when an insect pierces the surface. Now the skin-like effect of surface tension acts to prevent the creature from escaping. Surface tension is also responsible for the shape of liquid droplets.

- ***Can you work out what shape a water droplet would be in space?***

You may have been able to figure out that in the absence of gravity, the droplet would be spherical. On earth, the effect of gravity is to cause elongation of the droplet, and it becomes, well, droplet-shaped. The ability of water to form droplets is put to good use in **nebulisers**, which are discussed in Chapter 6. In a nebuliser, a solution of a drug in water is formed into small droplets (nebulised) that can then be inhaled. This is just one medical use that we make of surface tension. Another is outlined in Practice point 4.2, while surface tension in the body is considered in Practice point 4.3.

Practice point 4.2

Low surface tension and skin disinfection

It is worth noting that the surface tensions of different liquids are not the same. For example, the surface tension of the alcohol ethanol is less than a third that of water. Ethanol thus has a lower tendency to form droplets than does water and tends to spread out more when spilled; as a consequence, ethanol evaporates more readily than water. This rapid evaporation causes cooling, which you may have noticed when using cleansing alcohol hand rubs in hospital wards. The property of rapid evaporation is also put to use when antiseptics are presented as alcoholic solutions used to cleanse a patient's skin before a surgical procedure. They are often preferred to aqueous solutions, since they dry more quickly.

In addition, **antiseptics** and **disinfectants** also have lower surface tensions than water. As a consequence, they too spread out and more effectively wet tissues - clearly an important property, since to be effective such a solution has to have contact with the wound.

In-text review

- ✔ Matter exists in the solid, liquid and gaseous states.
- ✔ Water is a polar covalent compound.
- ✔ Each water molecule consists of two atoms of hydrogen and one of oxygen - H_2O.
- ✔ Ionic compounds readily dissolve in water; covalent compounds do not.
- ✔ Forces of cohesion are responsible for droplet formation and surface tension.
- ✔ In water, forces of adhesion are greater than forces of cohesion, and this is responsible for the formation of a bowl-shaped meniscus.

Practice point 4.3

Surface tension in the body – surfactant

We have already looked at surface tension in a number of practical situations, but now we turn to look at one important example of surface tension in the body. In the lungs, there are thousands of microscopic sac-like structures called **alveoli**. It is across these that gaseous exchange takes place. A single alveolus and capillary are illustrated in Figure 4.7.

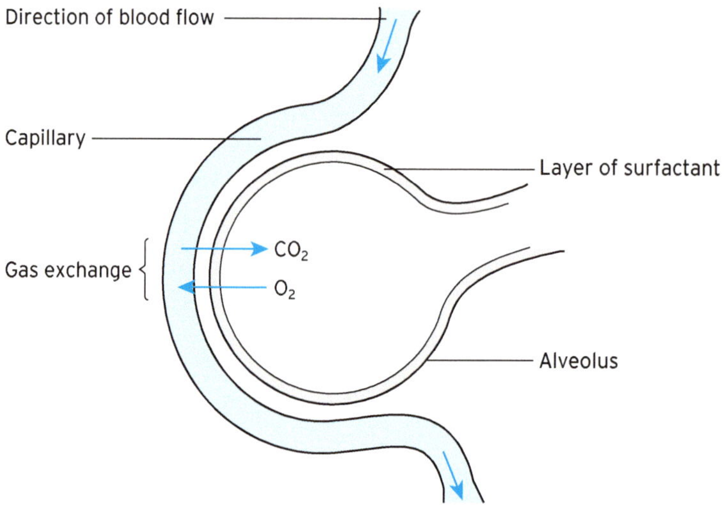

Figure 4.7
A single alveolus and capillary.

Each alveolus is lined with a film of fluid. We have already noted that water has a very high surface tension, and water is a major component of this fluid. The surface tension in alveolar fluid acts to reduce the alveoli to their smallest possible size. This is similar to the way in which the surface tension of a bubble tends to cause it to collapse. Indeed, if the alveolar fluid were pure water, then the alveoli would collapse (**atelectasis**). However, a **phospholipid** surfactant, which is secreted by the alveolar cells, is present in the fluid, and this reduces the cohesive forces between water molecules and, as a consequence, reduces the surface tension. Incidentally, the term 'surfactant' is a contraction of the expression surface-active agent, which means a substance that reduces surface tension.

Surfactant is present in foetal lungs from about 23 weeks' gestation, but before 28-32 weeks it rarely occurs in quantities sufficient to prevent alveolar collapse. This means that in babies born prematurely, the alveoli may collapse, causing the condition neonatal respiratory distress syndrome (RDS). In addition, some full-term infants also have a surfactant deficiency.

Aqueous mixtures

An aqueous mixture is simply a mixture of a substance in water. Nurses meet aqueous mixtures all the time. Cough linctus, antiseptic solutions and intravenous fluids are all obvious examples. However, there are a number of different kinds of mixture, as explained below.

Mechanical suspensions

This is the simplest type of aqueous mixture, which involves the dispersal of small particles of a solid in water. If a **mechanical suspension** is left to stand for any length of time, the solid will separate out and the mixture will need to be re-created by shaking. The use of the word 'small' in connection with the particles of a mechanical suspension is relative. They are small to the naked eye, but compared with water molecules they are very large indeed and can easily be removed from the water by filtering through paper or cloth. Muddy water is one example of a mechanical suspension, and on first examination this appears to have little to do with nursing. You might be surprised, however, to learn that one remedy for diarrhoea is a mechanical suspension of the clay **kaolin**, sometimes with the drug **morphine** added. Kaolin mixture is rather an old-fashioned remedy, but nonetheless it is effective and still available from pharmacies.

When presented as a paste - in other words, the amount of water present is less - kaolin can be used to make a hot poultice which, when applied to painful joints, may provide relief. Kaolin poultices have also traditionally been used in the treatment of infected wounds where there is a collection of pus into which antibiotics do not readily penetrate. The application of the hot poultice to the wound causes blood vessels to dilate and may cause pus to discharge through the wound. Once again, this is rather old-fashioned but still finds occasional use. **If you are involved in the application of hot poultices, you must ensure that the patient is not in danger of receiving a burn.**

Perhaps a more familiar mechanical suspension is that of zinc oxide (ZnO) in water, otherwise known as **calamine lotion**. This is used to gain relief from sunburn. As is the case with muddy water, the particles in kaolin mixture and calamine lotion separate out when left to stand. Consequently, it is important to shake the bottle before use.

Colloidal suspensions

The particles in a **colloidal suspension** are smaller than those in a mechanical suspension, being only 1-100 nm in diameter. Nonetheless, this is still larger than atoms and ions and, indeed, larger than many molecules too. The particles in a colloidal suspension consist of groups of ions or atoms or of large molecules such as starch and proteins. If a colloidal suspension is allowed to stand, the particles and water do not usually separate out; if they do, they do so only very slowly.

The small size of colloidal particles means that they pass through ordinary filters but not through biological membranes such as the **capillary endothelium** or the filtration membrane of the **nephron** of the kidney.

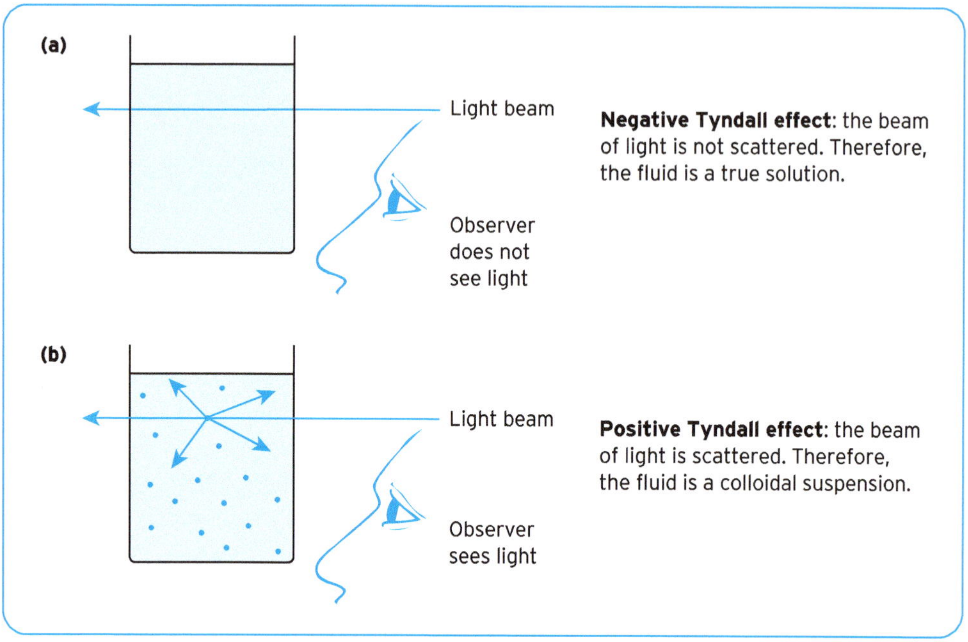

Figure 4.8
The Tyndall effect.

Along with mechanical suspensions, colloids show a positive **Tyndall effect**; that is, they scatter a beam of light shone through them. As a consequence, the beam can be seen from the sides of the container as well as from a position directly opposite the light source, as illustrated in Figure 4.8.

In addition, it is worth noting that there are a number of different types of colloidal suspension, which are described below.

Foams: these are produced when a large volume of air is dispersed through a smaller volume of liquid or solid. When we whip cream, we are in fact producing foam; other examples include shaving foam and the contents of foam fire extinguishers.

Emulsions: these are produced when one liquid is dispersed in another. You have probably heard of emulsion paint. French dressing (a combination of oil and vinegar) is another example. The emulsification of fats is considered in Practice point 4.4.

Sols: this term is applied to many different colloidal mixtures in which a solid is dispersed through another solid, a liquid or a gas. The latter is referred to as an aerosol, and these are encountered in both everyday life and nursing practice. For example, povidone-iodine dry powder spray is an aerosol used in the disinfection of minor skin wounds and infections.

Gels: these are colloidal mixtures of liquids dispersed in solids; they might be described as being on the borderline of solidity. They are not easily poured, but they are only semi-rigid. Examples include gelatine, which is used in the manufacture of jelly desserts, and **agar**, which is manufactured from seaweed. In Victorian times agar, was also used in making

Practice point 4.4

Emulsification of fats

We have already noted that a mixture of oil and vinegar is an example of an emulsion.

- ***What happens when the mixture is left to stand?***

They separate and have to be shaken together again.

- ***Couldn't we add something to cause them to remain in an emulsified state?***

Yes, we could: a pinch of mustard powder does the trick. Consequently, we might refer to the mustard as an emulsifying agent. Emulsifying agents are also important in the body. When food is ingested, fats form large droplets, which present a relatively small surface area to the fat-digesting enzyme **lipase**. **Bile** from the **gall bladder** passes into the **duodenum**, where bile salts emulsify the fats. That is, the fat is broken up into small droplets and an emulsion is formed. These emulsion droplets present a much larger surface area to lipase, so their digestion is facilitated. Note that bile salts are not enzymes: they do not digest the fat. Rather, their emulsifying action is required for the effective action of lipase. You will find out more about fat digestion in Chapter 7.

desserts, but it was subsequently chosen as a medium on which to grow bacteria and it is still employed for this purpose today. (Perhaps agar was initially chosen for this purpose because an early scientist noticed colonies of organisms growing on a dessert?) Gels are encountered in nursing practice as some are used as wound dressings. Hydrocolloids and hydrogels are occlusive or semi-occlusive dressings that adhere to dry skin but interact with moisture in a wound to form a gel. They have a number of advantages over traditional dressings; you might like to find out what these are.

True solutions

Perhaps you have noticed that when discussing aqueous mixtures, thus far we have used the term 'suspension' and avoided the term 'solution' where possible. This is because the mixtures described up to this point have not been true solutions. (Although note that in clinical practice, the word 'solution' is commonly applied to aqueous mixtures, regardless of whether they are true solutions.) True **solutions** are characterised by having components that exist almost entirely as individual ions, atoms or molecules rather than as groups of these. Consequently, the particles of a true solution are very small and do not settle when the solution is left to stand. In addition, solutions readily pass through filters and often through biological membranes too. The particles are also too small to show a positive Tyndall effect. The characteristics of different aqueous mixtures are summarised in Table 4.1.

In true solutions, two or more substances are mixed, so that their particles are distributed uniformly between each other. The most abundant substance is referred to as the **solvent** and the other substances are referred to as **solutes**. We do not simply describe solutes as being dispersed in the solvent; instead, we say that they are **dissolved** in it.

Table 4.1 Summary of characteristics of aqueous mixtures.

Characteristic	Mechanical suspension	Colloidal suspension	True solution
Particles	Visible lumps	Collections of ions, atoms or molecules or single large molecules	Single ions, atoms or molecules
Particle size	> 100 nm	1–100 nm	< 1 nm
Settling	Particles settle out quickly	Particles do not settle out, or do so only slowly	Particles never settle out
Separation by simple filters	Yes	No	No
Separation by semi-permeable membranes	Yes	Yes	No
Tyndall effect	Yes	Yes	No

For example, suppose you are asked to get a bag of normal saline. Normal saline is a solution of 0.9 g of sodium chloride (NaCl) dissolved in 100 ml of water.

● ***Which is the solute and which is the solvent?***

Sodium chloride is the solute and water is the solvent.

We can represent the formation of a true solution in the manner shown in Figure 4.9. Note that the solute particles are distributed evenly throughout the solvent, but because the proportion of solute particles is small there are many solvent particles that have no immediate contact with the solute.

Most of the different types of aqueous mixture are encountered in clinical practice. Practice point 4.5 deals with crystalloid and colloid intravenous fluids.

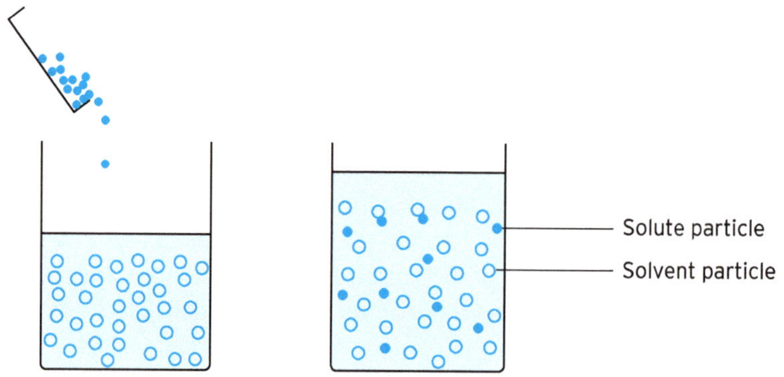

Figure 4.9
The formation of a true solution.

Practice point 4.5

Crystalloid and colloid intravenous fluids

Many patients in hospital have to be given fluids directly into a vein. This procedure is referred to as an **intravenous infusion**. There are many reasons for administering an intravenous infusion, and you might like to find out what some of these are. Some intravenous fluids are colloidal suspensions; these include **blood**, **albumin solution** (at least 95% of the protein present is albumin) and **plasma protein solution** (at least 85% of the protein present is albumin). The latter two are derived from human plasma. In addition, there are a number of plasma protein substitutes, such as suspensions of gelatine, starch and dextran.

Other intravenous fluids, for example sodium chloride and dextrose (glucose), are true solutions, although in clinical practice they are often referred to as **crystalloids** because of the ability of the solute to form crystals. This can be achieved by gently heating the solution so that the water is evaporated away to leave the solute crystals behind.

- ***Are there specific reasons for choosing one fluid for infusion rather than another?***

Yes, there are. You might like to find out more about this subject by consulting a nursing text. Briefly, crystalloid solutions are used to rehydrate a patient who has experienced prolonged vomiting and diarrhoea. On the other hand, a patient who has suffered severe bleeding will require a blood transfusion, since it is necessary to replace the lost red blood cells as well as the water and solutes contained within blood. Sometimes blood may not be available immediately - perhaps you are part of a team that has just arrived at the scene of a road traffic accident. In this case, plasma substitutes may be given until blood becomes available.

Plasma substitutes, such as those mentioned previously, have advantages over crystalloid solutions since they do not readily cross biological membranes and thus do not 'leak' out of the vascular compartment. Instead, they remain within the blood vessels and continue to exert an influence on blood volume. Consequently, they may be referred to as **plasma expanders**. There are many other uses of intravenous infusions, but greater detail is reserved for your further study. Whichever type of fluid is chosen, there are certain observations that you should make before connecting a bag of fluid to an infusion-giving set. You should, of course, note that it is the correct fluid for the patient concerned and that the concentration chosen is the concentration prescribed. You should note the expiry date of the fluid and the batch number. The hospital pharmacy and manufacturer will need to know these in the event of an untoward reaction to any fluid. You should not, of course, administer any fluid once its expiry date has passed.

Next, you should check that the bag and its packaging are intact. If not, the contents will no longer be sterile and they should be discarded. You should also check the fluid itself. Hold the bag up to the light. Remember that only colloidal suspensions should show a positive Tyndall effect; true solutions should not. In addition, colloidal suspensions often have a pale amber or straw colour, whereas true solutions are uncoloured. Finally, although true solutions are often referred to as crystalloids, there should be no particles of solid material in any type of intravenous fluid.

Electrolytes and non-electrolytes

Before defining these terms, we should look at solution formation in more detail, beginning with sodium chloride as an example. Sodium chloride is an ionic compound, and in the solid state it exists as a crystal lattice. This is explained more fully in Chapter 3. The ionic bonds between the positively charged sodium ions (Na^+) and the negatively charged chloride ions (Cl^-) are very strong. In order to break the ionic lattice and melt sodium chloride, the temperature would have to be raised to 804 °C. At this point, the ions would no longer be held in a fixed position but would instead become free to move. Consequently, whereas solid sodium chloride does not conduct electricity, molten sodium chloride does.

In view of this, you may now be surprised to learn that when ionic compounds are mixed with water, their component ions are pulled out of the lattice and become dissolved.

- ***How is this achieved so easily by water, when we have just noted that it requires a high temperature to break the ionic lattice of the solid compound?***

First of all, you need to recall that water is a polar molecule and that water molecules are attracted to each other. In a similar way, the hydrogen end of the water molecule (slightly positive) is attracted to negatively charged chloride ions (Cl^-) and the oxygen end of the water molecule (slightly negative) is attracted to positively charged sodium ions (Na^+).

- ***Surely these forces of attraction are relatively weak compared with the forces of attraction between ions in a crystal lattice?***

Yes, they are; but there are two more points that have to be considered here. First, ions located at the outside of a crystal lattice are not surrounded completely by other ions, and they are, therefore, held less securely. As a consequence, they are also pulled out of the lattice more readily by polar water molecules. Second, once an ion has been pulled free from the lattice, it immediately becomes surrounded by water molecules, each of which exerts forces of attraction upon the ion. Although each of these forces is relatively weak, the combined effects of the numerically superior water molecules is considerable. This is illustrated in Figure 4.10. The water molecules have, in effect, 'come between' the ions, and as a consequence the forces of attraction between the ions are very much reduced.

- ***What has this to do with the term 'electrolyte'?***

The point is that when an ionic compound is dissolved in water, the result is a solution of free ions. Such solutions are good conductors of electricity, and any substance that dissociates into ions when dissolved in water is referred to as an **electrolyte**.

By now you may have sufficient time to work out that although ionic compounds are soluble in water, they do not dissolve in non-polar solvents such as hexane. This is because such non-polar liquids do not exert forces of attraction upon ions in a crystal lattice. Perhaps you have also worked out that many covalent compounds do not dissolve in water.

- ***Why is this?***

These uncharged molecules cannot disrupt the forces of attraction between polar water molecules. In contrast, covalent compounds dissolve readily in non-polar solvents, since the

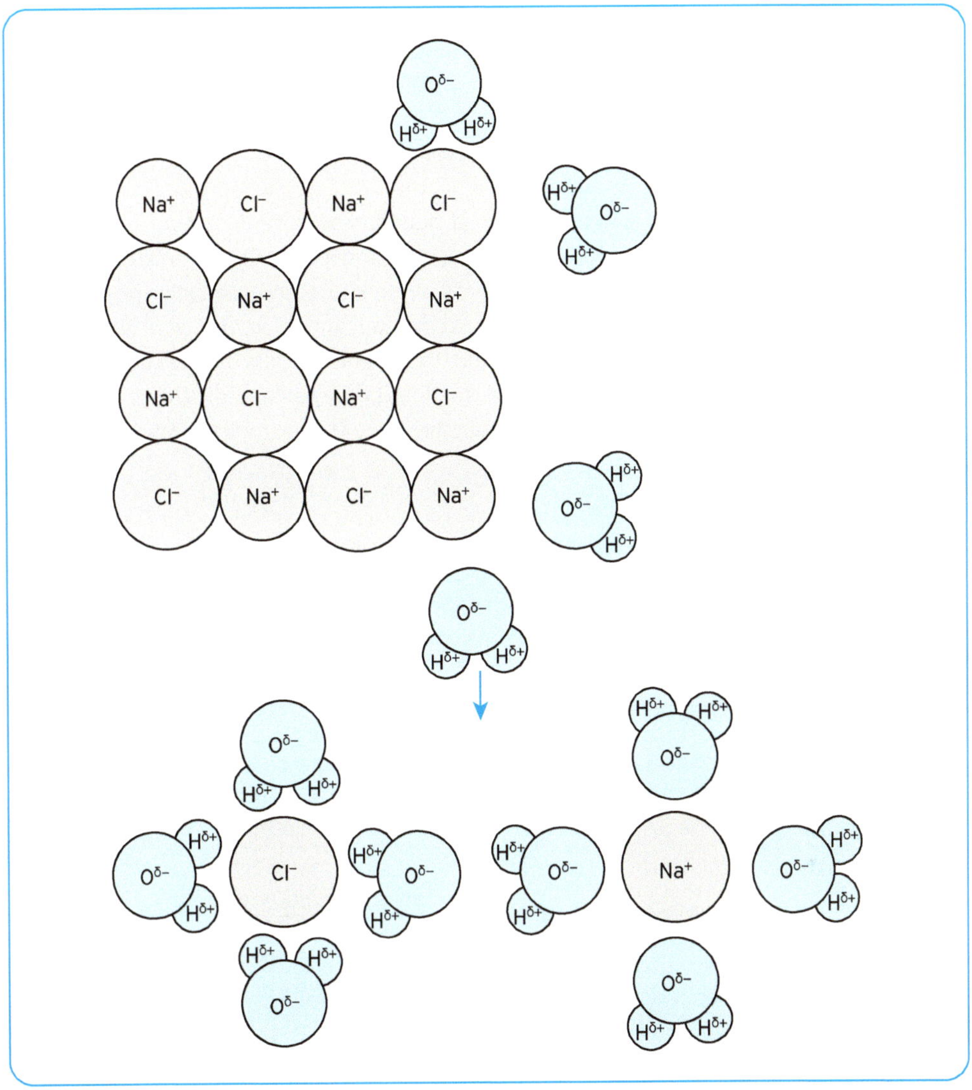

Figure 4.10
The effect of water on an ionic lattice.

forces of attraction between solvent and solute molecules are similar to those between solute molecules themselves.

However, some covalent compounds, such as glucose, amino acids and urea (the waste product of amino-acid metabolism), do dissolve in water.

● ***How can this be explained?***

Covalent compounds that do dissolve in water are always those with a polar nature, like water itself. Consequently, the forces of attraction between the different molecules in the mixture (solvent-solvent, solute-solute and solvent-solute) are of similar strength, and this allows polar covalent compounds to dissolve in water. However, since polar covalent compounds do not dissociate into ions upon dissolving, they are described as non-electrolytes.

The concept of concentration

Thus far, we have looked at different kinds of aqueous mixture, including true solutions. When we deal with such fluids, it may be important to know what kind of mixture it is. It will certainly be important to know the components of a mixture and probably the **concentration** too. There are a number of ways of describing concentration, but what this measurement tells us is the relative proportions of solute to solvent. It would of course be convenient if one unit of concentration could be used all the time, but unfortunately this is not the case. As nurses, we have to be familiar with a number of different units. Some of these are described below.

Percentage concentration

You will encounter this expression of concentration in a number of contexts, including the concentration of intravenous fluids. The most commonly used concentration of sodium chloride for intravenous infusion is 0.9% (w/v) and for dextrose (glucose) it is 5% (w/v).

- ***But what do these figures mean?***

The expression 'w/v' means weight per unit volume, and the percentage concentration (w/v) is defined as the mass of a solute dissolved in 100 ml of solution. It is given by the following formula below

$$\text{Percentage concentration (w/v)} = \frac{\text{mass of solute (g)}}{\text{volume of solution (ml)}} \times 100$$

Thus, a 0.9% solution contains 0.9 g of solute in every 100 ml of solution, while a 5% solution contains 5 g of solute in every 100 ml.

Percentage concentrations can also be expressed as the weight of solute per unit weight of solvent (w/w) or volume of solute per unit volume of solvent (v/v) if both solute and solvent are liquids. These two expressions are much less common. Nonetheless two examples are given here:

- Aluminium hydroxide mixture (non-proprietary) 4% (w/w) Al_2O_3 in water is used as an antacid (reduces stomach acidity).
- Pre-injection swabs are saturated with 70% (v/v) isopropyl alcohol.

Other expressions of concentration as a weight per unit volume

Instead of expressing concentration as a percentage, we could give the weight of solute in a different volume of solution, say in 5 ml instead of 100 ml.

- ***Can you think of occasions when this might be more convenient?***

One example would be liquid medicines - I doubt that 100 ml of a medicine would ever be required! The concentration of liquid medicines is usually given in terms of the number of milligrams (mg) per 5 ml of mixture. Take the example of pholcodine linctus, which is used to suppress a dry cough. This is commonly presented at a concentration of 5 mg/ml.

- ***Why is the 5-ml measure so important?***

Have you realised that this is the volume of a standard medicine spoon? It is also the approximate volume of a culinary teaspoon, but of course cutlery does not conform to a standard volume, and so special medicine spoons or graduated medicine pots should always be used to measure the volume of preparations containing drugs. The 5-ml measure is a matter not only of accuracy but also of convenience. A typical dose of the concentration of pholcodine mentioned is 5-10 ml (one or two spoons) three to four times each day.

This way of expressing concentration is also important when administering continuous infusions of drugs - perhaps solutions of **analgesics** in the management of postoperative pain.

Molarity

Another way of expressing concentration is in terms of **molarity** - that is, in terms of the number of moles of solute per litre of solvent (mol/l).

- ***Do you remember what the term 'mole' means?***

If you are unsure, go back to Chapter 3. You might have remembered, however, that a mole of a substance is its molecular mass in grams. For example, the molecular mass of glucose ($C_6H_{12}O_6$) is 180, so one mole of glucose weighs 180 g. The formula for this expression of concentration is given below:

$$\text{Concentration (mol/l)} = \frac{\text{number of moles}}{\text{solution volume in litres (l)}}$$

Even a concentration of 1 mol/l is quite high for most medical and nursing applications, however, and so concentrations are often measured in terms of millimoles per litre (mmol/l) instead. A solution of 1 mmol/l contains one-thousandth of a mole per litre of solution.

A number of applications of this measurement could be given. One such example is that of sodium bicarbonate (sodium hydrogen carbonate) 1.26% intravenous fluid, which contains 150 mmol/l each of sodium ions (Na^+) and bicarbonate ions (hydrogen carbonate ions, HCO_3^-). In addition, the concentration of substances dissolved in blood is usually given in terms of millimoles per litre. Practice point 4.6 covers how we express plasma concentrations.

Other units: the milliequivalent per litre

This unit is uncommon, but it is used in the USA and is described here for the convenience of any readers who might be employed there. The milliequivalent (meq) takes into account the charges carried by particles. The formula for milliequivalents per litre (meq/l) is given below:

$$\begin{array}{c}\text{Number of milliequivalents}\\ \text{per litre (meq/l)}\end{array} = \text{molarity (mmol/l)} \times \text{number of charges carried by particle}$$

For example, sodium ions (Na^+) carry a single charge, and the numerical value of their concentration in blood expressed in meq/l is therefore the same as that expressed in mmol/l

Practice point 4.6

Plasma concentrations

When caring for physically ill patients, we often need to make a note of the concentration of various electrolytes and non-electrolytes. Important electrolytes include sodium ions (Na^+), chloride ions (Cl^-), potassium ions (K^+), hydrogen carbonate ions (bicarbonate ions, HCO_3^-) and calcium ions (Ca^{2+}). Important non-electrolytes include glucose and urea.

You might like to consider the circumstances in which the concentration of these substances in blood are measured. Two examples include the plasma glucose concentration in diabetes mellitus and electrolyte concentrations during a period of prolonged vomiting and diarrhoea.

When completing laboratory request cards, doctors often use abbreviations for the tests they require. This is not always a good idea, but perhaps you will already be able to recognise that 'u's & e's & glc' is a request for the measurement of the concentrations of urea, electrolytes and glucose. The numerical values of some important solute concentrations are given below:

Na^+	135–145 mmol/l
K^+	3.5–5.0 mmol/l
Cl^-	100–106 mmol/l
Ca^{2+}	2.1–2.6 mmol/l
HCO_3^-	19–29 mmol/l
Glucose	3.9–5.6 mmol/l
Urea	2.9–8.9 mmol/l

Finally for this section, you should note that some blood values are not given in terms of mmol/l. The concentration of hydrogen ions (H^+) is described in terms of the pH scale (see Chapter 5) and haemoglobin concentration is given in terms of grams per decilitre (g/dl; that is, g/100 ml).

(within the range 135–145). The same is, of course, true of all ions that carry a single charge, such as potassium ions (K^+) and chloride ions (Cl^-). Magnesium ions (Mg^{2+}), however, carry a double charge, so the numerical value of their concentration in blood expressed in meq/l (2 meq/l) is twice that of the value expressed in mmol/l (1 mmol/l).

In-text review

- ✔ An aqueous mixture is a mixture of a substance in water.
- ✔ Mechanical suspensions, colloidal suspensions (including foams, emulsions, sols and gels) and true solutions are examples of aqueous mixtures.
- ✔ When an ionic compound is dissolved in water, the result is a solution of free ions.
- ✔ Any substance that dissociates into ions when dissolved in water is referred to as an electrolyte.
- ✔ Concentration is an expression of the relative proportions of solute and solvent.
- ✔ Concentration is measured as a percentage or in terms of molarity.

Diffusion and osmosis

Diffusion and **osmosis** are important physical processes that you may have experienced in everyday life without knowing it. If you have studied biological science before, you will certainly have encountered these processes and performed experiments to demonstrate their effects. Before we proceed, however, it might be worthwhile describing a very simple experiment to show the random movement of particles of a gas.

Imagine that you have a small glass container into which some smoke is blown. The container is then sealed. Smoke consists in part of small particles that result from the burning of a solid, and we could examine these by placing the small glass container under the light microscope.

- ***If we were to look down the microscope at the particles of smoke, what would we see? Would the particles be stationary?***

If you have decided that they would not, but would be seen to be moving randomly, then you are right.

- ***Why is this?***

The movement of the smoke particles is caused by the collisions that they experience with the molecules of the gases that form the air. We cannot see these molecules with the ordinary light microscope, but we can see their effects on the larger smoke particles. What this simple experiment demonstrates is that the molecules of the gases that form the air atmosphere are in constant random movement, and this is referred to as **Brownian motion**.

Diffusion

Now let us apply this understanding to a real-life example. Suppose someone were to allow a volume of a gas to escape into the corner of a room. Imagine that the door and windows are closed and that you are sitting in the opposite corner.

- ***Would the gas remain confined in the corner into which it was released?***

You obviously know from experience that it would not, but our observation of Brownian motion now enables us to explain why. The collisions that our mysterious gas molecules have with the molecules of the gases that form the atmosphere mean that they eventually become dispersed throughout the room. After some time, you might even detect them from your seat in the opposite corner - perhaps the gas has an unpleasant smell. Whether you realise it or not, you have just experienced diffusion - that is, the movement of a gas from an area of high concentration, down a **concentration gradient**, to an area of low concentration. The expression 'down a concentration gradient' refers to the fact that the concentration of gas particles is greater at the moment of their release into the room than after their dispersal. Diffusion is not, of course, confined to gases - it is a process that takes place in liquids too. Imagine that we take a small volume of ink and drop it into a glass of water.

- ***Would it remain confined as a small drop?***

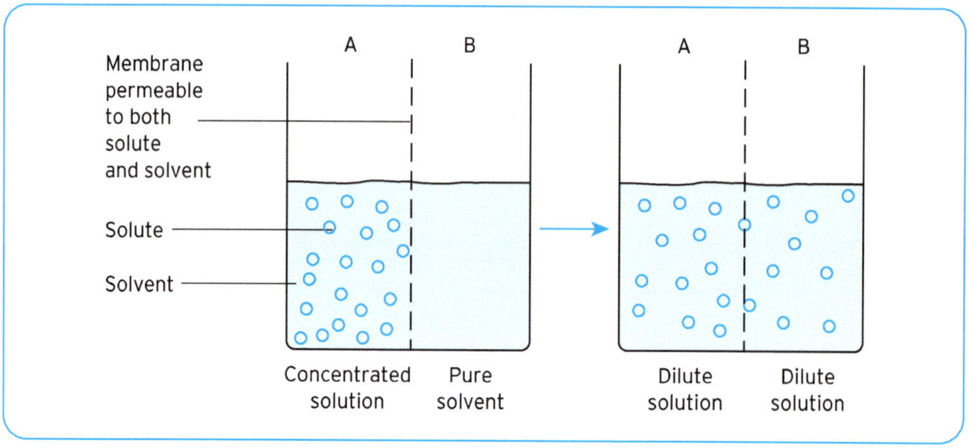

Figure 4.11
An experiment to demonstrate diffusion.

No - eventually, it would become dispersed in the water and we would have a dilute ink solution. Once again, the cause of this dispersal of the ink particles is collisions, this time with randomly moving water molecules.

- ***How could we speed up the process of the dispersal of the ink?***

We could agitate the glass or stir the water. This is an obvious but important point. Although the process of diffusion is quite capable of leading to a uniform dispersal of ink throughout the water, it does take some time. You should note, then, that diffusion is much more rapid in the gaseous phase.

When you study the human body, you will encounter diffusion again. It is one of the important processes by which substances move within the body. Here, however, diffusion often involves movement through a membrane such as the plasma (cell) membrane or the respiratory membrane of the lungs. You might wish to study these in more detail later, but we can simulate diffusion across a membrane in the experiment illustrated in Figure 4.11. In this experiment, a membrane divides a vessel equally into two compartments, A and B. An equal volume of fluid is poured into each compartment, but in A the fluid is a concentrated solution of some substance, let's say glucose or sodium chloride, while in B there is only pure water. The membrane separating the compartments has pores; the point you need to bear in mind is that the diameter of these pores is greater than that of the solute particles.

- ***So what happens next?***

Let us concentrate on just one solute particle. It suffers many collisions with solvent particles (water molecules) and with other solute molecules too. Consequently, it experiences the kind of random motion that we have described already. If we were to chart the course of just one solute particle, it would consist of a zigzag line, as represented in Figure 4.12.

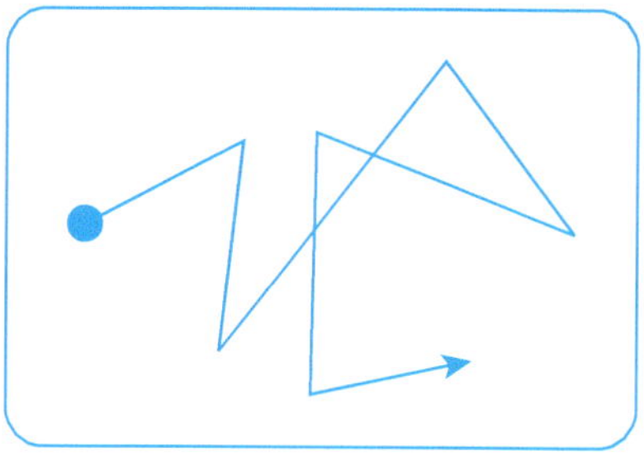

Figure 4.12
Representation of the movement of a single solute particle.

Each change of direction is the result of a collision - lesser changes by glancing blows and greater changes by near-head-on collisions. Sometimes the solute particles bounce off the sides or bottom of the container and off the membrane. If the course of a particle coincides with a pore, however, it will pass straight through into compartment B. Later on, it might pass back again. This pattern is repeated by all the solute particles. Given enough time, we would find that, on average, the solute particles are distributed equally between the two compartments, although at any one moment in time there might be more particles in one compartment. So, instead of A containing a concentrated solution and B containing pure water, both now contain dilute solutions. This is illustrated in Figure 4.11.

Now we are in a position to give a fuller definition of diffusion that takes into account the presence of a membrane:

> **Diffusion is the movement of solute particles from an area of high solute concentration, through a semi-permeable membrane, to an area of low solute concentration, until equilibrium is reached.**

Here, the phrase 'until equilibrium is reached' refers to the fact that after a sufficient period of time, the number of solute particles moving from A to B equals the number moving in the opposite direction. It would also be true to say that the average number of solute particles on either side of the membrane is the same, or that the concentrations of the solutions on either side are equal.

In addition, we should clarify the term 'semi-permeable'. This is applied to a membrane that has pores of a certain size and that therefore allows particles of a smaller size to diffuse through it. Not surprisingly, such particles are then referred to as diffusible particles and larger particles as non-diffusible. In the case of artificial membranes, the permeability of the membrane is fixed by the pore size and the term 'semi-permeable' is applied. In the body, however, the permeability of biological membranes can often be varied and the term 'selectively permeable' is applied.

● ***Are there factors that influence the rate of diffusion?***

Perhaps you already know that there are. A number are given below.

Surface area: the greater the surface area of the membrane, the greater the number of particles that come into contact with it, and the faster the rate of diffusion. This principle is employed in the body. For example, the alveoli of the lungs provide a surface area for gas exchange that is 1000 times the area of the surface of the body. If this sounds a lot, you should perhaps also know that the absorption of nutrients by the **ileum** of the gut is enhanced by **villi** and **microvilli**, which provide a surface area one million times that of the surface of the body.

Particle size: more energy is required to move larger particles than is required to move smaller particles. Consequently, the rate of diffusion of individual ions, such as electrolytes in plasma, is much greater than that of large molecules, such as plasma proteins.

Concentration: the greater the difference in concentration of two solutions, the greater the rate of diffusion between them. We refer to a difference in the concentration of two solutions as a **concentration gradient**.

Temperature: higher temperatures cause faster movement of particles and a greater diffusion rate.

Charge: some diffusible particles (ions) are charged, and you may already know that like charges repel each other while unlike charges attract. These electrostatic forces affect the diffusion rate. For example, in the resting state, the concentration of sodium ions inside nerve cells is much less than the concentration of the same ions outside the cell. In addition, the inside of the cell is charged negatively compared with the outside. We refer to this difference in charge as an **electrical potential difference**. Thus, there is not only a concentration gradient favouring the movement of sodium ions into nerve cells but also an electrical gradient. That is, the positively charged sodium ions (Na^+) are attracted to the negatively charged interior of the cell. When the nerve cell is in the resting state, however, sodium ions do not readily pass through the cell membrane.

- ***Do you remember that we said that biological membranes, such as the cell membrane, are selectively permeable?***

Perhaps you recall that this means that their permeability to a particular solute can be altered. When the nerve cell is stimulated, sodium channels through the cell membrane are opened, and now the rate of diffusion of the sodium ions into the cell is so great that textbooks often describe them as 'rushing' in. This influx of sodium ions is the first phase in the production of a nervous impulse and is dealt with in more detail in Chapter 11.

Pressure: an increase in pressure on one side of the membrane results in a greater rate of diffusion.

Osmosis

Now let us consider another experiment very similar to the diffusion experiment described previously. Our new experiment is illustrated in Figure 4.13. Here, as before, there is a vessel divided into two equal compartments, A and B, filled with the same liquids as before. The difference between this and the previous experiment is that the membrane has very small pores - too small, in fact, for the solute particles to pass through, but still larger than water molecules.

- ***If the solute molecules cannot pass from A to B, is there any change in the contents of the two compartments?***

To answer this question, we need to focus on the movement of solvent particles through the membrane, through which the solute particles can no longer pass.

- ***In which compartment is the solvent concentration the greatest?***

Note that we said 'solvent concentration' - this is greatest in compartment B. The concentration of solvent molecules in compartment A is in fact diluted by the presence of solute. We do not, of course, normally talk this way, but it is perfectly correct to do so. Solvent molecules move randomly and pass down concentration gradients, just as solute molecules do. Consequently, a sufficient lapse of time will reveal that there has been a net movement of water from compartment B to compartment A. This can be seen in the raised fluid level in A, as shown in Figure 4.13.

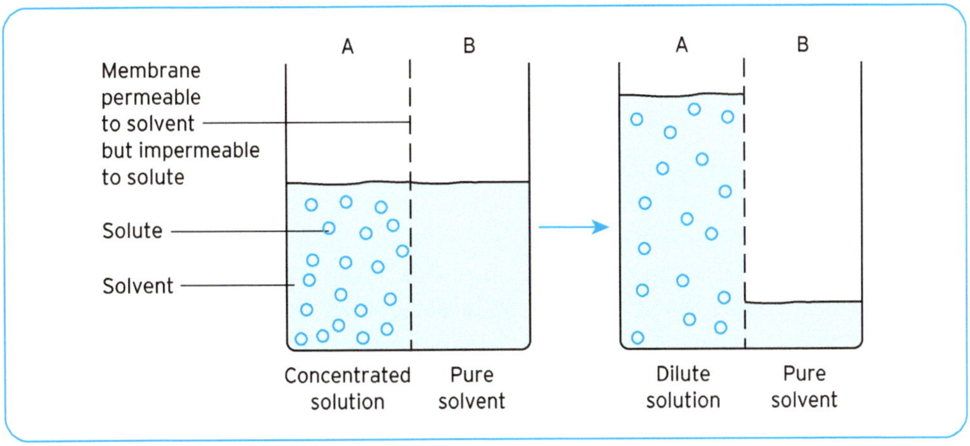

Figure 4.13
An experiment to demonstrate osmosis.

This movement of water is referred to as **osmosis**, which we are now in a position to define:

> **Osmosis is the movement of solvent molecules from an area of high solvent concentration, across a semi-permeable membrane, to an area of low solvent concentration.**

Note that in this definition the phrase 'until equilibrium is reached' does not appear. This is because an equal concentration either side of the membrane could never be achieved. No matter how much water were to move from compartment B to compartment A, the solute concentration in compartment A will always be greater than in compartment B. The factor that limits the net movement of water from B to A is the pressure developed by the expanded volume of fluid in A. This pressure serves to oppose the movement of water by osmosis. This does not mean that there is now no movement of water molecules at all. Indeed, the molecules are still moving randomly and experiencing collisions as they did before. Rather, it is that the rate of movement of water from A to B now equals the rate of movement in the opposite direction. Consequently, the volume of liquid in each compartment is stable, but A contains a greater volume than does B. This discussion leads us on to consider the concept of **osmotic pressure**.

Osmotic pressure

Osmotic pressure may be considered to be the pressure required to prevent the movement of solvent from a region of pure solvent and into a solution. The SI (Système Internationale) unit of pressure is the **pascal** (Pa), but sometimes the unit millimetres of mercury (mmHg) is used. You will find out more about measuring pressure in Chapter 6.

For now, the point to note is that the greater the concentration of solutes in solution, the greater the pressure required to stop the net movement of solvent into that solution by osmosis. When we consider osmotic pressure, however, we often think of it as a kind of water-pulling power. It is easy to see how this comes about, since water will move by osmosis from one solution and into another that has a greater concentration of solutes and, therefore, a higher osmotic pressure. It is worth bearing this in mind, since in practice you may hear the expression 'osmotic pull' being used as well as osmotic pressure.

Finally, the osmotic pressure of a solution depends upon the number of particles dissolved in solution. In the blood, sodium ions (Na^+) are the most abundant solute particles, and as a consequence they exert the greatest influence upon osmotic pressure. In addition, there are many other ionic and non-ionic solutes as well as larger suspended molecules, such as plasma proteins. Sometimes a distinction is made between the total osmotic pressure and that fraction of it for which the plasma proteins are responsible. When the latter is being referred to, the term **oncotic pressure** is used.

Osmolarity and osmolality

We have already noted that the osmotic pressure is dependent upon the number of particles in solution. Keep in mind that a particle could be an ion, an atom or a molecule. No matter how large or small, each of these counts as one particle as far as osmolarity is concerned.

- ***Perhaps we need a new unit to express concentration of solute in terms of the number of particles.***

What do you think? Can't we stick with using moles? After all, life is complicated enough already. On first examination, it may appear that there is no need to consider an additional unit. For example, suppose we dissolve 1 mole of glucose in water.

- ***How many particles do we have?***

To answer this question, you will need to remember that a mole is the molecular mass of a substance in grams (180 g in the case of glucose) and that one mole of a substance has the same number of particles as one mole of any other substance.

- ***Do you remember how many particles a mole of a substance contains?***

Perhaps you remember that a mole of any substance contains 6×10^{23} particles of that substance (Avogadro's number). If you are not sure about this, you may need to go back and look at Chapter 3.

Thus, there seems little need to consider additional units further. To work out the number of particles, we just need to know how many moles of a solute have been dissolved. It may look that way so far, but if you think carefully about electrolytes and non-electrolytes, you might realise that there is a problem.

- ***Is glucose an electrolyte or a non-electrolyte? Does it dissociate into ions in solution?***

Glucose is, indeed, a non-electrolyte and it does not dissociate into ions in solution.

- ***But what about sodium chloride (NaCl)?***

Sodium chloride is an electrolyte and dissociates into ions in solution. Consequently, if we take one mole of sodium chloride and dissolve it in water, we produce one mole of sodium ions (Na^+) and one mole of chloride ions (Cl^-) - that is, twice as many particles as one mole of glucose produces. Perhaps we had better consider another unit after all. Meet the **osmole**.

Osmolarity

To work out the number of osmoles in a solution, simply multiply the number of moles by the number of particles that a solute particle produces in solution. The mathematical formula for the osmole is

$$\text{Number of osmoles} = \text{number of moles} \times \begin{array}{c}\text{number of particles into which}\\ \text{a solute particle dissociates}\end{array}$$

Go back to glucose as an example, and you should see that since glucose does not dissociate in solution, one osmole of glucose has the same numerical value as one mole. In the case of sodium chloride (NaCl), however, one mole produces two osmoles in solution.

In addition, just as we often talk about molarity - that is, the concentration of a solution in mol/l or mmol/l - we also refer to **osmolarity** - that is, the number of osmoles per litre (osmol/l) or milliosmoles per litre (mosmol/l). The formula for osmolarity is

$$\text{Osmolarity} = \text{molarity} \times \text{number of particles into which solute particle dissociates}$$

Thus far, we have imagined aqueous solutions that consist of only one solute.

- ***But what about solutions with more than one solute? How would we work out their osmolarity?***

Let us imagine that we have 1 l of a solution in which there is dissolved 1 mole of glucose and 1 mole of sodium chloride (NaCl).

- ***What would be the osmolarity of this solution?***

From what has gone before, you should be able to work out the following. Since 1 mole of glucose in solution generates 1 mole of glucose, and 1 mole of NaCl generates 1 mole of sodium ions (Na^+) and 1 mole of chloride ions (Cl^-), the total number of particles generated is 3 osmol. The osmolarity of the solution is, therefore, 3 osmol/l.

At this point, you should also recognise that a solution with a greater osmolarity than another is referred to as being hyperosmotic and one with a lower osmolarity is described as hypo-osmotic. Two solutions that have the same osmolarity are described as being iso-osmotic.

It should be noted, however, that although iso-osmotic solutions have the same concentration of particles, they do not necessarily have the same particles.

- ***Remember that a particle could be an ion, an atom or a molecule. Each counts as one particle as far as osmolarity is concerned.***

Let us take a real-life example. When we compare intracellular fluid (inside cells) and extracellular fluid (outside cells), we discover that both have an osmolarity of approximately 280 mosmol/l - that is, they are iso-osmotic. However, they have very different solute concentrations (Table 4.2).

Table 4.2 Composition of intracellular and extracellular fluid.

Substance	Concentration (mosmol/l)		
	Plasma	Interstitial fluid	Intracellular fluid
Na^+	142.0	139.0	14.0
K^+	4.2	4.0	140
Ca^{2+}	1.3	1.2	0.0
Cl	108.0	108.0	4.0
(HCO_3^-)	24.0	28.3	10.0
Protein	1.2	0.2	4.0

Osmolality

It is also worth pointing out that we sometimes talk about **osmolality** instead of osmolarity. The formula for osmolality is

$$\text{Osmolality} = \text{molality} \times \text{number of particles into which a solute particle dissociates}$$

Molality differs from molarity in that it is the number of moles of solute per kilogram (kg) of solution rather than the number of moles of solute per litre (l) of solution. Consequently, osmolality gives the number of particles of solute per kilogram of solution rather than per litre. Since one litre of water weighs very nearly one kilogram, however, the units osmolarity and osmolality are almost identical.

Tonicity

In this section, we are going to consider the effect of different fluids on the movement of water in and out of cells. The erythrocyte (red blood cell) is commonly chosen as an example, since blood samples are easy to obtain. In addition, an effect upon blood cells in vitro (outside the body) may be reproduced in vivo (within the body) by the administration of fluid intravenously. This is clearly of interest to nurses who regulate the administration of infusions.

First, we need to remind ourselves that although intracellular fluid and extracellular fluid have different concentrations of solutes, they have the same osmolarity. In addition, the cell membrane is selectively permeable and regulates the movement of solutes across it. Water is able to move through the cell membrane freely, however.

- ***In the circumstances described above, is there a net movement of water in or out of the cell?***

If you think not, then you are right. The intracellular fluid and extracellular fluid are **iso-osmotic** and there is no net movement of water. Since this is the case, we also say that intracellular fluid and extracellular fluid are **isotonic**. This literally means that they have the same strength. The intracellular fluid cannot pull water into the cell from the extracellular fluid, and the extracellular fluid cannot pull water out of the intracellular fluid.

Now let us perform an experiment in order to determine the effect of **hyperosmotic** and **hypo-osmotic** solutions upon our red blood cells by placing some cells in each of the solutions and then examining them under the microscope. In each case, you should assume that the solute is non-diffusible - that is, it does not readily cross the cell membrane and enter the cell. Sodium chloride (NaCl) and glucose are examples of non-diffusible solutes.

- ***What would be the effect of placing the cells in a hyperosmotic solution?***

Water would move out of the cell by osmosis and the cell would shrink. This is illustrated in Figure 4.14 and is referred to as **crenation**. When a solution has the ability to draw water out of a cell in this way, it is described as being **hypertonic**.

- ***In contrast, what would happen to the cells placed in a hypo-osmotic solution?***

Water would be drawn into the cells by osmosis, and the cells would swell and rupture - a process referred to as **plasmolysis**. This is also illustrated in Figure 4.14. Solutions that cause plasmolysis are referred to as **hypotonic**.

So, isotonic solutions cause no net movement of water in or out of cells, hypertonic solutions cause crenation, and hypotonic solutions cause plasmolysis. Note that in our example, the

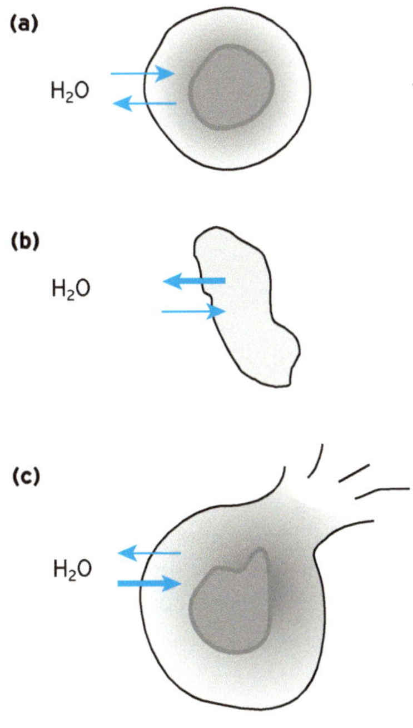

(a) Effect of an isotonic solution upon a red blood cell: there is no net movement of water, and the unique shape of the cell is maintained.

(b) The effect of a hypertonic solution upon a red blood cell: there is net movement of water out of the cell, which shrinks and loses its shape - crenation.

(c) The effect of a hypotonic solution upon a red blood cell: there is net movement of water into the cell, which swells. Eventually, the cell membrance ruptures - plasmolysis.

Figure 4.14
The effects of isotonic, hypertonic and hypotonic solutions on a red blood cell.

isotonic solution is also iso-osmotic, the hypertonic solution is hyperosmotic and the hypotonic solution is hypo-osmotic.

- ***So, then, isn't tonicity the same as osmolarity?***

You could be forgiven for thinking so, but in reality they are different. Osmolarity is concerned with the concentration of solute particles in solution, while tonicity deals with the tendency of a solution to cause crenation or plasmolysis. Although it is true that isotonic solutions are usually iso-osmotic, hypertonic solutions are usually hyperosmotic and hypotonic solutions are usually hypo-osmotic, it is not always the case.

- ***But how could it be otherwise?***

First, note that in our red blood cell experiment, we made a point of saying that the solute was non-diffusible.

- ***What would happen if we were to use a solution with a diffusible solute, such as urea?***

Suppose we place a sample of our red blood cells in an iso-osmotic solution of urea. Remember that iso-osmotic means the same concentration of particles, not necessarily the same particles. Urea molecules will diffuse into the cell, the contents of which now become hyperosmotic. Consequently, water is drawn into the cell by osmosis, and the cell swells and plasmolyses. Thus, osmolarity and tonicity are not the same thing at all.

- ***Are there any practical applications of this?***

We are sure that you will not be surprised that there are - have a look at Practice point 4.7.

Practice point 4.7

Tonicity, osmolarity and intravenous solutions

Suppose that we need to administer fluids intravenously to a patient.

- ***If crenation or plasmolysis of red blood cells is to be avoided, what type of fluid is usually administered?***

Isotonic solutions are chosen. The most commonly administered isotonic crystalloid solutions are sodium chloride 0.9% (w/v) and dextrose (glucose) 5% (w/v). (Incidentally, in some parts of the world the abbreviation D5W is used for dextrose 5% in water.) Both of these solutions are iso-osmotic with blood plasma. Remember that this does not mean that plasma is a 0.9% solution of sodium chloride and a 5% solution of glucose. Rather, it means that these solutions have the same concentration of particles as does plasma. It is just that plasma has very many different kinds of particle, whereas the infusion fluids mentioned are pure solutions of only one particle. Hypertonic and hypotonic solutions are occasionally administered intravenously, but the reasons for this are beyond the scope of this book. If you see them being used in clinical practice, however, you might like to have staff explain their use to you.

In-text review

- ✔ Diffusion is the movement of solute particles from an area of high solute concentration to an area of low solute concentration until equilibrium is reached.
- ✔ The greater the difference in concentration between two solutions (concentration gradient), the greater the rate of diffusion between them.
- ✔ Osmosis is the movement of solvent from an area of high solvent concentration, across a semi-permeable membrane, to an area of low solvent concentration.
- ✔ Osmotic pressure is the pressure required to prevent the movement of solvent by osmosis.
- ✔ The osmole is an expression of the number of particles of solute.
- ✔ The number of osmoles of a substance is calculated by multiplying the number of moles of solute by the number of particles into which the solute dissociates.
- ✔ Osmolarity is an expression of concentration in terms of the number of osmoles per litre of solution (osmol/l) or milliosmoles per litre (mosmol/l).
- ✔ Osmolality is an expression of concentration in terms of the number of osmoles per kilogram of solution (osmol/kg) or milliosmoles per kilogram (mosmol/kg).
- ✔ An isotonic solution is one that causes no net movement of water into or out of cells.
- ✔ A hypertonic solution is one that causes water to move out of cells, leading to crenation.
- ✔ A hypotonic solution is one that causes water to move into cells, leading to plasmolysis.

Filtration

At this point, it is worthwhile distinguishing diffusion and **filtration**. Filtration is the process whereby a liquid is forced through a porous membrane by a pressure difference on either side of the membrane. What filtration has in common with diffusion is that the size of some particles prevents their movement through the membrane. In reality, however, the two processes are quite different.

In the case of diffusion, the net movement of particles of a substance is from an area of high concentration to an area of low concentration as a consequence of the random motion of the particles. Particles actually move in both directions, as we have discussed previously; it is their **net movement** that in solution is down a concentration gradient. In filtration, particles are forced in one direction through a membrane by a pressure gradient.

In the body, the formation of interstitial fluid and its reabsorption involves filtration and the kidneys filter the blood – a process that leads to the production of urine.

The distribution of water within the body

We have already mentioned intracellular fluid and extracellular fluid, but in fact there are three fluid compartments within the body. The extracellular compartment can be divided further into the **intravascular fluid** (plasma) and the **interstitial fluid**. Interstitial fluid is the fluid found both outside cells and outside the circulation. It bathes cells and is the medium through which substances diffuse between cells and the blood. Interstitial fluid is formed from blood but contains only some of its constituents. For example, there are no cells or large molecules, such as plasma proteins, in interstitial fluid; these are simply too large to escape through blood vessels in normal circumstances. The electrolyte concentrations of plasma and interstitial fluid are very similar, since water and ions move freely across blood capillary walls. Table 4.3 shows the distribution of fluid between the three compartments as a percentage of body weight in adults.

Table 4.3 Distribution of water within the body as a percentage of total body weight.

	Percentage of body weight (%)
Total body fluid	60
Intracellular fluid	40
Extracellular fluid	20
Intravascular fluid (plasma)	4
Interstitial fluid	16

When we think of fluid in the body, our minds often turn first to blood. When looking at Table 4.3, however, you should note that although 60% of body weight is water, most of this water is inside rather than outside cells. Even when we consider extracellular fluid alone, we find that interstitial fluid accounts for the greatest proportion and that blood is only 4% of body weight.

This pattern is repeated for adolescents, but it is not the case for infants and children, as Table 4.4 illustrates. In the case of neonates, 80% rather than 60% of the total body weight is water, and the greater proportion of this is extracellular rather than intracellular.

The formation of interstitial fluid

Interstitial fluid is formed at the arterial end of capillaries and resorbed at their venous ends. The process of the formation of interstitial fluid is illustrated in Figure 4.15. **Capillaries** connect **arterioles** and **venules**. The driving force of the blood through the circulation is referred to as the **hydrostatic pressure** (blood pressure). Note that at the arterial end of a capillary, the hydrostatic pressure (blood pressure) is approximately 32 mmHg, while at the venous end it is only 12 mmHg.

Table 4.4 Distribution of fluid within the body for different age groups.

Age group	Percentage of body weight (%)	Extracellular (%)	Intracellular (%)
Puberty	60	20	40
1 year	70	25	45
Neonate	80	45	35

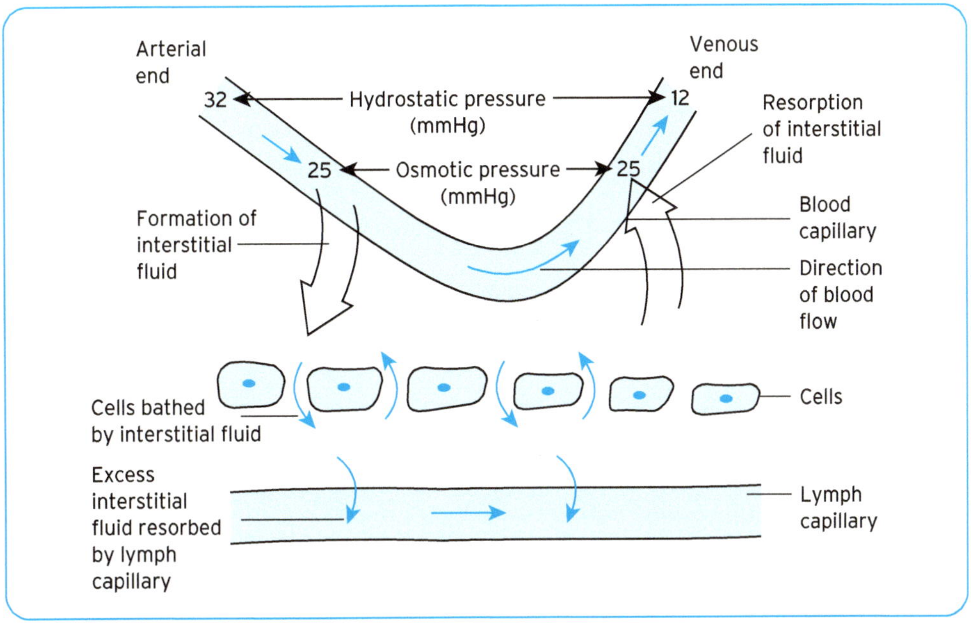

Figure 4.15
The formation of interstitial fluid.

- ***Why does the hydrostatic pressure fall along the length of the capillary?***

It falls because fluid is lost from the capillary as interstitial fluid is formed.

Hydrostatic pressure tends to force small molecules, such as water, through the capillary wall, but it is opposed by osmotic pressure that is approximately 25 mmHg.

- ***At the arterial end of the capillary, which is greatest: hydrostatic pressure or osmotic pressure?***

Hydrostatic pressure is greater than osmotic pressure, and there is a net pressure of 7 mmHg (that is, 32 – 25) in favour of the formation of interstitial fluid.

- ***But what about the venous end? Which is the greater pressure?***

At the venous end, the situation is quite different and hydrostatic pressure is less than osmotic pressure. Here, a net pressure of –13 mmHg (12 – 25) favours the resorption of water.

In summary, we can say that interstitial fluid bathes the cells of the body and that it is formed at the arterial end of capillaries but resorbed at their venous ends. Remember that in normal circumstances, only small molecules can escape through capillary walls, and so interstitial fluid contains no cells or large molecules, such as plasma proteins.

It is worth noting here, however, that not all the interstitial fluid formed at the arterial end of capillaries is in fact resorbed at their venous ends.

- ***What happens to the interstitial fluid that is not resorbed?***

If you have studied biology before, you will no doubt remember that interstitial fluid that is not returned immediately to the circulation is collected by lymph capillaries, as illustrated in

Figure 4.15. The lymph system is a very important system of vessels within the body with roles in both normal health and disease. When you have a moment, you might like to find out more about the lymph system. The condition of excess interstitial fluid (oedema) is considered in Practice point 4.8.

Practice point 4.8

Oedema

Let us begin this section by imagining that the capillaries of a patient have become excessively permeable or 'leaky', and as a consequence molecules that normally remain in the circulation, such as the protein **albumin**, are able to pass into the interstitium.

- ***What effect do you think this loss of albumin will have on capillary osmotic pressure and interstitial osmotic pressure?***

Capillary osmotic pressure will fall and interstitial osmotic pressure will rise.

- ***What will be the effect of these changes upon the formation of interstitial fluid?***

There will be an increase in the production of interstitial fluid. An excess of interstitial fluid is called **oedema**. Oedema may be a generalised or localised condition that is a common cause of swelling of the tissues. For example, oedematous ankles show an increase in girth, and gentle compression with the pads of the fingers will produce indentations referred to as pitting.

Increased capillary permeability may be caused by a lack of oxygen or by the release of **vasoactive substances** during an inflammatory reaction. Think about the swelling that occurs at the site of a wasp sting. The term 'vasoactive' literally means 'having an effect on blood vessels', and one effect is increased capillary permeability. **Histamine** is an example of a vasoactive substance that is important in local injuries, such as a wasp sting, in allergic reactions, such as hay fever, and in asthma. Some drugs that help to reduce swelling do so by blocking histamine and are referred to as **antihistamines**. One such drug is terfenadine, which is used in the treatment of hay fever and allergic skin conditions.

At this point, it is worth mentioning that in some patients, the symptoms of an allergy are widespread and include cardiovascular collapse and oedema of the airway that impairs breathing. This condition is called **anaphylactic shock** (allergic shock); a fuller discussion is beyond the scope of this book, but you may wish to find out more about this for yourself.

Increased capillary permeability is not the only cause of oedema. Raised hydrostatic (blood) pressure, reduced plasma osmotic pressure and lymphatic obstruction are other possible causes.

Raised hydrostatic pressure

Hydrostatic pressure may be elevated following the intravenous administration of an excessive volume of fluid. Therefore, care should be taken to regulate infusion rates accurately. The most serious effects are seen in the pulmonary (lung) circulation, where pulmonary oedema is responsible for impaired gas exchange and decreased lung compliance - that is, the lungs are stiff to inflate. Both contribute to **dyspnoea** (the experience of difficulty in breathing). **Tachypnoea** (fast respiratory rate), cough and the production of clear sputum, which may be blood-streaked, are other manifestations. Pulmonary oedema is managed by the intravenous administration of the **diuretic** (increases urine output) drug furosemide; in addition, the patient should be sat upright and given oxygen.

Pulmonary oedema may also occur when blood volume is normal but the pumping ability of the heart is impaired, such as is the case following a myocardial infarction (heart attack). Once again, the mechanism is raised pulmonary hydrostatic pressure, but the cause is a failure of the damaged left side of the heart to clear blood returning to it from the lungs - you might say that there is a backlog. Check this explanation with the simple diagram of the circulation given in Figure 4.16.

Backlogging of blood in the pulmonary circulation increases the workload of the right side of the heart, and eventually right heart failure may occur, with subsequent development of systemic oedema. This is often seen in elderly people as swollen ankles.

Much less serious is lower-limb oedema, which occurs when standing for prolonged periods. Standing causes venous congestion, since the compression of the veins of the leg by muscle contraction when walking is essential for the promotion of venous return. It may be prevented in people whose occupations require prolonged standing by periodic contraction of the leg muscles and by wearing support stockings that compress the limb with uniform pressure and so aid venous return. Resting with the affected limb on a stool above the level of the hips will relieve lower-limb oedema when it does occur, but this should be avoided when pulmonary oedema is present, since it will be exacerbated by the increased venous return.

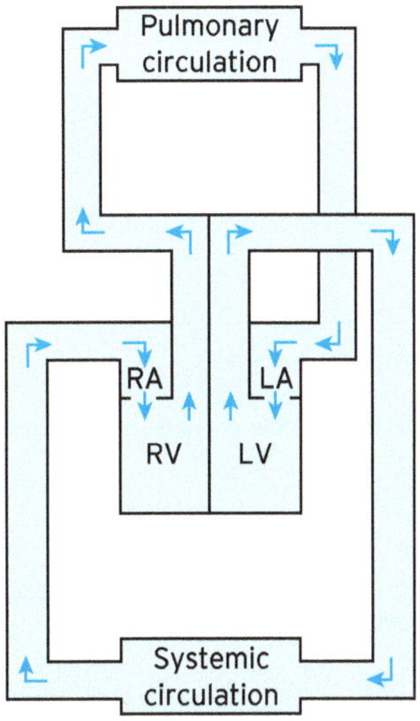

RA = right atrium
RV = right ventricle
LA = left atrium
LV = left ventricle

Figure 4.16
Diagram of the circulation.

Reduced plasma osmotic pressure

The importance of plasma proteins in the maintenance of blood osmotic pressure has already been noted. Consequently, **hypoproteinaemia** (low blood protein), such as occurs in starvation and liver disease (plasma proteins are manufactured in the liver), is another cause of oedema.

Lymphatic obstruction

Since lymphatic capillaries drain interstitial fluid that is not resorbed by blood capillaries, obstruction of these capillaries also causes oedema. Lymphatic obstruction may be caused by the growth of a tumour or, in tropical countries, by a type of worm (*Wuchereria bancrofti*). The resultant gross swelling of the lower limbs gives rise to the name **elephantiasis**.

Specialised body fluids

It is worth noting that a very small proportion of the fluid present in the body is localised in spaces where it performs specialised functions. For example, **cerebrospinal fluid** (CSF) surrounds and cushions the brain, **synovial fluid** is a lubricant in joints and **plural fluid** allows the two plural membranes to slide over each other during breathing. You will find a little more information on specialised fluids in Chapter 6, but for a fuller discussion you should refer to a physiology text.

The regulation of fluid balance within the body

The term 'fluid balance' implies the state in which fluid intake and output are equal. This is the normal state of the body over a period of time, as the figures in Table 3.5 show. Note that **insensible losses** are those of which we are not immediately aware, such as in sweat, faeces and breath.

- ***How is this balance achieved?***

When we consider fluid balance in the body, we are concerned primarily with plasma, since this is the only fluid that can be directly acted upon to control its volume and composition. Since water and ions move freely across capillary walls, however, when plasma is regulated the volume and composition of interstitial fluid are also regulated. The intracellular fluid is, in turn, influenced by changes in extracellular fluid, but this is limited by the selective permeability of the cell membrane.

- ***Control of sodium balance is important in regulating extracellular fluid volume.***

We have noted previously that sodium ions are the most abundant particles in extracellular fluid, and so they exert the principal influence upon osmotic pressure. We have also noted that osmotic pressure is sometimes referred to as a 'pull' on water and can be thought of as 'water-holding ability'. Consequently, the mass of sodium ions in extracellular fluid determines the extracellular fluid volume, and regulation of extracellular fluid volume depends upon controlling sodium balance.

- ***How is sodium balance regulated?***

An obvious point to note here is that in order to maintain sodium balance at a certain level, ingestion must equal excretion.

- ***So, do we regulate sodium intake?***

The answer to this question is that our sodium intake may vary, but we do not regulate it specifically to meet our needs at any particular point in time. We may add salt (sodium chloride) to our meals because we like the taste of it, or we may be unaware of the salt content of particular foods. Alternatively, we may avoid salt because we have heard that an excess

Table 3.5 Balance of water intake and output.

Fluid intake (ml)		Fluid output (ml)	
Drinking	1250	Insensible losses, e.g. sweat, faeces, breath	1100
Water in food	1000	Urine	1500
Water produced by metabolic reactions	350		
Total	**2600**		**2600**

intake of it may be associated with hypertension (high blood pressure). The point is that sodium intake is not regulated as such, and a typical daily intake of 10-15 g is very much in excess of the required 1 g. So, if we do not regulate sodium intake, we must regulate its excretion.

- ***How is sodium lost from the body?***

Sodium (in sodium chloride) is lost in sweat, but sweating is part of the thermoregulatory mechanism. We sweat because we need to cool down rather than because we need to control sodium balance. Similarly, the sodium lost in faeces is not controlled. The amount of sodium lost in urine, however, is regulated. The mechanisms are not dealt with here - you can find out more about them in a physiology textbook. The important thing to note is that our kidneys regulate salt balance and maintain the volume of extracellular fluid.

- ***Are there mechanisms that act upon water balance too?***

Yes, there are, as you will see from the example below.

Regulation of blood osmolarity by antidiuretic hormone and thirst

In the case of water, we regulate our intake, driven by thirst, and our excretion in urine too. Of course, there are water losses that we cannot control - the so-called **insensible losses**. These losses include water in sweat and faeces and water vapour in breath.

- ***So how does the body determine how much water to lose?***

A part of the brain called the **hypothalamus** monitors the osmolarity of blood passing through it. The cells that achieve this monitoring function are, not surprisingly, called **osmoreceptors**. Let us take the case of an elevated osmolarity as a means of illustrating what happens next. First, an elevated osmolarity stimulates thirst, and the individual seeks out a drink. The thirst centre of the brain is also located in the hypothalamus.

- ***Do you see how increasing fluid intake will tend to reduce osmolarity to normal again?***

But suppose that a drink is not available immediately - perhaps you are in the middle of a game of squash! In this case, water conservation is the priority. The hypothalamus is linked to the posterior lobe of the **pituitary gland**, which is located beneath the brain. From this gland, a hormone called **antidiuretic hormone** (ADH, vasopressin) is released.

- ***What does ADH do?***

Its name tells all - antidiuretic hormone reduces **diuresis** (urine output). So, increasing water intake and reducing water loss work together to restore blood osmolarity. These mechanisms are illustrated in Figure 4.17.

- ***Do you recognise the above as an example of a negative feedback mechanism? Now attempt to draw a similar diagram for reduced blood osmolarity.***

So, the body regulates the volume and composition of extracellular fluid primarily by regulating sodium and water excretion and water intake.

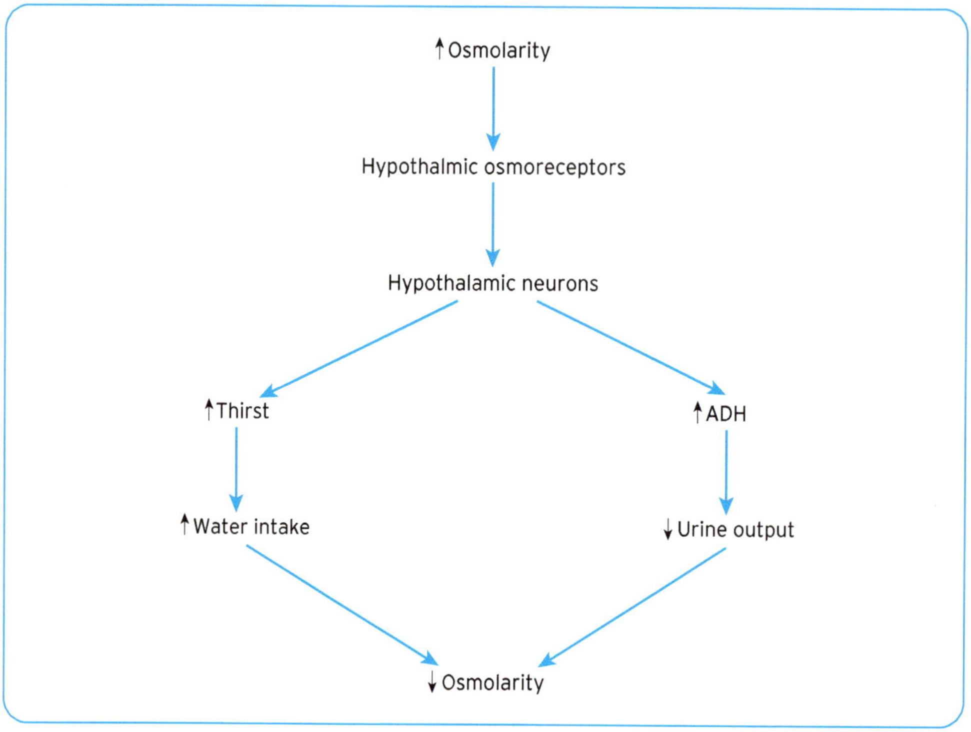

Figure 4.17
The control of water balance by thirst and antidiuretic hormone (ADH).

● ***Could something go wrong?***

It could. But this is not a pathology text, so we will consider just one example - that of dehydration (see Practice point 4.9).

Specific gravity

We have seen that in order to maintain fluid balance, the body is able to regulate sodium and water excretion. Consequently, samples of urine obtained from the same individual, but at different times of the day, differ in composition. Sometimes it is useful to determine whether there has been any gross change in the urine composition before resorting to expensive laboratory tests. One easily taken measurement is that of **specific gravity**, or relative density. This is the ratio of the density of a solution to that of water; the formula for it is

$$\text{Specific gravity} = \frac{\text{density of a substance}}{\text{density of water}}$$

Density is the mass of a substance per unit volume. The SI (Système Internationale) unit of density is the kilogram per cubic metre (kg/m^3). If you are unsure about this, see Chapter 1. The density of water is 1000 kg/m^3 and its specific gravity is, of course, 1.

Practice point 4.9

Dehydration

Dehydration may be described as a negative water balance - that is, the state in which losses exceed gains. Reduced water intake may accompany problems such as a swallowing defect, confusion in elderly people or perhaps the water jug simply being placed too far away from a frail patient. When you next visit a placement where frail, elderly or confused people or people with learning difficulties are cared for, think about basic physiological needs, such as that for water.

- ***List some possible causes of excessive water loss.***

Your list may include vomiting, diarrhoea and excessive urine production. The latter occurs in the conditions **diabetes insipidus** (a lack of ADH) and diabetes mellitus. Although it is true that many causes of dehydration involve water and electrolyte loss, water is often lost in a greater proportion.

- ***What effect would you expect this to have on blood osmolarity?***

You should be able to work out that blood osmolarity will rise.

- ***What will be the effect of this upon intracellular fluid?***

Water will be drawn out of the cells by osmosis. Consequently, we refer to this state as extracellular fluid hypertonicity. We might initially detect dehydration from the appearance of the tissues when water has been lost from the cells. For example, the eyeballs appear sunken, the tongue and mucous membranes are dry and the skin is inelastic. More serious effects are related to the shrinkage of brain neurons and range from confusion and irrational behaviour to convulsions and death. Incidentally, castaways on desert islands and shipwrecked mariners in open boats are sometimes portrayed as confused and irrational - at least in some rather bad films! No doubt this image is based partly on the real-life manifestations of severe dehydration.

- ***What about urine – what is its specific gravity?***

The first thing to note here is that urine is an aqueous solution and the presence of solutes means that it has a greater density than that of pure water. Consequently, its specific gravity will be above 1. Second, since urine composition changes with the body's fluid balance status, its normal specific gravity exists within a range, between 1.001 and 1.035.

In the modern health-care setting, the specific gravity of urine is measured easily using a reagent strip. This simple test is performed regularly as part of a general health check - perhaps when you register with a doctor for the first time or visit a hospital for almost any reason. A specific gravity outside the normal range may indicate the need for additional tests. The point to remember is that specific gravity may show that urine composition is abnormal, but it is a non-specific test - it does not indicate what the abnormality is. Furthermore, some changes in urine composition are not reflected in changes in specific gravity - it is a crude test.

Dialysis

In the presence of partial or complete kidney failure, the role of the kidneys in the maintenance of water, electrolyte and acid-base balance and in the elimination of waste may be undertaken by an 'artificial kidney' in a process referred to as **dialysis**. There are two forms of dialysis - **haemodialysis** and **peritoneal dialysis**.

Haemodialysis

In haemodialysis, blood is diverted from the circulation to an 'artificial kidney' (the dialyser) and then pumped back to the patient again as illustrated in Figure 4.18. A number of different designs of artificial kidney exist, but the principle of haemodialysis is the same in each case. Blood is passed over one side of a semi-permeable membrane, while a special fluid (dialysate) flows over the other side. A pressure difference is maintained on either side of the membrane, so that both water and solutes are filtered from the blood. In addition, the composition of the dialysate is such that a concentration gradient is also maintained across the membrane and solutes such as urea diffuse from the blood and into the dialysate. Finally, the composition of the dialysate determines its osmolarity, which in turn regulates the movement of water from the blood to the dialysate by osmosis. Despite great advances in the technology of dialysis, it is effective only during the time that it is performed, and the patient has to return for treatment frequently.

Peritoneal dialysis

In this procedure, the patient's own peritoneum serves as a membrane and dialysate is instilled into the peritoneal cavity, where it remains for a period of time before being drained

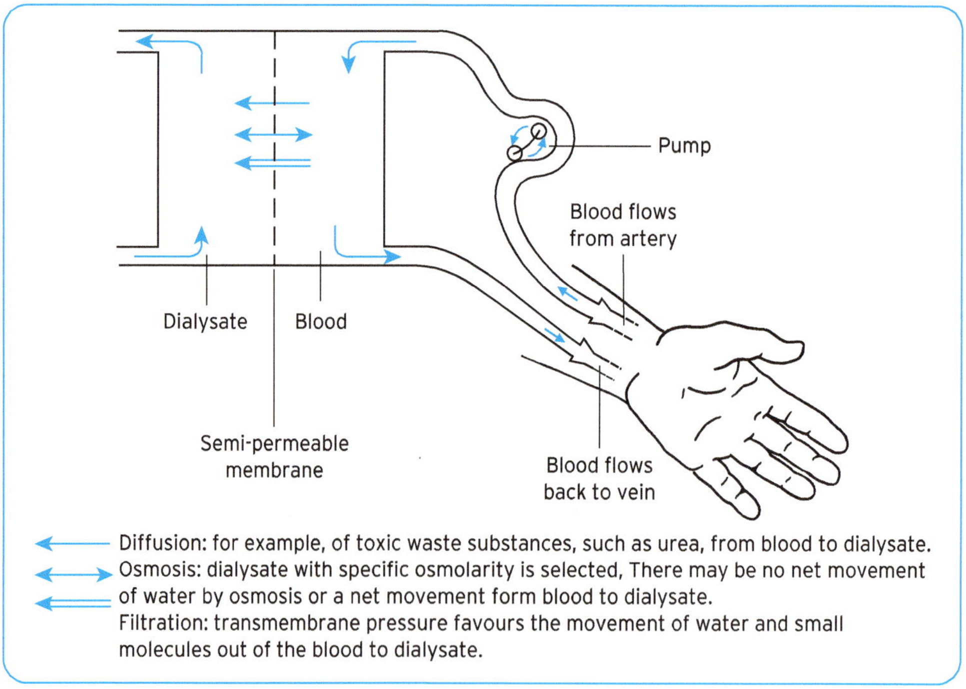

Figure 4.18
Diagram illustrating haemodialysis.

out. Patients in their own homes may perform one form of peritoneal dialysis, and consequently a good deal of independence is achieved.

In-text review

- ✔ Filtration is the process whereby a liquid is forced through a porous membrane by a pressure difference on either side.
- ✔ Within the body, water is found both within cells (intracellular compartment) and outside cells (extracellular compartment).
- ✔ The extracellular compartment is divided further into the intravascular compartment and the interstitial compartment.
- ✔ Interstitial fluid is formed at the arterial end of capillaries and resorbed at their venous ends.
- ✔ Oedema is an excess of interstitial fluid.
- ✔ Fluid balance is regulated by a number of hormones, including antidiuretic hormone (ADH), which reduces water loss by the kidney.
- ✔ Specific gravity (relative density) is the ratio of the density of a solution to that of water. Normal range is 1.001–1.035.
- ✔ Dialysis is the process of exchanging water and solutes across a semi-permeable membrane between blood and a specially prepared solution (dialysate).

Summary

This chapter began by looking at the structure of the water molecule before proceeding to consider different kinds of solution. Examples of the different types of solution used in clinical practice, such as intravenous infusions, were given. Although this chapter has dealt with science related to the water molecule, and we have looked at important physical processes such as diffusion and osmosis, these have been related to important clinical situations, such as water balance and conditions such as oedema. Finally, application to health care in terms of dialysis has been made.

Summary points

- → **Water is a polar molecule.**
- → **The shape of a meniscus is determined by the relative strengths of the forces of adhesion and cohesion.**
- → **Cohesive forces are responsible for surface tension.**
- → **Aqueous mixtures include mechanical suspensions, colloidal suspensions and true solutions.**
- → **True solutions consist of a solute and a solvent.**

- Solutes that dissociate into ions in solution are referred to as electrolytes.
- Ionic compounds and polar molecules dissolve in polar solvents.
- Non-polar covalent molecules dissolve in non-polar solvents.
- The concentration of a solution identifies the relative proportions of solute and solvent.
- Concentration may be expressed as a percentage or in terms of molarity.
- Diffusion is an important physical process that accounts for the movement of particles of a solute or of a gas.
- Osmosis is an important physical process that accounts for the movement of solvent particles.
- The number of particles of a solute is expressed in terms of osmolarity or osmolality.
- The tendency of a solution to produce plasmolysis or crenation is described in terms of tonicity.
- The control of sodium balance is important in the regulation of extracellular fluid volume.
- Antidiuretic hormone (ADH) and thirst regulate blood volume.
- Specific gravity is the ratio of the density of a liquid to that of water.
- The process of dialysis involves filtration as well as diffusion and osmosis.

Self-test questions

1 Which one of the following statements is true of water?
(a) It is an ionic compound.
(b) It is a polar molecule.
(c) It is an element.
(d) It is a non-polar molecule.

2 Match the substance on the left with the appropriate description on the right.

(a) Hexane	(i) Non-polar solvent
(b) NaCl	(ii) Ionic compound
(c) Glucose	(iii) Polar solvent
(d) Water	(iv) Polar solute

3 Which one of the following is an electrolyte?
(a) Urea.
(b) Glucose.
(c) Sodium chloride.
(d) Acetone.

4 Which one of the following saline concentrations (w/v) is described as isotonic?
(a) 0.09%.
(b) 0.9%.
(c) 0.5%.
(d) 5%.

5 Which one of the following glucose concentrations (w/v) is described as isotonic?
(a) 0.09%.
(b) 0.9%.
(c) 0.5%.
(d) 5%.

6 If a solution of sodium chloride has a concentration of 1 mol/l, what will be its osmolarity (in osmol/l)?
(a) 0.1.
(b) 1.0.
(c) 2.0.
(d) 10.0.

7 Which one of the following represents a normal specific gravity for urine?
(a) 1.020.
(b) 0.20.
(c) 1.050.
(d) 10.50.

8 Which one of the following is *not* a possible cause of oedema?
(a) Elevated blood osmotic pressure.
(b) Increased venous hydrostatic pressure.
(c) Increased capillary permeability.
(d) Lymphatic obstruction.

9 When a concentration is expressed as 5% (w/v), what volume of solution (in ml) contains 5 g?
(a) 1.
(b) 10.
(c) 100.
(d) 1000.

10 If blood osmotic pressure is 25 mmHg and hydrostatic pressure at the arterial end of a capillary is 32 mmHg, what is the net pressure leading to the formation of interstitial fluid (in mmHg)?
(a) 7.
(b) 25.
(c) 32.
(d) 57.

Further study/exercises

In giving practical examples relevant to this chapter, we have mentioned intravenous infusions and wound dressings.

1 **What care is required by the patient who has an intravenous infusion?**

Royal College of Nursing (2005) *Standards for Infusion Therapy*. www.rcn.org.uk/publications/pdf/standardsinfusiontherapy.pdf

2 **Identify examples of hydrocolloid, hydrogel and alginate wound dressings. How and when are they used?**

Fletcher, J. (2005) Understanding wound dressings: alginates. *Nursing Times*, 101(16), 53-4.

Fletcher, J. (2005) Understanding wound dressings: hydrocolloids. *Nursing Times*, 101(46), 51.

Jones, A. and Vaughan, D. (2005) Hydrogel dressings in the management of a variety of wound types: a review. *Journal of Orthopaedic Nursing*, 9(Suppl. 1), S1-11.

5

Acids, bases and pH balance

Learning outcomes

After reading the following chapter and undertaking personal study, you should be able to:

1 Define the terms 'acid' and 'base'.

2 Identify examples of acids and bases that are encountered in everyday life and clinical practice.

3 List the properties of acids and bases.

4 Outline the first-aid measures to be taken in chemical burns.

5 Describe the pH scale and identify clinical practice situations in which it is used.

6 Identify the products of a reaction between an acid and a base and give an example of this reaction in clinical practice.

7 Distinguish between the meaning of the terms 'strength' and 'concentration' when used in connection with acids and bases and relate this to clinical practice.

8 Define the term 'buffer' and give examples in the body.

9 Outline the regulation of acid-base balance in the body by reference to buffer systems, respiratory regulation and renal regulation.

10 Using the results of laboratory tests, identify an acid-base imbalance as either acidosis or alkalosis and distinguish the cause as either respiratory or metabolic.

Introduction

Students who have not studied science before may be unfamiliar with the terms '**base**' and '**alkali**'. (In this book, the terms 'base' and 'alkali' are taken to be synonymous.) However, few will not have heard of the term '**acid**'. Although this term may conjure up images of dangerous caustic substances that are best avoided, we often encounter acids and bases in our everyday lives. They are important substances in the environment, we use them as drugs and they have particular relevance to us in health or disease. Nonetheless, since some acids and bases are potentially dangerous, a brief explanation of the relevant first aid is given in Practice point 5.1.

- ***Identify some of the acids and bases that are important within the body or may be found in the home.***

Tables 5.1 and 5.2 identify some of the acids and bases that we meet regularly.

In this chapter, we consider what acids and bases are. If you have studied basic chemistry before, this will not present any problems. If not, you should first read Chapter 3. This chapter includes quite a lot of chemistry, but there is a reason for this. Flick to the end of the chapter and you will see that the information covered is applied to various conditions seen in patients. For the moment, we examine what acids and bases are.

Table 5.1 Some common acids.

Acid	Common name/function
Acetylsalicylic acid	Aspirin; a common analgesic and antipyretic
Amino acids	The group of acids that make up proteins
Ascorbic acid	Vitamin C
Carbonic acid	Formed from the reaction between CO_2 and water
Citric acid	Found in citrus fruits and important in the energy-producing reactions of the body
Deoxyribonucleic acid	Carries genetic information
Fatty acids	Important molecules in fats
Folic acid	One of the B group vitamins
Hydrochloric acid	Important in digestion in the stomach

Table 5.2 Some common bases.

Base	Common name/function
Aluminium hydroxide	Gastric antacid
Magnesium hydroxide	Gastric antacid
Magnesium sulphate	Epsom salts; a laxative
Magnesium trisilicate	Gastric antacid
Sodium hydrogen carbonate	Baking soda; a gastric antacid also used to correct acidosis
Sodium sulphate	Glauber's salt; a laxative

Acids

An acid is a substance (a **molecule** or an **ion**) that donates a **hydrogen ion** (H^+) to another substance during a chemical reaction. A hydrogen ion results when an **atom** of hydrogen loses an **electron**:

H	$\longrightarrow$	H^+	+	e^-
hydrogen atom		hydrogen ion		electron

- ***Of which subatomic particles does a hydrogen atom consist?***

A hydrogen atom normally consists of only one electron and one **proton**. If a hydrogen atom loses an electron, the resultant hydrogen ion is simply a proton. For this reason, acids may be defined as **proton donors**, as you will see as we move on to consider some examples in more detail.

Hydrochloric acid

Hydrochloric acid is an important acid found in the stomach, where it is responsible for turning **pepsinogen** into the protein-digesting enzyme **pepsin** and also for conferring a degree of protection against microorganisms, some of which are unable to survive the acidic environment of the stomach. Hydrochloric acid is an important substance in health, but if it is produced in excess or when the stomach is not protected adequately against its action, a gastric (stomach) **ulcer** may result. Hydrochloric acid exists only in the presence of water. In the absence of water, the substance is more correctly referred to as hydrogen chloride (HCl) - a gas formed from the **covalent bonding** of hydrogen and chlorine. The dry gas hydrogen chloride does not produce protons, and so it is not an acid. Hydrogen chloride, however, is highly soluble, and the dissolved molecules dissociate (break up) into hydrogen ions (H^+) and chloride ions (Cl^-) as shown below:

HCl	$\xrightarrow{H_2O}$	$H^+_{(aq)}$	+	$Cl^-_{(aq)}$
hydrogen chloride		hydrogen ion		chloride ion

The subscript (aq) means aquated and refers to the fact that ions in solution (dissolved in water) have a number of water molecules attached. For the reasons described above, we use the symbols $HCl_{(aq)}$ when referring to hydrochloric acid and HCl when referring to dry hydrogen chloride gas. Note that in the equation showing the dissociation of hydrochloric acid into hydrogen ions and chloride ions, the arrow indicating the direction of the reaction is from left to right. This is to show that in water, hydrochloric acid dissociates completely into ions. It is, therefore, referred to as a strong acid.

Ethanoic acid

Ethanoic acid is sometimes referred to as **acetic acid**, and the reader will certainly have encountered it in dilute solution - vinegar. Ethanoic acid belongs to a group of acids called **carboxylic acids**, and these may be represented by the general formula shown in Figure 5.1, where R represents either a hydrogen atom or a chain of carbon atoms.

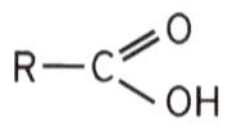

Figure 5.1
General formula of carboxylic acids.

Carboxylic acids are also important in health and illness, since they combine with **glycerol** to form **glycerides** (**neutral fats**). For this reason, carboxylic acids are also referred to as **fatty acids**. In your studies of health and diet, you will encounter fatty acids again, but for now let us return to ethanoic acid. Unlike hydrochloric acid, ethanoic acid is a weak acid, which means that it is not dissociated completely in water. Its dissociation is represented in the following way:

$$\underset{\text{ethanoic acid}}{CH_3COOH} \rightleftharpoons \underset{\text{ethanoate ion}}{CH_3COO^-} + \underset{\text{hydrogen ion}}{H^+}$$

Two arrows are used to represent the reaction, which can proceed from both left to right (ethanoic acid dissociating into ethanoate ions and hydrogen ions) and right to left (ethanoate ions and hydrogen ions combining to form ethanoic acid). Since at room temperature only 7% of the ethanoic acid molecules dissociate into ions, the arrow pointing from right to left is emphasised.

Hydrogen carbonate (bicarbonate) ion

The two previous examples of acids were covalently bonded molecules that dissociated in solution. Now we consider an ion that can act as an acid:

$$\underset{\text{hydrogen carbonate ion}}{HCO_3^-} \rightleftharpoons \underset{\text{hydrogen ion}}{H^+} + \underset{\text{carbonate ion}}{CO_3^{2-}}$$

We have emphasised the arrows equally to show that, in the body, the equilibrium of the reaction may be tipped to the left or to the right, depending upon the concentration of hydrogen ions. If in low concentration, the reaction equilibrium is tipped to the right and more hydrogen ions are generated. If hydrogen ions are in excess, then the reaction equilibrium will be tipped to the left and hydrogen ions will be removed by combination with carbonate ions.

Bases

A base is a molecule or ion that accepts a hydrogen ion during a chemical reaction. An older definition of a base is a substance that yields **hydroxide ions** (OH^-) in solution, but in reality the two definitions are saying the same thing. A small number of water molecules dissociate into hydrogen ions and hydroxide ions:

$$H_2O \rightleftharpoons H^+ + OH^-$$

Consequently, the addition of any substance that removes hydrogen ions leads to a relative excess of hydroxide ions.

Sodium hydroxide

Perhaps **sodium hydroxide** (NaOH) is unfamiliar to you, but you may have heard it referred to by its common name **caustic soda**. Indeed, you may have even bought products that contain this in order to unblock a drain or clean an oven. The use of sodium hydroxide in such products is related to its ability to dissolve fat; since cell membranes contain a high proportion of fat, sodium hydroxide is potentially dangerous to body tissue, especially if splashed into the eyes. Sodium hydroxide is an ionic compound. Even in the solid state, however, it does not exist as molecules of NaOH but rather as sodium ions (Na^+) and hydroxide ions (OH^-). Since it is the hydroxide ions that accept protons, we can for the moment ignore the sodium ions and demonstrate the action of sodium hydroxide as a base in the following way:

$$\underset{\text{hydroxide ion}}{OH^-} + \underset{\text{hydrogen ion}}{H^+} \rightleftharpoons \underset{\text{water}}{H_2O}$$

Sodium hydroxide is described as a strong base because it is dissociated completely into sodium ions and hydroxide ions.

Liquid ammonia

Ammonia is actually a gas (NH_3), but it dissolves in water to produce an opaque solution (cloudy ammonia) that may be used as a cleansing agent. You may have bought a product that contained ammonia for cleaning the toilet. Aqueous ammonia is a weak base - that is, only a small proportion of the ammonia molecules are ionised by the acceptance of hydrogen ions:

$$\underset{\text{aqueous ammonia}}{NH_{3(aq)}} + \underset{\text{hydrogen ion}}{H^+} \rightleftharpoons \underset{\text{ammonium ion}}{NH_4^+}$$

Hydrogen carbonate (bicarbonate) ion

The behaviour of the **hydrogen carbonate ion** as an acid has already been discussed, but it can also behave as a base according to the following equation:

$$\underset{\text{hydrogen carbonate}}{HCO_3^-} + \underset{\text{hydrogen ion}}{H^+} \rightleftharpoons \underset{\text{carbonic acid}}{H_2CO_3}$$

Note that the reaction direction arrows are emphasised equally to show that, in the body, the equilibrium reaction in which the balance may be tipped to the left or the right, depending upon the concentration of the reactants and products.

Properties of acids and bases

Those acids that are safe to taste are sour - think about citrus fruits such as lemons (**citric acid**) and vinegar (ethanoic acid). They turn blue **litmus** paper red (litmus is a vegetable dye, and paper impregnated with it can be used to detect acids and bases). Bases that are safe to taste have a bitter or metallic taste - think about the taste of soap. They turn red litmus paper blue. Both acids and bases may be caustic - they can cause burns and destroy body tissue. Acids and bases react together to form a **salt** (ionic compound) and water. For example:

$HCl_{(aq)}$	+	NaOH	$\rightarrow$	NaCl	+	H_2O
hydrochloric acid		sodium hydroxide		sodium chloride		water

In the above example, the salt is common salt (sodium chloride). The term 'salt', however, specifically refers to an ionic compound that dissociates into ions.

Practice point 5.1

First aid

The caustic (corrosive) nature of many acids and bases has already been noted. Burns that result from contact with them can be severe. For this reason, you should wear safety glasses (or shields if you already use spectacles) all the time you are in a science laboratory. When part of the body comes into contact with an acid or a base, the best first-aid measure is to wash the body part with plenty of clean water. If you are in a laboratory, the first-aid box will contain an eyewash bottle; you should find out where this is located before beginning any experiment involving acids. Alternatively, there may be taps set aside for eyewashing. Never attempt to neutralise an acid with a base or a base with an acid: you may do more harm than good. Once first-aid measures have been carried out, medical advice should be sought immediately.

Measuring acidity

Before considering how acidity is measured, it is important to clarify some terms. The terms 'weak' and 'strong' have already been used in connection with acids and bases. Here, the tendency for the acid or base to dissociate is being referred to. This should not be confused with the concentration. For example, hydrochloric acid is referred to as a strong acid, because in solution it dissociates completely into hydrogen ions and chloride ions. Conversely, ethanoic acid is described as a weak acid, because only a small proportion of the molecules of ethanoic acid dissociate in solution into yield hydrogen ions and ethanoate ions. In a similar way, sodium hydroxide is described as a strong base because it dissociates completely in solution into sodium ions and hydroxide ions, while ammonia is ionised incompletely in water and therefore is a weak base.

In contrast, concentration is concerned with the amount of a substance dissolved in a solvent. For example, a 1-M (1-molar) solution contains 1 mole of the solute dissolved in 1 l of solvent (1 mol/l); a 0.01-M solution contains 0.01 moles of a solute dissolved in 1 l of solvent (0.01 mol/l); and so on. Consequently, it is possible to have the following combinations:

- A concentrated solution of a strong acid, such as 10-M hydrochloric acid.
- A dilute solution of a strong acid, such as 0.05-M hydrochloric acid.

- A concentrated solution of a weak acid, such as 10-M ethanoic acid.
- A dilute solution of a weak acid, such as 0.05-M ethanoic acid.

Of course, it is also possible to have a range of concentrations for any named acid, and in a similar way we may talk of concentrated and dilute solutions of strong and weak bases.

- ***This can appear a little confusing at first, and you might need to read the last section again.***

Once you have grasped the idea that, as far as acids and bases go, concentration and strength are different things, you will probably realise that in describing acidity what we really need to know is the concentration of hydrogen ions - $[H^+]$. In chemistry, the use of square brackets refers to concentration, and so $[H^+]$ means the concentration of hydrogen ions. The hydrogen ion concentrations that we will consider are in the range 1–0.000 000 000 000 01 mol/l. Clearly, we are looking at some very low concentrations, and the use of mol/l is somewhat clumsy with all those zeros. We could instead use a logarithmic scale - that is, we could speak of the concentration in terms of the powers of 10. The range of concentrations would then be 10^0–10^{-14} mol/l. This is somewhat easier, but it can be made simpler still. Whenever acidity needs to be described, whether by scientists, nurses or even brewers, the **pH scale** is used (the letters pH stand for power of hydrogen). pH is the negative log of the hydrogen ion concentration and it enables us to describe acidity in terms of simple numbers. That is, a logarithmic scale gets rid of the powers of the zeros, and by defining the scale as a negative log the negative powers 10^0–10^{-14} are turned into positive figures. Table 5.3 is a comparison of $[H^+]$ and pH, while Table 5.4 gives the pH of various body fluids.

Table 5.3 Comparison of $[H^+]$ and pH.

$[H^+]$ (mol/l)	pH
10^0	0
10^{-7}	7
10^{-14}	14

Table 5.4 The pH of various body fluids.

Fluid	pH
Bile	7.6–8.6
Blood	7.35–7.45
Cerebrospinal fluid	7.35–7.45
Gastric secretions	1–3
Pancreatic secretions	8–8.3
Saliva	6–7
Semen	7.2–8
Urine	4.6–8

More about the pH scale

When using the pH scale, a number of points must be considered. First, since it is a logarithmic scale, every change of one unit in pH represents a tenfold change in hydrogen ion concentration, a change of two units in pH a 100-fold change in hydrogen ion concentration, and so on. For this reason, the normal range of blood pH (7.35–7.45) is not as narrow as it first appears, and apparently small changes in blood pH represent large changes in hydrogen ion concentration, which you may need to report. Second, the pH scale is a negative scale - that is, a falling pH represents a rise in hydrogen ion concentration and a rising pH represents a falling hydrogen ion concentration.

Pure water has a pH of 7 and an identical concentration of hydrogen ions and hydroxide ions, and therefore is referred to as **neutral**. If hydrogen ions are added, then $[H^+]$ rises and pH falls - that is, acids have a pH of less than 7. In contrast, if hydrogen ions are removed, then $[H^+]$ falls and pH rises - that is, bases have a pH of greater than 7.

Salts as acids and bases

When acids and bases react together, the salt (ionic compound) formed may be neutral, acidic or basic, depending on the strengths of the acid and base used in the reaction. If a strong acid is added to a strong base, or a weak acid is added to a weak base, then the resultant salt is neutral. In contrast, the reaction between a strong acid and a weak base results in the formation of an acidic salt, while the reaction between a weak acid and a strong base produces a basic salt.

In-text review

- ✔ Acids are substances that donate hydrogen ions during a chemical reaction.
- ✔ Bases are substances that accept hydrogen ions during a chemical reaction.
- ✔ Acids and bases are described as weak or strong, depending upon the extent of their dissociation.
- ✔ A solution of an acid or base can be concentrated or dilute, irrespective of whether the acid or base is strong or weak.
- ✔ Acids and bases react together to produce a salt and water.
- ✔ The concentration of hydrogen ions is described in terms of pH.

Acid–base balance

We have already looked at the concept of **homeostasis** in Chapter 2. We noted that the cells of the body require a stable environment in which to function and that this environment is comprised of such parameters as temperature and the concentration of various electrolytes, including hydrogen ions. The pH of intracellular fluid is not measured easily, but blood pH is often measured in clinical practice and the normal value is found to be within the range 7.35-7.45.

- ***Look at these figures again – note that blood is normally slightly alkaline.***

If the pH rises above 7.45, then the condition is referred to as **alkalosis** and we would describe the patient as being **alkalotic**. On the other hand, if the pH falls below 7.35, then the condition is referred to as **acidosis** and we would describe the patient as being **acidotic**. Since neutrality is 7, and the lower normal limit of blood pH is 7.35, the terms 'acidosis' and 'acidotic' are used even when the blood remains slightly alkaline - but less alkaline than usual. In fact, it is not usual for patients to survive if the pH is less than 7; similarly, a pH of 8 is usually fatal. Consequently, it is important for the body to regulate acid-base balance, which it does through the three mechanisms of buffer systems, respiratory regulation and renal regulation.

Buffer systems

A **buffer** system is a solution that resists a change in pH. That is, if an acid or base is added, then the change in pH that occurs is much less than that which might otherwise be expected to occur. Buffer solutions consist of a mixture of a weak acid and its basic salt. The weak acid dissociates partially to release hydrogen ions and tends to cause the pH to fall, while the basic salt removes hydrogen ions and tends to cause the pH to rise. The actual pH of the solution depends upon the ratio of weak acid to its basic salt in solution. Following the addition of hydrogen ions to a buffer solution, a fall in pH is resisted by the presence of the basic salt. Conversely, following the addition of a base, a rise in pH is resisted by the presence of the weak acid. As far as the body is concerned, a change in blood pH is resisted by a number of buffers.

The hydrogen carbonate buffer system

If a hydrogen carbonate buffer system is being prepared in the laboratory, a solution of carbonic acid (the weak acid) is added to a solution of sodium hydrogen carbonate (the basic salt). In the blood, carbonic acid is formed from the reaction of carbon dioxide (produced by cellular metabolism) with water. In addition, hydrogen carbonate ions are also present from the dissociation of this acid, and we can illustrate the reactions involved in the following way:

$$\underset{\text{carbon dioxide}}{CO_2} + \underset{\text{water}}{H_2O} \rightleftharpoons \underset{\text{carbonic acid}}{H_2CO_3} \rightleftharpoons \underset{\text{hydrogen ion}}{H^+} + \underset{\text{hydrogen carbonate ion}}{HCO_3^-} \rightleftharpoons \underset{\text{hydrogen ion}}{H^+} + \underset{\text{carbonate ion}}{CO_3^{2-}}$$

Remember that the hydrogen carbonate ion can act as an acid or a base, and consequently the presence of hydrogen carbonate ions in blood buffers a change in pH. Suppose for a moment that an acid is added to the blood, and the concentration of hydrogen ions begins to increase. These would be removed by combination with hydrogen carbonate ions to form carbonic acid - that is, the reaction equilibrium is tipped to the left. On the other hand, if a base is added to the blood and hydrogen ions are removed, then their concentration would be restored by the further dissociation of carbonic acid (which yields hydrogen ions and hydrogen carbonate ions) - that is, the reaction equilibrium is tipped to the right.

Later, we shall see the close relationship of this buffer system to the renal and respiratory systems. For example, the concentration of hydrogen carbonate ions is regulated by the kidneys, while in the lungs carbonic acid dissociates into water and carbon dioxide, which are eliminated through breathing. In this way, the body avoids a build-up of carbon dioxide that would otherwise push the reaction equilibrium to the right.

The phosphate buffer system

This system is similar to the hydrogen carbonate system. Two ions are important - the **dihydrogen phosphate ion** ($H_2PO_4^-$) and the **monohydrogen phosphate ion** (HPO_4^{2-}). Monohydrogen phosphate ions are able to combine with excess hydrogen ions to form dihydrogen phosphate ions:

HPO_4^{2-}	+	H^+	$\rightarrow$	$H_2PO_4^{2-}$
monohydrogen phosphate ions		hydrogen ions		dihydrogen phosphate ions

In contrast, the addition of hydroxide ions to dihydrogen phosphate ions results in the formation of monohydrogen phosphate ions and water:

$H_2PO_4^-$	+	OH^-	$\rightarrow$	HPO_4^{2-}	+ H_2O
dihydrogen phosophate ions		hydroxide ions		monohydrogen phosphate ions	water

The low concentration of these ions in blood means that the phosphate buffer system has little effect there. The concentrations are much higher, however, in the kidneys, where the system is important.

The protein buffer system

Proteins consist of chains of amino acids. Amino acids possess a weak acid group (the carboxyl group - COOH) and a weak basic group (the amino group - NH_2), as illustrated in Figure 5.2.

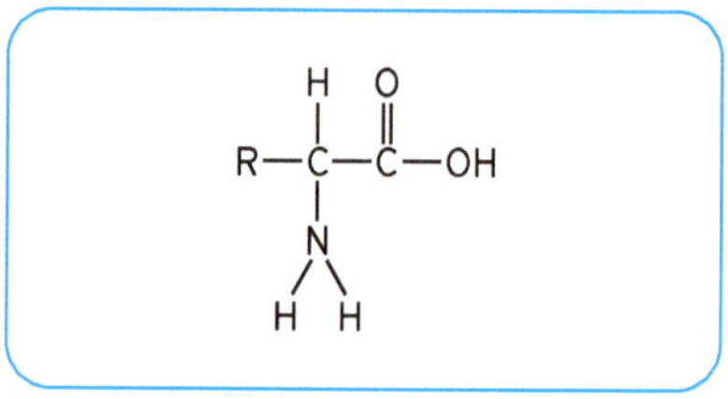

Figure 5.2
General formula of an amino acid.

The carboxyl group donates a hydrogen ion to the amino group to form a substance with two charged ionic regions (**zwitterions/dipolar ion**), as shown in Figure 5.3.

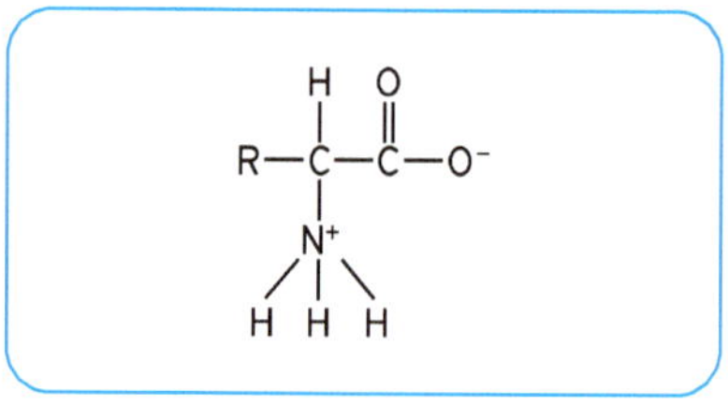

Figure 5.3
Formation of a zwitterion/dipolar ion.

Zwitterions can function as buffers in the following way. A fall in pH is resisted when an excess of hydrogen ions is removed by combination with the COO^- group, as shown in Figure 5.4.

Conversely, an excess of hydroxide ions results in the release of hydrogen ions from the amine group to form water, as shown in Figure 5.5.

The haemoglobin buffer system

Haemoglobin is the protein found in **erythrocytes** (red blood cells) that is responsible for the transportation of oxygen. Erythrocytes, and in particular haemoglobin, also play an important role in buffering pH change. In addition to the possession of haemoglobin, erythrocytes also have the enzyme **carbonic anhydrase**, which catalyses the reaction between carbon dioxide and water to yield carbonic acid. We have noted previously the dissociation

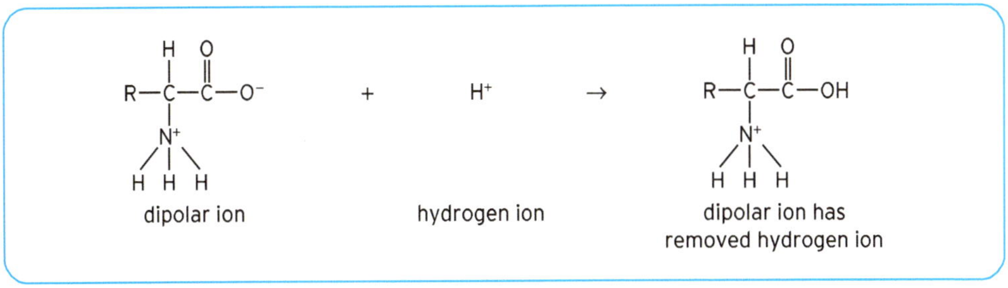

Figure 5.4
Removal of hydrogen ions by zwitterions.

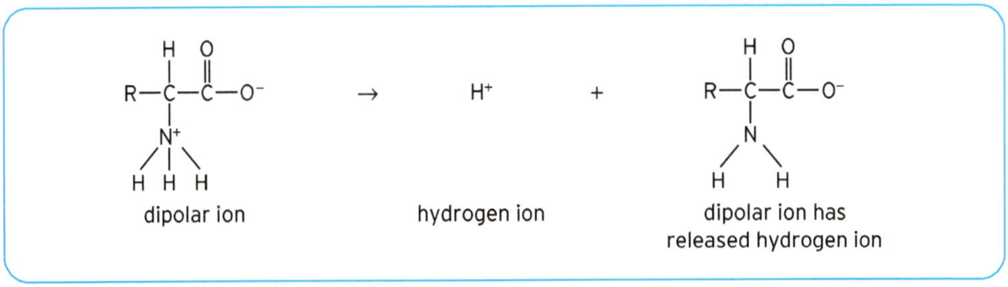

Figure 5.5
Release of hydrogen ions by zwitterions.

of carbonic acid into hydrogen ions and hydrogen carbonate ions, and it is the fate of these ions that concerns us here. Hydrogen carbonate ions formed within erythrocytes diffuse into the plasma (the liquid part of the blood); their role has already been discussed. The retention of hydrogen ions by erythrocytes might be expected to cause a fall in intracellular pH, but such a change is buffered as a consequence of the combination of hydrogen ions with haemoglobin. In fact, **reduced haemoglobin** (haemoglobin not combined with oxygen) has a much greater affinity for hydrogen ions than does **oxyhaemoglobin** (haemoglobin combined with oxygen). We might, therefore, regard the function of haemoglobin once it has delivered oxygen to the cells as transporting hydrogen ions from the cells to the lungs. Here, reduced haemoglobin combines with oxygen to form oxyhaemoglobin, from which hydrogen ions are released. In the plasma, these combine with hydrogen carbonate ions, and the carbonic acid that results dissociates into carbon dioxide and water, which are of course eliminated in the breath.

In summary, haemoglobin serves as a buffer by chemically combining with hydrogen ions and so temporarily removing them from the plasma.

The ammonia buffer system

This system operates in the kidneys. Each kidney contains over one million microscopic structures called **nephrons**. Each nephron consists of a **renal corpuscle** and a **renal tubule**. Identify these structures on the diagram in Figure 5.6. Note that each corpuscle consists of

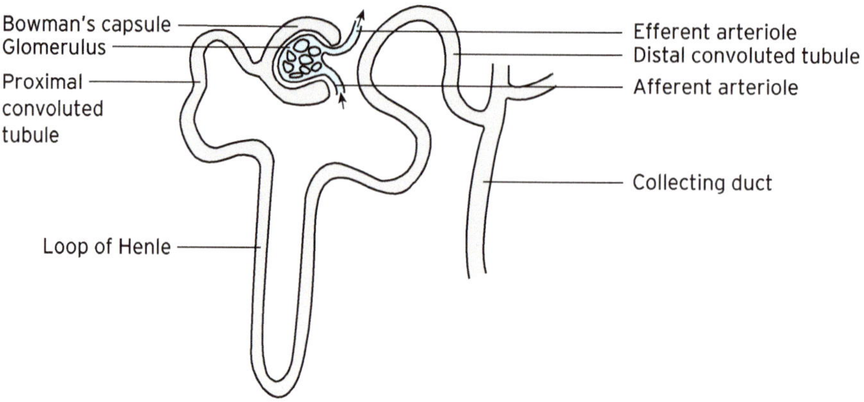

Figure 5.6
The nephron.

a capillary network call a **glomerulus**, surrounded by a capsule called the **Bowman's capsule**. Blood arrives at the glomerulus in the **afferent arteriole** and is drained in the **efferent arteriole**. As blood passes through the glomerulus, water and small dissolved molecules are forced out of the bloodstream and into the Bowman's capsule. In effect, the blood has been filtered; the resultant fluid is called **filtrate**. The filtrate passes through the tubule, where it is modified, eventually being excreted as urine.

Having explained this, we can now describe the ammonia buffer system. Amino acids are **deaminated** (broken down) in the cells of the renal tubule to form ammonia (NH_3), which diffuses into the renal filtrate. Ammonia molecules are then able to combine with free hydrogen ions to form ammonium ions (NH_4^+), thus:

$$\underset{\text{aqueous ammonia}}{NH_{3(aq)}} + \underset{\text{hydrogen ions}}{H^+} \rightarrow \underset{\text{ammonium ions}}{NH_4^+}$$

Ammonium ions combine with chloride ions (Cl^-), and the resultant salt, ammonium chloride (NH_4Cl), is eliminated in the urine. The presence of the phosphate and ammonia buffer systems means that excess hydrogen ions can be eliminated in the urine without high urine acidity.

Respiratory regulation

It is important to note that buffer systems do not actually remove hydrogen ions from the body - this role is performed by the respiratory and renal systems. Furthermore, the supply of buffers is not without limit, and it is possible to reach the maximum buffering capacity of the body. Consequently, other mechanisms are required to ensure acid-base balance.

We have noted already that carbon dioxide has a great influence on blood pH due to its reaction with water to form carbonic acid. Therefore, the extent to which carbon dioxide is eliminated by the lungs is a major factor in acid-base balance. Chemical-detecting cells called **chemoreceptors** (a contraction of the term 'chemical receptors') in the **aorta** and **carotid arteries** are sensitive to changes in the blood pH, while chemoreceptors in the respiratory centre of the brain stem (the lowest part of the brain) are highly sensitive to changes in the pH of **cerebrospinal fluid** (CSF - the fluid that surrounds the brain). Perhaps it is not surprising to discover that a falling pH detected by chemoreceptors is responsible for stimulating an increase in both the rate and depth of breathing (**hyperventilation**) and that this tends towards a restoration of acid-base balance by increasing the elimination of carbon dioxide. Conversely, when blood pH returns to normal, the respiratory stimulus is removed and the individual ceases to hyperventilate. If you have already read Chapter 2, recognise this as an example of homeostasis. Remember that all homeostatic control mechanisms regulate **controlled conditions.**

- ***What is the controlled condition in this case?***

It is the pH of the blood and cerebrospinal fluid. Homeostatic control mechanisms consist of three components.

- ***What are the components?***

Perhaps you recall that they are **receptors** (detectors), a **control centre** and **effectors.** In the above example, the receptors are chemoreceptors, the control centre is the brain stem and the effectors are the lungs.

- ***What kind of feedback mechanism is this?***

Since the response of the lungs is to reverse a change in pH, the above is an example of a negative feedback mechanism.

Renal regulation

Look again at Figure 5.6. We have noted that filtrate is formed from the blood in the corpuscle and that it then passes down the tubule, where some substances are resorbed from the tubule and others secreted into the tubule. Eventually, the modified filtrate is excreted as urine. The secretion of hydrogen ions into the filtrate and the resorption of hydrogen carbonate ions from it are important processes in the maintenance of pH balance. Cells in the distal (far) part of the renal tubule are sensitive to changes in blood pH. Carbonic anhydrase within these cells catalyses the reaction between carbon dioxide from blood and water to form carbonic acid, which dissociates into hydrogen ions and carbonate ions. The hydrogen ions are actively transported into the filtrate in exchange for sodium ions, which, along with hydrogen carbonate ions, pass into the blood. The secretion of hydrogen ions is accelerated by a falling pH, and this, together with the release of hydrogen carbonate ions into the blood, accounts for one way in which the kidney regulates acid-base balance. Once again, you should recognise this as an example of a negative feedback mechanism. It is, however, an interesting example of such a mechanism, since it operates at a local level without the involvement of the nervous system.

It should be noted that an increase in hydrogen ion secretion into tubular fluid does not cause the pH of filtrate to fall as much as might be expected. This is due to the effect of the phosphate and ammonia buffer systems described previously. In addition to the secretion of hydrogen ions into filtrate, hydrogen carbonate ions can be resorbed from filtrate when required to maintain acid-base balance. The size and negative charge of hydrogen carbonate ions, however, makes this difficult. Instead of being resorbed directly, they are converted to carbon dioxide in the following way: Hydrogen carbonate ions in the renal filtrate react with hydrogen ions to form carbonic acid, the dissociation of which yields carbon dioxide and water. The water is excreted in the urine, thus removing hydrogen ions from the body. The carbon dioxide diffuses into tubular cells, where it forms carbonic acid, which in turn dissociates into hydrogen ions and hydrogen carbonate ions, the fate of which has been described already. Although we have referred to renal regulation, it is important to note that the contribution of the kidneys to acid-base balance is itself controlled by hormones of the endocrine system. This is explained briefly in Practice point 5.2.

Practice point 5.2

Hormones and acid–base balance

The renal regulation of acid-base balance may be affected by **endocrine glands** (**hormone**-secreting glands). For example, the cortex (outer part) of the adrenal glands (situated just above the kidneys) produces the hormone **aldosterone**, which increases the rate of sodium resorption and potassium secretion in the tubule. When aldosterone levels are elevated, however, hydrogen ion secretion is also stimulated. Consequently, patients who produce aldosterone in excess (**aldosteronism**) may experience an elevated blood pH (alkalosis). Conversely, abnormally low levels of aldosterone (**Addison's disease**) may lead to acidosis.

Acid–base imbalance

An acid-base imbalance may be either acidosis or alkalosis.

- ***Remember that acidosis is a fall in pH below 7.35 and alkalosis is a rise above 7.45.***

An acid-base imbalance may be described further as either respiratory or metabolic. Respiratory disturbances involve carbon dioxide elimination, while metabolic disturbances involve acids normally excreted by the kidneys. It must be admitted, however, that this terminology is not ideal, since carbon dioxide is of course produced as a consequence of the metabolic activity of the cells.

Respiratory acidosis

This results whenever carbon dioxide retention occurs. The accumulation of carbon dioxide within the blood pushes the carbonic acid equilibrium to the right, resulting in an excess of hydrogen ions. The cause may be **hypoventilation** (inadequate ventilation of the lungs) following head injury or excessive use of sedating drugs, an excess of pulmonary secretions, a pulmonary infection, **asthma** or a **chronic obstructive pulmonary disease** such as **chronic bronchitis**. Other causes include collapsed alveoli (**atelectasis**) and pulmonary **embolism**. An embolism is a free-floating mass within the circulation. One form of embolism is a fragment of a clot (**thrombus**) formed within the circulation. You have probably heard about the dangers of a thrombus forming in the veins of the leg during a prolonged flight. Although the thrombus itself can be problematic and cause pain, it is when a part of it breaks free and becomes a mobile embolus that the condition may become life-threatening. This is because the embolus may obstruct the circulation to the lungs (pulmonary embolism).

Respiratory alkalosis

Respiratory alkalosis occurs when there is an increased elimination of carbon dioxide as a consequence of hyperventilation (excessive ventilation of the lungs). The cause may be hysteria or poorly adjusted mechanical (artificial) ventilation.

Metabolic acidosis

Metabolic acidosis results when the ability of the kidney to secrete hydrogen ions into filtrate is impaired, as is the case in chronic renal failure and Addison's disease. Another important cause is the production of acidic **ketones**, which may occur in **diabetes mellitus**. Whenever a lack of the hormone **insulin** results in a cellular deficiency of glucose, fats are used as a fuel instead. This process is explained more fully in Chapter 8, but for now it is sufficient to know that the metabolic pathway involved in fat metabolism results in an over-production of ketones (**ketoacidosis**). Finally, acidosis that occurs following excessive ingestion of acidic drugs such as **aspirin** (**acetylsalicylic acid**) and that which results from the loss of base from the body, such as diarrhoea, is also included here.

Metabolic alkalosis

Metabolic alkalosis may result from excessive loss of hydrogen ions from the body and may follow vomiting or administration of **diuretics** (drugs that increase urine output). Alkalosis in aldosteronism has already been mentioned; another cause may be the excessive ingestion of alkaline indigestion medication.

Recognising acid–base imbalance

Help in recognising acid-base imbalance is often required by both students and qualified staff. Recognition involves comparing laboratory data with normal acid-base laboratory values (such as those given in Table 5.5), as explained in Practice point 5.3. The management of acid-base imbalance is then discussed in Practice point 5.4.

Table 5.5 Normal acid-base laboratory values.

pH	7.35–7.45
$PaCO_2$	4.7–6.0 kPa
$[HCO_3^-]$	19–29 mmol/l
Base excess	–2 to +2

Practice point 5.3

Systematic assessment of acid–base balance

First of all, look at the patient's most recent blood laboratory results and check the pH. Now describe an imbalance as acidosis or alkalosis. Next, identify the cause as a respiratory or metabolic one. For respiratory imbalances, check the partial pressure of carbon dioxide in arterial blood ($PaCO_2$). The normal range is 4.7-6.0 kPa; a value above this is respiratory acidosis and a value below is respiratory alkalosis. For metabolic imbalances, check the hydrogen carbonate ion concentration ($[HCO_3^-]$). The normal is 19-29 mmol/l; a value above this is metabolic alkalosis and a value below is metabolic acidosis.

However, the $[HCO_3^-]$ is affected not only by metabolic disturbances but also by respiratory disturbances. For example, in respiratory acidosis, $[HCO_3^-]$ rises along with $PaCO_2$ according to the by now familiar equation

$$CO_2 + H_2O \rightleftharpoons H_2CO_3 \rightleftharpoons H^+ + HCO_3^-$$

The answer to this problem is, in reality, a simple one. Before the measurement of $[HCO_3^-]$ in the laboratory, the blood sample is artificially brought under standard conditions of $PaCO_2$ and temperature. For this reason, the measurement of $[HCO_3^-]$ is referred to as the standard hydrogen carbonate ion concentration. Perhaps you would like to attempt some examples. Consider the following:

Patient 1

pH = 7.33, $PaCO_2$ = 5.6 kPa, $[HCO_3^-]$ = 18 mmol/l

pH is low: acidosis.
$PaCO_2$ is normal.
$[HCO_3^-]$ is low.

Conclusion: metabolic acidosis.

Patient 2

pH = 7.47, $PaCO_2$ = 5.5 kPa, $[HCO_3^-]$ = 35 mmol/l

pH is high: alkalosis.
$PaCO_2$ is normal.
$[HCO_3^-]$ is elevated.

Conclusion: metabolic alkalosis.

Patient 3

pH = 7.31, $PaCO_2$ = 7.5 kPa, $[HCO_3^-]$ = 22 mmol/l

pH is low: acidosis.
$PaCO_2$ is high.
$[HCO_3^-]$ is normal.

Conclusion: respiratory acidosis.

Patient 4

pH = 7.51, $PaCO_2$ = 3.2 kPa, $[HCO_3^-]$ = 22 mmol/l

pH is high: alkalosis.

$PaCO_2$ is low.
$[HCO_3^-]$ is normal.

Conclusion: respiratory alkalosis.

When you next see some laboratory reports, work through them in a similar way. Perhaps you have seen such reports already. If so, you will no doubt have noticed results of another test used to assess the severity of a patient's metabolic disturbance - the **base excess**. This is a measure of the amount of acid that would need to be added to the sample of patient's blood to restore acid-base balance to normal. The normal value of base excess is, therefore, zero; in metabolic alkalosis it is positive and in metabolic acidosis it is negative. For the sake of simplicity, values of base excess have not been included in the examples given here.

So far, we have considered acid-base disturbances that affect only one system - the respiratory system or the kidneys. It is worth remembering that the body attempts to compensate for a disturbance in one system by a change in the other. Look at a further three examples:

Patient 5

pH = 7.32, $PaCO_2$ = 7.2 kPa, $[HCO_3^-]$ = 32 mmol/l
pH is low: acidosis.
$PaCO_2$ is high.
$[HCO_3^-]$ is high.

Conclusion: compensated respiratory acidosis.

Patient 6

pH = 7.35, $PaCO_2$ = 4.3 kPa, $[HCO_3^-]$ = 18 mmol/l
pH is on the low side of nomal: alkalosis.
$PaCO_2$ is low.
$[HCO_3^-]$ is low.

Conclusion: compensated metabolic acidosis.

Patient 7

pH = 7.37, $PaCO_2$ = 7.7 kPa, $[HCO_3^-]$ = 36 mmol/l
pH is on the low side of normal: acidosis.
$PaCO_2$ is high.
$[HCO_3^-]$ is high.

Conclusion: compensated respiratory acidosis.

Practice point 5.4

Managing acid-base imbalance

It is not within the scope of this book to give a comprehensive description of the management of acid-base imbalance. However, Table 5.6 summarises the interventions that might be made by the multidisciplinary team. Note that not all the interventions listed are appropriate in each case. Doctors, nurses and physiotherapists are all involved in the management of acid-base imbalance,

Table 5.6 Management of acid-base imbalance.

Disturbance	Aetiology	Intervention
Respiratory acidosis	CO_2 retention due to hypoventilation (central nervous system (CNS) depression or pain), excess of pulmonary secretions, pneumonia, atelectasis, chronic obstructive pulmonary disease (COPD)	Improve ventilation and gas exchange: coughing and deep breathing exercises, postural drainage, respiratory stimulants, narcotic antagonists, steam inhalations, nebulised saline, bronchodilators, pain control, artificial ventilation
Respiratory alkalosis	Excessive CO_2 loss due to hyperventilation in anxiety/hysteria or poorly adjusted mechanical ventilation	Sedation, relaxation exercises, adjust mechanical ventilation
Metabolic acidosis	Accumulation of ketones in diabetes (ketoacidosis), excessive loss of base in diarrhoea, failure to secrete H^+ in renal disease	Treat underlying cause
Metabolic alkalosis	Prolonged vomiting, nasogastric aspiration, excess intake of antacids	Antiemetics, reduce antacids

but some interventions are primarily the responsibility of a particular professional group - for example, the prescription of drugs by doctors.

Respiratory acidosis

There are many causes of respiratory acidosis, and the management depends on correctly identifying the cause. In each case, however, the aim is to improve ventilation and gas exchange. Perhaps the simplest way to do this is to help the patient to sit upright and perform deep breathing exercises. The patient may have a condition such as a chest infection that results in an excess of secretions, and clearly it is helpful if these are coughed up. When secretions are present, deep breathing often triggers coughing; a sputum pot with a lid and tissues should be placed within the patient's easy reach. If the patient is weak or coughing is ineffective, it may be necessary to remove secretions using a catheter attached to suction, but training in this procedure is required. Secretions can become thick and difficult to cough up in the dehydrated patient, so ensuring adequate fluid intake is also important. **Postural drainage** is a technique of positioning a patient so that a region of the lung is drained of secretions more effectively than it would otherwise. The advice of a physiotherapist is important in this therapy and some degree of coordination with other activities is required. For example, it would be thoughtless to position a patient in which it is difficult to eat at lunchtime.

Bronchdilators are drugs that dilate the airway and are important in asthma - a condition in which contraction of smooth muscle in the airway causes it to constrict. Bronchodilators are often administered via inhalers and sometimes as a mist of droplets via a **nebuliser**. This device is described in Chapter 6.

Hypoventilation may occur when pain is present - think about how difficult it is to breathe in the presence of a large chest or abdominal wound. Consequently, **analgesics** (drugs that relieve pain) may have a role to play. It is important to know, however, that some analgesics (for example, **narcotics**) produce sedation and may themselves lead to hypoventilation. It may even be necessary to reverse the effects of a narcotic using a narcotic antagonist.

Finally, a patient's respiratory status may become so poor that artificial ventilation is required. In this treatment, the action of inflating the lungs is performed by a machine (the ventilator), and air enriched with oxygen is delivered via a tube inserted into the trachea via the mouth (**endotracheal tube**) or via an incision into the front of the neck below the larynx (**tracheotomy**).

Respiratory alkalosis

Excessive CO_2 loss can occur during artificial ventilation, and it may be necessary to adjust the ventilator settings when respiratory alkalosis exists. The condition can also result from hyperventilation as a consequence of anxiety, and sedation or relaxation exercises may have a role to play. Perhaps you have heard of patients being encouraged to breathe in and out of a paper bag. This is not as crazy at it sounds - since respiratory alkalosis occurs through excessive CO_2 elimination, rebreathing exhaled breath from a paper bag addresses this imbalance. Incidentally, a rebreathing circuit can be included in artificial ventilators so that respiratory alkalosis is prevented in a similar way.

Metabolic acidosis

In cases of metabolic acidosis, treatment of the specific cause is required. For example, in poorly controlled diabetes mellitus, the use of fats as a source of energy leads to the accumulation of ketoacids (ketoacidosis). This is managed by the administration of infusions of glucose and the hormone insulin, which is responsible for the transport of the glucose into cells. This treatment would obviously by inappropriate in other causes of metabolic acidosis, such as excessive loss of base in diarrhoea. This requires fluid and electrolyte replacement, which can be achieved in mild cases using oral electrolyte solutions. However, in severe diarrhoea, such as occurs in cholera, an **intravenous infusion** (drip) is required. Failure to secrete H^+ in renal disease will require specialised treatment such as **dialysis** (see Chapter 4).

Metabolic alkalosis

Prolonged vomiting may cause loss of acid, and oral electrolyte solutions are of use once again. Excessive ingestion of antacid medication may occur when a patient who has pain from a gastric ulcer self-medicates. Treatment of the underlying cause of the ulcer is then required.

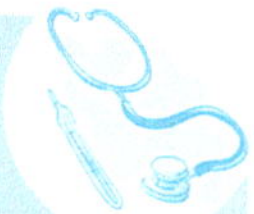

In-text review

- ✔ The maintenance of acid-base balance is an example of homeostasis.
- ✔ Homeostatic mechanisms serve to resist a change in acid-base balance and are, therefore, examples of negative feedback mechanisms.
- ✔ The body's acid-base balance is maintained by buffer systems, respiratory regulation and renal regulation.
- ✔ Buffers are substances that resist a change in the pH of a solution.
- ✔ Respiratory regulation is achieved by controlling the elimination of carbon dioxide (CO_2).
- ✔ Renal regulation is achieved when the kidneys control the elimination of hydrogen ions (H^+) and the resorption of hydrogen carbonate ions (HCO_3^-).
- ✔ Acid-base imbalances are either acidosis or alkalosis.
- ✔ The causes of acid-base imbalance may be respiratory or metabolic.

Summary

In this chapter, we have covered quite a lot of chemistry related to acids and bases and the reactions they undergo. This was done so that acid-base imbalance, such as occurs in a variety of conditions, could be addressed. You will have noticed that on several occasions, reference was made to Chapter 2, since acid-base balance is very much concerned with regulating the normal internal environment.

Summary points

- **Acids are substances that donate hydrogen ions during a chemical reaction.**
- **Bases are substances that accept hydrogen ions during a chemical reaction.**
- **Acids and bases are described as weak or strong, depending upon the extent of their dissociation.**
- **Acids and bases react together to produce a salt and water.**
- **The concentration of hydrogen ions is described in terms of pH.**
- **A buffer is a solution that resists a change in pH.**
- **The body's acid-base balance is maintained by buffer systems, respiratory regulation and renal regulation.**
- **Acid-base imbalances are either acidosis or alkalosis and may be described further as respiratory or metabolic.**

Self-test questions

1 Which one of the following acids does the stomach produce?
(a) Citric acid.
(b) Amino acid.
(c) Hydrochloric acid.
(d) Folic acid.

2 Which one of the following acids is *not* an important component of the diet?
(a) Folic acid.
(b) Amino acid.
(c) Ascorbic acid.
(d) Acetylsalicylic acid.

3 Which one of the following particles may also be referred to as a hydrogen ion?
(a) An electron.
(b) A proton.
(c) A neutron.
(d) An atom.

4 Match the acid on the left with the appropriate description on the right.

(a) Carboxylic acid
(b) Carbonic acid
(c) Ascorbic acid
(d) Deoxyribonucleic acid

(i) The substance formed from the reaction between carbon dioxide and water
(ii) A substance that is a component of fats
(iii) A substance that carries genetic information
(iv) A substance also known as vitamin C

5 Which acid has the chemical formula CH_3COOH?

(a) Ethanoic acid.
(b) Citric acid.
(c) Deoxyribonucleic acid.
(d) Hydrochloric acid.

6 Neutrality on the pH scale is taken to be which one of the following?

(a) 4.
(b) 14.
(c) 7.
(d) 17.

7 A fall in blood pH as a consequence of the excessive production of ketones in diabetes mellitus is described as which one of the following?

(a) Respiratory acidosis.
(b) Respiratory alkalosis.
(c) Metabolic acidosis.
(d) Metabolic alkalosis.

8 Which one of the following most closely represents normal $PaCO_2$?

(a) 4.0 kPa.
(b) 5.0 kPa.
(c) 7.0 kPa.
(d) 8.0 kPa.

9 Which one of the following most closely represents normal $[HCO_3^-]$?

(a) 10 mmol/l.
(b) 15 mmol/l.
(c) 25 mmol/l.
(d) 35 mmol/l.

10 Which one of the following group of figures represents compensated respiratory acidosis?

pH	$PaCO_2$/kPa	$[HCO_3^-]$/mmol/l
(a) 7.33	5.5	18
(b) 7.30	7.5	23
(c) 7.31	7.5	33
(d) 7.33	4.2	17

Further study/exercise

The next time you visit a clinical area where patient blood results are available, look over the values and determine whether there is an acid-base imbalance. Discuss what you decide with a clinical supervisor.

6

Pressure, fluids, gases and breathing

Learning outcomes

After reading the following chapter and undertaking personal study, you should be able to:

1. Define the term 'pressure'.
2. List some of the units used to measure pressure, especially those used in nursing practice.
3. Describe how to measure arterial blood pressure using a sphygmomanometer and stethoscope.
4. Apply an understanding of Pascal's principle to static fluids within the body.
5. Describe the factors that influence blood pressure.
6. Apply an understanding of Boyle's law to breathing.
7. Apply an understanding of the laws of Dalton and Henry to gas exchange in the lungs.
8. Outline the factors that influence blood flow through a vessel, and relate this to disease.
9. Describe oxygen therapy and distinguish between fixed- and variable-performance oxygen masks.
10. Describe the operation of a nebuliser.

Introduction

In this chapter, we consider the concept of **pressure** and apply an understanding of it to fluids in the body, such as blood, and to gases and breathing. Most people will have some idea that pressure has something to do with **force**. Even in everyday conversation, we say that someone who compels another to act in a certain way 'places pressure on them' or 'forces them'. So, even if you have not studied science before, perhaps the concept of pressure is familiar. When the word 'pressure' is used in a scientific context, however, something quite specific is meant. Pressure is defined as force per unit area:

$$\text{Pressure} = \frac{\text{force}}{\text{area}}$$

Pressure is not the same as force but depends upon both force and the area over which the force is applied. For example, it is not usual for an individual of average weight to damage a tiled floor simply by walking on it. This is because the body weight (force) is spread over the surface of the soles of the shoes. If stiletto heels are worn, however, the same force is applied over a much smaller area and the effect resembles small hammer blows to the surface of the tiles. In a similar way, the point of a hypodermic needle (injection needle) readily penetrates the skin, but the same force produces much less pressure when applied over the larger surface area of the fingers when examining the body.

Even such a simple understanding of pressure and its relationship to force and surface area has immediate practical applications for health practitioners. For example, suppose we take a solid block of wood some 70 kg in weight and place it on a table. If we now had some means of measuring the pressure beneath the block, we would find that, provided the surfaces of both block and table were smooth, the pressure would be the same at any point we might care to measure. Now let us compare this with a 70-kg patient lying supine (flat on the bed). The surface of the patient's body is certainly not flat, and some parts, such as the hollow of the back, are not in contact with the bed at all. This means that a much greater pressure than might otherwise be expected is exerted upon those parts of the body that do have contact. This is especially true of the bony prominences, as illustrated in Figure 6.1. When

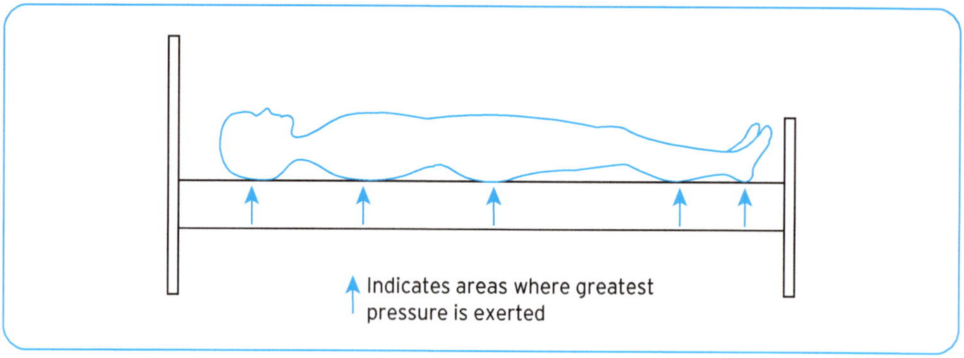

Figure 6.1
A patient lying in bed.

pressure is maintained against the tissue overlying such prominences, a wound called a pressure ulcer may result; pressure ulcers are discussed in Practice point 6.1.

Practice point 6.1

Pressure ulcers

Throughout both wakefulness and sleep, some part of the body is subjected to pressure from its own weight as a consequence of lying, sitting or leaning. Movement ensures that the pressure exerted upon the soft tissues does not remain over one area for very long. Indeed, even during sleep, the weight of the body against the skin is continually redistributed because of movement.

- ***What happens if mobility is restricted?***

Experience shows that one consequence of sustained low pressure against the body is damage to the integument and the development of a **pressure ulcer**.

- ***Write down some possible causes of reduced mobility.***

You may have realised that possible causes include physical illness that necessitates spending longer than usual in bed, and restricting therapies, such as **intravenous infusions** (drips). Some people may be too frail to move or find changing position too painful, while others may be sedated or unconscious.

- ***What do pressure ulcers look like?***

Like any other kind of wound, pressure ulcers can differ in severity. The word 'ulcer', however, implies erosion or wound in which there is tissue loss in contrast to a cut. Commonly, pressure ulcers extend through the **epidermis** and into the **dermis** (layers of the skin), although it is possible for them to extend deeper through fat and muscle to bone.

- ***How can the weight of our own bodies result in such severe wounds?***

To answer this question, go back and consider once again the individual lying in bed. Remember that bodies are not flat like a wooden block and that the pressure of the body against the bed is greatest over bony prominences, such as the **sacrum**, heels, elbows, shoulders and **occiput** (the back of the head). In fact, if we were to measure the pressure applied to the surface of the body by its own weight at such points, we would find it to be in excess of the pressure of blood in capillaries. This compresses them and deprives the soft tissue of a blood supply, causing it to die and resulting in a pressure ulcer. Thus, pressure ulcers do not result from the direct effects of pressure, but a low sustained pressure results in cell death through the mechanism of a compromised blood supply. There is a great deal more to learn about pressure ulcers, but for now this brief introduction has served to illustrate how important a consideration of pressure is to nursing practice.

Thus far, we have considered only pressure and solid objects, but when we consider pressure in the body we are often thinking about gases and breathing or liquids such as blood. In addition, we often want to know how to measure pressure. To do this, let us first think about atmospheric pressure.

Atmospheric pressure

Most people know something about atmospheric pressure, even if it is only through watching the weather forecast or from taking a trip in an aeroplane. We do not think too much about the pressure exerted by the atmosphere against our bodies because, for most of the time, we cannot feel it. Nonetheless, the mixture of gases that surrounds us and that forms the atmosphere does exert quite a pressure on our bodies. Perhaps the time when we do become aware of it is when the atmospheric pressure changes, as is the case when driving up or down a steep hill in a car or during take-off or landing in an aeroplane. At these times, we may feel uncomfortable because of the distortion of the **tympanic membrane** (eardrum) caused by a difference in pressure between the middle and outer ears. You can find a diagram of the ear in Chapter 13. The **eustachian tube** vents the middle ear; swallowing helps to open this tube and equalise the pressure in the middle ear, thus preventing the distortion of the drum, which can be painful.

- ***Can you think of a common cause of inability to vent the middle ear, which then results in considerable pain when flying?***

You may have worked out that the eustachian tube may become blocked if you have a cold. For this reason, flying is not then recommended. The purpose of noting this is simply to point out that we all have some experience of atmospheric pressure on our bodies. Practice point 6.2 deals briefly with relieving the pain of flying.

Practice point 6.2

Relieving the pain of flying

- ***If swallowing helps to vent the middle ear through the eustachian tube, what could be done to relieve the discomfort of take-offs and landings?***

You probably already know that sucking a sweet may help, but what about babies? Have you noticed that babies often wake up and cry during take-off and landing? This is because they are experiencing discomfort, but they cannot reach for a bag of sweets.

- ***What could you advise about this?***

If the baby can be encouraged to suckle, then the middle ear will be vented and the discomfort reduced.

Let us now return to our consideration of atmospheric pressure.

- ***If we wanted to measure this pressure, how could it be done?***

This problem faced Evangelista Torricelli in the seventeenth century. His solution was to take a glass tube filled with mercury and invert it into a container also containing mercury. This is illustrated in Figure 6.2. This experiment could easily be repeated today, but since mercury is poisonous its use is best avoided. (In developed countries, even closed systems such as mercury-in-glass thermometers have been replaced by devises that do not use mercury.) Examine Figure 6.2 and consider what happened. When inverted, the heavy column of mercury sank, creating a near-vacuum (V) in the closed end of the tube. The height of the column of mercury above that in the container is indicated by *h*.

- ***Why did the mercury column not fall further?***

You may have worked out that it was prevented from doing so by the atmospheric pressure (ap) pressing on the mercury in the container and pushing the column up.

- ***Work out what would happen if we were to take Torricelli's device up a mountain.***

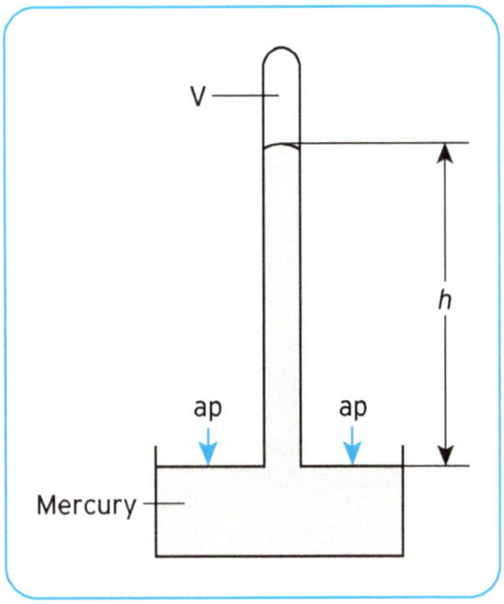

Figure 6.2
Torricelli's barometer.

As atmospheric pressure decreases with altitude, the mercury column would fall; consequently, we could measure atmospheric pressure in terms of the height of the column. Torricelli used millimetres (mm); since the chemical symbol for mercury is Hg, the unit mmHg (millimetres of mercury) was born. This is significant, since this unit of measurement of pressure is still used by health professionals today. It is worth pointing out, however, that pressure is not a length. The height of the column depends upon both the weight of the mercury being supported in the tube and the cross-sectional area of the tube. The height of the column is a measurement of the ratio of force to area.

Finally, suction (negative pressure) can be measured in terms of negative units. For example –50 mmHg suction may be applied to a chest drain in order to facilitate the evacuation of the **pleural space**. (This is described in a little more detail in Practice point 6.8 later in this chapter.)

Other units of measurement of pressure

The measurement of pressure is complicated by the use of a number of different units. For example, the unit mmHg is sometimes referred to as the torr after Torricelli (1 mmHg = 1 torr). When atmospheric pressure is measured at sea level, it is found to be 760 mmHg, and this value is sometimes referred to as a standard atmosphere (atm). Of course, water could be used in a measuring device instead of mercury, but since water is much less dense than mercury, a very tall tube would be needed to measure atmospheric pressure. The unit cmH_2O is sometimes used by health professionals, however, in the measurement of **central venous pressure** (pressure in the great veins, e.g. **vena cava**), which is much lower than arterial blood pressure. Other units of measurement of pressure include pounds per square inch (psi) and the SI unit of pressure the pascal (Pa). Since the pascal is commonly used in clinical practice, it is worth describing it in a little more detail.

The SI unit of area is the square metre (m^2) and that of force is the newton (N). At this point, it is not essential to understand how the SI unit of force came into being, but we measure pressure in terms of newtons per square metre (N/m^2 or Nm^{-2}) - a unit subsequently renamed the pascal in honour of the French scientist Blaise Pascal. This is, however, a very small unit of pressure, so in practice units of 1000 pascals (kilopascal, kPa) are used. We have spent some time looking at the units of measurement of pressure, since you will encounter them in clinical practice. Indeed, it is sometimes necessary to convert between units. With this in mind, the following data are given:

1 kPa = 7.5 mmHg = 10.2 cmH_2O
1 mmHg = 0.133 kPa = 1.36 cmH_2O
1 cmH_2O = 0.098 kPa = 0.735 mmHg

Pressure-measuring devices

The term **manometer** refers to a device in which pressure is measured by means of a vertical column of fluid. Therefore, Torricelli's device was a manometer, and health professionals commonly use manometers too. For example, central venous pressure is measured using a saline manometer, and arterial blood pressure can be measured using a mercury-filled **sphygmomanometer** (*sphygmo* is Greek for pulse), although again these have been replaced in developed countries by devices that do not contain mercury. Devices such as the sphygmomanometer measure pressure in reference to atmospheric pressure. Consequently, when we measure systolic blood pressure as 120 mmHg, what we really mean is that it is 120 mmHg above atmospheric pressure.

The term 'manometer' should not be confused with **barometer**, which is a device for measuring atmospheric pressure. Of course, a barometer may use a column of fluid, as is the case in Torricelli's device, but this is not necessarily so. For example, anaeroid barometers measure atmospheric pressure based upon the extent of the distortion of an evacuated box. Anaeroid devices may also be used to measure arterial blood pressure. They are easily identified by the presence of a dial and needle instead of a graduated mercury column. Strictly speaking, such devices are not manometers, but they are commonly referred to as such, since they perform the same role in the measurement of blood pressure. The method of blood-pressure measurement is explained in Practice point 6.3.

Practice point 6.3

Measuring blood pressure

Owing to the beating action of the heart, arterial blood pressure has two values - recorded during **systole** (contraction) and **diastole** (relaxation). Two pieces of equipment are needed to measure arterial blood pressure non-invasively (without inserting a needle into an artery): a sphygmomanometer and a stethoscope. The sphygmomanometer consists of a manometer, a cloth cuff enclosing an inflatable bladder and an inflating bulb with release valve, as shown in Figure 6.3.

Pressure created by the inflation of the bladder causes the needle of an anaeroid manometer to rotate, although the pressure is still measured in mmHg. It is a good idea to check the manometer before use. Before inflation of the cuff, the needle should be at zero and the cuff, bladder, tubing, connections, inflating bulb and valve should all be in good condition. Cuffs are available in different sizes for patients of different ages and different builds. The width of the inflatable bladder within the cloth cuff should be 40% of the circumference of the midpoint of the arm, while its

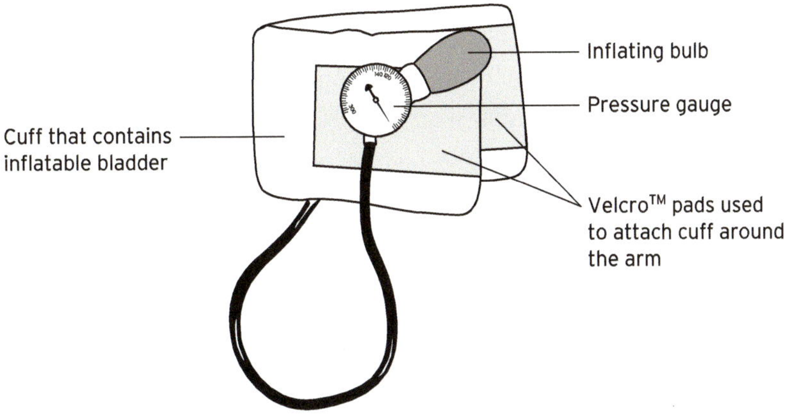

Figure 6.3
A spygmomanometer.

length should be at least 80% of the circumference. In children over 5 years old, the bladder should be over 12 cm long, while in normal and lean adult arms a bladder length of 35 cm is recommended as an alternative to the 23-cm-long bladders that are often used. A bladder 40 cm long is reserved for muscular and obese arms.

The stethoscope is a simple instrument for **auscultation** – that is, listening to sound waves originating from within the body. It is illustrated in Figure 6.4.

The stethoscope is basically a closed cylinder used to amplify the sound waves so that they can be heard more readily. After cleaning the earpieces with an antiseptic wipe and allowing them to dry, they are placed in the ears and angled forwards so that they follow the angle of the auditory

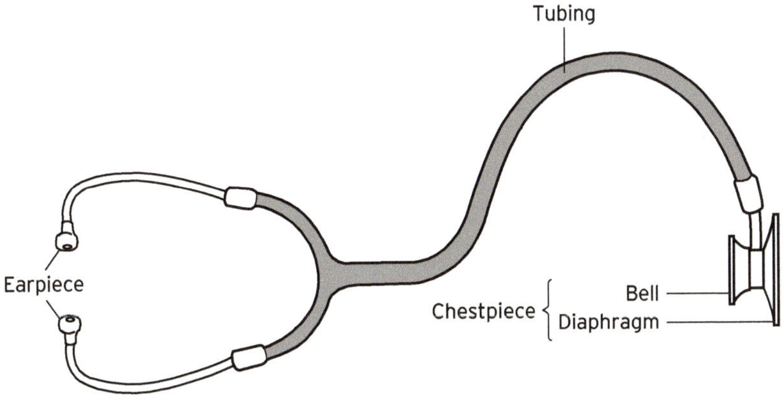

Figure 6.4
A stethoscope.

canal. The chestpiece is then placed against the body. This part of the stethoscope is so called because the instrument is commonly used to listen for respiratory sounds. In blood-pressure measurement, however, it is placed above the artery in which the pressure is to be measured. The diaphragm is the circular flat part of the chestpiece, which is covered by a plastic disc. This is good for listening to high-pitched sounds such as bowel and lung sounds. The bell transmits low-pitched sounds such as heart sounds.

● *Which shall I use here?*

The answer to this question is use whichever you can hear most clearly with. The operator should rotate the chestpiece so that the appropriate part is operational. Some simple stethoscopes, however, have no bell but only a diaphragm. In most cases, it makes little difference whether the patient is sitting or lying down during a blood-pressure measurement, but the patient should be at rest and not anxious or stressed by recent activity. Pregnant women sometimes experience a fall in blood pressure when lying supine (on the back) because raised abdominal pressure impairs venous return (return of blood to the heart); the blood pressure should then be taken with the woman sitting or lying on her side. Furthermore, some patients, such as those taking **antihypertensives** (medicines to treat high blood pressure), experience a fall in blood pressure when standing, and so measurement of blood pressure should be made in both supine and standing positions.

Whichever position is used, the arm should be supported in a comfortable horizontal position at heart level and the sphygmomanometer should be at the same level. If the arm is lower than the heart, the result will be artificially high; if the arm is above the heart, the measurement will be artificially low. The patient should be warm and restrictive clothing should be removed. The point of strongest pulsation of the **brachial artery** just above the **antecubital fossa** (inner aspect of the elbow) is identified and the appropriate size of cuff fitted to the upper arm so that the centre of the bladder lies over the line of the artery and the edge of the cuff 2–3 cm above the point where the pulse was felt. This is shown in Figure 6.5.

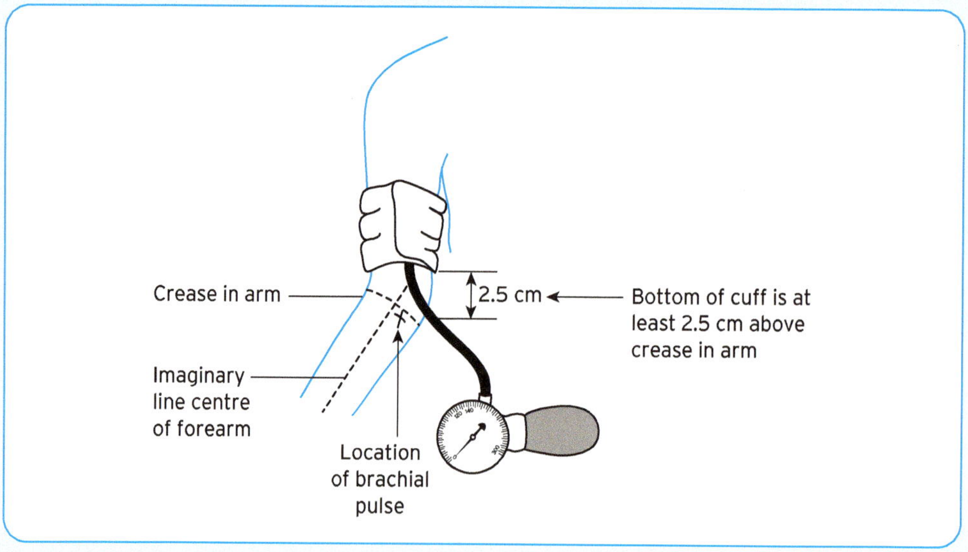

Figure 6.5
The positioning of the cuff in blood-pressure measurement.

Before using the stethoscope, however, an estimation of systolic pressure is made. This is achieved by palpating the brachial pulse and then inflating the cuff until the pulse disappears. The point at which it does so represents the approximate value of the systolic blood pressure.

- ***Work out why this is so?***

When the pressure in the cuff exceeds systolic blood pressure, blood flow in the artery ceases. Following this, an auscultatory measurement of systolic and diastolic blood pressure is made. The stethoscope is held gently over the brachial artery at the point of maximal pulsation. The cuff is now inflated to 30 mmHg above the estimated systolic blood pressure; following this, the valve is opened a little so that the cuff deflates slowly. The operator should now listen carefully. The point at which a tapping sound can be heard is an accurate measurement of systolic blood pressure.

- ***Can you work out why?***

As soon as the cuff pressure is reduced to systolic blood pressure, blood is forced through the compressed artery during systole. The tapping noise (the first **Korotkoff sound**, or phase one) is the result of this pulsating turbulence. A mental note of the systolic blood pressure is made as the cuff continues to deflate. The point at which the tapping sound disappears (the fifth Korotkoff sound, or phase five) is also noted, and this is an accurate measurement of diastolic blood pressure.

- ***Can you work out why this is so?***

When the pressure in the cuff reaches diastolic blood pressure, blood flows freely in the artery; therefore, the tapping sound disappears. In some people, however, such as children, pregnant women, **anaemic** people and elderly patients, the tapping sound never disappears completely. In these cases, the point at which the tapping sound becomes muffled (the fourth Korotkoff sound, or phase four) is recorded. The point of muffling is usually higher than the true diastolic pressure; thus, if this is recorded, it should be made clear that the second reading is phase four and not phase five. Phase four is, however, used routinely in pregnant women.

The values of blood pressure are usually recorded as though they are a fraction - for example, 120/80 mmHg. The first figure corresponds to the systolic measurement and the second to the diastolic measurement. If the first, fourth and fifth sounds are all recorded, then the result might be 120/100/80 mmHg.

You may be interested to note that the Korotkoff sounds are so called because a Russian surgeon of that name first noted them in 1905. Not all the sounds that he described have been noted here - only the first, fourth and fifth, which are important in blood-pressure measurement.

In-text review

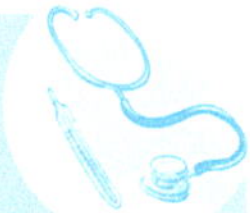

- ✔ Pressure is defined as force per unit area.
- ✔ The highest pressure will be created over the smaller of two areas when identical forces are applied to both.
- ✔ Pressure ulcers result from a compromised blood supply caused by the unrelieved pressure of the body against the object on which it is resting.

- ✔ A device that employs a column of fluid to measure pressure is referred to as a manometer.
- ✔ A barometer is a device for measuring atmospheric pressure.
- ✔ Commonly used units of pressure include pascals (Pa), millimetres of mercury (mmHg) and centimetres of water (cmH_2O).
- ✔ When blood pressure is measured using a sphymomanometer, the nurse uses a stethoscope to listen for the sound of blood flowing in the brachial artery.
- ✔ The normal arterial pressure during contraction of the heart (systole) and relaxation of the heart (diastole) is taken to be 120 mmHg and 80 mmHg, respectively.

Pressure in static liquids

The term 'static liquid' refers to fluid in an enclosed container. It does not mean that individual molecules are static, but rather that there is no net movement of the fluid. Individual molecules are indeed moving; by colliding with each other and with the sides of the container, the molecules exert a pressure. This pressure acts in all directions, and any change in pressure is transmitted to every part of the fluid (**Pascal's principle**). This behaviour of fluids has biological significance, since a number of body cavities contain fluid. An obvious example is **amniotic fluid** in the **amniotic cavity**, which surrounds the foetus (Figure 6.6).

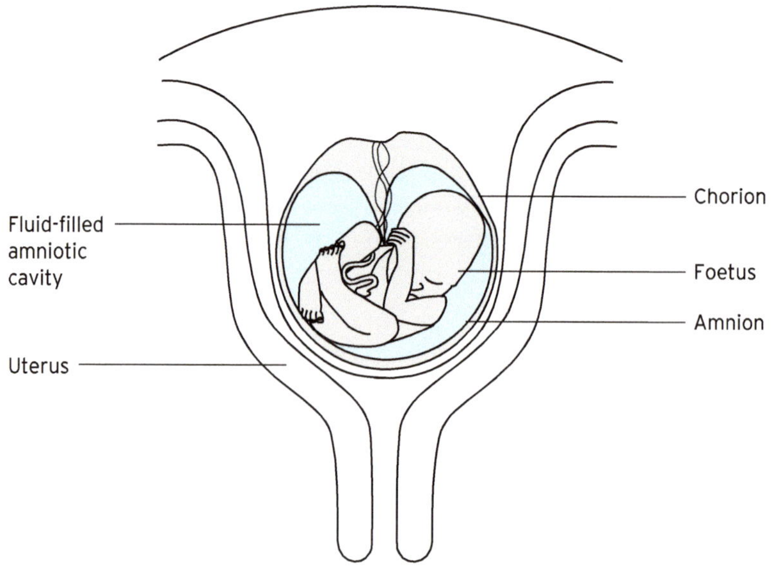

Figure 6.6
The foetus surrounded by amniotic fluid.

Clearly, a blow to the foetus could be damaging, but since the foetus is surrounded by amniotic fluid any rise in pressure is transmitted uniformly throughout the amniotic fluid (Pascal's principle), which serves to protect the foetus from localised damage.

Fluids in containers

Of course, the nurse is interested not only in fluid in compartments within the body - as nurses, we regularly have to deal with fluids in containers, and sometimes pressure is an important consideration here. The pressure at a point below the surface of a fluid in a container is dependent upon two factors. The first is the height of the column of liquid. Consider the diagram of a container with three holes (Figure 6.7).

- ***Through which hole is water flowing at the fastest rate?***

Water is flowing at the fastest rate through hole c - that is, the lowest hole.

- ***Why is this?***

This is because the pressure is greatest at this point, as this is the lowest hole and the height of the column of water is greatest above it. The other factor that determines the pressure of fluid in a container is the density of the fluid. Consequently, the pressure beneath a column of mercury is greater than that beneath a column of water of the same height.

The intravenous infusion (drip) is a method of administering fluid in a container directly into a vein. The regulation of the flow rate is described in Practice point 6.4.

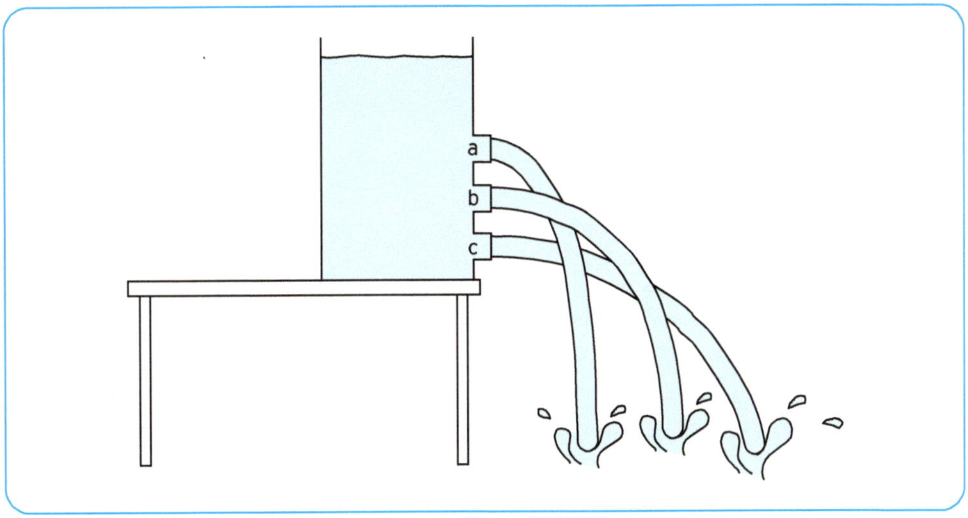

Figure 6.7
Fluid flowing out of a container with three holes.

Practice point 6.4

Regulating intravenous infusions

One obvious application to this understanding of the pressure of fluids in containers is in **intravenous infusions** (drips). A patient with an intravenous infusion is shown in Figure 6.8.

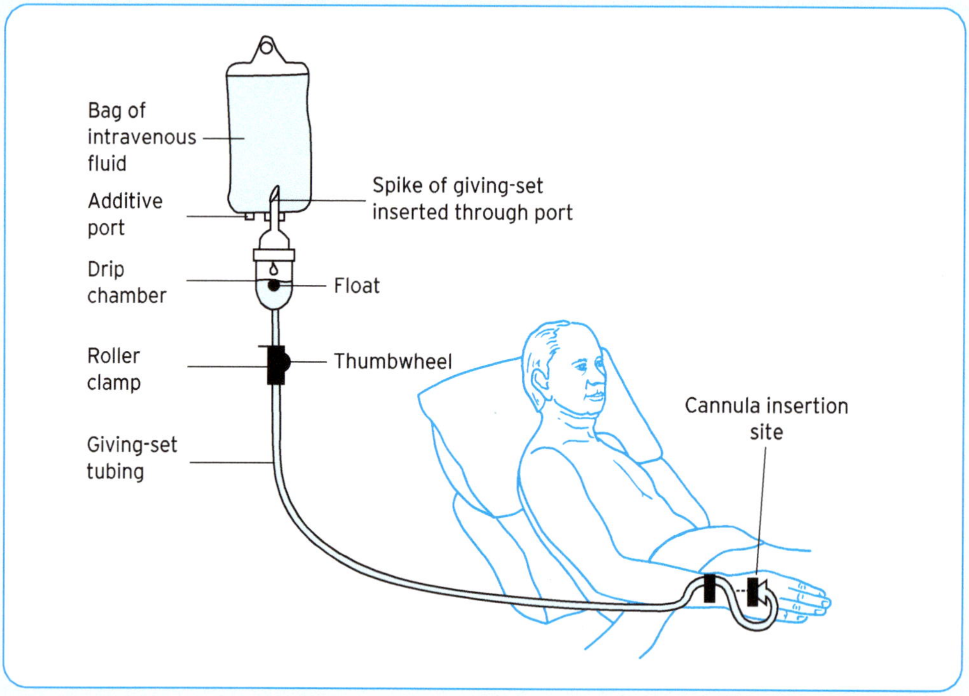

Figure 6.8
A patient with an intravenous infusion.

- ***What would be the effect upon the infusion flow rate if the height of the intravenous bag was raised?***

By raising the height of the intravenous bag, the pressure of fluid would rise at the point where the cannula enters the patient and the flow rate would increase. Perhaps this is a little obvious, but who said science had to be difficult? The important thing is to note that the height of the intravenous bag above the cannula is one factor that influences the intravenous flow rate. It is also worth noting another practical point: Suppose you have regulated the flow rate of an infusion so that the prescribed volume will be infused in the time desired but the patient now gets up from the supine position (lying flat on the back) and begins to walk around.

- ***How might this influence the flow rate?***

In the standing position, the height of the intravenous bag above the cannula is decreased, and so the flow rate will be reduced. For this reason, you will have to check the flow rate at intervals in order to ensure that the infusion is completed in the prescribed period of time.

Of course, to use variations in the height of the intravenous bag above the cannula as the means of controlling infusion rates would be a little inconvenient. Once the bag is hung from the drip stand, the flow rate is instead adjusted by a roller clamp, which compresses the intravenous tubing.

- ***So how is the flow rate actually determined?***

To work this out, you need to know how much fluid is to be given (for example, 500 ml in 4 hours) and how many drops of the drop counter of the giving-set there are to each millilitre. This information is given on the giving-set packaging. In an adult giving-set, it is usually 20 drops per 1 ml for clear fluids (such as dextrose or saline) and 15 drops per 1 ml for blood. Paediatric giving-sets usually give 60 drops per 1 ml. So, if we were to be giving 500 ml of normal saline in 4 hours through an adult giving-set, the drop rate calculation would be as follows:

$$\text{Drop rate (in drops per minute)} = \frac{\text{volume to be given} \times \text{number of drops per 1 ml}}{\text{number of hours} \times 60}$$

$$= \frac{500 \times 20}{4 \times 60}$$

$$= 42 \text{ drops per minute}$$

One other point to note is that we have moved from talking about static fluids to considering fluid flowing in an intravenous infusion. Although it is true that in the static state (when the fluid is not flowing) the pressure at a given point is proportional to the height of the column of fluid and the density of the fluid, there are other considerations when fluid flowing in a tube is considered. In the case of the intravenous infusion, there is a pressure drop between the beginning of the tubing and the point of attachment of the tubing to the cannula.

- ***Why is this?***

This drop in pressure is due to the friction between the fluid and the vessel walls.

- ***What factors influence the extent of this friction?***

You may have been able to work out that among the factors that influence the extent of friction between a fluid and the walls of a tube in which it is flowing are the viscosity of the fluid and the diameter of the tube. There are other factors too, as you will see when we move on to consider blood and blood vessels.

Blood flow

The circulatory system is the important transport system of the body. Like all transport systems, it has three components. First, there is a means of carrying the various substances that need to be transported; the blood performs this role. Then there is a means of propulsion; the heart undertakes this role. Finally, there is a system of structures through which the transport medium passes; these are the blood vessels.

- ***Why does blood flow?***

This may sound like an obvious question - you might say that blood flows because it is pumped by the heart - but let us look at blood flow in a little more detail. Fluids such as blood flow for one reason - there is a pressure gradient. Consider the arterial blood pressure for a moment.

- ***Remember that the normal is about 120/80 mmHg. What does this actually mean?***

Recall that the lower figure refers to the pressure in arteries during diastole - that is, when the heart is not contracting. The higher figure is the systolic pressure generated when the heart contracts (systole). So, blood flows from the heart during systole because the contraction generates a pressure gradient down which the blood flows. Note that it is not the blood pressure at a particular point but the difference in pressure between two points that determines blood flow.

Resistance to blood flow

We have already noted that friction between a fluid and the vessel in which it is flowing opposes the flow of blood, and we have noted some of the factors that account for this friction. We now consider blood viscosity, vessel length and vessel diameter in more detail.

Blood viscosity

The more viscous a fluid, the greater the friction between it and the vessel wall and the greater the resistance to blood flow.

- ***What factor influences blood viscosity the most?***

Blood is not a simple solution of dissolved substances. Blood is, in fact, a tissue and contains cells. It is the proportion of cells that has the greatest impact on blood viscosity, and since **erythrocytes** (red blood cells) are the most abundant type of blood cell it is these that are the most significant here.

- ***Can you think of situations in which the number of erythrocytes might vary?***

If you have not studied biological science before, you might have found this question difficult, but **anaemia** involves a reduced number of erythrocytes and, as a consequence, a reduced blood viscosity, which in turn results in rapid blood flow. In contrast, people with an excessive number of erythrocytes (**polycythaemia**) have an elevated blood viscosity and sluggish blood flow.

Vessel length

Note that the longer the vessel, the greater the inner surface and thus the greater the friction. For this reason, resistance to blood flow is directly proportional to the length of the vessel. This is illustrated in Figure 6.9. Here, there are three vessels of different lengths, and despite the fact that the pressure of fluid entering each vessel is the same the flow rates are different. In fact, the vessel that is three times the length of the shortest vessel has only a third of its flow.

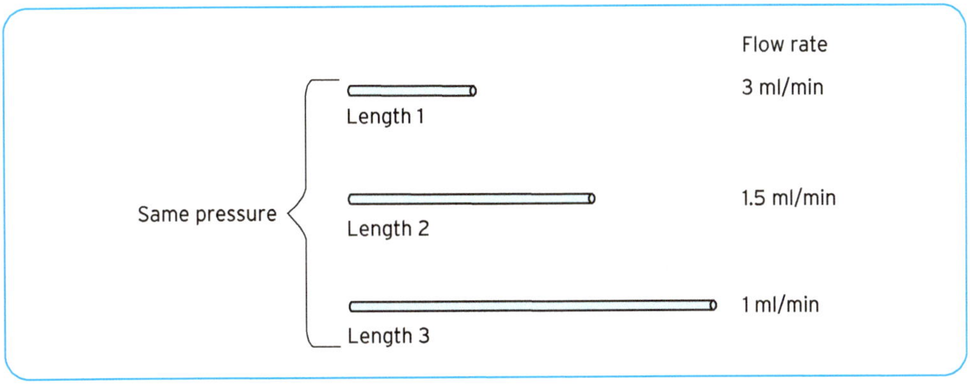

Figure 6.9
The effect of vessel length on flow.

Vessel diameter

The friction between a fluid and the vessel wall in which it is flowing is clearly an important consideration and leads to slow flow rates along the inner surface of the vessel. Fluid flowing down the middle of the vessel lumen, however, flows much faster. This effect means that flow in large-diameter vessels is very much greater than in narrow vessels, due to this rapid flow through the central portion of the vessel. In fact, flow rate is directly proportional to the fourth power of the diameter, provided that all other factors remain constant. This is illustrated in Figure 6.10. Note that the pressure of fluid entering the vessels is the same in each case. Note also that vessel b is twice the diameter of vessel a.

- ***How much greater is the flow rate in vessel b compared with that in vessel a?***

The flow rate in vessel b is 16 times that of the flow rate in vessel a.

Practice point 6.5 deals with atherosclerosis, a condition that affects the diameter of arteries and, as a consequence, the rate of blood flow through them. Practice point 6.6 explains briefly how the body regulates blood pressure, flow and resistance.

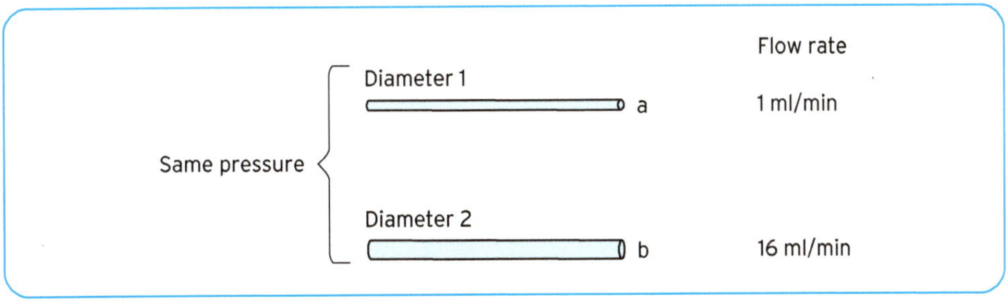

Figure 6.10
The effect of vessel diameter on flow.

Practice point 6.5

Atherosclerosis

Atherosclerosis is the accumulation of fats and other molecules in the walls of arteries, leading to the formation of plaques that reduce the internal diameter of vessels and, as a consequence, reduce blood flow. Atherosclerosis is associated with poor diet and smoking. Even a moderately narrowed lumen can result in a considerable reduction in flow rate.

- ***Can you recall why this is so?***

It is because the blood flow is proportional to the fourth power of the diameter. Therefore, if the diameter is reduced by half, the flow rate is reduced by one-sixteenth. Atherosclerosis can affect arteries in all sites of the body, but its effects on the **coronary arteries** (arteries that supply the heart) are probably most familiar to you.

- ***What are the effects of atherosclerosis on the heart?***

They include **angina** - crushing central chest pain associated with exercise and emotional stress. Angina results when the blood flow through atherosclerotic arteries cannot meet the heart's increased demand for oxygen when its workload is increased, as it is during activity. Consequently, when angina occurs, it is important to rest if the pain is to cease. The patient may also take the drug **glyceryl trinitrate** (GTN) as a tablet or spray under the tongue. This drug causes **vasodilation** (blood-vessel dilation), but not of the coronary arteries.

- ***How then does this help?***

The heart has less work to do when pumping against the reduced resistance offered by dilated arteries.

Practice point 6.6

The body regulates blood pressure, flow and resistance

We might summarise what we have said so far by saying that pressure tends to increase flow and resistance tends to decrease it. We can also state this as a formula:

$$\text{Blood flow} = \frac{\text{pressure}}{\text{resistance}}$$

We can see the body's attempts to regulate these three parameters in a number of different situations. For example, in the case of **pyrexia** (fever), the body attempts to increase heat loss.

- ***What change could be made to the resistance offered by vessels in the skin in order to increase heat loss?***

You have probably been able to work out that the resistance offered by the vessels in the skin is reduced by **vasodilation** (the muscles in the vessel walls relax and the vessels become wider). This increases the blood flow through the skin (as seen by flushing) and as a consequence heat loss is increased.

There are other applications too. Suppose an individual suffers considerable blood loss and arterial blood pressure starts to fall. Looking at our equation, we can see that if blood pressure starts to fall, then the blood flow will also fall, and the vital organs will be deprived of a blood supply. Clearly, the body needs to do something in order to maintain the blood pressure.

- ***But just what could the body do to maintain blood pressure?***

To answer this question, it might be helpful to rewrite our equation, this time making blood pressure the subject:

$$\text{Blood pressure} = \text{blood flow} \times \text{resistance}$$

In our current scenario, blood flow is reduced because of haemorrhage; therefore, in order to maintain blood pressure, resistance will have to rise - this is achieved through **vasoconstriction** (the muscles in the vessel walls constrict and the vessels becomes narrower). This sounds fine so far, but if the blood vessels to important structures such as the brain, heart and lungs were to constrict, thus maintaining the blood pressure, the blood flow to these organs would be reduced and the body's efforts would be thwarted.

- ***So just what could be done?***

If you think about this, you might realise that the response of the body to blood loss is to cause the blood vessels in certain areas such as the skin to constrict, thus helping to maintain the blood pressure, but the vessels to other structures remain unaffected so that blood flow to the brain, heart and lungs is ensured. This example of the importance of a consideration of pressure, flow and resistance is a little harder to understand than the first example, but no doubt it will begin to make a great deal of sense when you actually look after a patient who has suffered blood loss. Incidentally, not all blood loss is visible: It is possible to haemorrhage internally, and for this reason measuring the blood pressure even when there is no frank bleeding might be important.

- ***Are there other observations to be made too?***

Yes, there are a number. One is to look at the patient's complexion. We have seen that one method that the body employs to maintain blood pressure is to cause cutaneous vasoconstriction, and so **pallor** (pale complexion) may be a significant observation.

In-text review

- ✔ The protection afforded to various body structures by being surrounded by fluid is explained on the basis of Pascal's principle.
- ✔ Fluid flows between two points when there is a pressure difference between them.
- ✔ The flow rate of blood in a blood vessel is affected by blood viscosity, vessel length and vessel diameter.
- ✔ Resistance to the flow of a fluid is directly proportional to the length of the vessel in which the fluid is flowing.
- ✔ Flow rate is directly proportional to the fourth power of the diameter of a vessel, provided that other factors remain the same.
- ✔ The body alters the diameter of blood vessels in order to control blood pressure and the flow rate through the vessels.
- ✔ Narrowing of arteries in the vascular condition atherosclerosis accounts for the affect of this disease on blood flow.

Gases and breathing

The behaviour of gases is explained by a number of laws that are named after the scientists who first described them. Upon initial examination, you may not appreciate the relevance of these laws to nursing practice, but this section seeks to relate the laws to the function of the lungs and to interventions such as oxygen therapy.

Boyle's law

Boyle's law states that,

> **provided the temperature of a gas does not change, the pressure of a fixed amount of gas increases as the volume decreases (and vice versa).**

That is, pressure varies inversely with volume. This relationship may be given in the form of a formula (where the symbol $\propto$ means proportional to):

$$\text{Pressure} \propto 1/\text{volume}$$

Suppose we take a volume of gas in a sealed container at constant temperature and we have some means of changing the volume of the container – a piston perhaps. This arrangement is illustrated in Figure 6.11.

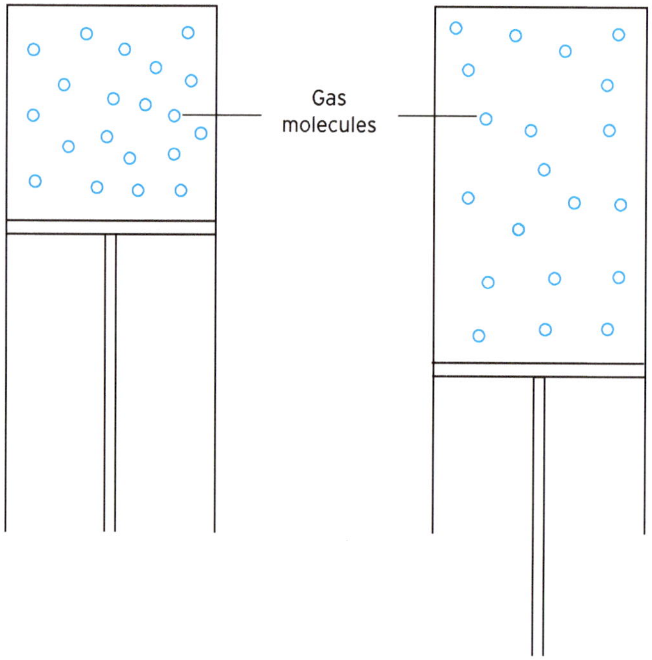

Figure 6.11
A simple apparatus for demonstrating Boyle's law.

- ***What happens to the pressure when pulling on the piston increases the volume of the sealed container?***

According to Boyle's law, it varies inversely - that is, the pressure falls. In Practice point 6.7, Boyle's law is related to breathing. In Practice point 6.8, Boyle's law is related to intercostal drains, a treatment for collapsed lung.

Practice point 6.7

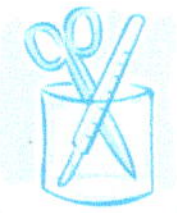

The mechanism of breathing

We could relate our consideration of Boyle's law to breathing. The chest is rather like our sealed container and has the capacity to change size, although not by the movement of a piston. Inspiration takes place when the **diaphragm** (the muscle that separates the chest from the abdominal cavity) contracts and becomes flattened, descending towards the abdomen. This results in an increase in the vertical dimension of the chest. At the same time, the external **intercostal muscles** (between the ribs) also contract and lift the ribs upwards, rotating them outwards. This results in an increase in the chest sideways and front to back, and the volume of the chest is increased.

- ***According to Boyle's law, what now happens to the pressure of gas inside the chest?***

Just like in the container in Figure 6.11, the pressure tends to fall. The expression 'tends to fall' is important here, because the chest is not actually a sealed box. There is one way in and out - the airway. Therefore, as the pressure begins to fall, air is drawn into the lungs via the mouth or nose until the increased space within the lungs is filled with air at atmospheric pressure. This sequence of events is illustrated in Figure 6.12.

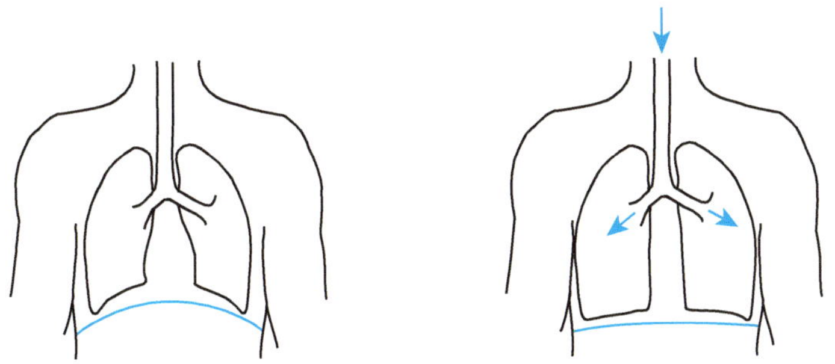

Figure 6.12
Inspiration.

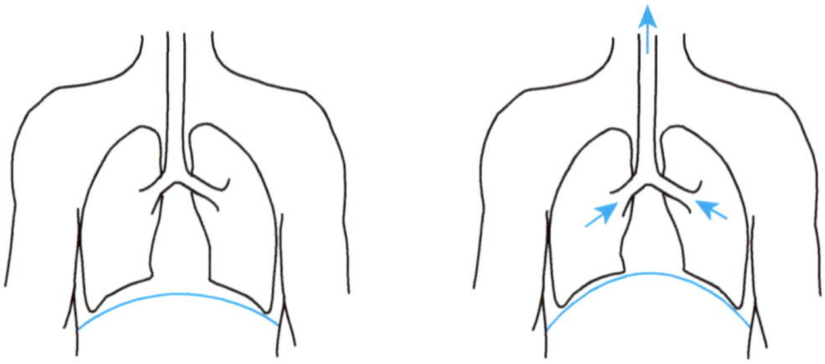

Figure 6.13
Expiration.

When inspiration ceases and expiration begins, the chest returns to its previous dimension by passive recoil. That is, it is not an active process - muscle contraction is not involved. As the volume of the chest falls you might have worked out from Boyle's law that the pressure in the lungs tends to rise and air is now forced out of the airway. Expiration is illustrated in Figure 6.13.

Practice point 6.8

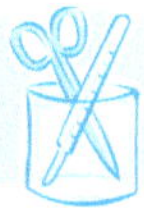

Intercostal drains

Intercostal drains are also referred to as chest drains, pleural drains and underwater seal drains, although this latter term refers to the type of drainage system rather than to the site of the drain. Intercostal drains present particular problems for nurses, who sometimes become confused about the management of such systems when they are uncertain about the science behind them. First, it is important to note that a membrane called the **pleura** covers the lung. This word may sound familiar if you have ever encountered someone with inflammation of the pleura (**pleurisy** or **pleuritis**) - perhaps because of an infection. The pleura is in fact a double membrane, as illustrated in Figure 6.14.

The innermost or visceral pleura is adherent to the lung surface, but at the point where the airway enters the lung (**hilum**) it is reflected back upon itself to form the outer pleura (**parietal pleura**). The parietal pleura is adherent to the chest wall, but the two layers of the pleura are not normally adherent to each other. In diagrams, the two membranes are often drawn as though there is a space between them, but this is not actually the case. In fact, there is a potential space between the two layers - that is, they touch but they are not stuck together, and they slide over each other but can be pulled apart. The pleura is described as a serous membrane - it secretes a fluid that resembles serum (fluid part of blood) and that helps the two membranes to slide over each other. As an illustration of how small the pleural space is, you might be interested to know that in adults, the volume of pleural fluid forming the film between the pleurae of one lung is only approximately 2 ml.

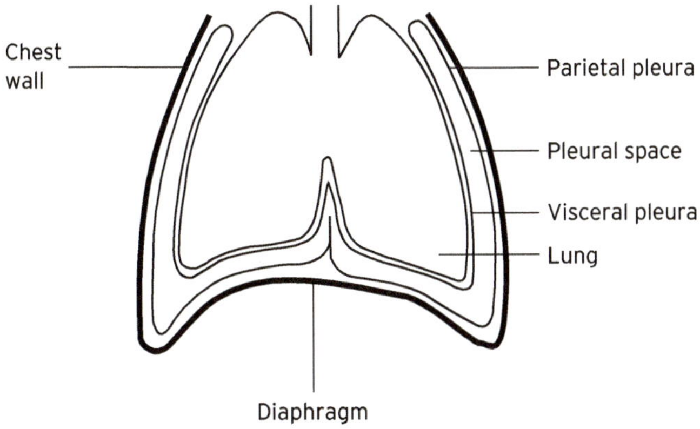

Figure 6.14
The pleura.

Next, it should be pointed out that the lung is filled with elastic tissue, which produces a tendency to collapse; since the visceral pleura is adherent to the lung, it is pulled away slightly from the parietal pleura.

- ***So what actually prevents the lung from collapsing?***

Let us think about this. Since the two pleurae are continuous, as the visceral is pulled away from the parietal the space between them is enlarged; according to Boyle's law, the intrapleural pressure drops. It is this slight negative pressure in the pleural space that just balances the tendency of the lung to collapse. We might say that the lungs are held up by suction.

Of course, since the pleural space is on the inside of the chest, it is subject to a change in pressure as we breathe in and out. Unlike the intra-alveolar pressure (pressure inside the **alveoli** – microscopic air sacs of the lungs), however, the intrapleural pressure does not oscillate between negative and positive but between more negative and less negative, as shown in the table below:

	Intra-alveolar pressure (mmHg)	Intrapleural pressure (mmHg)
Inspiration	$^{-3}$ mmHg	$^{-8}$ mmHg
Expiration	$^{+3}$ mmHg	$^{-3}$ mmHg

Now let us consider what would happen if either of the pleurae were to be breached. The visceral pleura might rupture as a consequence of a structural weakness, while trauma, such as a knife attack, may result in penetration of the parietal pleura and probably the visceral pleura and lung as well. The consequence would be that atmospheric air would enter the pleural space, and the negative pressure would be lost.

- ***What would happen now to the affected lung?***

Since there would no longer be a negative pressure in the pleural space of the affected lung, the natural elasticity of the lung would no longer be balanced and the lung would collapse, with consequent respiratory complications. This condition is referred to as **pneumothorax**, and you might like to read more about it in a nursing textbook.

It is not too difficult to work out that the treatment of pneumothorax must involve releasing air from the pleural space. The obvious way to do this is to place a tube within the space. There is a problem, however.

● ***Can you work out what it is?***

A simple tube passing from the outside and into the pleural space would allow air in as well as out. What is needed is some kind of valve that allows air to leave the pleural space but not to enter it. This is achieved most easily by connecting the drain to a tube, the end of which is dipped under water, as illustrated in Figure 6.15.

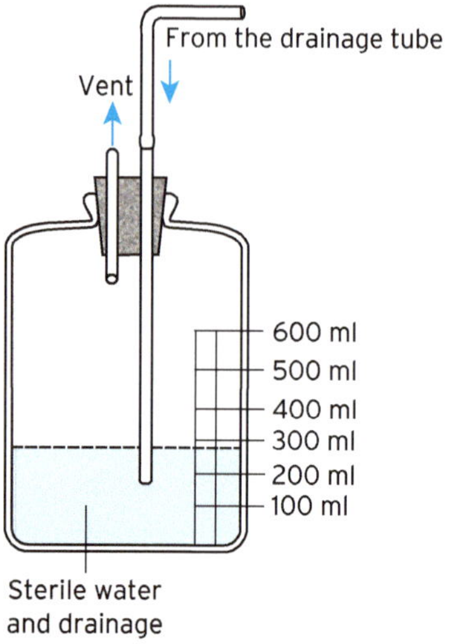

Figure 6.15
An underwater seal drainage system. (From Foss M. A. (1989) *Thoracic Surgery*. London: Austen Cornish.)

In this system, air is pushed out of the pleural space as it is compressed during inspiration. The air has only one route through which to pass, and it bubbles out in the water and escapes from the bottle via the vent. The air cannot re-enter the chest because of the presence of the water; hence, the term 'underwater seal' is used. In some cases, evacuation of the pleural space may be enhanced by attaching the vent to a vacuum and a pressure of up to $^{-13}$ kPa may be used.

Once again, you may like to look at a nursing textbook to find out more about intercostal drains. For now, it is sufficient to point out that a simple understanding of Boyle's law can help nurses comprehend normal physiology, altered physiology (such as pneumothorax) and interventions, such as intercostal drainage.

Dalton's law of partial pressures

Dalton's law helps us to understand mixtures of gases such as the atmosphere. The law states that **in a mixture of gases, the total pressure is a sum of the pressures exerted by each of the gases alone.**

That sounds like a bit of a mouthful, but let us see if we can make some sense of it. We have already thought about atmospheric pressure, and a value for it of 760 mmHg has been given. The air around us is a mixture of gases, mainly nitrogen, oxygen, carbon dioxide and water vapour.

● ***How much does each of these gases contribute to the net atmospheric pressure?***

Table 6.1 shows the typical figures for atmospheric air. The first column identifies the percentage of the atmosphere that the gas forms, while the second and third columns show the partial pressures of the individual gases in mmHg and kPa, respectively. Let us now

Table 6.1 The partial pressures of gases in atmospheric air.

Gas	Proportion of atmospheric air (%)	Partial pressure	
		mmHg	kPa
N_2	78.62	597	79.6
O_2	20.84	159	21.2
H_2O	0.5	3.85	0.51
CO_2	0.04	0.15	0.02

examine what these figures mean. For example, nitrogen is the most abundant gas in the atmosphere. In fact, 78.6% of the atmosphere is nitrogen, and it exerts 78.6% of the atmospheric pressure – that is, 79.1 kPa or 597 mmHg. This value is termed the partial pressure of nitrogen in atmospheric air. Therefore, a partial pressure is the fraction of the pressure of a mixture of gases exerted by one of the gases.

Henry's law

Gases such as oxygen and carbon dioxide are very important in the body. Oxygen is required for the energy-producing reactions of cellular respiration, while carbon dioxide is a waste product of these processes. Therefore, the body must be able to transport these compounds. You will probably realise that the principal transport system of the body is the bloodstream and that oxygen and carbon dioxide are not transported as free gases but instead are dissolved in solution. Oxygen is subsequently attached to a special carrier molecule – haemoglobin – while carbon dioxide undergoes a chemical reaction in the blood. Nonetheless, first of all both gases are dissolved in the plasma.

- ***What influences how much gas will dissolve in liquids such as water or plasma?***

The answer to this question is given by **Henry's law**, which states that **the mass of a gas that will dissolve in water at a given temperature is proportional to the partial pressure of the gas and to its solubility coefficient**. The solubility coefficient is a constant (unvarying property of the individual gas) – that is, some gases are more soluble than others. For a given gas, then, the higher the partial pressure, the greater the mass dissolved. The practical relevance of this is made clear in Practice point 6.9 (in relation to oxygen transport) and Practice point 6.10 (in relation to the effect of altitude).

Gases in solution and their movement

In order to have a fuller understanding of gases in solution and how they move between alveolar air and blood and between blood and the cells of the body, we have to think a little more about the physical principles of gases in solution and **diffusion**. Figure 6.16 shows a container half-filled with water, with atmospheric air above it. Molecules of the gases that form the atmosphere are continually bouncing against the surface of the water, and some

Practice point 6.9

Oxygen transport

We have just noted that some gases are more soluble than others. Let us look at a practical example in the body. Carbon dioxide is highly soluble in water, whereas oxygen is much less soluble. In fact, our blood cannot transport enough dissolved oxygen in order to meet the needs of our cells.

- ***So how does the blood transport oxygen?***

From what has been noted before, you will no doubt have realised that our bodies do not rely upon dissolved oxygen. Instead, once oxygen has been dissolved, it is in effect removed from solution by combination with the haemoglobin molecule. This then makes way for more oxygen to be dissolved, which in turn is bound to the haemoglobin molecule, and so on, until nearly all haemoglobin molecules have oxygen bound to them - that is, they have become **oxyhaemoglobin**. The proportion of the haemoglobin molecules that have oxygen bound to them is termed the **saturation**, which in arterial blood is normally 98-100%.

- ***When might you need to know the value of a patient's saturation?***

The saturation may fall when a patient has a respiratory disease that affects the ability of the lungs to take up oxygen from the atmosphere.

- ***Where in the blood is this important molecule haemoglobin found?***

It is found within erythrocytes (red blood cells), and so the amount of haemoglobin and the number of erythrocytes are also important measurements; you might like to find out what the normal values are.

- ***But what happens if an individual is deficient in haemoglobin or erythrocytes?***

This condition is called **anaemia** and it results in a reduced ability to transport oxygen, one manifestation of which is tiredness.

Having made these practical points, we do not need to consider the solubility coefficient in any more detail. It is sufficient to note that at a given temperature, the variable that influences how much of a gas dissolves is the partial pressure of that gas in the atmosphere. As the partial pressure increases, so does the amount of gas dissolved.

Practice point 6.10

The effect of altitude

We have noted previously that Torricelli found a fall in atmospheric pressure with increasing altitude: This is an effect of gravity - the atmosphere is most dense at sea level. The overall fall in net atmospheric pressure reflects a fall in the partial pressures of each of the atmospheric gases, including oxygen. If we now apply Henry's law, we are able to work out that the effect of this falling partial pressure is a reduction in the amount of oxygen that will dissolve in blood. It is this reduction that produces the effects of altitude sickness. This is clearly a potential problem for mountain climbers and people who travel to cities at high altitudes. Given time, the body adapts to high altitude by making more erythrocytes and so increasing the oxygen-carrying capacity of the blood.

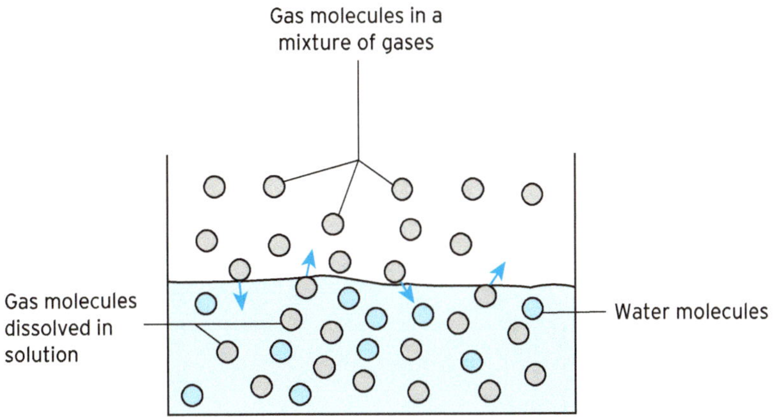

Figure 6.16
Gas molecules dissolving in water.

of them become dissolved in the water. These dissolved molecules continue to bounce among the water molecules and so exert a pressure against them. Some of these molecules then reach the surface of the water again and bounce back into the air. After some time, the number of gas molecules dissolving in the water becomes equal to the number moving in the opposite direction, and we say that a state of equilibrium has been reached.

An important point to note here is that molecules of gas dissolved in solution exert a pressure against water molecules just as they did against other gas molecules before they dissolved. This means that we can speak of the partial pressure of gases dissolved in solution as well as the partial pressure of gases in a gaseous mixture. The practical relevance of this becomes obvious when we consider the exchange of gases in the lungs. Figure 6.17 is a diagrammatic representation of a single **alveolus** and alveolar capillary on which is noted the partial pressures of oxygen and carbon dioxide in alveolar air, blood entering the capillary (venous blood) and blood leaving the capillary (arterial blood). The partial pressure of a gas in alveolar air is given as P_A, in venous blood entering the capillary as P_v and in arterial blood leaving the capillary as P_a.

It should be noted that the composition of alveolar air is not the same as that of atmospheric air, for a number of reasons. First, the air that we inhale is warmed and humidified on its passage through the upper airways, and this changes the gas composition. Second, the lungs eliminate carbon dioxide, and so the partial pressure of this gas is greater in alveolar air than it is in atmospheric air.

From Figure 6.17, we can see that the partial pressure of oxygen in alveolar air (13 kPa) is greater than that in venous blood (5 kPa). Consequently, oxygen diffuses from alveolar air and into the blood. In contrast, the partial pressure of carbon dioxide in alveolar air (5 kPa) is less than in venous blood (6 kPa), and so carbon dioxide diffuses from venous blood and into alveolar air. The net result of this diffusion of gases is that blood leaving the lungs has a partial pressure of oxygen of 13 kPa and of carbon dioxide of 5 kPa.

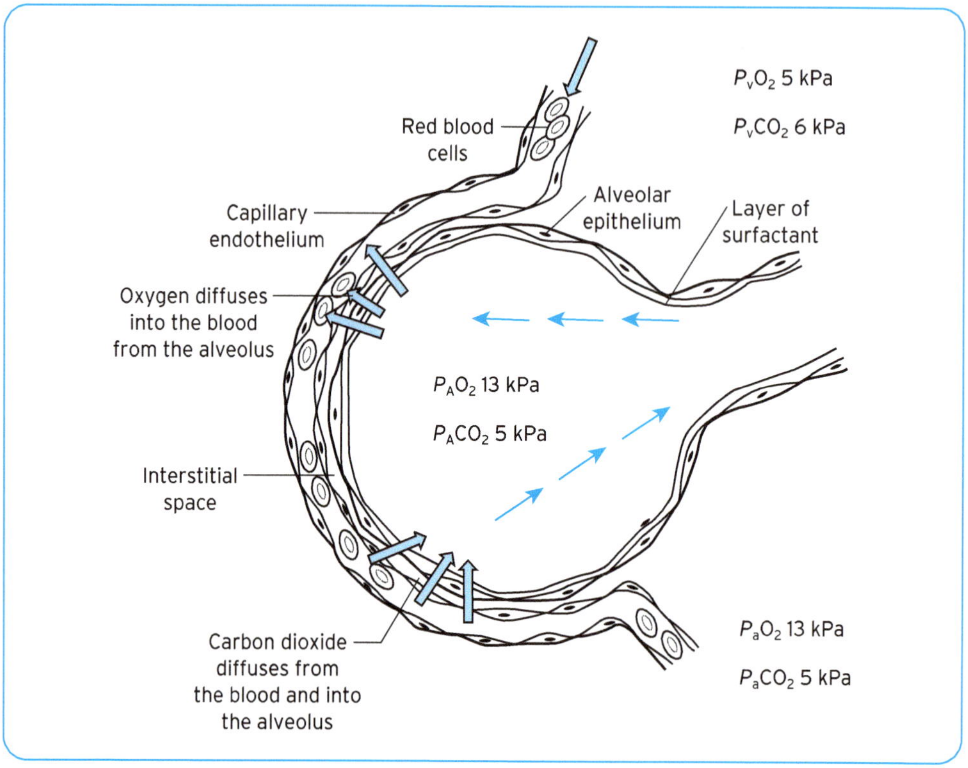

Figure 6.17
An alveolus and capillary. (From Foss M. A. (1989) *Thoracic Surgery*. London: Austen Cornish.)

Oxygen therapy

Oxygen therapy involves the administration of oxygen in concentrations higher than those in the normal atmosphere for the treatment of various conditions that result in **hypoxaemia**. Hypoxaemia is a state of reduced partial pressure of oxygen in arterial blood; it may be caused by a number of respiratory illnesses, such as chest infection, asthma and chronic bronchitis. Oxygen may be administered in a number of different ways, but the most obvious is the facemask, one example of which is illustrated in Figure 6.18.

- ***How is oxygen therapy effective?***

When an oxygen mask is applied over a patient's face, the mixture of gases that the patient inhales is changed. The proportion of oxygen given increases, and as a consequence the partial pressure of oxygen in the inhaled gas mixture increases. This is subsequently reflected in an increase in P_AO_2. In fact, if 100% oxygen is inspired, then P_AO_2 would rise from 13 kPa to 80 kPa.

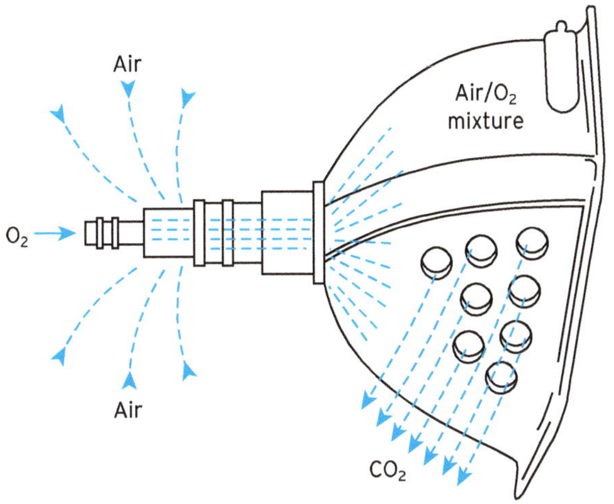

Figure 6.18
An oxygen mask. (From Foss M. A. (1989) *Thoracic Surgery*. London: Austen Cornish.)

The Bernoulli effect

It is worth considering the design of different oxygen masks, since their effectiveness varies. In order to do this, we need to understand the Bernoulli effect. In the eighteenth century, Daniel Bernoulli made the experimental observation that the pressure in flowing liquids is lowest where the speed of flow is fastest. This observation subsequently became known as the Bernoulli effect, and it is illustrated in Figure 6.19.

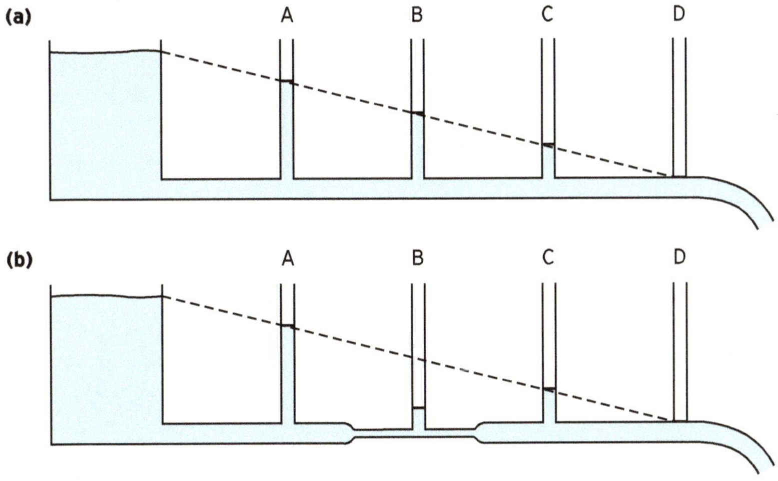

Figure 6.19
An experiment to demonstrate the Bernoulli effect.

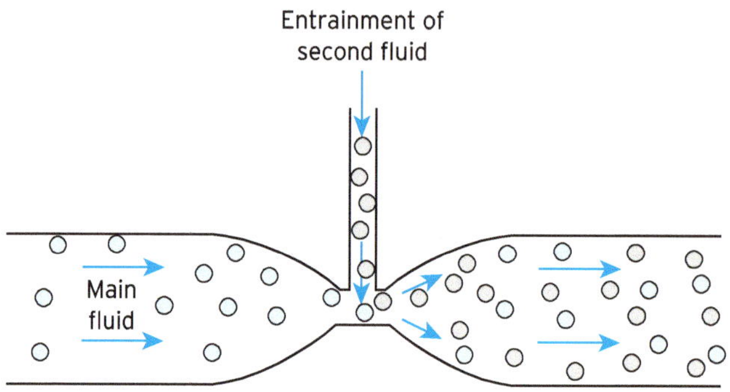

Figure 6.20
The principle of entrainment.

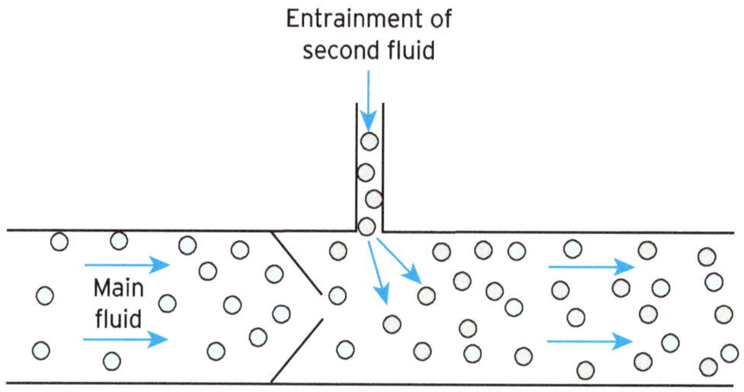

Figure 6.21
Entrainment through a Venturi nozzle.

Note that in Figure 6.19a, fluid is flowing at a constant rate in a horizontal tube. A fall in pressure can be seen between points A to D, as shown in the diminishing heights of the columns. Now consider Figure 6.19b. Here, there is a constriction that causes a drop in pressure at point B. This drop in pressure can be used to draw in (**entrain**) a second fluid, as illustrated in Figure 6.20.

Later experiments by Giovanni Venturi led to the development of a nozzle for the purpose of entrainment; Figure 6.21 shows how such a nozzle works.

The importance of this is that the Bernoulli effect can be used not only to entrain one fluid into another but also to entrain one gas into another or a fluid into a jet of gas. These latter two examples are illustrated in the case of oxygen masks and nebulisers.

Oxygen masks

When a patient uses an oxygen mask, the gas inspired consists of a mixture of oxygen, air from outside the mask and (carbon dioxide-rich) exhaled breath retained in the body of the mask. Furthermore, this mixture depends upon the flow rate created when the patient inspires, and this is not constant - it varies with each breath. The inclusion of a **Venturi barrel** is an attempt to deal with this problem. In a Venturi barrel, a relatively low flow rate of oxygen is forced through a narrow opening, which results in a very fast jet of gas entering the mask. The barrel has side holes; the fast-moving jet of oxygen causes a drop in pressure, and air from outside the mask is drawn in through these holes at a fast rate. The resultant gas mixture created by the mask is at a rate above inspiration, and so the gas mixture is constant. Slight differences in jet design produce different gas mixtures, and so it is possible for the oxygen concentration required by an individual patient to be specified.

Nebulisers

Nebulisers are devices in which a pressurised gas, such as oxygen or air, is used to create droplets of a fluid, perhaps containing a drug, which are then inhaled. The use of nebulisers in order to administer drugs is common in patients with respiratory diseases. Figure 6.22 will be used to illustrate how nebulisers work.

The pressurised gas is forced into the nebuliser through a narrow opening, through which it accelerates, creating a drop in pressure inside the nebuliser - the Bernoulli effect once again. As a consequence of this, droplets of fluid are drawn into this stream of gas, which then leaves the nebuliser and is inhaled by the patient. The fluid used in the nebuliser might be normal saline, which may be of use in loosening tenacious secretions, or a drug for the

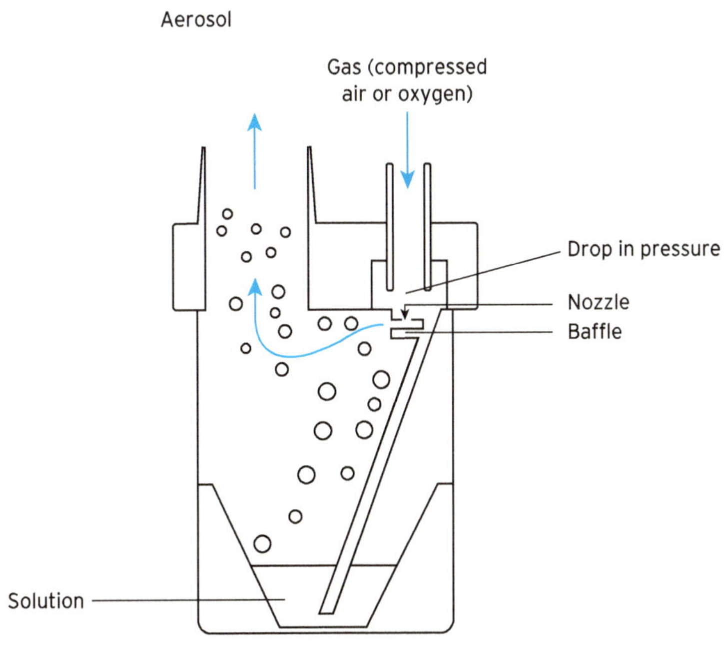

Figure 6.22
A nebuliser.

treatment of a respiratory illness. You might like to find out more about the kinds of drug that are used in nebulisers when you meet a patient using such a device. For now, it is sufficient to note that an understanding of the Bernoulli effect will help you to understand how two common items of medical equipment function.

In-text review

- ✔ Boyle's law (provided the temperature of a gas does not change, the pressure and volume of a fixed amount of gas are related inversely) is used to explain normal breathing.
- ✔ Inspiration results from an increase in the volume of the chest, which causes the pressure within it to fall.
- ✔ Expiration results from a decrease in the volume of the chest, which causes the pressure within it to increase.
- ✔ Henry's law identifies the importance of the partial pressure of a gas in determining the mass of gas that will dissolve in water at a given temperature.
- ✔ Gas exchange in the lungs can be explained in terms of the partial pressure of oxygen and carbon dioxide in alveolar air and venous blood.
- ✔ Oxygen moves down a pressure gradient from inhaled air to the blood.
- ✔ Carbon dioxide moves down a pressure gradient from the blood to inhaled air.
- ✔ The Bernoulli effect, in which the pressure in a liquid is lowest when the speed of flow is fastest, is used to explain the operation of a nebuliser.
- ✔ The Bernoulli effect is used to produce entrainment in the Venturi barrel of an oxygen mask.

Summary

If you look back over this chapter, you will see that we have considered the meaning of pressure and applied this to gases and fluids. A number of aspects of science have been considered, including the gas laws. This has not been simply an academic study, however. We have applied the topics covered to diverse clinical issues such as pressure ulcers, measuring blood pressure and the administration of oxygen. When you next visit a clinical area for a practice placement, identify any of the treatments or procedures mentioned in this chapter and review the science behind them.

Summary points

- → **Pressure is defined as force per unit area.**
- → **Pressure ulcers result from a compromised blood supply caused by the unrelieved pressure of the body against the object on which it is resting.**

- Commonly used units of pressure include pascals (Pa), millimetres of mercury (mmHg) and centimetres of water (cmH_2O).
- Normal arterial blood pressure is considered to be 120/80 mmHg.
- The protection afforded to various body structures by being surrounded by fluid is explained on the basis of Pascal's principle.
- Fluid flows between two points when there is a pressure difference between them.
- Resistance to the flow of a fluid is directly proportional to the length of the vessel in which the fluid is flowing.
- Flow rate is directly proportional to the fourth power of the diameter of a vessel, provided that other factors remain the same - an important consideration in the vascular condition atherosclerosis.
- Pressure = flow × resistance.
- Boyle's law, which states that provided the temperature of a gas does not change, then the pressure and volume of a fixed amount of gas are related inversely, is used to explain normal breathing.
- Henry's law identifies the importance of the partial pressure of a gas in determining the mass of gas that will dissolve in water at a given temperature.
- Gas exchange in the lungs can be explained in terms of the partial pressure of oxygen and carbon dioxide in alveolar air and venous blood.
- The Bernoulli effect, in which the pressure in a liquid is lowest when the speed of flow is fastest, is used to explain the operation of a nebuliser.
- The Bernoulli effect is used to produce entrainment in the Venturi barrel of an oxygen mask.

Self-test questions

1 Suppose that 20% of a gas mixture is oxygen and the pressure of the mixture of gases is 50 kPa. Which one of the following is the partial pressure of oxygen?

(a) 1 kPa.
(b) 10 kPa.
(c) 20 kPa.
(d) 50 kPa.

2 Which one of the following would be considered to be a normal value for systolic blood pressure in mmHg?

(a) 60.
(b) 80.
(c) 120.
(d) 240.

3 When using a sphygmomanometer and stethoscope to measure blood pressure, which one of the following points is considered to be the diastolic pressure?
(a) There is a continuous rushing sound.
(b) A tapping sound can first be heard.
(c) Muffling of the sound.
(d) Disappearance of the sound.

4 According to Boyle's law, pressure is proportional to which one of the following (T = temperature; V = volume)?
(a) 1/T.
(b) 1/V.
(c) V.
(d) VT.

5 Which one of the following represents a normal PaO_2 in kPa?
(a) 30.
(b) 3.
(c) 1.3.
(d) 13.

6 In the case of a container of liquid, which of the following statements about pressure at a point in the liquid are true?
(a) It depends upon the depth of the point below the surface.
(b) It acts in all directions.
(c) It depends upon whether the point is in the middle of the container or near the sides.
(d) It depends upon the volume of liquid above the point.

7 A patient with an intravenous infusion is prescribed 1 l of fluid to be administered over 8 hours. Assuming that there are 20 drops to a millilitre, to which one of the following rates (in drops per minute) should the infusion be regulated?
(a) 12.
(b) 24.
(c) 32.
(d) 42.

8 Suppose that the diameter of a blood vessel is reduced to half. Provided the blood pressure remains the same, to which one of the following fractions would flow through the vessel be reduced to:
(a) 1/4.
(b) 1/2.
(c) 1/8.
(d) 1/16.

9 Concerning gaseous exchange in the lungs, which of the following are true?
(a) P_AO_2 is greater than P_vO_2.
(b) P_vO_2 is greater than P_aCO_2.
(c) P_vCO_2 is greater than P_aCO_2.
(d) P_aO_2 is greater than P_AO_2.

10 Concerning an oxygen mask with a Venturi barrel, which of the following statements are true?
(a) Atmospheric air is entrained through the Venturi barrel.
(b) The mask may be described as a variable performance device.
(c) Relatively low oxygen flow rates produce a high flow rate through the mask.
(d) The gas mixture delivered to the patient is constant in composition.

Further study/exercises

1 **Suppose you wish to identify which of your patients are at risk of developing pressure ulcers. How could this be done?** (Hint: find out about pressure ulcer risk calculation scores such as those of Norton and Waterlow.)

2 **How are pressure ulcers prevented?**

European Pressure Ulcer Advisor Panel: www.epuap.org
Pressure Ulcer Prevention Guidelines: www.epuap.org/glprevention.html
NHS National Institute for Health and Clinical Excellence (NICE): www.nice.org.uk
Pressure ulcers: www.nice.org.uk/page.aspx?o=20052
Royal College of Nursing (RCN): www.rcn.org.uk
Pressure Ulcer Risk and Prevention: www.rcn.org.uk/publications/pdf/guidelines/pressure_ulcer_implement_audit_protocol.pdf
Waterlow Score: www.judy-waterlow.co.uk

7

Biological molecules and food

Learning outcomes

After reading the following chapter and undertaking personal study, you should be able to:

1. Identify the seven components of the diet.
2. Outline the chemical structure of carbohydrates, fats and proteins.
3. Describe how carbohydrates, fats and proteins are digested and outline their use within the body.
4. Outline the roles of vitamins and minerals within the body.
5. Describe a healthy diet.
6. Outline the relationship between the different nutritional groups, health and illness.

Introduction

If you were to list the most important health issues affecting our society, what would you include? There are many, but within any list of health threats some, such as heart disease and obesity, are related to diet. If you have read Chapter 3, you may have wondered how quickly you would be able to relate chemistry to health care. Healthy eating is one example of a subject in which knowledge of chemistry is helpful, since foods are chemicals. To begin with, we return to a distinction made in Chapter 3 - **organic chemistry** and **inorganic chemistry**. Organic chemistry is the study of compounds that contain carbon; this is important here, since most components of the diet are organic compounds. Inorganic chemistry is the study of substances that do not contain carbon; some nutrients are inorganic substances.

Diet and food

The components of the diet may be divided into seven groups:

- **carbohydrates**
- **proteins**
- **lipids** (fats)
- **vitamins**
- **minerals**
- **water**
- **fibre** (roughage/non-starch polysaccharide).

All of these are important substances in food, but there are significant differences between them. For example, not all are organic compounds. Water is not, and neither are the minerals. Some, such as the carbohydrates, proteins and lipids, have to be digested (broken down) before they can be absorbed, while vitamins, minerals and water are absorbed unchanged. Finally, fibre is neither digested nor absorbed but provides bulk to food and is important in the maintenance of formed faeces that pass readily through the intestines.

Carbohydrates

The word 'carbohydrate' indicates that this type of substance contains carbon, hydrogen and oxygen. There are three classes of carbohydrate:

- **monosaccharides** (simple sugars)
- **disaccharides** (double sugars)
- **polysaccharides** (complex sugars).

Monosaccharides

The word 'monosaccharide' means 'one sugar', and it is used to indicate those compounds that cannot be broken down into more simple sugars. The ratio of carbon, hydrogen and oxygen in monosaccharides is 1 : 2 : 1, as is the case in **glucose** - $C_6H_{12}O_6$. Glucose is found naturally, in honey along with another monosaccharide, **fructose**, which is the sugar found in fruit. Indeed, the word 'fructose' means 'fruit sugar'. **Galactose** is a monosaccharide found in milk; like fructose and glucose, its molecular formula is $C_6H_{12}O_6$. If you have read Chapter 3, you will realise that these three sugars are **isomers** - compounds with the same **molecular formula** but different **structural formulae**. The structural formulae of all the monosaccharides are not given, but that of glucose can be seen in Figure 7.1.

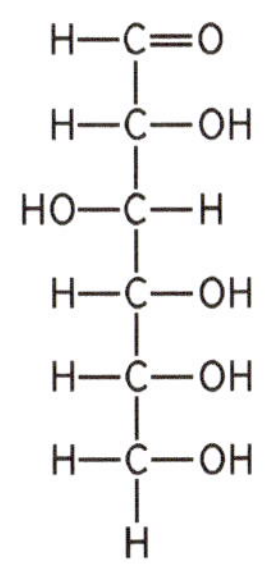

Figure 7.1
The structural formula of glucose.

When ingested, glucose, fructose and galactose are absorbed into the body through the **ileum** of the gut (Figure 7.2) without the need to be broken down into simpler substances. Fructose and galactose, however, are subsequently converted into glucose, since only glucose can be used as a source of energy.

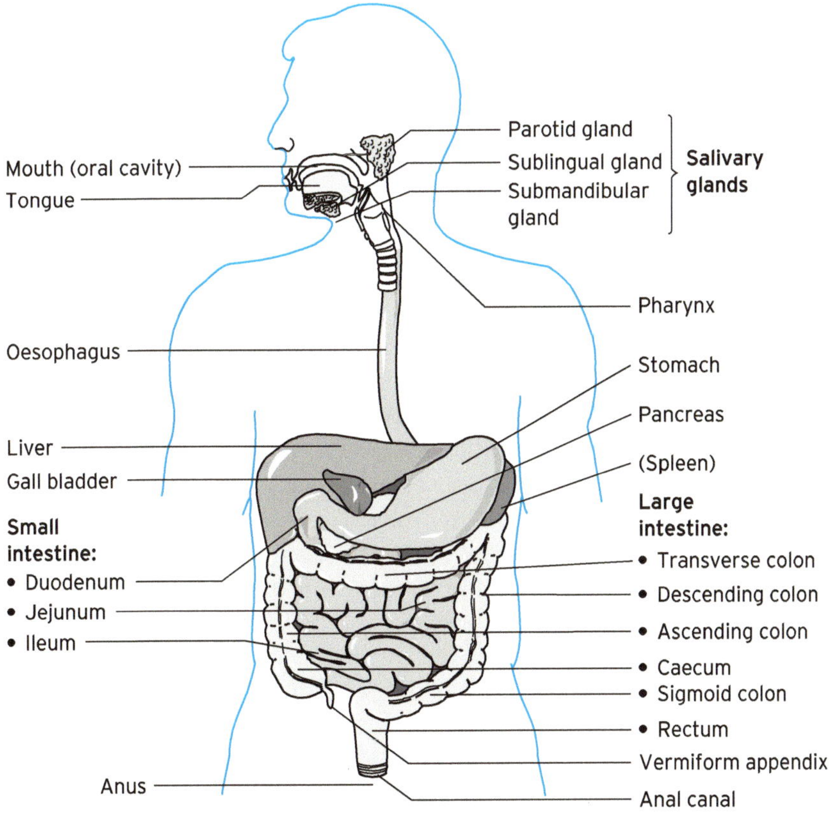

Figure 7.2
The gastrointestinal tract. (From Coleman G. J. and Dewar D. (1997) *The Addison Wesley Science Handbook for Students*. Don Mills, Ontario: Addison-Wesley.)

The cells of the body are dependent upon receiving a constant supply of glucose. Sometimes a pinprick sample of blood is obtained from a patient and tested for glucose concentration. The normal range is 3.9-5.6 mmol/l. In the condition **diabetes mellitus**, blood sugar is elevated (**hyperglycaemia**) and the body begins to excrete glucose in the urine (**glycosuria**). Glucose is not normally present in the urine, but if diabetes is suspected a patient's urine may be tested for its presence. Since one form of diabetes can go undetected for years, testing the urine of apparently healthy individuals is a useful health-screening measure. The traditional test for glucose involves a laboratory procedure in which a colour change is observed. In the clinical setting, however, we do not have to resort to using test tubes and reagent solutions, since the reagents are presented in pads on a plastic strip. In the analysis of urine (**urinalysis**), the reagent strip is dipped into a fresh sample of urine and the colour change is read after a given period of time. The amount of glucose present is determined by comparing the colour of the reagent pad against a colour chart. Urinalysis reagent strips contain a number of different reagent pads, so tests for a number of substances can be undertaken at the same time. It is important when undertaking such tests to follow the instructions of the manufacturer of the brand of reagent strips being used. Reagent strips are also available for testing blood sugar levels.

Disaccharides

Disaccharides are formed from a condensation reaction between two monosaccharides. A **condensation reaction** is one in which water is eliminated from the following reaction:

$$C_6H_{12}O_6 + C_6H_{12}O_6 \rightarrow C_{12}H_{22}O_{11} + H_2O$$

Three disaccharides are important. **Sucrose** is what we buy in packets at the shops. It is supplied as crystals of different sizes (table sugar, icing sugar, and so on), but it is all sucrose. Sucrose was first extracted from sugar cane and brought to Britain in the eighteenth century following the colonisation of the West Indies. Today, however, it is extracted from sugar beet. **Maltose** is the sugar that results when a plant seed converts its long-term energy store of **starch** for the purposes of germination and growth. Maltose is what makes bean sprouts taste sweet and the sugar manufactured by grains such as barley when they are given warmth and moisture in the malting house. You will have seen this process if you have ever visited a brewery or distillery. Finally, **lactose** is the disaccharide found in milk. It is possible to break these disaccharide molecules to form two monosaccharides by boiling them with acid - a reaction referred to as **hydrolysis** (meaning 'to break with water'):

$$C_{12}H_{22}O_{11} + H_2O \rightarrow C_6H_{12}O_6 + C_6H_{12}O_6$$

Since disaccharides are too large to be absorbed, the body also has to perform hydrolysis, but it uses **enzymes** rather than boiling with acid. Remember that enzymes are protein catalysts that speed up chemical reactions by reducing the amount of energy required to get the reaction started (**activation energy**). The enzymes involved in disaccharide digestion are found in the **duodenum** - part of the **small intestine**. The resultant monosacharides are then absorbed in the ileum, another part of the small intestine (see Figure 7.2).

In the naming of enzymes, the prefix identifies the **substrate** (substance acted upon) and the suffix 'ase' indicates that an enzyme is being referred to. Consequently, **maltase**, **sucrase** and **lactase** are the enzymes that act upon maltose, sucrose and lactose, respectively. These enzymatic reactions are given below:

$$\text{Maltose} \xrightarrow{\text{maltase}} \text{glucose} + \text{glucose}$$

$$\text{Sucrose} \xrightarrow{\text{sucrase}} \text{glucose} + \text{fructose}$$

$$\text{Lactose} \xrightarrow{\text{lactase}} \text{glucose} + \text{galactose}$$

Note that in the digestion of one disaccharide molecule, two monosaccharide molecules result; one of these is always glucose. In addition, maltose yields a second glucose molecule, sucrose a molecule of fructose, and lactose a molecule of galactose. At this point you might begin to wonder what would happen if one of the aforementioned enzymes was not present. This happens rarely, but lactase can be absent, as Practice point 7.1 explains.

Practice point 7.1

Lactose intolerance

If you are involved in caring for infants, you may look after babies who fail to produce lactase and who cannot, therefore, digest lactose. This condition is known as **lactose intolerance** and it is characterised by diarrhoea and failure to thrive. Lactose intolerance is a serious illness, since lactose is present in all animal milk, which of course is the only source of food in early life.

- ***What might affected infants be given instead?***

Soya milk is used.

Polysaccharides

Polysaccharides consist of chains of monosaccharides - poly means 'many'. The polysaccharide chain may be elongated and the molecule described as **fibrous**. Such chains are often employed for the purpose of giving strength and support. An example is the plant polysaccharide **cellulose**, which is important in plant cell walls. Alternatively, the polysaccharide chain may be wound up like a ball, when the expression **globular** is used. Examples of globular polysaccharides are energy-storage molecules such as **starch** in plants and **glycogen** in animals. The naturally occurring **anticoagulant** (impairs blood clotting) **heparin** is also a globular polysaccharide.

After ingestion, polysaccharides are broken down in the gastrointestinal tract. The digestion of cooked starch, such as in bread and potatoes, begins in the mouth with the enzyme salivary **amylase** (from the salivary glands). Since food spends relatively little time in the mouth, the process is not completed there. The effect of salivary amylase is to convert some of the starch in a meal to substances called **dextrins**, which are intermediate molecules between starch and maltose. You may have performed a simple test using iodine to show this. Iodine turns cooked starch blue/black. Try it on some bread. Now take another piece of bread and chew it for a while before repeating the test. You will now find iodine produces a red colour, indicating the presence of dextrins. Carbohydrate digestion does not continue in the stomach because of the low pH there. The environment in the duodenum, however, is alkaline, and the conversion of starch to maltose is completed by further amylase - this time from the **pancreas** (see Figure 7.2). Finally, the maltose that results is digested into two molecules of glucose, as described previously.

In summary, disaccharides and polysaccharides are broken down into the three monosaccharides, which are absorbed via the cells of the ileum. Here, fructose and galactose are converted into glucose before absorption into the blood. Therefore, glucose is the end product of carbohydrate digestion. Glucose is important because it is the body's principal source of energy. The body regulates the blood glucose level very carefully, as Practice point 7.2 explains.

Practice point 7.2

How does the body keep a constant blood glucose level?

After glucose has been absorbed into the blood, it travels in the **hepatic portal vein** to the **liver**. Some of this glucose is converted by **hepatocytes** (liver cells) into the storage product glycogen. This process is known as **glyconeogenesis** (literally 'making glycogen'). The hormone **insulin** (from the pancreas) and a number of enzymes are important in this process. If blood sugar subsequently becomes lowered (**hypoglycaemia**), glycogen in the liver can be broken down into glucose once more in a process called **glycogenolysis**. **Epinephrine** (adrenaline) and **glucagon** (also from the pancreas) are important hormones in this process. In addition, the body is able to manufacture glucose from non-carbohydrate sources such as **amino acids**. This process is described as **gluconeogenesis**, meaning 'making new glucose'.

Energy production

Of course, the ultimate fate of glucose in the body is to be broken down (**glycolsis**) so that the energy locked in its molecules is released. This is described in Chapter 8. Before we leave this topic, we consider an important problem of carbohydrate metabolism - diabetes mellitus - in Practice point 7.3.

Practice point 7.3

Diabetes mellitus

Diabetes mellitus is a disorder of carbohydrate metabolism, one form of which (type I) is characterised by an inadequate production of the hormone insulin by the beta cells of the **islets of Langerhans** in the pancreas. Insulin is required for the uptake of glucose by most cells of the body, except brain cells. Therefore, when insulin production is inadequate, the cells are supplied inadequately, no matter how much carbohydrate is eaten. One of the features of diabetes mellitus is **hyperglycaemia**.

- ***Work out the reason for this.***

In the absence of insulin, glucose absorbed into the blood has nowhere to go, and consequently the blood sugar level rises. This high blood sugar level has a number of effects, including increasing the susceptibility to infection. In the long term, there may be damage to capillaries, such as those of the **retina** at the back of the eye; after many years, blindness could result. While the blood sugar level is high, however, the cells do not have access to this source of energy due to the lack of insulin. Not surprisingly then, the patient often complains of weakness. The blood glucose level may rise so high that glucose begins to appear in the urine (glycosuria). In **glomerular filtrate** (the fluid produced when the kidney filters the blood), glucose exerts an **osmotic** effect, which results in increased urine output. You may need to think about this point a little more, but for now it is enough to know that **polyuria** (increased urine output) is another feature of diabetes mellitus.

- ***Can you work out what might be the effect of an elevated urine output on thirst?***

Perhaps this question is a little more obvious. The patient complains of thirst and drinks a lot (**polydipsia**). There is, of course, much more to learn about diabetes mellitus, but in summary it is characterised by a lack of insulin, which leads to hyperglycaemia, weakness, susceptibility to infection, polyuria, polydipsia and, in the long term, possibly blindness.

In-text review

- ✔ The seven components of the diet are carbohydrates, proteins, lipids, vitamins, minerals, fibre and water.
- ✔ The process of digestion of carbohydrates, proteins and lipids is enzymatic hydrolysis.
- ✔ Carbohydrates are divided into three classes - monosaccharides (simple sugars), disaccharides (double sugars) and polysaccharides (complex sugars).
- ✔ Glucose, fructose and galactose are monosacharides found in the diet.
- ✔ Maltose, sucrose and lactose are disaccharides found in the diet.
- ✔ Disaccharide-digesting enzymes are maltase, sucrase and lactase.
- ✔ Starch is the digestible plant polysaccharide found in the diet.
- ✔ Starch is digested by the enzyme amylase.
- ✔ All carbohydrates are digested to form simple sugars, which can then be absorbed.
- ✔ Diabetes mellitus is characterised by hyperglycaemia, caused by a lack of the hormone insulin necessary for the cellular uptake of glucose.

Proteins

Proteins consist of chains of molecules called **amino acids**. Like carbohydrates, proteins contain carbon, hydrogen and oxygen, but amino acids also contain nitrogen. The general structure of amino acids is given in Figure 7.3, in which R represents a hydrogen atom or chain of carbon atoms with hydrogen attached.

In proteins, amino acids are joined together by **peptide bonds** formed following a condensation reaction, as illustrated in Figure 7.4. The molecule formed from the combination of up to ten amino acids is termed a **peptide**, while longer chains are referred to as **polypeptides**. Only chains of more than 100 amino acids are called proteins. Twenty different amino acids are important in health. Non-essential amino acids are those that can be synthesised by the body (provided other amino acids are present), and as a consequence they do not need to be present in the diet. However, eight amino acids cannot be synthesised and so must be present in the food we eat. These are termed **essential amino acids**.

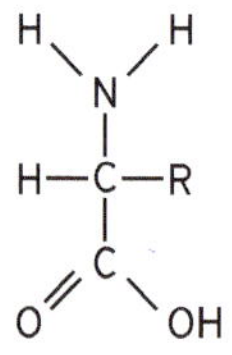

Figure 7.3
The general structure of amino acids.

Based upon the relative amounts of amino acids that they contain, proteins in the diet are classified as complete (high-quality) or incomplete (low-quality). Complete proteins provide all the essential amino acids in adequate amounts and are obtained only from animals (meat, fish, eggs and dairy products). In contrast, plant proteins are incomplete, as they are deficient in one or more amino acids. Because different plant proteins lack different essential amino acids, however, they can be combined in the diet so as to complement each other. When all sources of animal protein are avoided (pure vegetarian/vegan diet), the consumption of a combination of vegetables, grains, nuts and seeds ensures that sufficient quantities of all the essential amino acids are consumed.

Protein structure

The order of amino acids in a protein chain is termed the **primary structure** (Figure 7.5a). We might draw an analogy between this and the order of coloured beads in a child's necklace. Few proteins, however, exist as simple chains. The **secondary structure** of a protein results from **hydrogen bond** formation between different areas of the chain. The most common

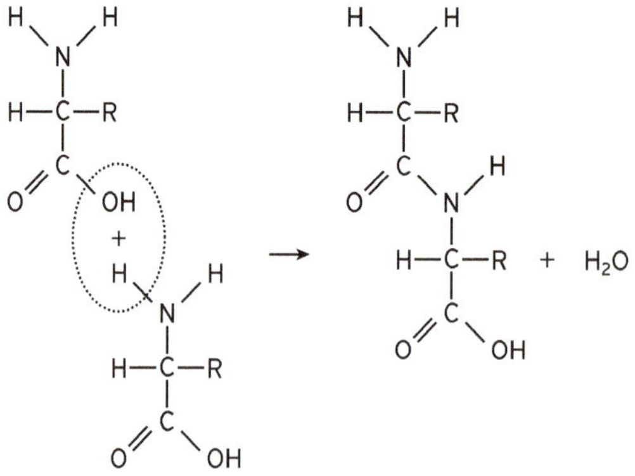

Figure 7.4
The formation of a peptide bond.

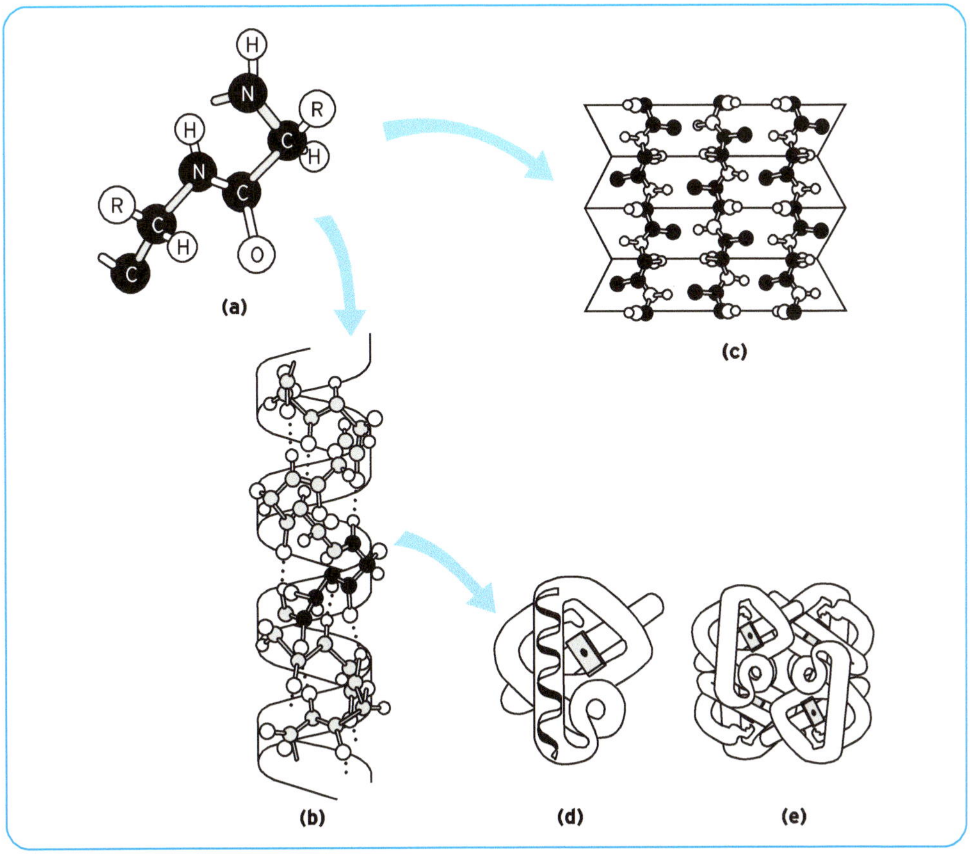

Figure 7.5
The (a) primary, (b) secondary, (d) tertiary and (e) quaternary structure of proteins. (Adapted from Sackheim G. I. (1996) *An Introduction to Chemistry for Biology Students*, 5th edn, Belmont, CA: Benjamin/Cummins.)

form of secondary structure is the alpha-helix (Figure 7.5b), which results from a tight coiling of the amino acid chain. In contrast, the beta-pleated sheet results when hydrogen bonds link chains that lie side by side (Figure 7.5c). A higher level of complexity, referred to as the **tertiary structure**, occurs when alpha-helices or beta-pleated sheets fold upon one another to produce a globular (ball-like) molecule (Figure 7.5d). Finally, when several protein units, each with its own primary, secondary and tertiary structure, combine to form a more complex molecule, the term **quaternary structure** is applied (Figure 7.5e). For example, the protein **haemoglobin** (responsible for oxygen transport) has a quaternary structure of four subunits.

Proteins can also be classified as globular or fibrous in a similar way to carbohydrates described previously. The chains of globular proteins are wound up like a ball. They have functional rather than structural uses – that is, they perform functions other than forming part of the structure of the body. Enzymes are globular proteins, as are the **plasma** (liquid part of blood) proteins **albumin** and **fibrinogen** and the **erythrocyte** (red blood cell) pigment haemoglobin. In contrast, the chains of fibrous proteins are extended like fibres in a rope, and these have important structural functions. For example, the protein **keratin** confers the property of impermeability on the **epidermis** (outer layer of the skin). Compare the appearance of the inside of your mouth with the skin covering your body. The skin covering your body is keratinised and is much tougher and less permeable than the mucous membrane of the mouth. Keratin is also an important component of hair and nails. Other examples of fibrous proteins include the helical molecules **collagen** and **elastin**. These are also important in the skin, but this time in the **dermis** (lower layer of the skin). Collagen confers toughness, while elastin ensures that the dermis has a degree of elasticity. To check this out, pinch a fold of skin and note how quickly it springs back when you let go. If you were to repeat this simple test on the skin of an elderly person, the fold would remain for some moments after pinching. This is because there is less elastin in the skin of elderly people compared with young people; as a consequence, the skin of elderly people is more susceptible to trauma. You will need to understand this when caring for elderly people.

Protein digestion

Protein digestion begins in the lumen of the stomach, where the enzyme precursor **pepsinogen** is converted into the active enzyme **pepsin** by **hydrochloric acid**. Pits in the lining of the stomach (**gastric pits**) contain a number of secretory cells. Some produce mucus to protect the tissues, while **zymogenic** (chief) cells secrete pepsinogen and **oxyntic** (parietal) cells secrete hydrochloric acid.

- ***Why is pepsin itself not secreted but instead formed from the action of hydrochloric acid on pepsinogen?***

Since pepsin is a protein-digesting enzyme, secretion of it in its active form may result in the digestion of the stomach cells themselves. When performing laboratory experiments with pepsin, take care not to splash it into your eyes. **Wear safety glasses or shields whenever you perform an experiment involving chemicals**.

The action of pepsin upon protein chains is to break them down into a number of smaller (peptide) chains. The peptides that result from the digestion of a protein are sometimes referred to as **peptones**. This process may be summarised as follows:

$$\text{pepsinogen} + HCl_{(aq)} \rightarrow \text{pepsin}$$
$$\swarrow$$
$$\text{protein} \rightarrow \text{peptides}$$

Protein digestion continues in the duodenum with two enzymes from the pancreas - **trypsin** and **chymotrypsin**. Trypsin breaks down peptide chains into smaller peptide chains. Like pepsin, trypsin is not secreted in an active form but results from the action of the enzyme **enterokinase**, found in intestinal secretions, upon the enzyme precursor **trypsinogen**:

$$\text{enterokinase}$$
$$\downarrow$$
$$\text{trypsinogen} \rightarrow \text{trypsin}$$
$$\swarrow$$
$$\text{peptides} \rightarrow \text{smaller peptides}$$

Furthermore, trypsin itself activates another enzyme precursor present in pancreatic secretions - **chymotrypsinogen**:

$$\text{chymotrypsinogen} \xrightarrow{\text{trypsin}} \text{chymotrypsin}$$

Chymotrypsin has a similar action to trypsin. Finally, a group of enzymes called **peptidases**, some of which are present in pancreatic secretions and some in intestinal secretions, break off amino acids from the small peptide chains. These amino acids then diffuse into the bloodstream via the intestinal **villi** and pass to the liver in the hepatic portal vein.

Amino acids and the liver

The liver uses its supply of amino acids to synthesise a number of proteins, including the serum (liquid part of blood) proteins **albumin**, **fibrinogen** and **prothrombin**. The latter two are important in blood clotting. Other amino acids are circulated and used by cells elsewhere in the body, while the liver also plays a role in breaking down unwanted amino acids. Damaged components of the body are constantly being replaced, and this includes protein.

What happens to unwanted amino acids?

In the liver, the nitrogen-containing part of amino acids (amino group) is removed - a process known as **deamination**. This leads to the formation of **ammonia**, which is extremely toxic, but the liver converts ammonia into the less toxic substance **urea**, which is eventually excreted in the urine along with **creatinine** - the waste substance produced from the breakdown of muscle protein.

Before we leave this topic, we consider disturbances of protein metabolism in Practice point 7.4.

Practice point 7.4

Disturbances of protein metabolism

A number of conditions affect our ability to digest or use protein. For example, **cystic fibrosis** is a genetic disease in which the pancreas and other exocrine glands become blocked with abnormally viscous mucus. Consequently, pancreatic enzymes cannot reach the duodenum and protein digestion is impaired. Fortunately, these enzymes can be added to food just before eating, but this does not prevent the effects of the disease elsewhere in the body.

Second, **phenylketonuria** is a condition caused by an enzyme deficiency that results in failure to break down the amino acid **phenylalanine**. The accumulation of phenylalanine in infants leads to mental retardation, so a diet low in this amino acid must be consumed by infants with the enzyme deficiency.

Nitrogen balance

The term 'nitrogen balance' refers to the state in which the intake of nitrogen (protein) equals its loss. A negative nitrogen balance is the state in which protein intake is less than expenditure, as is the case in starvation and **anorexia nervosa**. In contrast, conditions affecting the liver or kidneys, in which the ability to metabolise and eliminate amino acids is impaired, require the intake of protein be restricted.

Lipids

The terms 'lipid' and 'fat' are used synonymously for a group of substances that contain the elements carbon, hydrogen and oxygen but not in a fixed ratio, as is the case in monosaccharides. Lipids often contain phosphorus. A number of different molecules are classified as lipids because they share the common physical property of being insoluble in water but soluble in organic solvents such as **acetone**. Four classes of lipid are described: **glycerides**, **sterols**, **phospholipids** and **prostaglandins**. Each will be examined here, but we shall concentrate on the most abundant group - the glycerides.

Glycerides

Glycerides are also known as neutral fats and are the substances that first come to mind when the word 'fat' is used. Glycerides are stored in **adipose tissue** (fat tissue) of the body, where they form an important long-term energy store and act as an insulator. Adipose tissue also gives shape to the body and provides protection for vital structures such as the kidneys. Glycerides are composed of two types of molecule - **carboxylic acids** (fatty acids) and **glycerol**. You have already encountered carboxylic acids in previous chapters. They conform to the general formula RCOOH and undergo a reaction with alcohols to form **esters**. Glycerides are esters of the alcohol glycerol and different carboxylic acids. Remember that glycerol possesses three **hydroxyl groups** with which to react with carboxylic acids. If only one hydroxyl group reacts with a carboxylic acid, then the resultant ester is referred to as a **monoglyceride**. If two hydroxyl groups react, a **diglyceride** results, and if all three react the result is a **triglyceride**. Most of the fat within the body occurs as triglycerides. The formation of triglycerides is illustrated in Figure 7.6.

Saturated and unsaturated fats

If you are to understand health-promotion advice relating to **saturated** and **unsaturated** fats, then you must first understand the meaning of these terms and something of the chemistry of fats. Saturated fats are those in which all the carbon atoms of the component carboxylic acids have the maximum number of hydrogen atoms attached - that is, there are no double bonds in the molecule. An example is palmitic acid ($C_{15}H_{31}COOH$), the structure of which is shown in Figure 7.7.

Saturated fats are solid at room temperature and are mainly of animal origin (think of lard and butter). Some plants, however, such as coconuts and palms, also produce saturated fats. Unsaturated fats are those in which double bonds occur in the carboxylic acid chain, and

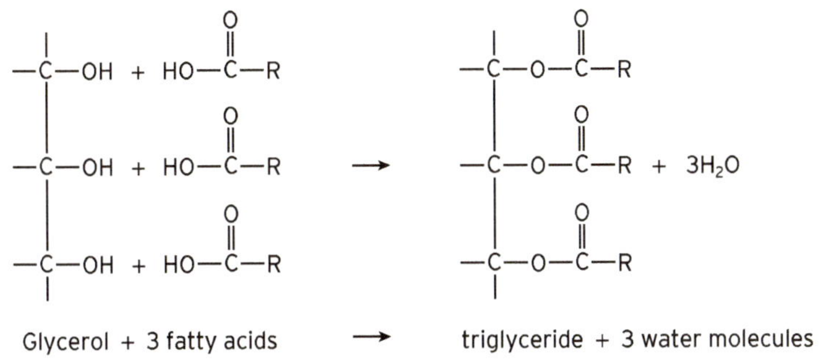

Figure 7.6
The formation of a triglyceride.

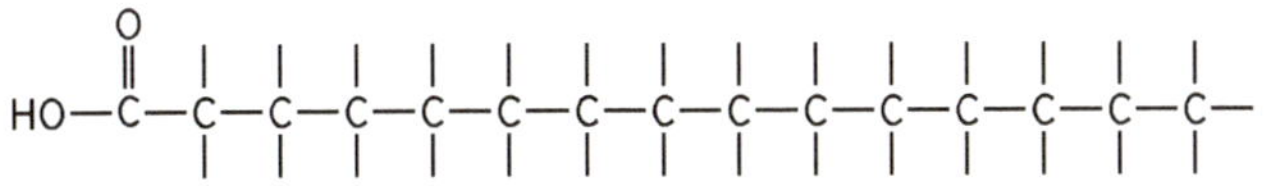

Figure 7.7
The structure of palmitic acid.

therefore the molecules have fewer than the maximum number of hydrogen atoms. The terms **monounsaturated** and **polyunsaturated** are used to distinguish between those fats with carboxylic acid chains that have one double bond (monounsaturated) and those with more than one double bond (polyunsaturated). An example of a polyunsaturated carboxylic acid is linolenic acid ($C_{18}H_{29}COOH$), the structure of which is shown in Figure 7.8.

Unsaturated fats are liquids or soft solids at room temperature and are of plant extraction (think of sunflower oil and vegetable oil). Sometimes a more solid presentation of vegetable fat is required, as is the case in margarine. In order to achieve this, hydrogen atoms are added to the carboxylic acid molecules, which are then described as **hydrogenated**. Indeed, if you look at the information on margarine cartons, you will often find this referred to.

For most people, a consideration of saturated and unsaturated fat becomes important only when they think about their health and whether they are too fat. But how do we determine who is too fat or thin? We consider this in Practice point 7.5. Why some people remain fat and others become lean is discussed in Practice point 7.6.

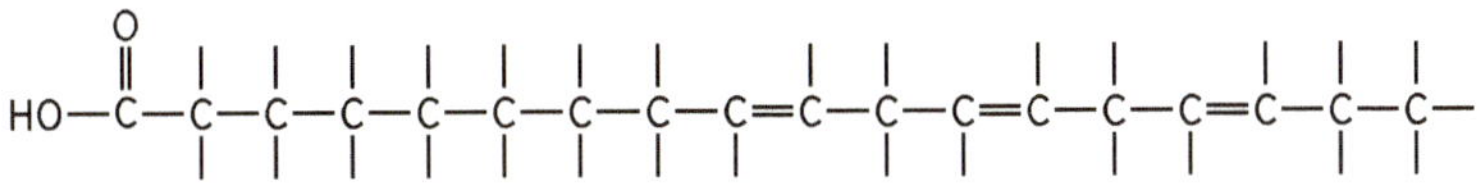

Figure 7.8
The structure of linolenic acid.

Practice point 7.5

Who is too fat or too thin?

Most people believe that there is a weight that is 'about right' for them and that being either excessively underweight or overweight is unhealthy. Nonetheless, they may be unsure as to what their ideal weight is.

- ***How do we determine who is too fat or too thin?***

Clearly, we cannot rely upon what we intuitively think is acceptable, since this would be influenced by social expectations and have more to do with what we perceive as attractive. When we want a realistic idea of the appropriateness of a person's weight, we have to compare the weight with height in the calculation of the **body mass index** (BMI):

$$\text{Body mass index} = \frac{\text{weight in kg}}{(\text{height in m})^2}$$

Body mass index	Description
20-25	Ideal
30	Obese
40	Gross obesity

- ***Why do we consider a body mass index of 20–25 to be ideal?***

The reason is that a body mass index of 20-25 is associated with the lowest risk of illness, while outside this range the risk is elevated. We use body mass index in a number of different situations, including promoting health in patients who are obese or who have diseases that are associated with obesity (such as type II diabetes mellitus). Some patients may be undernourished - they might have a serious acute illness such as cancer of the **oesophagus** or perhaps they have mental health problems such as **anorexia nervosa** or **bulimia nervosa**. Finally, assessing the risk of **pressure ulcers** involves determining whether the patient is overweight, and body mass index is useful in this situation.

Practice point 7.6

Why do some people become fat and others remain lean?

We have looked previously at how we decide whether a person is overweight by using body mass index. Now we look briefly at obesity itself.

- ***Is obesity a disease?***

If obesity is a disease, then it should be possible to formulate a theory that would explain why it develops in certain people and not in others. For our theory to be accepted, it must be reliable - that is, it must explain all cases of obesity. No such single theory for obesity exists, and therefore we cannot consider obesity to be a disease. Nonetheless, there are some endocrine conditions, such as **hypothyroidism** (low levels of the hormone **thyroxine**) and **Cushing's disease** (increased secretion of hormones of the **adrenal cortex**), that do involve weight gain. The important thing to note here is that when such conditions exist, weight gain is not the only symptom. Whatever the cause of obesity, the following equation must be true:

$$\text{Energy intake} = \text{energy expenditure} \pm \text{changes in body energy stores}$$

Since obesity represents an increase in the body's energy stores (that is, fatness), then it must result from either an excessive energy intake or reduced energy expenditure.

- ***So does obesity result from overeating?***

Surprisingly, most large-scale surveys have failed to demonstrate overeating by obese people, although we might question the reliability of the dietary record as a method of investigation. It is possible that those people who take part in such surveys simply under-report what they eat, or perhaps they actually eat less for the period of investigation.

- ***What about energy expenditure? Are obese people simply underactive?***

Once again, research has failed to demonstrate conclusively that this is the case. Perhaps you are beginning to realise that obesity is more complicated than it first appears and that different people are obese for different reasons. Nonetheless, overeating and too little exercise are possible causes. In fact, whatever the cause of obesity, and provided disease is absent, reducing the amount of food consumed and increasing the amount of exercise taken must result in weight loss.

- ***Does the type rather than the amount of food eaten influence the development of obesity?***

'Empty-calorie' foods (those that have no additional nutritional value) such as sugar provide a lot of energy in a small volume and so fail to fill you up. In addition, sugar actually stimulates the appetite. Perhaps that's why desserts appear so 'moreish', even when we feel full after a main course. In contrast, sources of complex carbohydrates, such as wholemeal bread and potatoes, provide calories in a much more filling form. In addition, they also contain other nutritional substances, such as vitamins, minerals and fibre. Finally, studies suggest that we fat faster when more of the energy is provided as fat than as carbohydrate.

- ***How is this related to health promotion?***

It makes sense to recommend that if the amount of energy consumed by the individual is about right, then most of this energy is provided in the form of carbohydrate and not as fat.

- ***What kind of carbohydrates would you recommend to replace fat?***

You will probably have worked out that complex carbohydrates rather than empty-calorie foods should be chosen.

Digestion and absorption of glycerides

The small intestine is the only site of fat digestion, since the pancreas is the only source of the fat-digesting enzyme **lipase**. Since glycerides and their breakdown products are all insoluble in water, however, special treatment is necessary before digestion can take place. In water, fats aggregate in large globules, with a relatively small proportion of molecules on the surface and exposed to water-soluble lipase. Upon entry to the duodenum, however, fat globules are acted upon by **bile salts**. Bile salts are molecules with a **hydrophobic** (water-repelling) end and a **hydrophilic** (water-attracting) end. The hydrophobic end adheres to glyceride molecules, while the hydrophilic end repels other bile salt molecules. The result is that small droplets of lipid are pulled away from larger globules and, as a consequence, many more glyceride molecules are exposed to lipase. Such a solution of small suspended droplets is called an **emulsion**. You might wonder what would happen if bile was not present. This is considered in Practice point 7.7.

Practice point 7.7

Biliary obstruction

Bile is produced by the liver and stored in the **gall bladder**, where it is concentrated before being passed through a series of ducts referred to as the **biliary tree**. Sometimes its components solidify and form **gall stones**. These may obstruct the biliary tree, preventing the passage of bile to the duodenum.

- ***How would this affect the patient?***

Without bile, lipids present in the diet are not emulsified and digestion is impaired. As a consequence, undigested fat is passed in the faeces.

- ***How is this identified?***

First, the faeces tend to be bulky and pale. Remember, too, that fat floats on water, and so another effect is that the faeces float. Finally, the gall bladder is stimulated to contract by the presence of a meal containing fat, but when the biliary tree is obstructed this results in pain.

- ***How might this pain be alleviated?***

The patient may be advised to adhere to a low-fat diet.

The action of lipase upon triglycerides is to break off two of the carboxylic acid chains, thus yielding free carboxylic acids and monoglycerides, both of which are insoluble in water. Free carboxylic acids and monoglycerides quickly become associated with bile salts and **lecithin** (a phospholipid in bile) to form **micelles**. These are collections of insoluble substances surrounded by bile salts, with the hydrophilic ends oriented towards the outside. The hydrophobic core consists of monoglycerides, carboxylic acids, **cholesterol** and fat-soluble vitamins. Micelles are similar to, but much smaller than, emulsion droplets and can diffuse between the **microvilli** (small finger-like projections) of the cells of the ileum. When in close contact with the cells, the lipids, their breakdown products and fat-soluble vitamins diffuse through the lipid-containing plasma membrane and enter the cells of the intestinal epithelium (lining). Here, the free carboxylic acids and monoglycerides are turned back into triglycerides. The triglycerides are then combined with small amounts of phospholipid, cholesterol and free carboxylic acids and are coated with protein to form water-soluble lipoprotein droplets called **chylomicrons**. Chylomicrons are too large to enter blood capillaries and so diffuse into the more permeable lymph capillaries (**lacteals**). Thus, the route for the absorption of the end products of lipid digestion is quite different from that for glucose and amino acids, which are small enough to enter blood capillaries. Chylomicrons appear in the circulation, eventually, however, as they drain in turn through lymph vessels and the **thoracic duct**, which empties its fatty milky contents (**chyle**) into the left **subclavian vein** in the base of the neck.

Sterols

The structure of this group of lipids is based around the circular sterol molecule. Included in this group are cholesterol and steroid hormones such as **progesterone**, **testosterone**, **cortisone** and **aldosterone**. (Note that the names of steroid hormones usually end in 'one'.)

Phospholipids

Phospholipids are similar to glycerides, but a molecule containing phosphate replaces one of the carboxylic acid molecules. You will encounter phospholipids as important components of cell membranes.

Prostaglandins

Prostaglandins are lipids produced by most cells of the body. They may be released as part of a response to injury (inflammation) and they play an important role in pain perception and temperature regulation. **Aspirin** (**acetylsalicylic acid**) inhibits prostaglandin synthesis and is therefore important as an anti-inflammatory drug, as an **analgesic** (reduces pain) and as an **antipyretic** (reduces fever).

Before we leave this topic, Practice point 7.8 explains some important points about fats and health.

Practice point 7.8

Fats and health

The transportation of fats as **lipoproteins** has been described already. Lipoproteins may be classified according to density. **Low-density lipoproteins** (LDL) and **very low-density lipoproteins** (VLDL) have a greater proportion of lipid than do **high-density lipoproteins** (HDL). LDL and VLDL are implicated in the development of the arterial disease **atherosclerosis**. The term 'atherosclerosis' means 'porridge-like hardening' and refers to the focal accumulation of lipids and other large molecules in artery walls. The consequence is a narrowed vessel lumen (opening) and compromised blood supply. If the **coronary arteries** are affected, then **angina** (heart pain) and **myocardial infarction** (heart attack) may result. Atherosclerosis of **cerebral arteries** may lead to a **cerebrovascular accident** (CVA, stroke).

A number of factors contribute to the development of atherosclerosis, including high circulating levels of LDL and VLDL, which are associated with a diet high in saturated fat. Consequently, current health-promotion advice is to reduce the amount of animal fat in the diet and to consume unsaturated fat instead. In contrast, HDL appears to be protective against atherosclerosis - removing fat from arterial walls and transporting it to the liver for metabolism and excretion in the bile. The discovery that fish oil is associated with increased HDL levels has added a new impetus to recommending its consumption.

In-text review

- ✔ Proteins consist of chains of amino acids joined together by peptide bonds.
- ✔ Proteins have primary, secondary, tertiary and quaternary structures.
- ✔ Proteins are digested to form amino acids, which can then be absorbed.
- ✔ All lipids share the property of insolubility in water and solubility in organic solvents.
- ✔ Important classes of lipid include glycerides, sterols, phospholipids and prostaglandins.
- ✔ Glycerides are esters of the alcohol glycerol and carboxylic acids (fatty acids).
- ✔ Depending on whether glycerides have one, two or three carboxylic acid chains, they are described as monoglycerides, diglycerides or triglycerides.
- ✔ Glycerides are digested to form glycerol and carboxylic acids.
- ✔ Lipids may be described as saturated, monounsaturated or polyunsaturated.

Vitamins

The word 'vitamin' is derived from the Latin word for 'life' and serves to indicate the importance to health of this group of organic molecules. Vitamins must be obtained from food, since few are synthesised in the body or at least not in sufficient quantities. Having noted this, the amount of each vitamin needed daily is very small. Vitamins are often destroyed by heat, but they are not broken down in the digestive tract and are absorbed unchanged. The body uses vitamins in their original or slightly modified forms. They function as **cofactors** for enzymes important in regulating metabolic reactions. Despite the fact that what we now know as vitamin C was a key factor in the investigation into the treatment of scurvy conducted by Lind on HMS *Salisbury* in 1747, no vitamin was isolated until the twentieth century. Indeed, vitamin C was not isolated in its pure form until 1932. The system of identifying vitamins devised by Hopkins involves identifying each by a letter, vitamin A being the first to be discovered. Subsequently, this simple system became more complex, with some vitamins being identified by a letter unrelated to the order of discovery and some being referred to more commonly by name. In addition, some vitamins are actually a group of closely related substances that are referred to collectively, while in other cases the individual substances are distinguished by a letter and a number. The first step in classifying vitamins, however, is to distinguish two groups on the basis of solubility in fat or water.

Fat-soluble vitamins

The fat-soluble vitamins are A, D, E and K. They are not absorbed directly into the gut but pass first into the lymphatic system. Since they are not soluble in water, they can be transported only as components of lipoproteins. Fat-soluble vitamins are readily stored by the body and do not need to be consumed every day. The principal sites of storage are the liver and adipose tissue. If consumption is excessive, then fat-soluble vitamins are not readily eliminated; toxicity may thus be a problem if dietary supplements are used excessively. This is especially true of vitamins A and D.

Vitamin A (retinol)

Vitamin A was identified in 1913. The alternative name **retinol** is derived from the name of the structure in which it plays a major role - the **retina** of the eye. Retinol is a pigment important in night (black-and-white) vision. In its preformed state it is found only in animal foods, especially liver. The body can synthesise vitamin A from a number of pigments (**carotenes**) found in plants, however. Carotenes are yellow pigments, their name indicating the vegetable (carrot) in which they are clearly visible. Carotenes are present in a number of vegetables, however, but the darker green pigment chlorophyll often masks their colour. Sources of carotenes include leafy vegetables, broccoli, carrots, peaches and apricots. In addition, vitamin A is added to margarine.

The presence of vitamin A in a wide range of foods means that nutritional deficiency in developed countries is unlikely. Even if vitamin A were eliminated from the diet, extensive stores mean that manifestations of deficiency would not become obvious for a number of years. When vitamin A is lacking, **night blindness** and **xerophthalmia** may result. In addition to its role as a visual pigment, vitamin A is important for the health of secreting **epithelia** (lining and covering tissue). Xerophthalmia is the name given to the ulceration of the **conjunctiva** and **cornea** of the eye, which occurs mostly in eastern Asia and Africa. Subsequently, the cornea becomes scarred and opaque, and blindness ensues. Despite the fact that the association between eye lesions and nutritional deficiency in African people was first made by David Livingstone as long ago as 1857, and that xerophthalmia is relatively easy to prevent with high-dose vitamin A capsules, many people are affected each year.

In developed countries, the problem of vitamin A toxicity related to the consumption of supplements may occur. Manifestations range from dry skin, brittle nails and hair loss to liver damage. Finally, the consumption of liver by pregnant women is best avoided, since the large amounts of vitamin A concentrated in the liver by herbivores fed animal products pose a threat to the normal development of the foetus.

Vitamin D

Dietary sources of vitamin D are few but include liver, fish-liver oils and eggs. Vitamin D is also added to margarine. In contrast to other vitamins, most vitamin D is synthesised in the body - a process that involves the skin, the liver and the kidneys. Vitamin D is essential for the absorption of calcium from the gastrointestinal tract and for the effective use of calcium in bone formation. Vitamin D deficiency results in loss of bone density, leading to the deformity **rickets** in children and **osteomalacia** in adults. The amount of vitamin D synthesised depends upon the area of the skin exposed, the length of exposure and the characteristics of the skin (light-coloured skin synthesises vitamin D more readily than dark-coloured skin). Consequently, dark-skinned people who live in cities of the northern hemisphere are particularly susceptible. Rickets and osteomalacia may be prevented by exposure to sunlight and by dietary supplements. Excessive consumption of vitamin D also presents a danger, however. Overdose leads to **hypercalcaemia** (elevated blood calcium), the manifestations of which include thirst, **polyuria** (increased urine output), renal **calculi** (stones) and renal damage.

Vitamin E

Vitamin E is a group of related substances called **tocopherols** that are important in maintaining cell-membrane integrity. These are found in vegetable oils and margarine; animal fats are poor sources. Compared with vitamins A and D, vitamin E appears relatively non-toxic, which is perhaps fortunate, since unsupported claims for its efficacy have led to its consumption as a remedy for conditions as different as heart disease, cancer, infertility and skin disorders.

Vitamin K

The designation of the letter K to this vitamin is based upon its role in blood coagulation (German *koagulation*). Two forms of vitamin K exist - K_1 is found in dark-green vegetables while K_2 is synthesised by intestinal bacteria. Animal foods provide both forms. The regular consumption of vitamin K in the diet is important, since intestinal synthesis alone is inadequate to meet the body's needs and stores of vitamin K in the liver are not large. Nonetheless, deficiency is uncommon, except where malabsorption exists, such as in biliary obstruction. Since vitamin K is important in the synthesis of the coagulation protein prothrombin, deficiency is manifest by **hypoprothrombinaemia** (low blood prothrombin level) and bleeding. Consequently, patients who are to have surgery for biliary obstruction receive a supplement of vitamin K; in some countries, it has become customary for the prevention of **haemorrhagic disease of the newborn** to administer a dose of vitamin K to the infant at birth. Haemorrhagic disease of the newborn is caused by vitamin K deficiency as a consequence of a sterile gut and low levels of vitamin K in breast milk.

The anticoagulant **warfarin** owes its therapeutic action to its antagonism of vitamin K. Therefore, vitamin K injection is the antidote to overdose and should be kept in stock wherever warfarin is administered.

Water-soluble vitamins

The water-soluble vitamins are the B group and vitamin C. Water-soluble vitamins are absorbed directly into the bloodstream through the gut wall, without the need for specialised carrier molecules. They are readily filtered by the kidney and lost in the urine when consumed in excess. The body is unable to store large quantities of water-soluble vitamins, and therefore they should be supplied daily in the diet.

Vitamin B_1 (thiamine)

Thiamine is abundant in unrefined grains and cereals, pulses, seeds and nuts, but it is present in other vegetables and in meats too. Thiamine is an important component of an enzyme involved in the conversion of glucose to energy. It is also needed for protein and fat metabolism and the normal function of the nervous system. Severe thiamine deficiency, known as **beri beri**, is now rare, but it may occur where people are reliant upon milled rice as a principal component of the diet if they have no other source of thiamine. Rice is not deficient in thiamine, but refining of rice reduces the thiamine content. The effects of thiamine deficiency are also seen with excessive alcohol consumption, as Practice point 7.9 explains. Beri beri is characterised by fatigue, muscle weakness (including heart failure), paralysis, irritability, emotional instability, depression and confusion.

Practice point 7.9

Wernicke–Korsakoff syndrome

It is unlikely that many people reading this book will witness beri beri at first hand, but thiamine deficiency related to alcohol abuse is more common. Chronic excessive use of alcohol affects the intake, absorption and metabolism of thiamine and results in Wernicke-Korsakoff syndrome. In 1880, Wernicke described alcoholic **encephalopathy** (brain disease) characterised by apathy, stupor and loss of balance. In 1887, Korsakoff described memory problems and confusion. The combination of observations made by Wernicke and Korsakoff provides a picture of the typical chronic excessive alcohol abuser.

Vitamin B_2 (riboflavin)

There are no body stores of this vitamin, and so it must be supplied in the diet on a daily basis. Riboflavin is distributed widely in foods, but only in small amounts. Much of the riboflavin in the British diet is supplied in milk and cheese, but it is also found in meat and fish. Riboflavin is a component of enzymes involved in the energy-producing reactions of the cells, but its biochemical functions do not explain easily the manifestations of deficiency. These include **dermatitis** (inflammation of the skin), normocytic **anaemia** (low erythrocyte number, but the cells are normal), **cheilosis** (cracks in the lips), angular **stomatitis** (cracks in the skin in the corners of the mouth) and **glossitis** (inflammation of the tongue). The recognition of deficiency is complicated by the fact that many of the manifestations also occur in other deficiency states, but fortunately riboflavin is rarely absent from the diet. People at risk of inadequate intake of riboflavin are those whose calorie intake is poor, including adolescent females, elderly people and alcoholics. In addition, some specific groups of people have increased riboflavin requirements, including pregnant women and people with **thyrotoxicosis** (elevated production of the hormone **thyroxine**). Riboflavin is used pharmacologically only to treat deficiency states.

Vitamin B_6 (pyridoxine)

A number of closely related substances are included under the name of this vitamin. The substances are found widely in meat and fish and in wholegrain cereals, peanuts and eggs. Consequently, deficiency is rare, although in 1954 an outbreak of convulsions in babies was attributed to insufficient pyridoxine in a modified cow's milk formula. Pyridoxine forms part of a co-enzyme involved in amino-acid metabolism, and so the body's requirement for it is related directly to protein intake.

Vitamin B_{12} (cobalamin)

This vitamin is found only in animal products, a fact that is of special importance to vegans. Food sources rich in vitamin B_{12} are offal, meat, eggs, fish and dairy products. Vitamin B_{12} plays a role in the synthesis of **ribonucleic acid** (RNA) and **deoxyribonucleic acid** (DNA), and it is required for the growth and maturation of erythrocytes (red blood cells). Primary dietary deficiency is rare, except in vegans who fail to take oral vitamin B_{12} supplements. Even then, the signs of deficiency may take many years to develop due to the presence of extensive B_{12} stores in the body. Vitamin B_{12} is absorbed in the final part of the ileum. Vitamin B_{12} deficiency caused by an inadequate intake can be corrected by oral supplements, but deficiency due to impaired absorption requires intramuscular B_{12} injections. Pernicious anaemia is the type of anaemia caused by the absence of vitamin B_{12}. This is described in Practice point 7.10.

Practice point 7.10

Pernicious anaemia

Even when vitamin B_{12} is present in the diet, its absorption in the ileum requires the presence of **intrinsic factor** secreted by the stomach. Consequently, the absence of intrinsic factor leads indirectly to B_{12} deficiency. Regardless of whether B_{12} deficiency results from a dietary deficiency or lack of intrinsic factor, the consequence is the condition **pernicious anaemia**. This is characterised by hyperchromic megaloblastic anaemia (the erythrocytes are large and have an abundance of the pigment haemoglobin). Signs include pallor, dyspnoea (the subjective experience of difficulty breathing), weakness, fatigue, and gastrointestinal symptoms such as glossitis (inflammation of the tongue), anorexia (loss of appetite) and indigestion.

Gastrectomy (surgical removal of the stomach) and surgical removal of the ileum are both **iatrogenic** causes (caused by medical intervention). Gastrectomy removes the site of the production of intrinsic factor and resection of the ileum removes the site of B_{12} absorption.

Niacin (nicotinic acid)

Although there are few body stores of this vitamin, it is found in a wide variety of foods, including meat, fish, milk, yeast and wholemeal grains. In addition, niacin can be synthesised by the body from the amino acid **tryptophan**. Consequently, niacin deficiency is rare, but it does occur in parts of Africa, where maize is the staple food. Niacin forms parts of a number of co-enzymes required by all living cells for the release of energy from carbohydrates, proteins and fats, including **nicotinamide adenine dinucleotide** (NAD - see Chapter 8). Early manifestations of deficiency include anorexia, apathy, weakness and indigestion. Severe deficiency is called **pellagra** (literally 'rough skin'), and classic symptoms are the four ds: dermatitis, diarrhoea, dementia and, if untreated, death. Niacin deficiency is treated readily with supplements, although toxicity can occur and includes flushing, itching, nausea, vomiting, diarrhoea, hypotension, tachycardia, fainting, hypoglycaemia and liver damage.

Folic acid (folate)

The name of this vitamin comes from the Latin for 'leaf', but it is found in a wide range of foods that come from both animal and plant sources. Body stores are not extensive, and so if the diet is deficient symptoms can develop quickly. Deficiency because of malabsorption or drug antagonism is more common, however. Alcohol is the most common antagonist. Deficiency results in a macrocytic (large cell) anaemia and consequent fatigue, weakness and pallor. Other symptoms include weight loss, diarrhoea and glossitis. Treatment is undertaken with folic acid supplements.

Vitamin C

This is almost certainly the most familiar vitamin to lay people, and most people will be able to identify blackcurrants and citrus fruits as good sources. Potatoes also provide a large percentage of the vitamin C intake in Britain - not because potatoes are especially rich in this vitamin but because large quantities of potatoes are eaten. A number of vegetables, such as cauliflower and broccoli, are also sources of vitamin C, as are liver and milk. Vitamin C is required for **collagen** synthesis; symptoms of deficiency (**scurvy**) reflect defects in the manufacture of this important body component, including inflamed gums that bleed easily, pinpoint haemorrhages in the skin, malformations of bone and fractures, and delayed wound healing. Vitamin C deficiency can be treated with oral supplements. In addition, some people advocate taking supplements of vitamin C at considerably greater than nutritional levels as a means of preventing common colds.

Minerals

Important minerals include sodium, potassium, calcium, iron, phosphorus and iodine. Minerals are inorganic substances necessary for the normal function of the body. Some are present in the body as ions dissolved in solution, and in this state they are referred to as electrolytes.

Sodium (Na/Na^+)

The element sodium is a highly reactive soft grey metal, while the sodium ion found widely in fruits, vegetables, meats and fish is stable and unreactive. The compound sodium chloride (common salt, NaCl) is used as a preservative in tinned foods and cured meats and is often added to food at the table. Consequently, the average daily intake in British diets of 10-15 g is considerably in excess of the required 1 g per day. The normal blood concentration of sodium is 135-145 mmol/l, and in the blood sodium ions function as an important osmotic regulator. In addition, sodium ions also play important roles in the generation of electrical impulses in nerves (**action potentials**) and in muscle contraction.

Low serum sodium is referred to as **hyponatraemia** and elevated serum sodium as **hypernatraemia**. Sodium and water are usually gained and lost together, however. For example, both are lost in excessive sweating, vomiting, diarrhoea and increased **diuresis** (urine output). If sodium and water depletion is excessive, then there is a reduction in the volume of extracellular (outside cells) fluid, which leads to reduced cardiac output and low blood pressure. Fatigue and faintness then occur. In contrast, sodium and water retention leads to an expansion of the blood volume and **oedema** (excess of **interstitial fluid**). This is common in cardiac, kidney and liver disease. The swollen ankles of elderly people (due to oedema) are commonly a manifestation of sodium and water retention caused by heart failure.

Potassium (K/K^+)

Potassium is another highly reactive metal with a stable and unreactive ion. Potassium is the principal **intracellular** (inside the cell) ion; blood levels are low, at only 3.0-5.5 mmol/l.

Potassium plays an important role in nerve conduction and muscle contraction. A low plasma potassium level (**hypokalaemia**) may result from diarrhoea and the use of certain **diuretics** (drugs that cause an increase in urine output). It manifests with weakness and mental symptoms such as apathy and confusion. High serum potassium (**hyperkalaemia**) occurs in kidney failure, when there has been excessive consumption of potassium supplements or when an intravenous infusion containing potassium is allowed to run too quickly. Elevated serum potassium may result in cardiac arrest (the heart stops effective pumping).

Calcium (Ca/Ca^{2+})

Calcium is found in cereals, vegetables and fish, and dairy products are very good sources. The absorption and use of calcium requires vitamin D, while the hormones **calcitonin** and **parathormone** (from the thyroid and parathyroid glands, respectively) are responsible for regulating the blood calcium level (normally 2.0–2.5 mmol/l). Calcium is an important component of bones and teeth and plays an important role in blood coagulation, the conduction of nervous impulses and muscle contraction.

A low serum calcium level (**hypocalcaemia**) may result when there is a deficiency in parathormone. An example of such a deficiency occurs when the parathyroid glands (which are embedded in the thyroid glands) are removed as part of a **thyroidectomy** (surgical removal of the thyroid gland). Hypocalcaemia may result in **tetany** – sustained involuntary muscular contraction, such as that of the wrist and ankle (**carpo-pedal spasm**). In the case of a longstanding deficiency of calcium, the body attempts to maintain serum calcium levels at the expense of calcium stores in the bones. This results in a negative calcium balance and loss of bone mass, referred to as **osteoporosis**. Osteoporosis is also associated with a lack of physical activity and a reduction of **oestrogen** in post-menopausal women. A high serum calcium (**hypercalcaemia**) may be recognised by nausea, vomiting, weakness, constipation, polydipsia (increased thirst) and polyuria (increased urine output). If present over a prolonged period, hypercalcaemia may result in renal calculi (kidney stones). Possible causes of hypercalcaemia include excessive ingestion of vitamin D and tumours of the parathyroid glands, with excessive production of parathormone.

Iron (Fe/Fe^{2+} and Fe^{3+})

The body contains about 3–5 g of iron, most of which is in the haem part of the haemoglobin molecule (the pigment of erythrocytes/red blood cells). Iron in the diet is present in two forms. That which forms part of the haem molecule is referred to as haem iron, and meat is a good source. Non-haem iron is obtained from plant sources, such as grains, vegetables and nuts. Only 10% of the iron in the diet is absorbed, and sometimes nurses have to consider how a patient may be helped to improve the availability of this important mineral. Haem iron is better absorbed than non-haem iron, but the latter accounts for a larger percentage of the total iron intake. In addition, the rate of haem iron absorption (about 15–35%) varies only with the body's need, while the rate of absorption of non-haem iron (about 3–8%) is increased by vitamin C. Consequently, when patients have an iron deficiency and are taking iron supplements, nurses traditionally have encouraged the consumption of a diet rich in vitamin C. Iron deficiency anaemia is described in Practice point 7.11.

Practice point 7.11

Iron deficiency anaemia

An important measurement that you should be familiar with is the amount of haemoglobin in the blood. This is approximately 11-13 g/dl (a decilitre (dl) is 100 ml) in women and 13-16 g/dl in men. Iron deficiency leads to a form of anaemia (the condition of a reduction in the amount of haemoglobin or the number of erythrocytes). In iron deficiency anaemia, the problem relates to a lack of haemoglobin because of the deficiency of this important component of the haemoglobin molecule. Therefore, erythrocytes are deficient in pigment (**hypochromic**) and as a consequence they are small (**microcytic**). Affected patients complain of pallor, fatigue and breathlessness. **Glossitis** (inflammation of the tongue), **gingivitis** (inflammation of the gums) and angular **stomatitis** (inflammation of the corners of the mouth) may also occur. Have you seen these features in elderly people? They are not at all uncommon, and you should be alert for them. Dietary deficiency of iron may also occur in prolonged breast-feeding of infants because milk is a poor source of iron. Other causes of iron deficiency anaemia include chronic blood loss in stomach and duodenal ulcers, **haemorrhoids** and heavy menses. In addition, pregnancy may result in an increased requirement for iron, and iron supplements may be prescribed. In the case of severe anaemia, a blood transfusion may be given. You might like to find out about this procedure and the role of the nurse by studying a nursing textbook.

Toxicity due to excessive consumption of iron supplements can occur, but it is children who are usually affected. Important advice to parents who are prescribed iron supplements is to store them where children cannot reach them. Manifestations of iron poisoning include gastrointestinal pain, nausea, vomiting, convulsions and coma.

Phosphorus (P)

This is the second-most abundant mineral in the body; fortunately, it is widespread in the diet too. Along with calcium, phosphorus forms the mineral matrix of bone. It is not surprising, therefore, that 85% of the body's phosphorus is found in bone. Nonetheless, phosphorus is important elsewhere too - for example, it combines with lipids to form phospholipids. These are important in all cells, where a double layer of phospholipids (**phospholipid bilayer**) is responsible for determining the characteristics of the cell membrane. Phosphorus also forms an important part of our genetic makeup, where it forms part of the sugar-phosphate backbone of DNA (deoxyribonucleic acid). The phosphate ion is formed from phosphorus and oxygen (PO_4^-), and phosphate ions are also important in the body's chemical form of energy **adenosine triphosphate** (ATP). More about ATP can be found in Chapter 8. Phosphorus is also an important component of the **monohydrogen phosphate ion** (HPO_4^{2-}) and the **dihydrogen phosphate ion** ($H_2PO_4^-$), the two of which form an important buffering system of the kidney. You will find more about this in Chapter 5.

Iodine (I)

Iodine is found in a number of different body tissues, but it is perhaps most familiar as an essential component of the thyroid hormone thyroxine. Seafood is a good source of iodine, as are plants grown in iodine-rich soils. When iodine is deficient, goitre may result, as Practice point 7.12 explains.

Practice point 7.12

Goitre

A deficiency of iodine leads to underproduction of thyroxine; in response, the thyroid gland swells - a condition known as **goitre**. Thyroxine production is triggered by a hormone from the **pituitary gland** (the hormone gland at the base of the brain) called **thyroid-stimulating hormone (TSH)**. When thyroxine levels are low, more TSH is produced in an attempt to stimulate the thyroid gland. However, thyroxine levels remain low due to iodine deficiency. The continued high level of TSH also stimulates the thyroid gland to grow, and goitre results. In the past, goitre in Britain was sometimes referred to as 'Derbyshire neck' because the low levels of iodine in the water of this hilly county meant that goitre was common there.

- ***Can you work out why this is no longer the case?***

You may have worked out that in developed countries, people are no longer confined to eating local produce.

Apart from its role in the diet you may encounter iodine in antiseptic solutions and hand-washing preparations, but be aware that some people are allergic to iodine and this should be ascertained before its use. This is especially important when **radio-opaque** (opaque to X-rays) iodine solutions are injected into the blood as part of a radiological investigation (investigation using X-rays). Finally, radioactive iodine preparations may be used in the investigation and treatment of thyroid disorders.

Fibre (roughage/non-starch polysaccharide)

The words 'fibre' and 'roughage' are often used without precise definition. They are commonly used synonymously for plant non-starch polysaccharide that cannot be digested by human enzymes. This material includes cellulose (a component of plant call walls), and **pectins** and **mucilages**, which give some fruits the ability to hold a lot of water. Of these molecules, only cellulose has a fibrous structure, and so the use of the term 'fibre' is perhaps not strictly accurate. Fibre can be divided into two types on the basis of its water solubility. Soluble fibre includes mucilages and pectins, while cellulose is an example of insoluble fibre. The effects of these two groups of substances are summarised in Table 7.1.

The two different types of fibre are found in different proportions in different types of plant material, but a diet that contains a variety of vegetables and fruit will ensure that both soluble and insoluble fibres are consumed. The consumption of both types of fibre is important for health. For example, both types decrease intestinal transit time (the length of time

Table 7.1 Effects of soluble and insoluble fibre.

Soluble fibre	Insoluble fibre
Decreases intestinal transit time	Decreases intestinal transit time
Slows gastric emptying	Absorbs water
Lowers serum cholesterol	Increases faecal bulk
Delays glucose absorption	Reduces pressure in colon

that ingested material remains in the gut), but insoluble fibre has the additional effect of absorbing water and increasing faecal bulk. The larger, softer stools are moved more readily through the gut by **peristalsis** (the wave-like contraction of the intestine), and this reduces the incidence of constipation. In contrast, soluble fibre influences the absorption of cholesterol and glucose. The former is an important consideration in dietary advice for the reduction of atherosclerosis, while the delayed absorption of glucose may help diabetic people.

In-text review

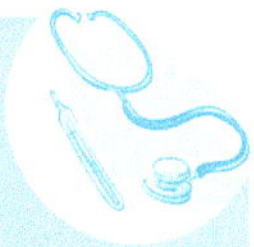

- ✔ Vitamins are organic compounds that function as cofactors for enzymes.
- ✔ Vitamins are either fat-soluble or water-soluble.
- ✔ The fat-soluble vitamins are A, D, E and K.
- ✔ The water-soluble vitamins are C and the B group.
- ✔ Minerals are inorganic substances that are necessary for the normal function of the body.
- ✔ Important minerals are sodium, potassium, calcium, iron, phosphorus and iodine.
- ✔ The terms 'roughage' and 'fibre' refer to plant material that cannot be digested by human enzymes.
- ✔ Cellulose is an example of insoluble fibre, and pectins and mucilages are examples of soluble fibre.

Summary

In this chapter we have introduced the seven nutritional groups and described the chemistry of carbohydrates, proteins and lipids. The digestion and absorption of different nutritional groups has been explained and relationships to health and illness have been made. An understanding of the contents of this chapter will be of use when giving health advice regarding obesity or the prevention of disease such atherosclerosis.

Summary points

- There are seven important components of the diet.
- Carbohydrates are divided into three classes - monosaccharides, disaccharides and polysaccharides.
- Diabetes mellitus is an example of a disorder of carbohydrate metabolism.
- Proteins consist of chains of amino acids joined together by peptide bonds.
- Proteins have primary, secondary, tertiary and quaternary structures.
- Important classes of lipid include glycerides, sterols, phospholipids and prostaglandins.
- Glycerides may be described as monoglycerides, diglycerides or triglycerides.
- Lipids may be described as saturated, monounsaturated or polyunsaturated.
- The process of digestion of carbohydrates, proteins and fats involves enzyme hydrolysis.
- Vitamins are organic compounds that function as cofactors for enzymes.
- Vitamins are either fat-soluble or water-soluble.
- Minerals are inorganic substances that are necessary for the normal function of the body.
- The terms 'roughage' and 'fibre' refer to plant material that cannot be digested by human enzymes.

Self-test questions

1 Match the substances on the left with the appropriate descriptions on the right.

(a) Glucose	(i) Monosaccharide
(b) Lactose	(ii) Table sugar
(c) Glycogen	(iii) Disaccharide found in milk
(d) Sucrose	(iv) Polysaccharide

2 Match the minerals on the left with the appropriate descriptions on the right.

(a) Sodium	(i) Involved in oxygen transport
(b) Calcium	(ii) The most abundant extracellular ion
(c) Iron	(iii) Important in the formation of thyroxine
(d) Iodine	(iv) Important component of bone

3 Match the vitamins on the left with the appropriate descriptions on the right.

(a) B1 (thiamine)	(i) Not present in any plant source
(b) D	(ii) Deficiency common in alcohol abuse
(c) K	(iii) Required for the formation of prothrombin
(d) B_{12}	(iv) Made in a process involving sunlight

4 Match the enzymes on the left with the appropriate descriptions on the right.

(a) Pepsin	(i) Responsible for starch digestion
(b) Amylase	(ii) Secreted by stomach
(c) Lipase	(iii) Proteolytic enzyme of the pancreas
(d) Trypsin	(iv) Responsible for fat digestion

5 Match the substances on the left with the appropriate descriptions on the right.

(a) Amino acid	(i) Vitamin C
(b) Carboxylic acid	(ii) Building block of protein
(c) Ascorbic acid	(iii) B-group vitamin
(d) Folic acid	(iv) Building block of triglycerides

6 Match the substances on the left with the appropriate descriptions on the right.

(a) Mucilages	(i) Consist of long chain of amino acids
(b) Cellulose	(ii) Soluble fibre
(c) Tocopherols	(iii) Vitamin E
(d) Polypeptides	(iv) Insoluble fibre

7 Match the substances on the left with the appropriate descriptions on the right.

(a) Minerals	(i) Always contain nitrogen
(b) Carbohydrates	(ii) Elements or inorganic substances
(c) Vitamins	(iii) Organic substances absorbed undigested
(d) Proteins	(iv) Contain only carbon, hydrogen and oxygen

8 Match the structures on the left with the appropriate descriptions on the right.

(a) Stomach	(i) B_{12} is absorbed here
(b) Terminal ileum	(ii) Pepsinogen is secreted here
(c) Colon	(iii) Contains enzymes secreted by parotid glands
(d) Mouth	(iv) The principal site of water absorption

9 Which one of the following best describes the effect of consuming a diet rich in marine fish oil?

(a) Reduces the serum level of low-density lipoprotein.
(b) Increases the serum level of low-density lipoprotein.
(c) Increases the serum level of high-density lipoprotein.
(d) Reduces the serum level of high-density lipoprotein.

10 Which one of the following best describes the effect of consuming a diet high in polyunsaturated fat and low in saturated fat?

(a) Reduces the serum level of low-density lipoprotein.
(b) Increases the serum level of low-density lipoprotein.
(c) Reduces the serum level of high-density lipoprotein.
(d) Increases the serum level of high-density lipoprotein.

Further study/exercises

1 **When you next sit down for a main meal, consider the foods that you are about to eat. Identify the sources of carbohydrates, fats, proteins, vitamins, minerals and roughage. Later, reminder yourself of the processes involved in the digestion of carbohydrates, fats and proteins. Is your diet a healthy one?**

NHS Direct On Line: www.nhsdirect.nhs.uk
How can I eat healthily at home?: www.nhsdirect.nhs.uk/articles/article.aspx?articleId=1134
How can I make healthy meals?: www.nhsdirect.nhs.uk/articles/article.aspx?articleId=1135

2 **We have seen that body mass index can be used to determine whether a person is overweight, but how can weight be lost safely?**

NHS Direct On Line: www.nhsdirect.nhs.uk
How can I lose weight safely?: www.nhsdirect.nhs.uk/articles/article.aspx?articleId=851

8

Energy in the body

Learning outcomes

After reading the following chapter and undertaking personal study, you should be able to:

1. Define the term 'energy'.
2. List various forms of energy and distinguish between kinetic and potential energy.
3. Describe the principle of the conservation of energy and identify examples of energy conversions.
4. Identify the units used to measure energy and use kilojoules (kJ) to compare the energy values of different foods and the energy expended in different activities.
5. Describe the adenosine triphosphate (ATP) molecule and identify its importance in the body.
6. Outline the energy-producing reactions of the body (cellular/internal respiration), including glycolysis, the conversion of pyruvic acid to acetyl co-enzyme A (acetyl-CoA), the Krebs cycle and the electron-transport chain.
7. Outline fat and protein catabolism and briefly describe some of the potential consequences of using fat as a principal source of energy.

Introduction

Health-care professionals sometimes use the expression 'malaise' to describe the experience of feeling generally unwell. Patients, however, often use more straightforward language and complain of having 'no **energy**'. We often refer to energy, such as the 'energy value' of foods when trying to control our weight, but if we had to define energy most of us would find it difficult. The concept is familiar and yet intangible. We seem to know what people mean when they use the word, but a convincing definition is elusive. When introducing new ideas, it is usual to begin with a definition of the topic, but in the case of energy it is probably the definition that is the trickiest part of the study. Perhaps one of the reasons for this is that it is difficult to come up with a definition of energy that takes into account all its different forms. We have to apply a definition to such diverse forms as light, heat, sound, a moving object and the energy locked up in a chemical such as glucose. This chapter begins with a general consideration of energy before moving on to look at energy in the body and especially at the energy-liberating reactions of cells.

Defining energy

Scientists define energy as the ability to do work. After what has been said previously about the difficulties of definition, the above seems extraordinarily simple. Perhaps it even appears unsatisfactory. After all, such a definition does not tell us anything about the nature of any specific form of energy such as light or heat, but this is to be expected when dealing with such a broad concept. Perhaps an example will illustrate how our definition holds true. Take the case of someone pushing a wheelchair uphill. Energy is being expended in muscular contraction and work is being done - perhaps the patient is heavy and it feels like hard work. This is using everyday language of course. To the scientist, the word 'work' has a specific meaning - it is the product of force and distance moved. So we can apply our definitions of energy and work to the case above.

- ***What about heat and light? How does our definition apply to them? How do they do work?***

The validity of the application of our definition of energy to heat and light becomes clear when we think of these forms of energy being converted into other forms. The steam engine is a good example of a device that uses heat to produce movement through the expansion of steam. Consider, too, the solar panel. Here, light is converted into electrical energy, which may be used to perform all kinds of work - power a water pump, perhaps. So, then, the scientist's definition of energy appears disappointing at first, but it can be applied to energy in all its forms.

Forms of energy

We have already noted the fact that energy exists in a number of forms, examples of which are given in Table 8.1.

Table 8.1 Different forms of energy.

Form of energy	Example
Mechanical	The moving parts of any machine - the engine of an ambulance for example
Heat	Heat is very familiar to us, but we sometimes make use of it in unusual ways. For example, the heat generated by a **diathermy** probe in the operating theatre is used to cut through tissue and to seal bleeding vessels
Electromagnetic, e.g. visible light, ultraviolet light, infrared light	We make use of visible light in a number of devices, including **endoscopes**, which enable the operator to examine inside the body
Chemical	Batteries are examples of this form of energy. Large batteries are used to power devices such as motorised wheelchairs, while very small batteries power **pacemakers** - implantable devices used to control the heart rate
Electrical	Electric motors are used in many applications, such as motorised beds and large scanners that move around the patient in order to produce an image of the body
Nuclear	Nuclear power stations are familiar to us, but nuclear medicine is also important in producing images of the body and in treating cancer

Some energy forms, such as light, heat and sound, are very familiar to us because we experience them in everyday life. There are separate chapters on each of these later in this book and indeed on other forms, such as electricity. In fact, since most chapters of this book refer to energy to a lesser or greater degree, you could say that much of this book is actually about energy. Some forms of energy are less tangible than others, and perhaps we don't think about them very often. After all, when did you last have a conversation about infrared radiation? Still other forms are given attention only when our perspective is changed by some event. For example, when out shopping, we are certainly concerned about the freshness and price of food. If we have to lose weight, however, energy value becomes important too. Similarly, the prospect of a holiday in a hot country may prompt us to think about **ultraviolet radiation**, sunburn and skin cancer. Thus, energy is definitely important in our bodies.

- ***Make a list of different forms of energy in the body.***

Now compare your notes with Table 8.2.

Table 8.2 Different forms of energy in the body.

Form of energy	Example in the body
Mechanical	Muscle contraction when walking, the pumping of the heart
Heat	Temperature homeostasis
Electromagnetic	Light and vision, ultraviolet light and tanning, sunburn and skin cancer
Sound	Hearing
Chemical	The energy value of food
Electrical	Nervous impulses

Kinetic and potential energy

When we consider forms of energy, they seem quite different. Think once again about pushing a patient uphill in a wheelchair. It is obvious to us that energy is being used. In contrast, when a cardiac (heart) pacemaker is held in the palm of the hand, it is difficult to see that energy is involved at all. In the first example, it is clear that energy is being used to perform work, since the wheelchair is being moved. In the case of the pacemaker, the batteries have the potential to do work, but they are not doing so at present. We have just made an important distinction between the energy of movement, which is called **kinetic energy**, and **potential energy**.

In order to distinguish these forms, we shall think about the patient in the wheelchair a little more. Suppose you arrive at the top of the hill and stop to admire the view. The wheelchair is no longer moving - it has zero kinetic energy.

- ***What about its potential energy? How has that changed?***

At the bottom of the hill, the wheelchair was unable to do any work - it had zero potential energy. Now it has been pushed to the top, its potential energy has increased. In order to demonstrate this, think about what would happen if you forgot to put on the brakes. Of course this would be a serious omission - the wheelchair would roll quickly down to the bottom of the hill, taking the patient with it. You could say that you have recouped some of the energy expended in dragging the wheelchair to the top in the first place. It is an example of a conversion from potential to kinetic energy.

The energy locked in a chemical is another example of the potential kind. For example, when plants make **carbohydrates** (such as **starch** in potatoes) from carbon dioxide and water, they use energy from the sun in the form of light. If we eat these plant products, our bodies are able to break the bonds between atoms of the carbohydrate molecules in order to release the energy for our own use. In other processes, there is a very long time between the manufacturing process by the plant and human use. For example, when we burn fossil fuels, such as coal or peat, we are making use of the remains of plants that died thousands of years ago. In each of these examples, energy is neither being created nor used - it is simply being converted from one type to another. We describe this as the **conservation of energy**.

The conservation of energy

We are not referring to a 'green' issue here but to the important principle that, in ordinary chemical reactions, energy cannot be created or destroyed, although it may be changed from one form to another. Consequently, if we talk about 'using' energy or the energy-'producing' reactions of the body, we are not strictly correct. Rather, one form of energy is being converted into another. The expression 'ordinary chemical reactions' is used here in order to exclude certain nuclear reactions in which energy and matter are interconverted.

Energy is converted from one form to another in our bodies and in devices made by us for this very purpose.

● *Think of some examples?*

Now check your list with Table 8.3.

Note that in some examples, a number of energy conversions actually take place. For example, in a gas-burning power station, the chemical potential energy of the gas molecules is converted to heat, which is used to produce steam, which in turn is used to drive a turbine to produce electricity. In a similar way, the energy produced from the breakdown of food in our bodies is actually used to regenerate a molecule called **adenosine triphosphate** (ATP), which is the source of energy for activities such as muscle contraction. We should also note that energy-converting reactions are generally inefficient. For example, the lightbulb produces a good deal of heat as well as light, while electric heaters commonly produce light too. The heat produced by the lightbulb and the light produced by the heater might be regarded as a kind of waste. Similar observations can also be made of the body. If you are not sure about this, simply perform a few minutes of vigorous exercise. What do you feel like? Hot and sweaty and possibly exhausted. Intensive muscular activity generates an excess of heat, and we have to lose this to the environment if we are to avoid overheating - more about this in the following chapter. For now, it is enough to note that we too produce waste energy.

Table 8.3 Examples of energy conversions.

In the body
Chemical → heat: all cells, especially liver cells
Light → electrical: the eyes
Sound → electrical: the ears
Chemical → mechanical: muscles
Artificial devices
Mechanical → electrical: generator
Electrical → mechanical: electric motor
Electrical → heat: electric heater
Chemical → electrical: battery
Electrical → light: lightbulb

Now let us further apply the principle of the conservation of energy to our bodies. In view of what we have learned so far, energy taken into our bodies in terms of the food we consume cannot disappear. It must be expended in some form of work or otherwise stored (mostly as fat). Consequently, the following equation must be true:

$$\text{Energy intake} = \text{energy expenditure} \pm \text{changes in body energy stores}$$

From the above, you will see that if energy intake exceeds energy expenditure, then there will be an increase in energy stores; the reverse must also be true. We might even begin to talk about the body's energy balance in a similar way to that of water balance, and this is clearly important when we consider weight control. Furthermore, if we are to consider the body's energy balance, we must have some way of measuring energy. This is what we consider next.

Units of energy

When we are concerned about the energy value of particular foods and ask how many **Calories** it contains, we clearly expect a numerical answer. We obviously assume that energy can be measured.

- ***What is a calorie? Are there other units of energy?***

The Calorie (spelled with a capital letter and abbreviated Cal) is mentioned here because, even if you have not studied science before, you will probably have heard of it. The **calorie** (without a capital letter and abbreviated cal) is the amount of energy required to raise the temperature of 1 g of water by 1 °C. It is a rather small unit of energy, and so the unit **kilocalorie** (kcal - 1000 calories) is more convenient. The energy value of food is sometimes given in nutritional Calories, which are actually the same as kilocalories. Apart from having the potential to confuse, calories are a rather old-fashioned unit and we shall use the SI unit of energy, the joule (J).

- ***Do you remember how we defined energy?***

We said that it is the ability to do work, and we defined work as the product of force and distance. We could express this in the form of a formula:

$$\text{Work} = \text{force} \times \text{distance}$$

Distance is no problem - we know that the SI unit of distance is the metre.

- ***What about force – how is it measured?***

The SI unit of force is the **newton** - it is named after Sir Isaac Newton. We shall consider this further in Chapter 10. For now, it is enough to know that force has units of newtons and distance has units of metres. If we now look back at our equation, we should be able to work out that the SI unit of work is, therefore, the newton metre. This sounds a little cumbersome, so you will be glad to know that is has been renamed the **joule**, after James Joule. In order to have some idea as to the magnitude of the joule, it is perhaps worth knowing that it takes 4183 J to raise the temperature of 1 kg of water by 1 °C. Once again, 1 J is therefore a rather small unit of energy, and it is more convenient to use the larger unit of 1000 J - the **kilojoule** (kJ).

- ***How many kilojoules would it take to raise the temperature of 1 kg of water by 1 °C?***

It would take 4.183 kJ. If you need to use both calories and joules, you should find it accurate enough to consider that 1 cal = 4.2 J.

- ***But do we use joules in clinical practice?***

As you might expect, the answer is yes - that is the reason for explaining this unit here. Have a look at Table 8.4. You will see that the energy value of some foods is given in kilojoules per 100 g (kJ/100 g). The energy value of food is considered further in Practice point 8.1.

Now have a look at Table 8.5, which shows energy consumption in kilojoules per minute (kJ/min) for various activities.

- ***Are the figures much as you expected? Work out the length of time it takes in moderate exercise (e.g. 20 kJ/min) to expend the energy contained in 100 g of flaky pastry compared with 100 g of grapefruit.***

You should obtain approximate figures of 2 hours for the pastry and 4.5 minutes for the grapefruit. Clearly, exercise may play an important role in the control of weight, but it may

Practice point 8.1

The energy value of food

Consider Table 8.4.

- ***Which foods have the lowest energy value?***

Fruit and vegetables have the lowest energy values, but their values depend upon how they are cooked. Compare boiled potatoes and chips, for example.

- ***Which foods have the highest energy value?***

High-energy value foods include chocolate and pastry.

- ***Are there any energy-value surprises?***

Look at butter and margarine - their energy values are similar. The important thing to note here is that the value to health of foods cannot simply be equated with their energy value. Margarine is said to be a healthy substitute for butter because it is made from **unsaturated fats** rather than **saturated fats**. Fats have already been discussed in Chapter 7.

- ***What about meat and fish?***

Fish, chicken and turkey have the lowest energy values. Nonetheless, there are a few surprises here too - stewing beef has a lower energy value than herring. Once again, do not confuse energy value with value to health. Fish oils have particular health benefits, while the consumption of high levels of animal fat poses a challenge to health.

Table 8.4 The energy values of selected foods.

Food	Energy value (kJ/100 g)	Food	Energy value (kJ/100 g)
Cornflakes	1523	Boiled potatoes	356
Porridge	197	Chips	1100
Chocolate biscuits	2239	Rice	544
Digestive biscuits	2026	Spaghetti	511
Brown bread	984	Butter	3097
White bread	1030	Margarine	3051
Chapattis	1461	Cheddar cheese	1716
Flaky pastry	2394	Cottage cheese	276
Milk chocolate	2252	Stewing beef	712
Apples	150	Beef sausages	1272
Bananas	360	Lamb chops	1569
Grapefruit	92	Liver	632
Oranges	167	Chicken	607
Brussels sprouts	75	Turkey	444
Cabbage	33	Cod	310
Carrots	92	Trout	569
Cauliflower	59	Herring	1000

(Taken from Bender D. A. (1997). *Introduction to Nutrition and Metabolism*, 2nd edn. London: Taylor & Francis, pp. 314-323.)

take a good deal of exercise to burn off the energy contained in higher-energy foods. It is also worth pointing out that we have considered the energy value of foods with energy reduction in mind. This is because excess energy consumption in relation to activity is a problem in developed countries and is part of the cause of obesity. On the other hand, if you work in a developing country, the opposite problem often exists, and you may need to consider ways of increasing energy intake.

Table 8.5 **Energy expended various exercises.**

Activity level	Example	Energy expended (kJ/min)
Very light	Typing, driving	< 10
Light	Bed-making	10–20
Moderate	Cycling, gardening	20–30
Heavy	Digging, football	30–40
Very heavy	Boxing, using an axe	40–50

(From Barker H. M. (1991). *Beck's Nutrition and Dietetics for Nurses*, 8th edn. Edinburgh: Churchill Livingstone.)

If you read over the section above again, you will notice that we have referred to energy in the body in terms of the potential energy in the foods that we eat. The body takes many steps to break down our food in order to release the energy it contains. The final step in this process is an important molecule called adenosine triphosphate (ATP).

In-text review

- ✔ Energy is defined as the ability to do work.
- ✔ Energy exists in a number of forms, such as light and heat.
- ✔ Each form may be classified as potential (e.g. the energy locked in chemicals) or kinetic (the energy of movement, e.g. muscle contraction).
- ✔ Energy cannot be created or destroyed, but it can be converted from one form to another.
- ✔ Various units are used to measure energy, the SI unit being the joule (J).
- ✔ The energy value of foods is given in kilojoules (KJ).

The ATP molecule

Adenosine triphosphate (ATP) is often described as the 'energy currency of the cell'.

- ***What is this term trying to express?***

Clearly, the body gains all of its energy from the food we eat, but breaking down nutrient molecules to release energy is quite a complex biochemical process, and the energy is not available immediately. What is required is a molecule that is able to temporarily store energy but that is then able to release that energy quickly in a one-step reaction. This is the role of ATP. It is an organic compound consisting of **adenine** (an organic compound also found in

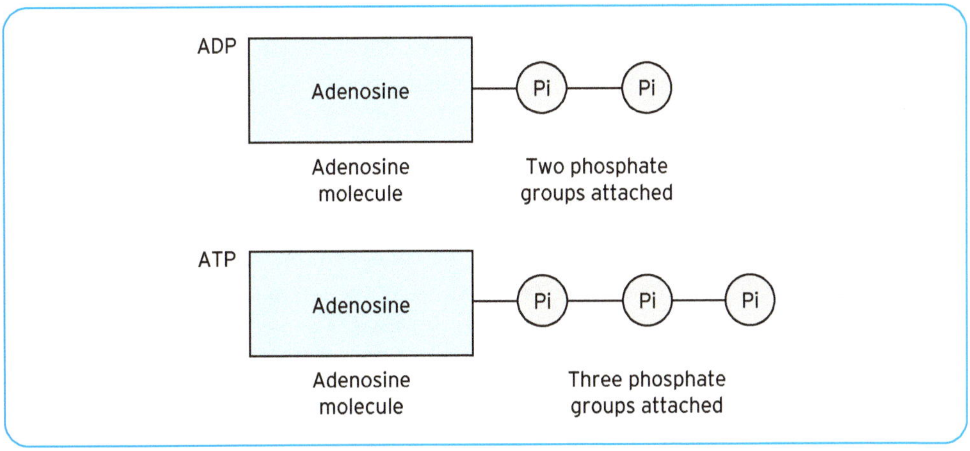

Figure 8.1
Representations of adenosine diphosphate and adenosine triphosphate.

deoxyriboucleic acid (DNA) and **ribonucleic acid** (RNA)) and a **pentose** (five-carbon-atom) sugar. ATP also contains three inorganic phosphate groups (Pi). ATP is synthesised from **adenosine diphosphate** (ADP) in all cells of the body. ATP and ADP are represented in Figure 8.1. Note that these are for the purpose of illustration - they do not represent the molecular structure of these compounds.

- ***How many phosphate groups does ADP possess?***

It has two; the conversion of ADP to ATP, therefore, requires the addition of one phosphate group - a process called **phosphorylation**. This process requires energy (e.g. from the breakdown of glucose), and it can be summarised in the following way:

$$\text{ADP} + \text{Pi} \xrightarrow{\text{energy}} \text{ATP}$$

Incidentally, because the energy for the above reaction is derived from the **oxidation** of food, the term 'oxidative phosphorylation' is applied.

The third phosphate group is readily removed from ATP to recycle ADP and Pi. In this process, energy is released again, as shown below:

$$\text{ATP} \longrightarrow \text{ADP} + \text{Pi} \quad (\searrow \text{energy})$$

Of course, in neither of these processes is energy actually being created or destroyed. Remember the important principle of the conservation of energy. Rather, the energy released by the breakdown of glucose is used to synthesise ATP; when ATP is itself broken down, the energy released is used to perform some form of work, such as muscular contraction. We are now in a position to begin to consider the processes by which glucose is broken down to provide the energy for the synthesis of ATP.

The energy-liberating reactions of cells

There are many reactions taking place within the body, and the word '**metabolism**' is used in reference to them all. Some of these reactions are of the synthesis type and are described as **anabolic**, while others involve breaking down substances and are denoted **catabolic**. The catabolic cellular reactions that result in the liberation of energy are also referred to as internal or cellular respiration. In carbohydrate catabolism, the starting point is glucose, which may be derived from carbohydrates in the diet or from the carbohydrate storage molecule **glycogen**. (The liver and muscle manufacture glycogen by joining together many glucose molecules.) In the breakdown of glucose, each glucose molecule is oxidised completely to carbon dioxide and water, and in the process a maximum of 38 molecules of ATP are generated. We can summarise the reaction as shown in the equation below:

$$C_6H_{12}O_6 + 6O_2 \rightarrow 6CO_2 + 6H_2O$$
$$38\ ADP \qquad\qquad 38\ ATP$$

The chemical potential energy of the products of this reaction is considerably less than that of the original glucose molecule. Clearly, some energy has been lost along the way.

- ***In what form has this energy been lost?***

You may have realised that this energy has been lost as heat. Keep this in mind when you study the next chapter. In order to proceed further, we need to review some of the points covered in Chapter 3.

- ***What is oxidation?***

Oxidation is a reaction involving the loss of hydrogen or an **electron**.

- ***What about reduction – how is it defined?***

Reduction is a reaction involving the gain of hydrogen or an electron. Oxidation and reduction always occur together. In a reaction that involves the oxidation of one substance, another substance is reduced.

In the reactions that are described later, two molecules (co-enzymes) appear a number of times. They are **nicotinamide adenine dinucleotide** (NAD), a derivative of the vitamin niacin, and **flavin adenine dinucleotide** (FAD), a derivative of vitamin B_2. From now on, we shall refer to them only by their abbreviations NAD and FAD - the full names are too long to fit easily into diagrams. Let us make life even simpler and not look at their chemical formulae - we do not need to for our purpose here. What we do need to know is that both of these molecules exist in two forms - the oxidised form and the reduced form. The oxidised form of NAD is NAD^+, which reacts with two hydrogen atoms to form NADH (reduced form) and H^+ (hydrogen ion/proton). This reaction is shown below:

NAD^+	+	2H	→	NADH	+	H^+
oxidised form		2 hydrogen atoms		reduced form		hydrogen ion

- ***Why do we say that NAD^+ has been reduced to NADH?***

It is because the molecule has gained a hydrogen atom and an electron. FAD behaves in a similar way, as shown below:

FAD	+	2H	→	$FADH_2$
oxidised form		2 hydrogen atoms		reduced form

If both NAD^+ and FAD are reduced as part of the energy-liberating reactions of the cell, then other substances are being oxidised, as will be seen below.

Overview of carbohydrate catabolism

There are four stages involved in the catabolism of carbohydrates (see Figure 8.2):

1 Glycolysis.

2 Conversion of pyruvic acid to acetyl co-enzyme A (acetyl-CoA).

3 Krebs cycle.

4 Electron-transport chain.

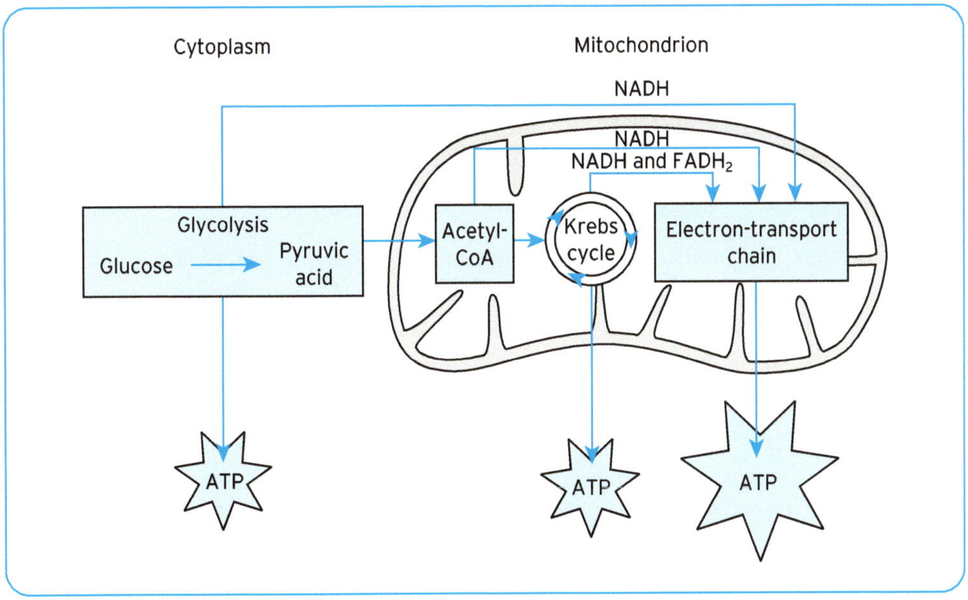

Figure 8.2
Summary of carbohydrate catabolism. (Adapted from Sockhevi G. I. (1996) *An Introduction to Chemistry for Biology Students*, 5th edn, Belmont, CA: Benjamin/Commins.)

Study Figure 8.2 for a moment. The cells of the body are bound by a membrane called the cell membrane. The contents of the cell are, collectively, called **cytoplasm** (literally, 'cell substance'). Within the cytoplasm are structures that undertake specific functions for the cell, and these are called **organelles** (literally, 'little organs'). One type of organelle, the **mitochondria**, is important in the production of energy. Note that glycolysis occurs in the cytoplasm, while the Krebs cycle and the electron-transport chain both take place in the mitochondria. The conversion of pyruvic acid to acetyl-CoA is an intermediate stage that also takes place in the mitochondria but that does not involve the liberation of energy. Glycolysis is described as an **anaerobic** process, meaning that it does not require oxygen. In contrast, the electron-transport chain requires oxygen and is described as an **aerobic** process.

- ***What about the Krebs cycle?***

The Krebs cycle itself does not require oxygen, but since it is linked closely to the electron-transport chain the two are often dealt with collectively and described as aerobic cellular respiration. You need to bear this in mind when looking at different textbooks, as it is a point at which students can become confused.

Let's have a brief look at all the stages in energy production – you will need to refer to Figure 8.2 in order to work out what is happening. In glycolysis, the starting point is glucose.

- ***To what is glucose converted?***

In glycolysis, glucose is converted to **pyruvic acid**.

- ***Is there anything else produced by glycolysis?***

Yes – ATP (remember that this is the body's chemical form of energy) and NADH. NADH transfers hydrogen elsewhere in the cell.

- ***To where does NADH transfer hydrogen?***

Follow the arrows in Figure 8.2 and you will see that NADH transfers hydrogen to the electron-transport chain of the mitochondria.

- ***What happens to pyruvic acid?***

In the second stage, pyruvic acid diffuses into the mitochondria, and here it is converted to acetyl-CoA, which enters the Krebs cycle. Note that this conversion also produces NADH, and guess where this goes? Yes, to the electron-transport chain. In Practice point 8.2 the fate of pyruvic acid is related to exercise and training and the symptom 'stitch'.

The Krebs cycle is the third stage; it leads to the production of $FADH_2$ and further ATP and NADH. The fourth stage, the electron-transport chain, is a series of reactions that lead to the production of many more molecules of ATP than does glycolysis or the Krebs cycle. Consequently, Figure 8.2 shows a larger 'explosion' symbol at this point.

Practice point 8.2

Exercise and training

Although what we have said so far is quite true, the actual fate of pyruvic acid depends upon the availability of oxygen at the time it is produced. If sufficient oxygen is not available (e.g. in muscle cells during vigorous exercise), then aerobic cellular respiration cannot proceed and NADH is unable to deliver its hydrogen atoms to the Krebs cycle and the electron-transport chain. Instead, the hydrogen atoms are offloaded to pyruvic acid, which is reduced to **lactic acid** and which causes the symptoms of fatigue and a burning or aching pain that we call 'stitch'. One effect of training (taking vigorous exercise regularly) is an improvement in blood supply, so that the individual becomes able to endure longer periods of vigorous exercise.

- ***So what do we do when someone has stitch?***

Stitch is painful, so the affected person rests, which restores the balance between oxygen supply and demand. When this happens, lactic acid is converted back to pyruvic acid, which then enters the aerobic pathway.

Fat catabolism

Thus far, we have concentrated upon carbohydrate catabolism and the release of energy from the oxidation of glucose. Although brain cells use glucose exclusively, most cells are able to metabolise other molecules, including fats. The first step is the hydrolysis (breakdown) of fat in fat cells. This leads to the production of **glycerol** and **carboxylic acids**. Glycerol enters glycolysis and ATP is produced as a consequence. Carboxylic acids are metabolised in the liver in a process called **beta oxidation** - the result is acetyl-CoA, which enters the Krebs cycle in the mitochondria.

- ***How much energy is available from the metabolism of fat?***

The answer to this question is that it depends upon the length of the fatty-acid chain. All fatty-acid chains have more carbon atoms than glucose and consequently yield more acetyl groups than does glucose. This may create something of a problem - the liver converts an accumulation of acetyl-CoA molecules to **ketones**. These are molecules that contain hydrocarbon groups (CH) attached to a carbonyl group (CO). One example, acetone, is shown below:

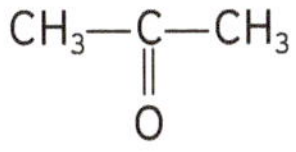

Other examples also possess a carboxyl group (COOH) and are referred to as **ketoacids**. Ketones and ketoacids are metabolised in muscle cells to produce energy, but an accumulation in excessive quantities (**ketoacidosis**) is detrimental (see Practice point 8.3).

Practice point 8.3

Ketoacidosis

Ketoacidosis refers to the blood becoming more acidic as a consequence of the production of ketones and ketoacids. It occurs when the availability of carbohydrates is reduced and the body begins to draw on its stores of fat.

- ***What circumstances might lead to fat being used as the principal source of energy?***

It is when there is a reduced availability of carbohydrates, such as occurs during prolonged fasting or starvation and in **diabetes mellitus**. In the most familiar form of diabetes mellitus (type I), the hormone **insulin** is deficient; since most cells require insulin for the transport of glucose across cell membranes, there is a cellular deficiency of carbohydrate. Consequently, fats are used as a source of energy, and this leads to the production of ketones and ketoacidosis.

- ***What are the effects of ketoacidosis?***

Whole books and journals are devoted to diabetes mellitus, so we're just skimming the surface here. First, remember that acids liberate hydrogen ions and lower blood pH (see Chapter 5). This pH is the principal stimulation of respiration and leads to a characteristic deep, fast respiratory pattern called **Kussmaul's respirations**. Second, ketones such as acetone produce a characteristic smell of pear drops on the breath. Third, ketones are eliminated in the urine and can be detected by **urinalysis** (testing urine with a reagent strip). Finally, high levels of ketones in the blood may eventually lead to coma. Clearly, understanding ketosis has important practical implications. For details of nursing care, you will need to consult a nursing textbook.

Protein catabolism

When other sources of energy are unavailable, for example in starvation, proteins may be catabolised and used to provide energy. In the liver, the amino group (NH_2) is removed from amino acids in a process called **deamination**. This NH_2 group is then converted to **ammonia** (NH_3) and finally to **urea**, which is excreted in the urine. The fate of the remaining part of the molecule depends upon which amino acid is being catabolised, but it is converted to one of the substances in the Krebs cycle. For example, following deamination, the amino acid alanine is converted to pyruvic acid, while leucine is converted to acetyl-CoA. The important thing to note is that the body's primary source of energy is glucose, but fats and proteins may both be catabolised when required.

Basal metabolic rate

The metabolic rate is the rate at which energy is expended by the body. It is measured in kilojoules per hour (kJ/h). A range of different conditions affect metabolic rate.

● ***Can you think of some of them?***

Your list might include the sleep-wake cycle, exercise, hormones, the feeding-fasting state, stress and illness. Clearly, if we are to compare the metabolic rates of different individuals, recordings must be made under identical conditions. In fact, basal conditions are chosen – hence, the term basal metabolic rate (BMR). 'Basal' refers to the state in which the individual is fasted, rested and inactive but awake. It is not the lowest metabolic rate that the body experiences, since that occurs during sleep. We do not describe the measurement of metabolic rate here, but it is important to understand the concept of metabolic rate because it is referred to in clinical practice. For example, BMR is influenced by the hormone **thyroxine**, which is secreted by the **thyroid gland** in the neck. Consequently, abnormal variations in BMR may reflect under-secretion or over-secretion of thyroxine. You might like to find out more about this hormone in a physiology textbook. You could follow this up by considering nursing care in thyroid dysfunction.

In-text review

- The body derives its energy from the oxidation of nutrient molecules.
- The body's principal source of energy is glucose.
- The body's chemical form of energy is adenosine triphosphate (ATP).
- There are four main stages of glucose catabolism: (i) glycolysis, (ii) conversion of pyruvic acid to acetyl-CoA, (iii) Krebs cycle and (iv) electron-transport chain.
- The breakdown of glucose to liberate energy may be summarised in the following way:

$$C_6H_{12}O_6 + 6O_2 \rightarrow 6CO_2 + 6H_2O$$

$$38\ \text{ADP} \qquad\qquad 38\ \text{ATP}$$

- Fats and proteins may, at times, be catabolised to liberate energy.
- The use of fat as a source of energy may lead to ketoacidosis.

Summary

We began this chapter by comparing the way in which we use the term 'energy' in everyday language with the scientist's concept of energy. We identified the different forms of energy and described the conversion of one form into another in various devices such as lights and heaters. This was used to introduce the energy conversions that take place in the body when it puts to use the food we eat. Energy could be considered a rather impersonal, scientific subject, but we have related its study to the energy value of foods, exercise and illness such as diabetes mellitus.

Summary points

- Energy is defined as the ability to do work.
- Energy exists in a number of forms, such as light and heat.
- Each form of energy may be classified as potential (e.g. the energy locked in chemicals) or kinetic (the energy of movement, e.g. muscle contraction).
- Energy cannot be created or destroyed, but it can be converted from one form to another.
- Various units are used to measure energy, the SI unit being the joule (J).
- The energy value of foods is given in kilojoules (kJ).
- The body derives its energy from the oxidation of nutrient molecules.
- The body's chemical form of energy is adenosine triphosphate (ATP).
- There are four main stages of glucose catabolism: (i) glycolysis, (ii) conversion of pyruvic acid to acetyl-CoA, (iii) Krebs cycle and (iv) electron-transport chain.
- The breakdown of glucose to liberate energy may be summarised in the following way:

$$C_6H_{12}O_6 + 6O_2 \rightarrow 6CO_2 + 6H_2O$$

$$\text{38 ADP} \qquad\qquad \text{38 ATP}$$

- Fats and proteins may, at times, be catabolised to liberate energy.

Self-test questions

1 Which of the following are examples of kinetic energy?
(a) A glucose molecule.
(b) Contracting heart.
(c) A compressed spring.
(d) Oxygen molecules diffusing in to blood.

2 Which of the following are examples of potential energy?
(a) The ATP molecule.
(b) Flowing blood.
(c) A stationary car at the top of a hill.
(d) Muscle contraction.

3 Which of the following statements about energy are true?
(a) It is impossible to change one form of energy into another.
(b) In ordinary chemical reactions, energy cannot be destroyed.
(c) One form of energy may be transformed into another.
(d) In ordinary chemical reactions, energy cannot be created.

4 Match the energy conversion on the left with the appropriate device on the right.

(a) Light → electrical	(i) Vacuum cleaner
(b) Chemical → electrical	(ii) Speaker
(c) Electrical → mechanical	(iii) Solar panel
(d) Electrical → sound	(iv) Artificial heart pacemaker

5 Which of the following statements are true?

(a) The calorie is the amount of energy required to raise the temperature of 1 kg of water by 1 °C.

(b) Calorie = 1000 calories.

(c) 1 calorie = 4.2 J.

(d) 1 Calorie = 42 J.

6 Which of the following statements about glycolysis are true?

(a) Pyruvic acid is the end product.

(b) It occurs in mitochondria.

(c) It begins with glucose.

(d) It results in the production of ATP.

7 Which of the following statements about the Krebs cycle are true?

(a) Pyruvic acid is the end product.

(b) It occurs in mitochondria.

(c) It begins with glucose.

(d) It results in the production of ATP.

8 Match the substance on the left with the appropriate description on the right.

(a) Acetyl-CoA	(i) The product of glycolysis
(b) ATP	(ii) Enters the Krebs cycle
(c) NAD	(iii) Referred to as 'energy currency'
(d) Pyruvic acid	(iv) A derivative of niacin

9 Match the reaction on the left with the appropriate description on the right.

(a) ADP → ATP	(i) Hydrolysis
(b) $NAD^+ \rightarrow NADH + H^+$	(ii) Oxidation
(c) $FADH_2 \rightarrow FAD$	(iii) Reduction
(d) Fats → fatty acids + glycerol	(iv) Phosphorylation

10 Match the reaction on the left with the appropriate description on the right.

(a) Removal of NH_2 group	(i) Reduction
(b) Metabolism of carboxylic acids	(ii) Ketoacidosis
(c) Production of molecules with a carbonyl group (CO) and a carboxyl group (COOH)	(iii) Beta oxidation
(d) NAD → NADH	(iv) Deamination

Further study/exercises

1 We have looked at the energy-liberating reactions of the body, but how do the energy requirements of individuals vary? To answer this question, compare the energy requirements of the following groups:

- A 6-month-old baby.
- A child 5 years old.
- Male and female adolescents.
- A pregnant woman.
- A lactating woman.
- An elderly person.

Barker H. M. (2002). *Nutrition and Dietetics for Health Care*, 10th edn. Edinburgh: Churchill Livingstone.

Dudek S. G. (2007). *Nutrition Essentials for Nursing Practice*. Philadelphia: Lippincott; Williams and Wilkins.

Truswell A. S. (2003). *ABC of Nutrition*, 4th edn. London: BMJ Books.

2 Clearly, the energy requirements of individuals depend not only upon their age and lifestyle but also on the presence of illness. How do the following influence the energy requirements of the body?

- Elective surgery.
- Major trauma.
- Extensive burns.

Barker H. M. (2002). *Nutrition and Dietetics for Health Care*, 10th edn. Edinburgh: Churchill Livingstone.

Dudek S. G. (2007). *Nutrition Essentials for Nursing Practice*. Philadelphia: Lippincott; Williams and Wilkins.

9

Heat and body temperature

Learning outcomes

After reading the following chapter and undertaking personal study, you should be able to:

1. Distinguish between heat and temperature.
2. Define the terms 'latent heat of fusion' and 'latent heat of vaporisation'.
3. Outline the Celsius and Kelvin scales for the measurement of temperature.
4. Describe various temperature-measurement devices used in clinical practice, including the mercury-in-glass thermometer, the thermistor and the tympanic membrane thermometer.
5. Distinguish between core and peripheral body temperature and give examples of importance to clinical practice.
6. Discuss some of the factors that influence body temperature in health.
7. Describe the procedure for taking body temperature with a thermistor and a tympanic membrane thermometer, and discuss the effects of site and duration of measurement upon the value obtained.
8. Describe four physical processes by which heat is transferred, and relate these to the body.
9. Describe the mechanisms of temperature homeostasis.
10. Discuss the causes, effects and management of pyrexia, heat exhaustion, heat stroke and hypothermia.

Introduction

Heat and temperature are important topics of study for health-care professionals. Indeed, one of the first clinical skills acquired by student nurses is the measurement of body temperature. Until recently, this was an uncomplicated task, there being only one device - the clinical (mercury-in-glass) thermometer - available for this purpose. Today, however, you will also need to be familiar with **thermistors** and **tympanic membrane thermometers**. Patients' problems remain the same as ever - for example, the elderly person with hypothermia (low body temperature) or the **febrile** (feverish) child with an infection. In contrast, situations such as the infant in whom profound **hypothermia** has been induced purposefully during a heart operation have become more common only in recent years.

The cases noted above illustrate the fact that a greater understanding of the science of heat and temperature and its measurement is currently demanded of health-care professionals than in the past. Let us begin our study of these topics by asking a question:

- ***What is the difference between heat and temperature?***

Heat and temperature

If you have read the previous chapter, you will already know that heat is a form of energy. Consequently, it might surprise you to learn that, until the end of the eighteenth century, heat was thought of as a material substance. Although we now know that this is not the case, we still speak of heat being transferred from one object to another. It is fine to talk this way, as long as we remember that what is being transferred (heat) is a form of energy. Temperature is not the same as heat; instead, it may be regarded as the degree of hotness.

- ***But don't two objects with the same temperature have the same amount of heat energy?***

If you are not sure about the answer to this question, think about the following illustration. Imagine two containers of water at room temperature (20 °C). Suppose one contains 1 kg and the other 2 kg of water. Now imagine that the same amount of energy is delivered to them both - 4.2 kJ (kilojoules) perhaps.

- ***Will the temperature of the water in both containers rise by the same degree?***

Intuitively, you might predict that the smaller volume will be hotter. If you go back to Chapter 8, you will be reminded that 4.2 kJ is sufficient energy to raise the temperature of 1 kg of water by 1 °C and so conclude that it would take twice as much energy to raise 2 kg of water to the same degree. Actually, we have not taken into account the amount of energy required to heat the container and the energy losses while heating takes place. The point of this discussion is not to work out the actual temperature rise but simply to show that heat and temperature are not the same thing at all. This difference is illustrated further when we consider the concept of latent heat.

Latent heat and changes in state

Let us think again about the experiment involving the heating of ice that we introduced at the beginning of Chapter 4. In this experiment, we noted that as the ice is heated, the temperature initially rises but remains stable for a time as the ice melts. Once melted, the temperature rises again but becomes stable as the water boils. These changes are illustrated by the graph in Figure 9.1.

- ***What is happening between points b and c?***

The ice is melting and there is no rise in temperature, despite the fact that heating continues.

- ***What is happening between points d and e?***

The water is vaporising (boiling); once again, there is no temperature rise despite the fact that heating continues.

- ***So how much energy does it take to get from a to b, compared with b to c, c to d, and d to e?***

Suppose we start with 1 kg of ice at –10 °C. It takes only 42 kJ of energy to raise the temperature of the ice from –10 °C to 0 °C (a to b). Surprisingly, it then takes a further 330 kJ to melt the ice (b to c). To raise the temperature of 1 kg of water from 0 °C to 100 °C then requires 420 kJ (c to d), but very much more (2260 kJ) to vaporise the water.

You may recall that the heat supplied during the melting of ice is used to enable water molecules to partially escape the strong attraction that they have for each other in solid

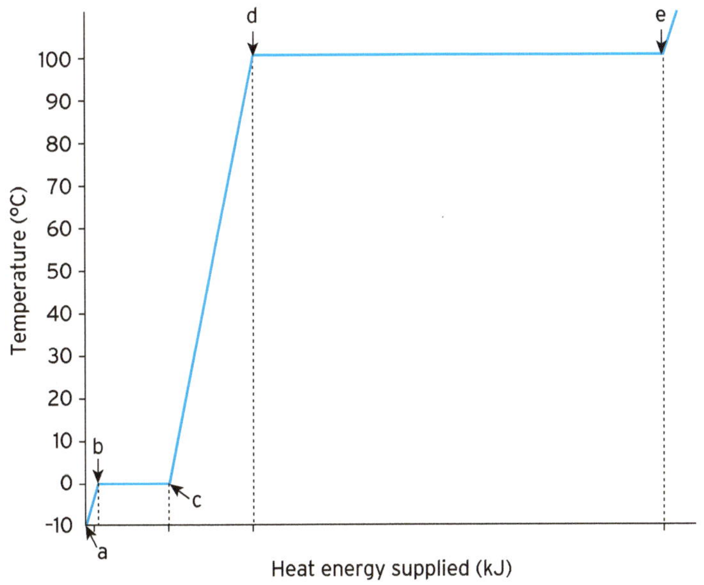

Figure 9.1
The rise in temperature as ice is heated.

state. The heat required for this process of melting is referred to as the **latent heat of fusion**. Here, the term 'latent' may be interpreted as 'hidden', since the heat cannot be detected with a thermometer. Similarly, the heat supplied during boiling enables water molecules to escape the weak attraction they have for each other in the liquid state and so enter the gaseous state. The heat required to vaporise the water is, not surprisingly, referred to as the **latent heat of vaporisation**.

- ***Can we make use of latent heat?***

Yes we can, as Practice point 9.1 demonstrates.

Practice point 9.1

Latent heat and ice packs

One example of the use we make of latent heat of fusion is the application of ice packs to the body for the purpose of cooling.

- ***What advantage does ice have over water for cooling?***

It isn't just a matter of temperature. Remember those figures quoted earlier? It takes relatively little energy to raise the temperature of 1 kg of ice by 10 °C (42 kJ) compared with the latent heat of fusion (330 kJ). When ice packs are applied to the body, there is initially no change in the pack temperature as the ice melts, but there is a considerable cooling of tissues to which the ice is applied.

- ***To what use might this be put?***

One application is the reduction of swelling and pain following injury, of joints for example, through the mechanism of **vasoconstriction** (constriction of blood vessels). Our bodies also make use of the latent heat of vaporisation, but we shall consider this later when we discuss sweating.

Temperature scales

The measurement of energy (including heat) in joules has already been described, so this chapter will focus upon temperature. One temperature scale has already been mentioned, and it is probably the one that is most familiar to you - the **Celsius** scale. Fortunately, this is also the scale used in clinical practice. It is named after Anders Celsius who, in the eighteenth century, proposed a scale based upon 100 divisions between the melting point of ice and the boiling point of water. Consequently, ice melts at 0 °C and water boils at 100 °C.

- ***What is normal body temperature in degrees Celsius?***

It is 37 °C, but there are other scales too. Although we have stressed the need to use SI units, the SI unit of temperature is the **Kelvin** (K, not °K) rather than the degree Celsius. The Kelvin scale is so named because William Thomson, who subsequently became Lord Kelvin, proposed it. In this scale, each division is equal to a division on the Celsius scale; to convert from Celsius to Kelvin, simply add 273.

- ***What are the melting and boiling points of water in Kelvin?***

They are 273 K and 373 K, respectively.

- ***How did this scale come about?***

It relates to the predicted temperature at which particles of matter have the lowest kinetic energy. This is –273 °C, which is taken to be the zero point on the Kelvin scale - sometimes called **absolute zero**.

Finally, you may have heard of the Fahrenheit scale, but this is now rarely used and certainly not in clinical practice. Its use should be avoided, but for the sake of completeness we note that ice melts at 32 °F and water boils at 212 °F. One degree Fahrenheit is not, therefore, equal to one degree Celsius. The following shows how the two units are converted:

$$°C = °F - 32 \times 5/9$$

$$°F = °C \times 9/5 + 32$$

Temperature-measurement devices

If we wanted to devise a means of measuring changes in temperature, we might think of making use of a substance, some physical property of which changes with temperature. A good choice would be mercury, which expands uniformly as temperature rises, is a good conductor of heat (see later) and is opaque and, therefore, visible. The **mercury-in-glass thermometer** makes use of these properties of mercury; this is such an effective device that it still finds use today - 350 years after it was invented.

The mercury-in-glass thermometer

This type of thermometer is illustrated in Figure 9.2. In this device, the mercury is located in a bulb but may expand up a fine tube that runs the length of the thermometer. In **clinical thermometers** (used to measure body temperature), this tube is very fine indeed. The tube has to be fine, since the degree of expansion of mercury over the range of variation in body

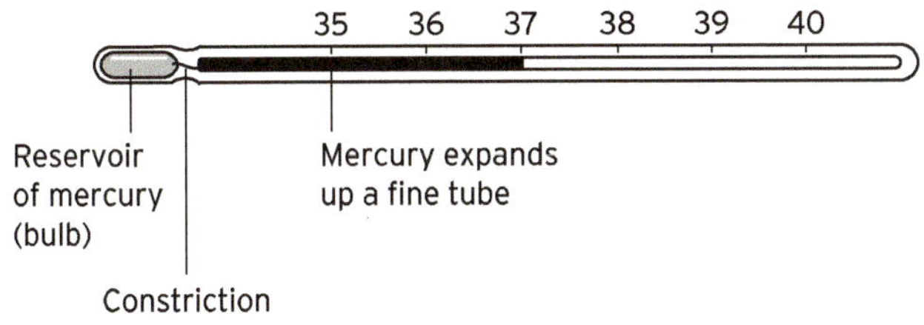

Figure 9.2
A mercury-in-glass thermometer.

temperature is slight. The fineness of the tube makes the mercury column within it difficult to see. The trick is to rotate the thermometer between the fingers and thumb while holding it horizontally at eye level. At a certain point, the glass of the thermometer will magnify the fine column and a reading can be taken from the scale.

- ***While I am doing this, will the mercury not contract again? Do I have to rush to get a reliable reading?***

Clinical thermometers have a special feature that ordinary mercury-in-glass thermometers do not possess - a constriction just above the bulb. This does not impede the mercury as it expands but it does prevent it from receding once the thermometer has been taken from the body. It is, therefore, an example of a maximum-reading thermometer.

- ***So how do I get the mercury column down again?***

It has to be shaken down - some care needs to be taken, since glass thermometers are easy to break and mercury is toxic. In the UK, mercury-in-glass thermometers have, for reasons of safety, been replaced by other methods of measuring temperature. The above description of the mercury-in-glass thermometer has been included for those whose work takes them into countries where it is still used.

The thermistor

This is an example of an energy-converting device - **thermistors** convert heat into electrical energy and give a digital readout of temperature. In the continuous monitoring of temperature, a thermistor consists of a heat-sensitive probe connected to a recording device. The probe is flexible and blunt and can be inserted into a body orifice. It may be passed into the **rectum** via the anus or into the **nasopharynx** or **oesophagus** via the nostril. It has to be said that this is not entirely comfortable! Consequently, thermistors are generally used in unconscious and more seriously ill patients, such as in critical care units. Although it is not difficult to pass a probe into the rectum, some skill is required to pass a probe into the oesophagus, especially if the patient is unconscious.

Thermistors are also available for recording a single measurement of temperature. A number of different designs are available, one of which is illustrated in Figure 9.3. In everyday language, health-care workers do not usually use the term 'thermistor' but instead refer to 'temperature probes' or 'electronic thermometers'.

Liquid-crystal thermometers

The term '**liquid crystal**' sounds like a contradiction in terms, but it refers to liquids that possess properties of certain crystals, such as colour change associated with temperature variation. Plastic strips impregnated with liquid crystals can be used to indicate temperature by placing the strip on the forehead. They have the advantage of requiring no skill in use, and this may be important in the home. However, they record the peripheral skin temperature only, and this may be considerably lower than the core temperature (see later). They therefore have limited use.

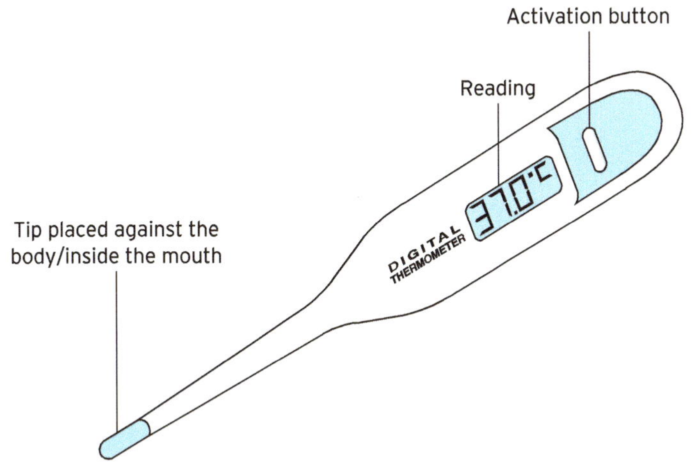

Figure 9.3
A thermistor (electronic thermometer).

Tympanic membrane thermometers

Tympanic membrane thermometers measure temperature indirectly from the intensity of **infrared radiation** (IR) emitted from the **tympanic membrane** (eardrum). Infrared radiation consists of energy in the form of rays that form part of the **electromagnetic spectrum**. Perhaps you are already familiar with infrared radiation, but if not it may help you to know that visible light is also part of this spectrum. We shall consider it in more detail in Chapter 12. An example of a tympanic membrane thermometer is illustrated in Figure 9.4. Such devices are quick, simple to operate and accurate. Consequently, they are gaining use in a variety of care settings and at home. We describe the procedure for taking temperatures in Practice point 9.2 later in this chapter, but first let us consider body temperature in a little more detail.

Body temperature

The temperature of the body at any one time depends upon the amount of heat generated by cellular metabolism and exchanged with the environment. At first sight, the term 'body temperature' appears self-explanatory, but if you study Figure 9.5 for a moment you will see that the value recorded varies according to the site at which the measurement is taken. The implication is that we have to clarify what we mean by the term.

Core temperature is that of the organs of the body cavities – the brain in the cranium, the heart and lungs in the chest, and the liver in the abdomen. In normal health, the resting core temperature varies from 37 °C by less than 1 °C, and it is this value that is most useful in clinical practice. Core temperature varies with activity level, and it may rise to 40 °C during

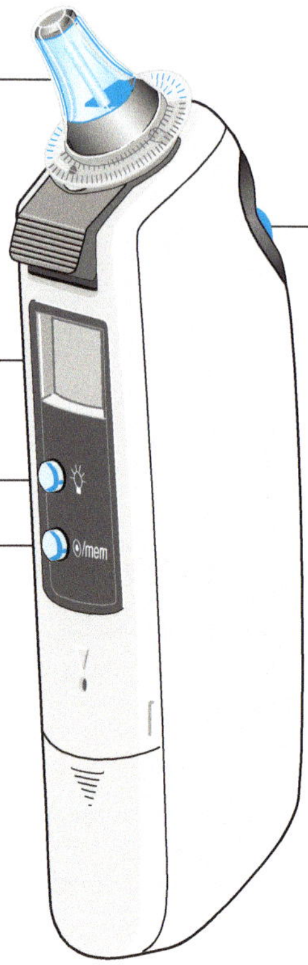

Figure 9.4
An infrared tympanic membrane thermometer.

vigorous exercise. Table 9.1 shows the normal range of body temperature for various activity levels. **Peripheral temperature**, sometimes called **shell temperature**, is the temperature of the surface of the body; it has a lower value than core temperature. At certain sites, for example the feet, peripheral temperature is considerably below the core value.

Table 9.1 Approximate core temperature at different activity levels.

Temperature (°C)	Activity level
40	Momentarily during vigorous exercise
39	
38	Moderate exercise
37	Normal at rest
36	On waking

The progressive fall in temperature as blood flows through the limbs, illustrated in Figure 9.5, indicates that an important heat-conserving mechanism is in operation. As blood flows away from the torso in the arteries of the limbs, heat is lost to the blood flowing in the opposite direction in adjacent and parallel veins. This means that blood returning to the torso is re-warmed, as is shown in Figure 9.6. This is an example of a counter-current mechanism that results in relatively stable temperatures at

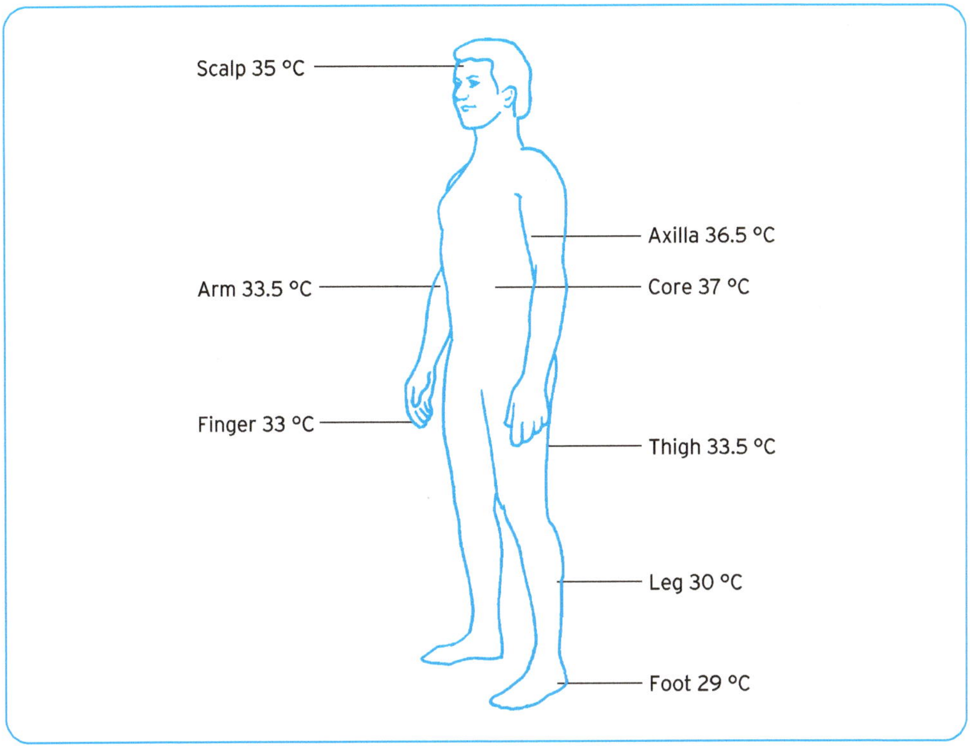

Figure 9.5
Approximate shell temperature recorded at various sites in a thermoneutral environment.

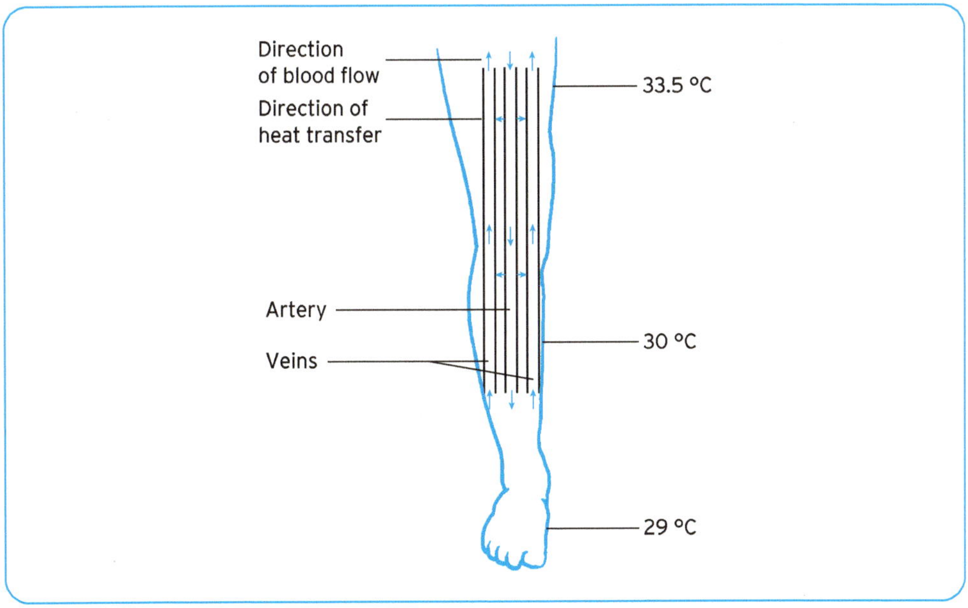

Figure 9.6
Counter-current heat transfer.

each point along both vessels. Were this mechanism not in operation, blood would cool as it passed through the arterial system and not be re-warmed as it returned in the venous system. This would tend towards a reduction in core temperature.

The above considerations help us to interpret the meaning of a body temperature value measured at different sites with different measurement devices. Further explanation is given in the following two Practice points. Practice point 9.2 deals with measuring body temperature with an electronic thermometer and 9.3 with a tympanic membrane thermometer.

Practice point 9.2

Measuring body temperature with an electronic thermometer

Electronic thermometers are simple to use, but there are a number of different designs. Become familiar with the type used in clinical areas where you have placements. Some electronic thermometers are self-contained units, the tip of which is applied to the point on the body where temperature is to be measured. In other designs, the temperature-sensing probe is separate from the power source and read out. Operation usually involves pressing a button and waiting for an audible signal that means the temperature value can be read. The ability to measure body temperature accurately is an important skill.

- ***How do I ensure that an accurate measurement of core temperature is obtained?***

The answer is to choose an appropriate site. The oral cavity is an obvious choice, but the tip of the device has to be placed adjacent to the **sublingual artery** at the base of the tongue. This ensures that the temperature of blood that has travelled only a short distance from the heart is recorded. Even so, the value obtained will be a little below that of the actual core temperature, since the sublingual pocket is not completely isolated from environmental influences. The difference may be about 0.4 °C.

- ***Are there any problems with the use of the oral cavity?***

Yes, but they are not difficult to perceive. The patient has to be conscious and cooperative. Do not use the oral cavity in infants or young children; many patients with learning disabilities are also unsuitable. In addition, no foods or fluids should have been consumed or cigarettes smoked in the 15 minutes before a measurement is taken, since these affect accuracy significantly. Cleanliness is also important if cross-infection is to be avoided; thus a fresh, disposable plastic sheath must be used to cover the tip of the device for each patient.

An alternative to the oral cavity is the **axilla** (armpit), but the depth of this cavity in elderly and emaciated patients may mean that it is difficult to keep the thermometer in place adjacent to the **axillary artery**. Even when this is achieved, the value of the measurement may be 1 °C lower than the value recorded in the oral cavity. Clearly it is important to record the site of measurement as well as the value itself. In addition, the axilla is unreliable when hypothermia is present. Unfortunately, in this case, the oral site may also be contraindicated, since the patient may not be fully conscious.

A solution is then to use a tympanic membrane thermometer, as accurate results can be obtained without disturbance to the patient.

Practice point 9.3

Measuring body temperature with a tympanic membrane thermometer

The tympanic membrane thermometer is a self-contained unit that may be rechargable or powered by replaceable batteries. The first thing to do is check the batteries or charge level. If you arrive on duty one morning and find that none of the thermometers is working, you will understand how important this basic point is. Before a typanic membrane thermometer can be used, a new plastic shield must be applied over the tip of the probe. Changing the shield between each patient reduces the risk of transmitting an ear infection. The unit is switched on and the probe inserted a little way into the **external auditory canal** (ear canal). A button is pressed to give an almost instant digital readout.

- ***It is simple and uncomplicated, then?***

Actually, no. Although typanic membrane thermometers can be very accurate, in the practice setting they may be much less accurate than we imagine. The reason for inaccuracy is almost always operator error. Earlier in this chapter, we described a thermometer as a device that uses a change in a physical property of a material to measure temperature. We illustrated this with the example of the clinical thermometer that uses the expansion of mercury in a thin glass tube. In contrast, the typanic membrane thermometer detects infrared radiation - strictly, it is not a thermometer. The point to note is that all surfaces of the body emit infrared radiation, including the external auditory canal. The intensity of the infrared radiation coming from the canal will be much less than that radiating from the tympanic membrane (eardrum).

To obtain an accurate reading of temperature, the detector head must then be directed towards the typanic membrane, but there is a problem: The external auditory canal is not straight, and its shape differs between infants and adults.

- ***What procedure should then be followed?***

Ideally, the patient should be sitting, although clear access to the side of the head can be gained in other positions too. An ear-tug needs to be performed to straighten the canal so that the probe is pointing towards the tympanic membrane. 'Ear-tug' is an unfortunate expression, but it is commonly used. It refers to gently pulling on the **pinna** (external ear). In infants up to 1 year old, gently pull the ear straight back; in adults, pull the ear up and back, as illustrated in Figure 9.7. The probe should now fit snugly into the external auditory canal and the activation button can be pressed. The thermometer then gives an almost instant digital readout of temperature.

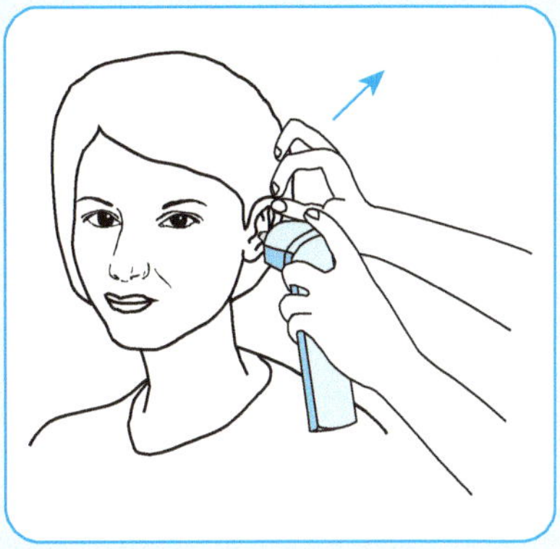

Figure 9.7
Performing an 'ear-tug' before using a tympanic membrane thermometer.

Cyclical variations in body temperature

Body temperature is not constant throughout the day but varies in a rhythmical fashion. Such body rhythms are referred to as **circadian rhythms**; those that occur on a daily basis are referred to as **diurnal**. The highest body temperature is recorded between 16:00 and 20:00 and the lowest value between 02:00 and 06:00. The difference is in the range 0.5–1.0 °C and should be borne in mind when interpreting a temperature record. In Practice point 9.4, the use of a measurement of body temperature as part of a method of natural birth control is outlined.

Practice point 9.4

Body temperature and natural birth control

In addition to the diurnal variation of body temperature noted above, that of the female also varies with the **menstrual cycle**. Daily measurements of body temperature may be used to indicate the onset of the absolutely infertile period - that is, the part of the menstrual cycle when intercourse will not lead to conception.

The **ovary** secretes the hormone **progesterone** following **ovulation** (the release of the **oocyte**/egg cell). This hormone is responsible for the peak in body temperature that remains until one or two days before the next period. The absolutely infertile phase is considered to have begun once three high temperatures have been recorded. Once progesterone levels begin to fall, the temperature also drops, but it is worth noting that the variation of body temperature attributable to progesterone is generally less than one-half of one degree Celsius. Consequently, as accurate a measurement as possible should be made. It is a good idea to use the same thermometer for each measurement and to take the temperature at the same time of day - ideally first thing in the morning. The measurement of body temperature in an attempt to determine when intercourse will not lead to conception is one aspect of a natural means of birth control. Women who practise natural birth control also make other observations, and you might like to find out more about what is involved. As you might expect, the reliability of this method is not high. It may, however, be chosen by women who do not require a high level of protection or who do not wish to use hormone-based contraception.

The transmission of heat

We have noted already that heat may be transmitted from one object to another; we are so familiar with this that we think little about it. After all, when we are cold it is the most natural thing in the world to stand by a heater. In the following section, we examine the physical processes involved in the transmission of heat and then apply this understanding to practice.

Conduction

Conduction is the process whereby heat is transmitted from one object to another in contact with it. If we go to pick up a spoon that has been resting for some time in a hot drink, we are not surprised to discover that the spoon is hot.

- ***What has actually occurred to make the spoon hot?***

Remember that we described previously how the kinetic energy of water molecules increases as water is heated. The high kinetic energy water molecules of the hot drink collide with, and so lose energy to, the atoms of the metal spoon; as a consequence, the temperature of the spoon rises. When we try to pick up the spoon, some of this energy is also transmitted to us, and our fingers also become hot. The important thing to note with regard to this form of heat transmission is contact between objects.

- ***Does all matter conduct heat equally well?***

We often make decisions about conductivity that show this is not the case.

- ***For example, what do we really mean when we say that we need a warm coat for winter?***

For a start, we do not mean that the coat itself is warm. The coat may be warm or cold, depending upon where it is at the time. What we mean is that the coat keeps us warm by not allowing heat to escape readily from our bodies. To put it another way, we could say that the coat is a poor conductor or a good insulator. In everyday language, we often make the mistake of referring to temperature when actually we are commenting upon a material's conductivity. For example, we may use the term 'cold steel', but actually we are indicating that metals are good conductors of heat. Consequently, even when metal is at room temperature, if we touch it with bare skin heat is readily conducted away from our body, and we detect this as a peripheral cooling. Similarly, if we walk barefoot on a tiled floor, we might describe the floor as cold, when in reality it is simply a better conductor of heat than carpet. An occasion when we do use the proper terminology is when we talk of insulating the loft. Here, we acknowledge that we are using a poor conductor - we do not usually say that we are warming the loft.

Convection

In our definition of conduction, we spoke of heat being transferred from one object to another. Here, the word 'object' stands for any form of matter - living organisms, solids, liquids and gases. In fact, heat is conducted from hot objects to a cooler atmosphere around them.

- ***Now work out what happens to the density of the air surrounding a hot object.***

Perhaps you have figured out that as air is heated, the kinetic energy of the gas molecules increases, and they move further apart. Consequently, the air becomes less dense and rises. Its place around the hot object is taken by denser, cooler air, which then becomes heated, and the process, called **convection**, is repeated. In this way, a hot object placed in a room in which the air is still begins to produce currents of air - we call them **convection currents**. Indeed, the expression is used to describe heaters - convector heaters or convectors. The important thing to note is that convection is a further physical process by which hot objects lose heat.

Radiation

You will no doubt have realised that one thing that conduction and convection have in common is that heat is lost from matter to matter. Now think about the warming of the earth by the sun.

- ***Is matter involved in the transmission of heat in this case?***

Clearly not, since the earth is separated from the sun by the vacuum of space. Another process must be involved here, and it is this that we refer to as **radiation**. Once again, the language used here should be familiar - we refer to some heating devices as radiators. The word 'radiation' actually refers to something diverging from a point. In this case, that something is energy in the form of rays - infrared rays in fact. Incidentally, dark objects absorb infrared radiation more readily than light ones, and silvered surfaces reflect infrared just as they reflect light. Consequently, you may have noticed that black cars become very hot in summer, but this is less of a problem in white cars. You may also have worked out that there is a good reason why Mediterranean houses are often painted white.

Evaporation

Wet objects lose heat as water changes from the liquid to the gaseous state - remember the latent heat of vaporisation? This occurs at much lower temperatures than the boiling point, since not all water molecules have the same kinetic energy and some higher-energy molecules will escape the attraction of others at temperatures below 100 °C. We call this process **evaporation**, and we are quite familiar with it in everyday life. Evaporation is the reason why puddles dry up after a shower of rain. We should also note that although all four processes that we have described depend upon a temperature gradient (heat is lost from hot objects to cooler ones), evaporation also depends upon a vapour pressure gradient. This means that for evaporation to be effective, the atmosphere must be dry. If the air around a wet object is saturated with water vapour, so that it is impossible for the air to take up any more water, evaporation will not occur. You may have experienced this if you have visited a tropical country and found that wet clothing takes a long time to dry.

- ***Is there anything that promotes the evaporation of water?***

You might have figured out that an air current does, since air with a higher water vapour pressure (that is, containing more water vapour) around the wet object is replaced by drier air, which can then take up more water by evaporation. This is, of course, the reason that washing dries more quickly on a windy day. We shall note the importance of this to the body later on.

Preventing heat losses: the vacuum flask

If we understand the mechanisms by which heat is transmitted, we can also work out how heat losses can be reduced. Take the example of the vacuum flask illustrated in Figure 9.8. Heat exchange between liquids placed in the flask and the environment is kept to a minimum by a number of features. First, the inner part of the flask consists of a double-walled glass bottle, the two walls of which are separated by a vacuum. This prevents heat losses by conduction and convection. In addition, the silvered surface of the glass bottle is reflective, and this reduces heat losses by radiation.

- ***What about heat exchanges and the body?***

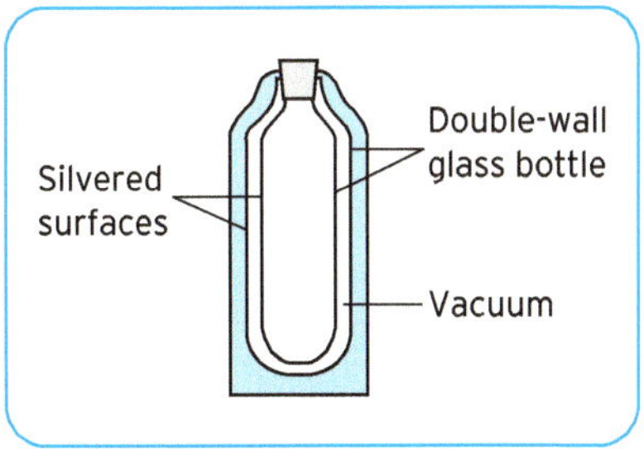

Figure 9.8
A vacuum flask.

Heat exchanges and the body

The exchange of heat between the body and the environment occurs by the same four physical processes that we described earlier and that affect inanimate objects. They are illustrated in Figure 9.9. Ordinarily, some 60% of the heat loss of the body occurs by the process of radiation, although it should be borne in mind that the body may also gain heat by this process. An

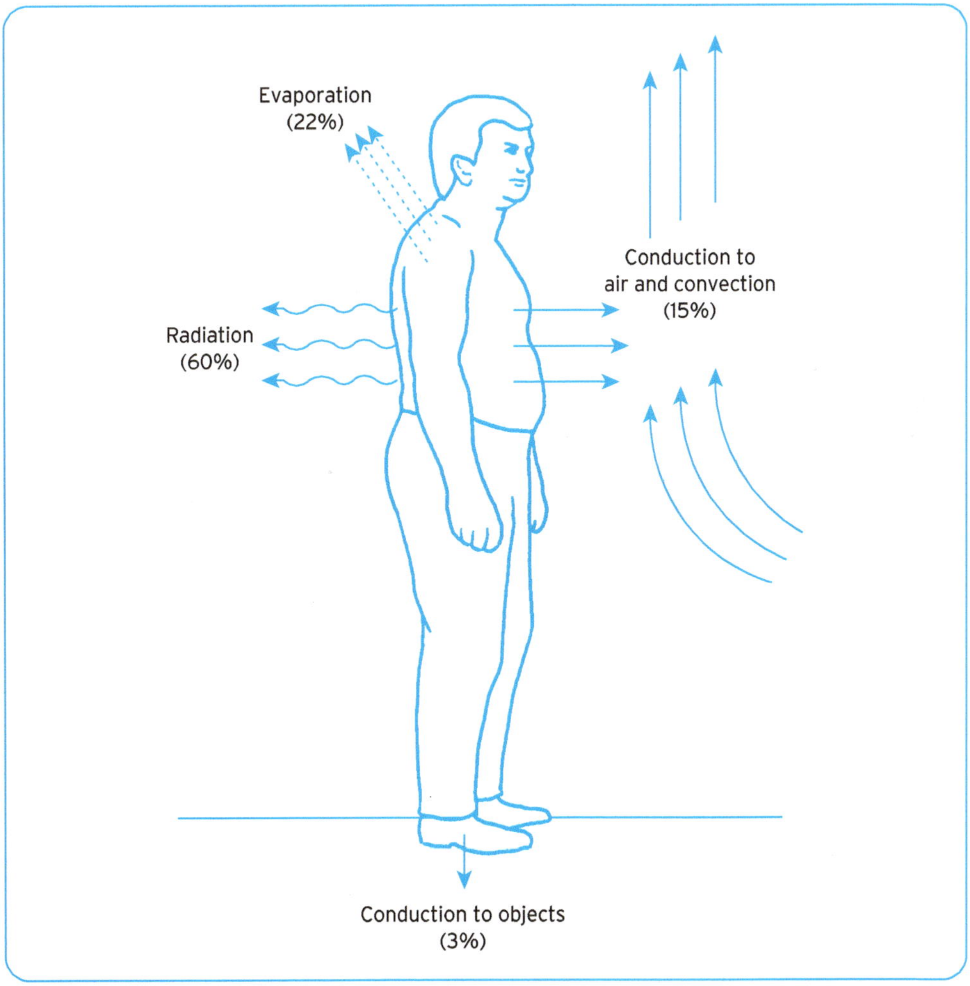

Figure 9.9
Heat losses from the body.

example is the warming produced by sunbathing. It is, of course, possible that this will eventually lead to hyperthermia (elevated body temperature), but do not confuse this with sunburn, which is caused by **ultraviolet radiation**. This is discussed in Chapter 12.

Much less body heat is lost by conduction and convection, since, for most of our lives, we are fairly well insulated, either by our clothing or by our bedclothes when asleep. When these are removed, it is usually in circumstances where the environmental temperature is quite high - a sunny day or after the bathroom heater has been on for a while. Once again, it is possible for the body to gain heat by conduction - a hot bath is a good example. There are some obvious practical applications here. The temperature of any clinical environment in which patients have to undress should take into account the increased heat loss. This invariably means that it is too hot for the staff, and thus uniforms should be of a suitable, lightweight design. In addition, patients who require assistance to get out of the bath should not be unattended for significant periods of time. Note that water has a much greater conductivity than that of air and, as the water temperature decreases, considerable cooling may result. Taken together, conduction and convection account for about 20% of the body's heat losses, but this figure can be increased when air is moved rapidly across the surface of the body, such as occurs in draughts and when fans are used.

Heat is lost from the body by evaporation at a basal level affecting the lungs and mucous membranes of the mouth and nose. During exercise, however, when sweating occurs, the latent heat of vaporisation accounts for a considerable increase in heat loss by this process.

- ***Can you think of other, perhaps less obvious, examples of increased heat loss through evaporation?***

You may have worked out that preventing water loss from the body is one of the functions of the skin. Therefore, patients who have extensive burns experience excessive heat loss and a warm environment will help prevent this. Surgery in which body cavities are opened also results in considerable cooling; unless hypothermia is to be induced as part of the procedure, operating theatres are usually kept quite warm. Indeed, this, together with the use of sterile gowns, sometimes presents a problem for students, who have to get used to the heat and restrictive clothing. It is probably this, rather than the sight of blood, that makes some people feel unwell at the operating table. On average, the evaporation of sweat accounts for about 20% of the heat lost from the body.

There are practical situations in which a consideration of the mechanisms of heat loss from the body become important. The example of the fallen elderly person is given in Practice point 9.5.

Practice point 9.5

Heat loss in the fallen elderly

Let us now put to use some of our knowledge of the physical processes by which heat is lost from the body. The case history of an elderly person who falls in the home, is unable to get up without assistance and subsequently is admitted to hospital with hypothermia (low body temperature) is not at all unusual. The individual may be unable to rise from the floor because of a **cerebrovascular accident** (CVA, stroke) or a fractured neck of **femur** (more common in elderly females). If any lengthy period is spent in inactivity, metabolic rate will fall and, along with it, body temperature. Hypothermia is dealt with a little later, but for now let us concentrate on the processes by which heat is lost.

Heat loss by radiation will continue much as before, but losses by conduction may be considerably increased due to contact between the body and the floor. Carpeting will provide some degree of insulation, but heat loss through tiled floors and floors covered with linoleum will be great. In houses without double-glazing, there may be draughts, which often are worse at floor level because of gaps under doors. Losses through evaporation will be increased if the individual is wet - an example is falling while getting out of the bath.

One practical thing that can be done is to assess the home for a risk of falling. Causes of falls include uneven floors, badly fitting carpets, rugs and slippery floors. In addition, the patient might have intrinsic factors that make a fall more likely, such as periods of low blood pressure (**hypotension**) or slow pulse (**bradycardia**) associated with fainting. Although it is not always possible to predict and prevent falls, it is possible to ensure that help can be called using devices that are worn as a pendant and that transmit a call for help when pressed.

In-text review

- ✔ Temperature and heat are not the same thing. Heat is a form of energy, while temperature is the degree of hotness of an object.
- ✔ The SI unit of temperature is the Kelvin, but degrees Celsius (°C) are used in clinical practice.
- ✔ The amount of heat required to melt a solid is referred to as the latent heat of fusion, and the amount of heat required to vaporise a liquid is referred to as the latent heat of vaporisation.
- ✔ Currently, the two most important temperature-measurement devices in clinical practice are the thermistor and the tympanic membrane thermometer.
- ✔ The temperature of organs within the body is referred to as the core temperature, while the temperature at the surface of the body is the peripheral temperature.
- ✔ Normal core temperature is taken to be 37 °C.
- ✔ The most reliable site for recording body temperature with an electronic thermometer is the sublingual pocket of the oral cavity.
- ✔ The tympanic membrane thermometer gives an immediate and accurate value of core temperature.
- ✔ The transfer of heat occurs by conduction, convection, radiation and evaporation.

Temperature homeostasis

The body strives to maintain core temperature by keeping heat production and heat loss in balance. This is an example of **homeostasis** (see Chapter 2). There are essentially three components to the mechanism by which this is achieved - detectors, control centre and effectors. Temperature detection is performed by structures of the nervous system called **thermoreceptors**, some of which are located in the skin and mucous membranes (peripheral), while others are found deep within the body (central). Impulses from thermoreceptors travel along nerves to the brain, where a structure called the **hypothalamus** functions as a control centre, interpreting the input from thermoreceptors and determining what the response should be. The hypothalamus initiates a response in various body systems. Structures responsible for the response are called effectors (simply meaning structures that have an effect). The hypothalamus strives to maintain a set point of core temperature, and for this reason it has sometimes been described as the body's thermostat.

- ***Which body systems play a part in temperature homeostasis? How does the body respond to a disturbance in temperature?***

After you have thought about this answer to this question, have a look at Figure 9.10. The hypothalamus possesses both heat-promoting and heat-losing centres. It is these areas that

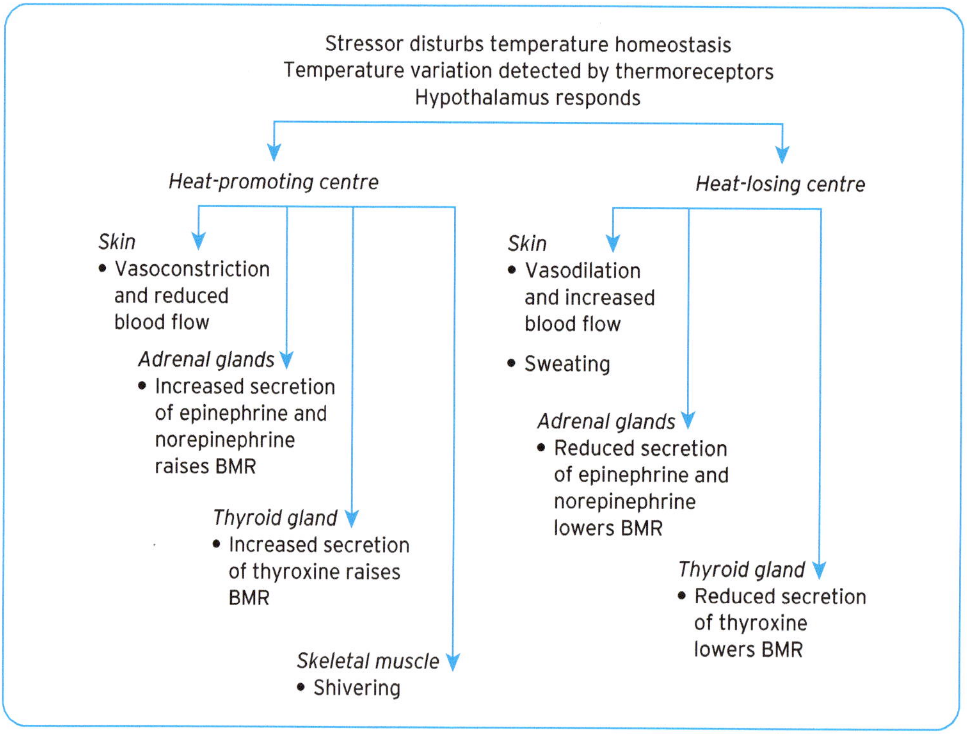

Figure 9.10
The mechanism of temperature homeostasis.

determine the response of the body to a disturbance in temperature. The body systems mainly affected are the skin, skeletal muscle, adrenal glands (situated above the kidneys) and the thyroid gland (situated in the neck).

Let us first consider a decrease in temperature. Nervous impulses to the skin induce cutaneous **vasoconstriction** (blood-vessel constriction in the skin), which results in a decrease in blood flow to the periphery; as a consequence, less heat is lost to the environment by conduction, convection and radiation. This is the reason why we look pale when cold. In addition, vasoconstrictor nerves are concentrated in the distal ends of limbs, and so the greatest effect is in the hands and feet. Other responses are concerned with increasing heat production. For example, the involuntary contraction and relaxation of skeletal muscle (shivering) generates considerable additional heat. Furthermore, the effect of the increased secretion of **epinephrine** (adrenaline) and **norepinephrine** (noradrenaline) from the adrenal medulla and **thyroxine** from the thyroid gland is to raise metabolic rate.

In contrast, when temperature is increased, the response of the body is essentially the opposite of that described above. Blood vessels in the skin dilate (cutaneous **vasodilation**) and heat losses by conduction, convection and radiation are increased. At the same time, the evaporation of sweat results in considerable heat loss through the latent heat of vaporisation, while a reduction in metabolic rate leads to decreased heat production.

One aspect of temperature regulation that we have not mentioned is that of a behavioural response. We change our behaviour with temperature fluctuations, since we find such fluctuations uncomfortable. Perhaps this sounds like stating the obvious, but there is an important point here: it is not always possible for patients to respond appropriately to temperature fluctuations – they may be immobile, may be unable to talk and express their needs, or may be unconscious. Of course, infants require special consideration, as do people with learning disabilities and people with mental health problems. For example, a profoundly depressed patient may simply lack the motivation to respond to cold.

Thermoregulation abnormalities

Thermoregulation abnormalities involve either a raised body temperature (**hyperthermia**) or a reduced body temperature (**hypothermia**). In addition, the terms '**pyrexia**' and 'fever' are also used when body temperature is elevated. These should not be considered to be synonymous with hyperthermia, however, as you will see below.

Conditions in which body temperature is raised

The term 'elevated body temperature' appears self-explanatory, but at what point do we regard a temperature rise to be abnormal? Commonly, it is when there is a persistent elevation above 37.5 °C. The key word here is 'persistent', since although the normal diurnal variation of body temperature is less than one degree Celsius, a healthy individual may have a recorded value of body temperature of between 36 °C and 40 °C, depending upon activity level. Consequently, we would not describe a body temperature of 40 °C as abnormal if it occurred immediately after vigorous exercise. On the other hand, a temperature of 38 °C that persisted for several hours would be considered abnormal.

● ***Are there problems associated with an elevated body temperature?***

First, the individual feels unwell; second, metabolic rate rises by 10% for every 1 °C rise in body temperature. The consequent increase in heat production then contributes to a further rise in metabolic rate, and so on. If body temperature exceeds 41 °C, physiological regulatory mechanisms are overwhelmed and the temperature will then continue to rise to the upper lethal limit of 44 °C.

Conditions in which body temperature is raised fall broadly into two groups - impaired heat dissipation and increased heat production. Impaired heat dissipation occurs when environmental temperature is high, especially if this is combined with high humidity. Possible consequences are heat exhaustion and the more serious heat stroke (see later).

Increased heat production may have one of a number of causes. Drugs may induce heat production or it may be due to excessive secretion of the hormone thyroxine (thyrotoxicosis). Another cause is damage to the heat-regulating mechanism itself, which may occur in head injury or cerebrovascular accident (CVA, stroke). Perhaps the most common cause of increased heat production, however, is the release of **pyrogens** into the bloodstream. These may be infective organisms, toxins or substances released from damaged cells that have the effect of raising the set point of temperature that the hypothalamus strives to maintain. Since infections are commonly accompanied by increased heat production, body temperature is often measured when infection is suspected or a possible complication of an intervention such as surgery. Since pyrogens may be released from damaged cells when no infection is present, however, temperature may also be elevated in disease processes that are not infective; **myocardial infarction** (heart attack) is an example of this.

Hyperthermia

The use of this term should be confined to conditions in which temperature is elevated because of impaired heat dissipation or when there is increased metabolic heat production. The patient commonly complains of feeling hot and will sweat and appear flushed (cutaneous vasodilation). Suitable interventions involve measures to increase heat loss from the body.

● ***What are these?***

Have a look at Table 9.2.

Table 9.2 Methods employed to cool the body.

Means by which heat losses due to conduction, convection and radiation may be increased	Means by which heat losses due to evaporation may be increased
Reducing environmental temperature	Washing with tepid water (27-30 °C)
Removing excessive clothing	
Creating gentle currents of air with electric fan	

- ***If we want to increase heat loss, why do we not direct electric fans towards the patient, use cold water in washing and apply ice packs?***

The answer to this is that such aggressive measures induce cutaneous vasoconstriction and shivering and would be counter-productive.

Heat exhaustion

We have noted that the response of the body to a hot environment includes sweating. If sweating is excessive or prolonged (perhaps when the individual is working or playing sport), then fluid and electrolyte losses can be considerable. This may lead to heat cramps. In addition, cutaneous vasodilation predisposes the individual to **orthostatic hypotension** (low blood pressure when standing) because blood becomes pooled in the lower extremities. This may result in fainting (heat syncope). Note that in such an individual, the skin feels cool and wet because of the evaporation of sweat, and this is important in preventing the temperature from becoming dangerously high. In fact, body temperature may be only a little above normal in this case. Treatment includes allowing the individual to rest in a cool place, using gentle cooling measures and giving cool drinks. Tomato juice replaces salt as well as fluid and may be considered to have an advantage over fruit juices. In addition, sachets of electrolyte powders that are diluted in water are available for the purpose of rehydration and treatment of electrolyte depletion.

Heat stroke

This is a much more serious condition than heat exhaustion, although it has the same causes. In heat stroke, the individual's ability to respond to a high environmental temperature is impaired and, as a consequence, core temperature rises dramatically. In this case, the individual does not sweat and the skin is hot and dry. Predisposing factors include dehydration, lack of acclimatisation, obesity and excess intake of alcohol. It is more common in elderly people. Cooling measures should be implemented and cool drinks given, but a rapid temperature rise to the upper lethal limit may occur before treatment can be instituted.

Pyrexia

This term is synonymous with fever, and its use should be confined to temperature increases that result from the resetting of the set point of the hypothalamus by pyrogens. It is important to understand the mechanism of action of pyrogens so that appropriate nursing interventions can be made. When the set point of temperature that the hypothalamus strives to maintain is raised, heat-conserving and heat-generating responses come into play.

- ***What does the patient feel like at this stage?***

The patient feels cold and generally unwell, appears pale due to cutaneous vasoconstriction, shivers and has an increased metabolic rate. As a consequence, the patient's core temperature will rise until it reaches the new set point.

- ***Are there any benefits to developing pyrexia?***

There may be some benefits. The immune system may be more effective when temperature is raised, and an elevated metabolic rate may be helpful in the healing process. You can find out more about this in a physiology textbook.

- ***What can the nurse do to help the patient with pyrexia? Should measures be taken to cool the patient?***

The answer to this question is not quite as obvious at it may seem. Initially, when the patient feels cold and unwell, the patient will almost certainly seek a warm bed. Even though the core temperature is raised, attempts to cool the patient will be counter-productive, since they will initiate further shivering and vasoconstriction. **Antipyretic** drugs may be given; these include **aspirin**, other **non-steroidal anti-inflammatory drugs** (NSAIDs) and **paracetamol**. Since 1986, the use of aspirin in children under 12 years of age has ceased because of its association with a serious condition called Reye's syndrome. If you care for children, you might like to find out more about this. A paediatric paracetamol preparation should be used instead.

After a period of time, the hypothalamic set point returns to normal. This may be part of a natural recovery process, may follow the administration of an antipyretic or, in the case of a bacterial infection, may follow the use of antibiotics. At this point, the core temperature will now be above the set point, and heat-losing responses will be initiated. The patient will feel hot, appear flushed (cutaneous vasodilation) and perspire. Interventions aimed at promoting heat loss, such as those discussed earlier, are now appropriate.

Malignant hyperpyrexia

This is the rapid and extreme rise in temperature associated with drugs such as the **muscle relaxant suxamethonium chloride** and the general anaesthetic **halothane**. A full discussion of the causes and management of this condition is beyond the scope of this book, but if you have a clinical placement in operating theatres you might like to find out more about it.

Hypothermia

Hypothermia is the state of an abnormally low body temperature. It may be described as mild, moderate or severe, but different authors ascribe different values to these descriptions. Consequently, we identify clinical signs for different values of core temperature for adults in Table 9.3. The principal cause of hypothermia is a low environmental temperature, and so the condition is more common in the winter months.

- ***Who is most at risk of accidental hypothermia?***

You should have been able to work out that those people at risk include individuals taking part in outdoor activities such as hill-walking, elderly people and infants. Elderly people are at risk of hypothermia for physiological and social reasons. Physiological reasons include reduced **adipose** (fat) tissue and an impaired shivering response. Elderly people also tend to be less active than younger people. Social reasons include poor housing and low incomes. Infants are at risk of hypothermia because of a high surface area to volume ratio, which results in greater heat losses. Infants are also reliant upon adults to provide suitable clothing and shelter.

- ***How should the patient with hypothermia be helped?***

Clearly the interventions made in hypothermia are aimed at re-warming the patient. These may be divided into passive techniques (preventing further heat loss) and active techniques (involving the transfer of heat to the body).

Table 9.3 Clinical signs of different core body temperatures.

Core temperature (°C)	Clinical signs
36-35	Cutaneous vasoconstriction Shivering Increased blood pressure
34-33	Poor coordination Confusion Normal blood pressure Clouded consciousness
32-31	Reduced shivering Low blood pressure Reduced heart and respiratory rates
30-29	Loss of consciousness Muscular rigidity
Below 28	Risk of cardiac arrest

Passive techniques include insulating the patient with blankets and increasing the environmental temperature. Ambient room temperature is taken to be 21 °C, and so the temperature of the environment in which the hypothermic individual is treated should be maintained above this - up to 30 °C. Reflective blankets (foil or space blankets) should be avoided if a suitable environmental temperature can be maintained, since they will reflect infrared radiation from the patient. They do, however, have a use in preventing hypothermia in a low environmental temperature, such as occurs when hill-walkers are stranded on a mountainside. In this case, they function to reduce heat loss from the body by radiation. Passive techniques are suitable for use in all hypothermic patients and are the main treatment when the temperature is above 32 °C.

If the patient's temperature is below 32 °C, however, active re-warming techniques may be employed. These include the administration of warmed intravenous fluids and gastric **lavage** with warmed saline (passing warmed saline into the stomach via a nasogastric tube). More dramatic is the establishment of an **extracorporeal** circulation. This involves an artificial circulation outside the body: Blood is re-warmed by passage through a heat exchanger and then pumped back into the patient.

- ***Why not simply apply heat to the surface of the body?***

This could indeed be done, but there are a number of problems. First, surface heating may prevent shivering, since the muscles are warmed before the core. Second, if the skin is warmed first, blood flow to the extremities will increase, and this may result in a fall in blood pressure. Such a fall is tolerated poorly in elderly people, who may have pre-existing heart disease. Third, as peripheral circulation is increased, cold blood is returned to the heart, and this may cause a drop in core temperature, which may precipitate **ventricular fibrillation** (a form of cardiac arrest). This may be the explanation for sudden death that occurs after treatment has begun. There is much more that can be said on this subject, and you might consider looking at this topic in more detail.

Other uses of heat and cold

Sterilisation

Sterilisation refers to the elimination of all living organisms from an object. Heat, in one form or another, is often used to achieve this. Heating has a number of advantages, including controllability and the rapidity and certainty of its effects. In addition, unlike chemical methods, heating leaves behind no potentially harmful substances. Heat sterilisation may involve dry or moist heat. Examples of dry heat include the incineration of contaminated disposables, such as dressings. Moist heat sterilisation includes the use of steam under pressure and is used in a device called the **autoclave**. You can read more about this is Chapter 16.

Induced hypothermia

In heart surgery, hypothermia is induced using topical and systemic techniques as a means of protecting the heart from a lack of oxygen - oxygen requirements are much lower in cold tissues. Only a small number of students who read this book will visit units in which such techniques are used, but you will realise that one aspect of the postoperative care of such individuals is the re-warming of the patient.

In-text review

- ✔ Temperature regulation is an example of homeostasis.
- ✔ In keeping with other homeostatic mechanisms, three aspects are important: detectors (thermoreceptors), control centre (hypothalamus) and effectors (cutaneous blood vessels, sweat glands and skeletal muscle).
- ✔ The body's response to elevated temperature is cutaneous vasodilation and sweating.
- ✔ The body's response to reduced temperature is cutaneous vasoconstriction and shivering.
- ✔ Thermoregulation abnormalities include hyperthermia, heat exhaustion, heat stroke and hypothermia.

Summary

In this chapter we have distinguished between heat and temperature and have described the different methods used to measure body temperature. We discussed the physical mechanisms by which heat is lost and subsequently applied these to patient examples. Finally we described temperature homeostasis and outlined how thermoregulation abnormalities are managed.

Summary points

- → Temperature and heat are not the same thing. Heat is a form of energy, and temperature is the degree of hotness of an object.
- → The SI unit of temperature is the Kelvin, but degrees Celsius (°C) are used in clinical practice.
- → The amount of heat required to melt a solid is referred to as the latent heat of fusion, and the amount of heat required to vaporise a liquid as the latent heat of vaporisation.
- → Currently, the two most important temperature-measurement devices in clinical practice are the thermistor and the tympanic membrane thermometer.
- → The temperature of organs within the body is referred to as the core temperature, while the temperature at the surface of the body is called the peripheral temperature.
- → Normal core temperature is taken to be 37 °C.
- → The most reliable site for recording body temperature with an electronic thermometer is the sublingual pocket of the oral cavity.
- → The tympanic membrane thermometer gives an immediate and accurate value of core temperature.
- → The transfer of heat occurs by conduction, convection and radiation.
- → Temperature homeostasis involves the skin and the nervous, endocrine and cardiovascular systems.
- → Thermoregulation abnormalities include pyrexia, heat exhaustion, heat stroke and hypothermia.

Self-test questions

1 Match the value on the left with the appropriate description on the right.

(a) 330 kJ	(i) Amount of energy required to raise the temperature of 1 kg of ice from –10 °C to 0 °C
(b) 2260 kJ	(ii) Amount of energy required to raise the temperature of 1 kg of water from 0 °C to 100 °C
(c) 42 kJ	(iii) Amount of energy required to vaporise 1 kg of water
(d) 420 kJ	(iv) Amount of energy required to melt 1 kg of ice

2 Which one of the following is considered to be the normal body temperature in degrees Celsius?

(a) 35.
(b) 43.
(c) 37.
(d) 40.

3 Which one of the following sites is considered to give the most accurate value of core body temperature?
(a) Sublingual pocket.
(b) Axilla.
(c) Rectum.
(d) Tympanic membrane.

4 Which of the following are true statements regarding an elderly patient who has fallen on a dry cold floor?
(a) Heat loss by conduction will increase.
(b) Heat loss by convection will be increased.
(c) Heat loss by radiation will be increased.
(d) Heat loss by evaporation will be increased.

5 Which of the following is considered to be the normal diurnal variation of body temperature in degrees Celsius?
(a) Less than 0.5.
(b) 0.5-1.0.
(c) 1.0-2.0.
(d) Greater than 2.

6 By which one of the following processes is most heat lost from the body of an individual at rest at normal room temperature?
(a) Conduction.
(b) Convection.
(c) Radiation.
(d) Evaporation.

7 Which one of the following is considered to be the best definition of a raised body temperature?
(a) A temperature of 39 °C or above.
(b) A persistent elevation of 37.5 °C or above.
(c) A temperature of 41 °C or above.
(d) A persistent elevation of 40 °C or above.

8 You observe that an individual suspected of a pyrogenic infection looks pale, shivers, is cold to touch and has an oral temperature 39 °C. He complains of feeling cold and takes to his bed, asking for another blanket. Which one or more of the following interventions would be appropriate?
(a) Administer prescribed antipyretic drugs.
(b) Tell the patient that he has a fever and that he should not have an extra blanket.
(c) Give him an extra blanket.
(d) Turn on an electric fan.

9 It is a hot day, and after a game of beach volleyball a friend complains of feeling unwell. He appears flushed and is sweating profusely. His oral temperature is 38.5 °C. Which one or more of the following interventions would be appropriate?

(a) Take your friend to a shaded place.
(b) Suggest that he recline and rest.
(c) Provide cool drinks and fan him gently.
(d) Suggest that he take some aspirin.

10 An elderly person is admitted to hospital after neighbours find him sitting in a chair in a cold flat. He is conscious, but his coordination is poor and he appears confused. His temperature taken by an infrared tympanic membrane thermometer is 33 °C. Which one or more of the following interventions would be appropriate?
(a) Check his temperature frequently.
(b) Cover him with plenty of blankets.
(c) Try to raise his temperature with hot water bottles.
(d) Check his pulse and blood pressure.

Further study/exercises

1 Suppose that you are a practice nurse involved in visiting housebound elderly people. What practical advice could you give regarding keeping warm in the winter?

Neno R. (2005). Hypothermia: assessment, treatment and prevention. *Nursing Standard*, 19(20), 47-52.
Wallis L. (2003). Cold comfort. *Nursing Standard*, 88(3), 14-15.
Wilkinson P., Pattenden S. and Armstrong B. (2004). Vulnerability to winter mortality in elderly people in Britain: population based study. *British Medical Journal*, 329(7467), 647-51.

2 Pyrexia in children may give rise to concern because of the possibility of febrile convulsions. What are febrile convulsions, and how should the child with pyrexia be cared for?

Hawksworth D. (2000). Simple febrile convulsions: evidence for best practice. *Journal of Child Health Care*, 4(4), 149-53.
Purssell E. (2000). The use of antipyretic medications in the prevention of febrile convulsions in children. *Journal of Clinical Nursing*, 9(4), 473-80.

10

Force, mechanics and biomechanics

Learning outcomes

After reading the following chapter and undertaking personal study, you should be able to:

1. Distinguish between scalar and vector quantities.
2. Define the terms 'speed', 'velocity', 'acceleration', 'mass', 'weight' and 'momentum'.
3. Define the term 'force' and distinguish between balanced and unbalanced forces.
4. Define the term 'friction' and relate it to the structure of synovial joints and to lubrication.
5. State Newton's laws of motion and relate these to the body.
6. Describe what is meant by 'force of gravity' and relate this to prolonged standing and the effects of immobility.
7. State what the term 'centre of gravity' means and relate this to the stability of the body and to lifting.
8. Describe three forms of lever and give examples of each within the body.
9. Relate an understanding of levers to lifting techniques and back injury.
10. Distinguish between fixed and moveable pulleys and describe their operation.
11. Draw vector diagrams in order to resolve two forces acting simultaneously upon an object.
12. Relate pulleys and vectors to orthopaedic traction.

Introduction

An aspect of nursing courses that has expanded and become more formalised in recent years is that of moving and handling training. Even the vocabulary has changed - we no longer speak of 'lifting training', for example. The reasons for this include the high level of back injury in nurses and the possibility of litigation as nurses seek to obtain compensation for injury sustained during employment. Of course, poor moving and handling techniques also present a danger to patients. One example is dislocation of the shoulder when the patient in bed is pulled forwards by the arm. This is especially likely following **cerebrovascular accident** (stroke). Consequently, you will undoubtedly be required to attend mandatory moving and handling training throughout your career as well as during your initial nursing training.

- ***So does this training begin here?***

Not exactly - this is not a moving and handling text. We shall, however, deal with some prerequisite knowledge that will help you to understand the topic. In this chapter, we will consider how things move (mechanics) and, in particular, how our bodies move (biomechanics). To begin with, however, we need an explanation of some important terms. The quantities to which we will refer may be described as either scalar or vector quantities. The difference between them is simple: **scalar** quantities have size only, while **vector** quantities have both size and direction. The significance of this distinction will become clear as you work through this chapter.

Speed and velocity

We know that **speed** is a measure of how fast something is travelling; it is expressed as the distance travelled per unit of time, as shown below:

$$\text{Speed} = \frac{\text{distance}}{\text{time}}$$

The SI unit of distance (length) is the metre, and we commonly express speed in terms of the number of metres travelled in one second (ms^{-1} or m/s). For example, nervous impulses travel as fast as 120 ms^{-1} in some **neurons** (nerve cells). When referring to objects such as cars and trains, however, it is obviously more convenient to use kilometres per hour (kph) or miles per hour (mph). The same units are also used to measure **velocity**.

- ***How does velocity differ from speed?***

The term 'velocity' is used only when an object is travelling in a straight line - that is, velocity is a **vector** quantity, while speed is a **scalar** quantity. Consequently, we cannot describe an electron orbiting the nucleus of an atom at constant speed as having constant velocity, since its direction of movement is changing constantly - it is circling around the nucleus.

Acceleration

When the velocity of an object is changing, we might describe it as accelerating (getting faster) or decelerating (getting slower). **Acceleration** is defined as the rate of change of velocity:

$$\text{Acceleration} = \frac{\text{velocity (ms}^{-1}\text{)}}{\text{time (s)}}$$

Consequently, the units of acceleration are metres per second per second (ms^{-2}).

- ***Think about this for a moment.***

Suppose an object at rest started to accelerate at a rate of 1 ms^{-2}.

- ***What would be its velocity after 3 seconds?***

It would be 3 ms^{-1}. This increase in velocity is referred to as a positive acceleration. If an object is slowing down, scientists tend to refer to negative acceleration rather than deceleration. The term 'acceleration' is also used of an object whose speed is constant but whose direction of travel is changing. Consequently, in the example of the atom used above, electrons are constantly accelerating, since their direction of travel is not linear.

- ***What would cause a moving object to change its direction or speed?***

Clearly, some force must have acted upon it. We shall consider the concept of force a little later, but first let us deal with mass and weight.

Mass and weight

Most people use these terms interchangeably, but to the scientist they mean two quite different things. **Mass** is the amount of matter contained in an object, and it is measured in kilograms. It is, therefore, a scalar quantity and also a **fundamental** quantity. This latter term refers to the fact that the mass of a stationary object does not change with its position. A 1-kg bag of flour has the same mass on earth, on the moon and in a rocket travelling between them.

- ***What about weight?***

Weight is not the same as mass – it is a **force**, and the weight of our 1-kg bag of flour is certainly not the same in all circumstances. For example, it weighs less on the moon than on the earth, and even less in space, where it becomes weightless. Clearly, we need to say more about this concept of force and (since we have mentioned planets, space and weightlessness) more about **gravity** too. Before we do so, we should note that, unlike mass, weight is a vector quantity, since a force always acts in a particular direction. For example, weight on earth always acts towards the centre of the earth.

Momentum

The term '**momentum**' is used to mean the product of the mass and velocity of an object.

- ***So, if a lorry and a car are both travelling at the same speed, which would have the greater momentum?***

The correct answer is the lorry, since although both vehicles have the same velocity, the lorry has the greater mass. On the other hand, a moving car has greater momentum than a stationary lorry, which, because it has zero velocity, has zero momentum. You will also no doubt realise that objects with the greatest momentum are most difficult to stop.

Force

We commonly use the word 'force' in everyday language to refer to some form of compulsion. For example, if our car develops a fault, we might say 'I was forced to stop.' When applied to physical objects, we recognise that a force involves some kind of push or pull. The SI unit of force is the **newton** (N), named after Sir Isaac Newton. One newton is the force that, when applied to a mass of 1 kg, produces, in the absence of **friction**, an acceleration of 1 ms^{-2}. This means that if a force of 1 N is applied to a stationary mass of 1 kg, the mass would be travelling at 1 ms^{-1} after 1 second, 2 ms^{-1} after 2 seconds, and so on. This definition specifies 'in the absence of friction', and friction makes a very great difference to the force required to move an object.

Friction

When two surfaces that are in contact are moving over each other, there is a force that resists this movement, and it is this force that we call **friction**. The amount of friction depends upon the nature of the two surfaces. For example, friction is greatest between rough surfaces and less between polished surfaces. Even highly polished surfaces appear rough, however, when viewed under a microscope, and so friction is always present between surfaces in contact.

- ***Is friction a good or bad thing?***

As you might expect, this depends on many things. The ability to walk depends upon friction between our shoes and the floor, and a walking frame without friction-producing rubber pads on the legs would be positively dangerous. On the other hand, friction between an object that you want to move and the floor increases the effort that you need in order to move it. Other problems with friction are that it produces heat and wears away surfaces that are rubbing against each other.

- ***If we wanted to reduce the friction between two surfaces, what methods could we use?***

One obvious thing that we could do is to fit one of the objects with wheels. Hospital beds are an example, since these frequently have to be moved, often with patients still in them.

Another solution is to use a lubricant - car engine oil is a good example. It might be more useful, however, to think instead about friction and the body as explained in Practice point 10.1.

Practice point 10.1

Friction and the body

An obvious site where friction occurs is within a joint. Figure 10.1 is an illustration of the structure of a **synovial joint**. Examples of synovial joints include the knee, elbow, shoulder and hip.

- ***So are there any wheels here?***

Obviously not, but synovial joints do contain very smooth surfaces that pass across each other. Upon examination, one might almost imagine that the ends of articulating bones have been polished. In fact, this polished-surface effect is produced by **cartilage**, which covers the ends of long bones where a joint is formed. In addition, the joint space between the bones contains a viscous fluid - **synovial fluid** - and this lubricant reduces friction still further. Of course, joints may be damaged by friction, and this is essentially the cause of **osteoarthrosis** (osteoarthritis). In this condition, the cartilage has become worn away and there is inflammation of the joint. Osteoarthrosis is more common in elderly people because they have experienced a greater period of wear and tear, but it is also associated with causes of increased wear and tear, such as obesity and playing sport.

- ***What are the effects of osteoarthrosis?***

Pain results from the wearing away of the joint surfaces and the range of movement of the joint decreases. As you can imagine, this may significantly reduce mobility and result in a reduced quality of life for the sufferer. **Analgesics** and anti-inflammatory drugs may help, but ultimately the sufferer requires a new joint - and that is exactly what is offered. One of the most common operations is the total hip replacement, in which both articulating surfaces are replaced by metal implants (**prostheses**). More recently, hip resurfacing has become common. In this case, surfaces of the bones that form the joint are resurfaced with metal.

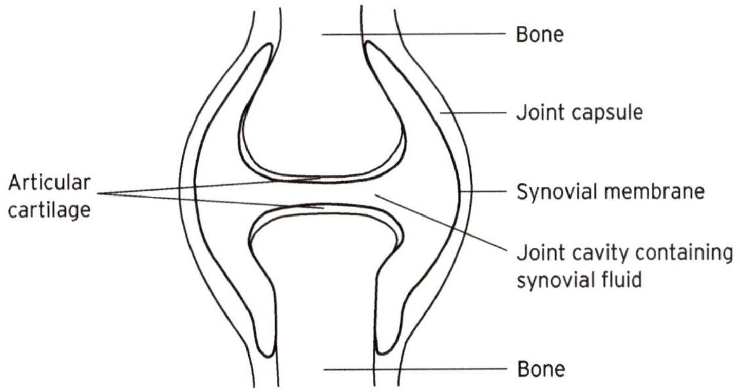

Figure 10.1
The generalised structure of a synovial joint.

Friction must also be considered when inserting instruments (**intubation**) or catheters (tubes) into the body. One example is the intubation of the urinary bladder (**catheterisation**) - a procedure that nurses commonly perform. In this procedure, a sterile catheter is passed into the urinary bladder via the urethra. If trauma to the urethra is to be avoided, a lubricant jelly is required. The procedure is more uncomfortable for male patients - the catheter causes pain at the point where the urethra passes through the **prostate gland**. For this reason, a preparation of lubricant containing a local **anaesthetic** (drug that blocks sensation) is used in males.

The concept of balanced and unbalanced forces

Imagine a man trying to push a very heavy object that is resting on the floor. Despite applying a great deal of force to the object, it just does not move.

- ***Why not?***

Is the answer that the object is too heavy? That is what we would say in everyday language, but we might also explain that the man cannot overcome the force of friction. When he pushes against the object, the force that he applies is opposed by friction. We might also say that the forces are balanced, since there is no movement of the object. Now imagine that the object has wheels. It is the same weight as before, but now when the man pushes against it friction has been very much reduced and there is much less opposition to the force he applies. The forces are unbalanced and the object moves. Forces are unbalanced when there is net force acting in a particular direction that produces movement. Sir Isaac Newton described the motion of objects in three laws, which we consider next.

Newton's laws of motion

When we speak of laws in science, reference is being made to rules about the universe that hold true in all circumstances. You may have learned these laws in school science, but we will repeat them here. Of course, we subsequently want to apply these rules to clinical issues, such as rapid deceleration injury, rather than to illustrations used in the physics laboratory.

Newton's first law (law of inertia)

This may be stated in the following way:

> **All objects remain at rest or in a state of uniform motion unless acted upon by an unbalanced force.**

This law simply states that objects continue to do the same thing unless a force compels them to do otherwise. For example, if an object is stationary, it does not move unless an unbalanced force compels it to do so; if in motion, the object does not change speed or direction unless an unbalanced force acts upon it. This is exactly what the expression 'uniform motion' refers to - constant speed and direction. This law is sometimes called the law of **inertia**. Inertia is essentially the tendency of a body to resist a force that is applied to it. Let us think a little more about this in the context of rapid deceleration injuries (see Practice point 10.2).

Practice point 10.2

Rapid deceleration injuries

It may be stating the obvious to note that these are injuries that result from the rapid deceleration of the body without impact with another object. One possible cause is a car crash. Among the most common rapid deceleration injuries are whiplash injuries to the neck; in order to work out what happens, imagine that you are driving at modest speed when your car is in a head-on collision with another.

- ***What happens next?***

Your car decelerates very quickly because of the impact.

- ***But what about you? Remember Newton's first law?***

Your body continues to travel forwards, and if you are not wearing a seatbelt you may strike on the steering wheel or be thrown through the windscreen. However, let us assume that you are wearing a seatbelt - your chances of survival are now much better.

- ***But what about your head – it isn't restrained, is it?***

Not initially, and your head continues to travel forwards so that your neck becomes bent forwards at an extreme degree (hyperflexion). Remember, though, that your body is held in place in the seat, so your head is now jerked backwards and becomes hyperextended - ouch! The description of this type of injury as whiplash is quite graphic, and you will no doubt understand that the alternate hyperflexion and hyperextension of the neck may result in muscular and **ligamentous** injury to the neck. You might imagine that muscle and ligament injury are not to be compared to fractures and penetrating injury, but this would not be entirely the case. Muscle and ligament damage produce a great deal of pain and recovery may take a long time. Whiplash injury is illustrated in Figure 10.2.

- ***Are there any features of car design that help to prevent whiplash?***

The main problem is hyperextension of the neck as the head is jerked back. A properly adjusted headrest limits this movement and helps to reduce neck injury. This is also illustrated in Figure 10.2. It is worth noting, however, that a headrest positioned too low may actually make the neck injury worse by acting as a point about which the head pivots. Consequently, headrests should be positioned so that the pad is behind the head and not the neck.

Whiplash is not the only injury to be caused by rapid deceleration. Another structure that may be affected is the **aorta** - the artery that leaves the heart to carry oxygenated blood to the body. The heart is located in the centre of the chest and, like the head in the above example, it too swings forwards and then backwards when the body is stopped suddenly. In contrast, the aorta is held more rigidly, and the force of the swinging action of the heart may be sufficient to cause the aorta to rupture. Needless to say, the affected individual usually bleeds to death rapidly. The crash position shown on airline safety cards is an attempt to reduce this type of injury, and it has been suggested that lives could be saved in air crashes if aircraft seats faced backwards. In this position, the swinging action of the heart within the chest is prevented.

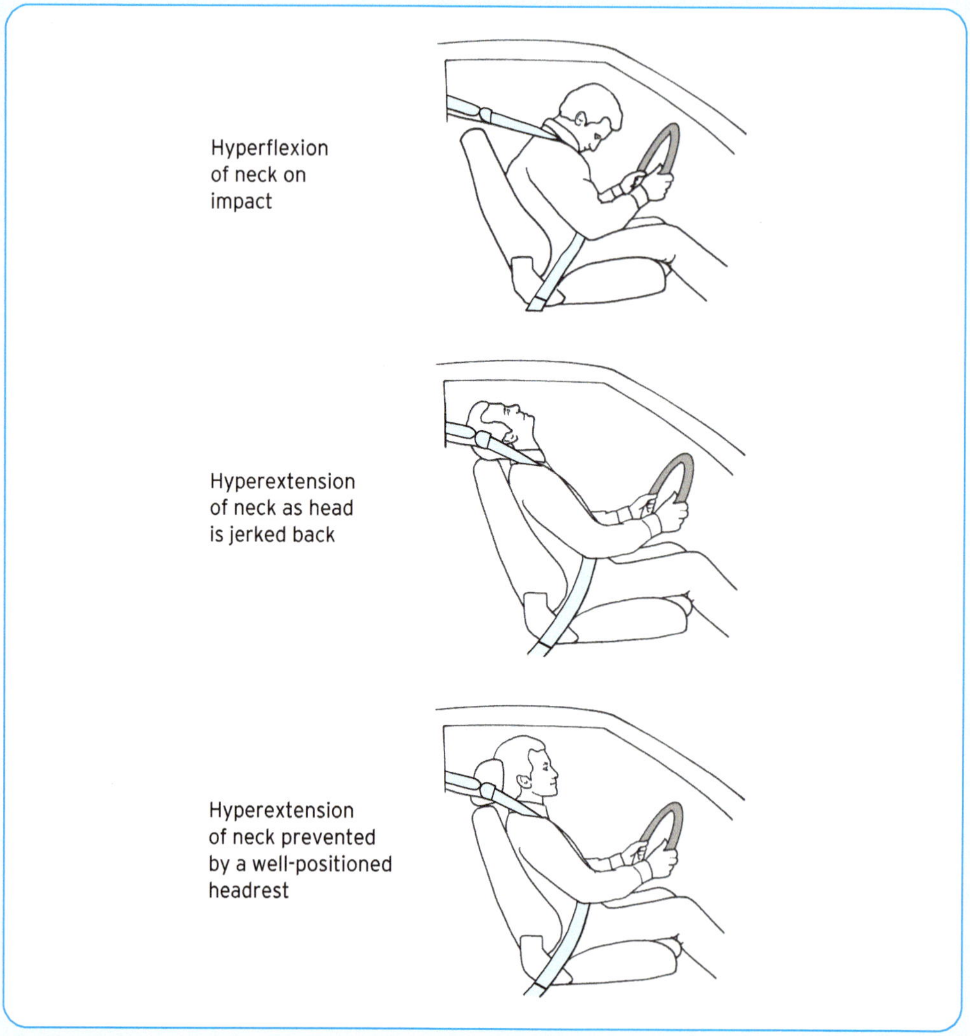

Figure 10.2
Demonstration of how a whiplash injury occurs.

Newton's second law

Newton's second law can be stated in the following way:

> **The acceleration of a fixed mass is proportional to the force applied to it.**

One application of this law is that the acceleration of a wheelchair that we are pushing is proportional to the force we apply to it. This example may appear too obvious, but science does not have to be difficult all the time.

Newton's third law

This law is often stated in the following way:

To every action, there is an equal and opposite reaction.

This is certainly a simple formulation, but perhaps a better one would be:

When an object exerts a force upon another, the second object exerts an equal force on the first but in the opposite direction.

Stated in this way, it becomes clear that two objects are involved. Consider walking as an example. In this case, the two objects are the individual and the earth. The act of walking involves the application of a force to the earth, but this is opposed by equal force exerted by the earth against the individual. Of course, in this case the two objects have different masses, and so it is the individual who is pushed forwards, not the earth. It is quite often the case, as in the example here, that the opposing force is friction, which we have thought about already.

What happens when friction is removed?

In the case of walking, our feet would not grip, the force we exert would not be opposed and we would slip over. Remember that many objects used in health care, such as wheelchairs, commodes, beds and bed tables, have wheels, which reduce friction and remove opposing force. It is, of course, important to lock these wheels when patients are using these devices, otherwise an accident may result. Once again, this is a rather obvious point, but it is not at all uncommon to find accident reports that cite failure to lock wheels or ineffective brakes as a cause of injury to the patient or carer. The next time you are involved in assisting a patient to move - perhaps a simple bed-to-chair transfer - make a point of checking that the brakes hold under modest force. If they do not, you and the patient may be at risk of injury. Needless to say, defective equipment should be labelled as such and not used until it is repaired.

In-text review

- ✔ Scalar quantities, such as mass and speed, have only size, while vector quantities, such as weight, velocity, acceleration and force, have both size and direction.
- ✔ An knowledge of friction is of help in understanding the structure of a synovial joint.
- ✔ The behaviour of objects in motion is described in Newton's three laws.
- ✔ Newton's first law helps us to understand what happens in rapid deceleration injuries.

The force of gravity

Most people know the story of the apple that Newton saw fall and that led him to describe gravity. Consequently, the idea that the earth attracts all objects to itself is a familiar one. In fact, experiments have demonstrated that every object exerts a force of attraction on every other object, and this attraction is proportional to the mass of the two objects added together and inversely proportional to the square of the distance between them. At first, this may be difficult to believe. When a brick is dropped from a building, it is quite obvious that it is attracted to the earth, since it accelerates downwards. What is not obvious is that the earth is attracted towards the brick with equal force, but this is actually what is happening. Of course, the earth is massive compared with the brick, and so its acceleration is effectively zero.

- ***Does gravity affect our bodies?***

Yes, as Practice point 10.3 makes clear.

Practice point 10.3

Gravity and the body

We have noted that all objects are attracted towards the earth; in this context the word 'object' includes the blood in our bodies. When we get up from lying down, there is a tendency for blood to pool in the legs. This is not normally a problem, since a reflex **vasoconstriction** (blood-vessel constriction) affecting the legs reduces this tendency. If someone has to stand for a long time, however, especially if it is hot, then there may be a reduction in the volume of blood returning to the upper body from the legs and, as a consequence, of blood flow to the brain too. The effect of this is that the person experiences a momentary loss of consciousness, commonly called a faint (**syncope**).

- ***So what is the first-aid measure in fainting?***

Quite simply, we make gravity work in favour of cerebral blood flow and lie the individual flat, with the legs slightly elevated. It is worth noting that the reflex vasoconstriction noted above becomes impaired following prolonged lying down. In the case of patients standing after a period of bed rest, it would be unwise to expect them to rise from the bed and stand in one movement - they may faint otherwise. Instead, ask the patient to sit on the edge of the bed and become used to the legs hanging down for a moment. This way, if they feel faint, they can simply lie back on the bed. If they feel no ill effects, however, they can stand, but they should not walk away from the bed immediately.

Bed rest has a number of unhelpful effects upon the body, and you may be interested to know that research in this field has been conducted by various space agencies. Researchers used bed rest to simulate a loss of gravitational stress on the upright body. Consequently, we now know a great deal about the effects of bed rest, one of which is a change in the balance of activity between bone-forming cells (**osteoblasts**) and bone-resorbing cells (**osteoclasts**). As a consequence of the loss of force exerted longitudinally through the bones, bone resorption is accelerated, bone density decreases and renal excretion of the important bone mineral calcium increases. Few illnesses require complete bed rest, and encouraging the patient to stand for periods during the day may prevent loss of bone density.

Centre of gravity

The centre of gravity of an object of uniform density and simple shape, such as a cube, is the geometric centre of the space that the object occupies. This is illustrated in Figure 10.3. The idea of the centre of gravity may be a familiar one.

Of what significance is this point?

The centre of gravity is a point within an object at which the entire weight of the object can be thought of acting for the purpose of considering **torque**. Torque is the tendency of a force to produce rotation about a pivot point (**fulcrum**). If an object is supported under its centre of gravity, it can be balanced so that it is not subject to any turning force. This is best illustrated in Figure 10.4, in which the object is a plank.

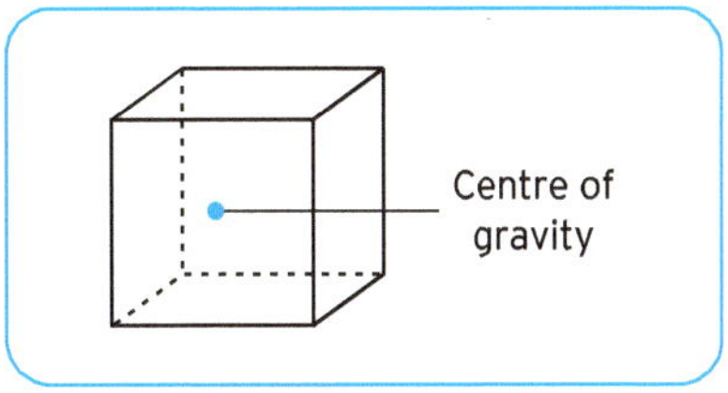

Figure 10.3
The centre of gravity of a cube.

The plank is a simple shape; if it has uniform density, its centre of gravity is its geometric centre, marked by X. When the plank is supported below the centre of gravity, it is not subject to a net turning force, and the condition of **static equilibrium** exists. A static equilibrium exists when an object is at rest and remains in a fixed position. In everyday language, we say that the plank is balanced. In contrast, the same plank supported at any other point will not be in a static equilibrium. It will be subject to a turning force and will, therefore, tip over. Having noted this, we can now move on to relate an understanding of the centre of gravity to our bodies (see Practice point 10.4).

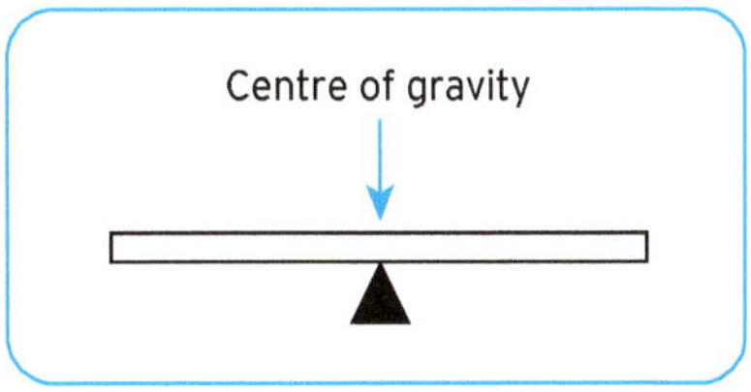

Figure 10.4
A plank balanced by being supported under its centre of gravity.

Practice point 10.4

Centre of gravity and our bodies

The first thing to note is that our bodies do not have uniform shape and density, and so the position of the centre of gravity is not immediately obvious. The centre of gravity in an individual standing with their arms at their sides is illustrated in Figure 10.5.

In what structure is the centre of gravity located?

It lies within the pelvis. The point to note here is that the centre of gravity is in the lower torso, thus producing stability. Consequently, standing requires little muscular effort.

What about infants – is the centre of gravity in the same place?

You have probably realised that it is not (see Figure 10.6).

Take the example of a child who is beginning to walk. Because the head of an infant is large in proportion to the body, the centre of gravity is above the pelvis, and this produces instability. Adults can simulate this instability by raising the arms above the head, which raises the centre of gravity. Walking also requires a movement of the centre of gravity - this time to one side of the pelvis in order to allow the non-weight-bearing leg to be swung forward.

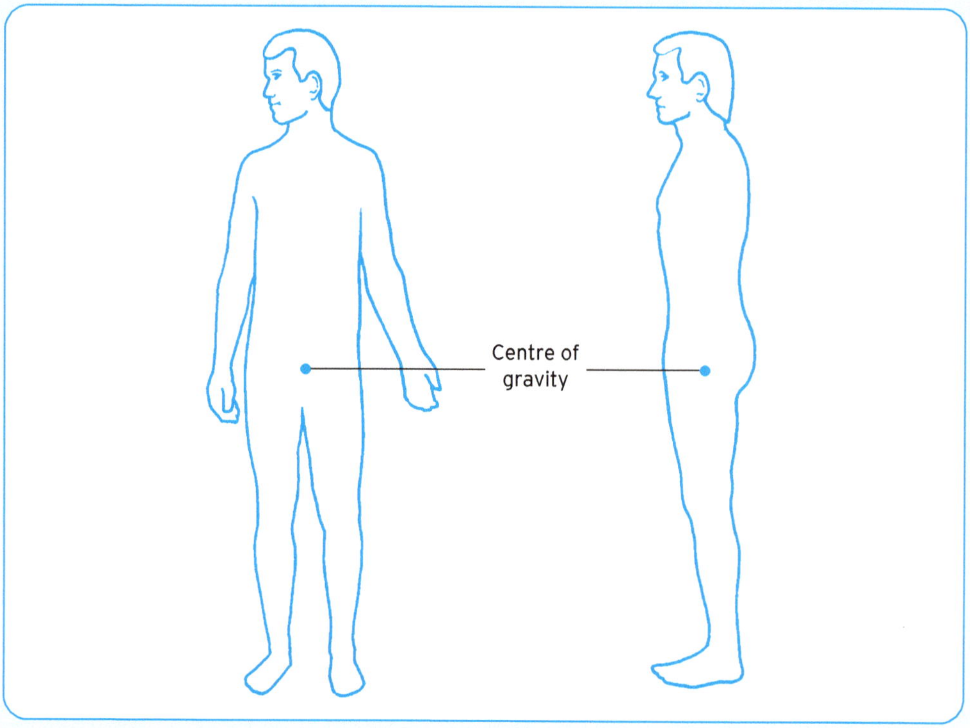

Figure 10.5
The centre of gravity of an individual, standing with arms at the sides.

● ***So what about the centre of gravity in the sitting and lying positions?***

Figure 10.7 shows that when a person is sitting, the centre of gravity lies outside the body. This makes getting up from this position difficult, and the way in which we normally deal with this is to bend forwards towards the edge of the seat, thus moving the centre of gravity closer to the body.

Nonetheless, the action of standing still involves some effort and contraction of the muscles of the abdomen.

● ***Can you work out which individuals might find this difficult?***

Perhaps you have noted this in frail elderly people, pregnant women, obese people and patients with abdominal wounds.

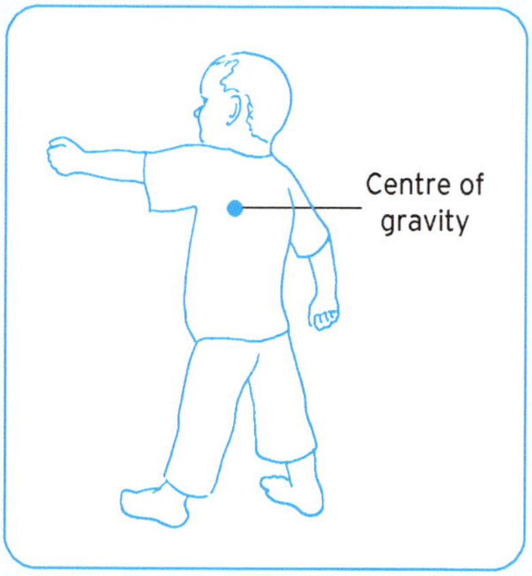

Figure 10.6
The position of the centre of gravity of an infant.

● ***What could be done to help?***

It is not difficult to work out that upright but comfortable chairs with armrests are generally easier to rise from; there are also chair models with electric motors that lift the seat for people with special difficulties. The next time you visit a placement where frail elderly people are cared for, examine the types of seating available and assess its suitability. Ask the patients what they think about it.

When lying recumbent, the centre of gravity is within the pelvis, and moving the pelvis will turn the body over. We make use of this fact when turning an unconscious patient into the recovery position. You might like to find out about this if you are not familiar with this aspect of first aid. Of course, when the patient is sitting in bed, the centre of gravity is outside the body, and this makes the patient more difficult to move.

The centre of gravity is also affected by body weight, as Figure 10.8 shows. In obesity, the additional body weight is not distributed evenly throughout the body - the abdomen is one important site for the deposition of fat. Consequently, obesity results in a forward displacement of the centre of gravity, and this may contribute to back strain, as will be explained later.

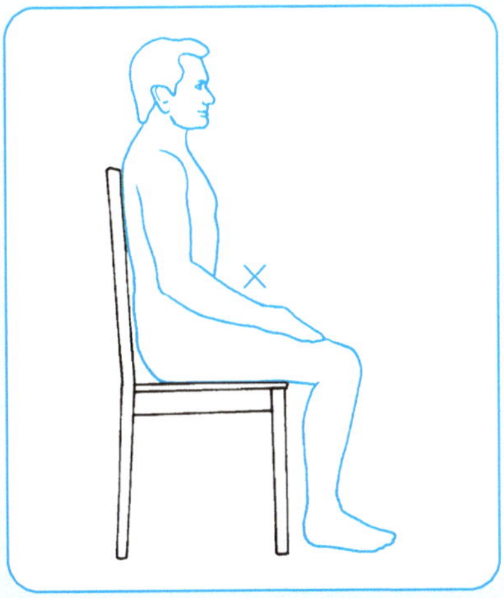

Figure 10.7
The position of the centre of gravity when sitting.

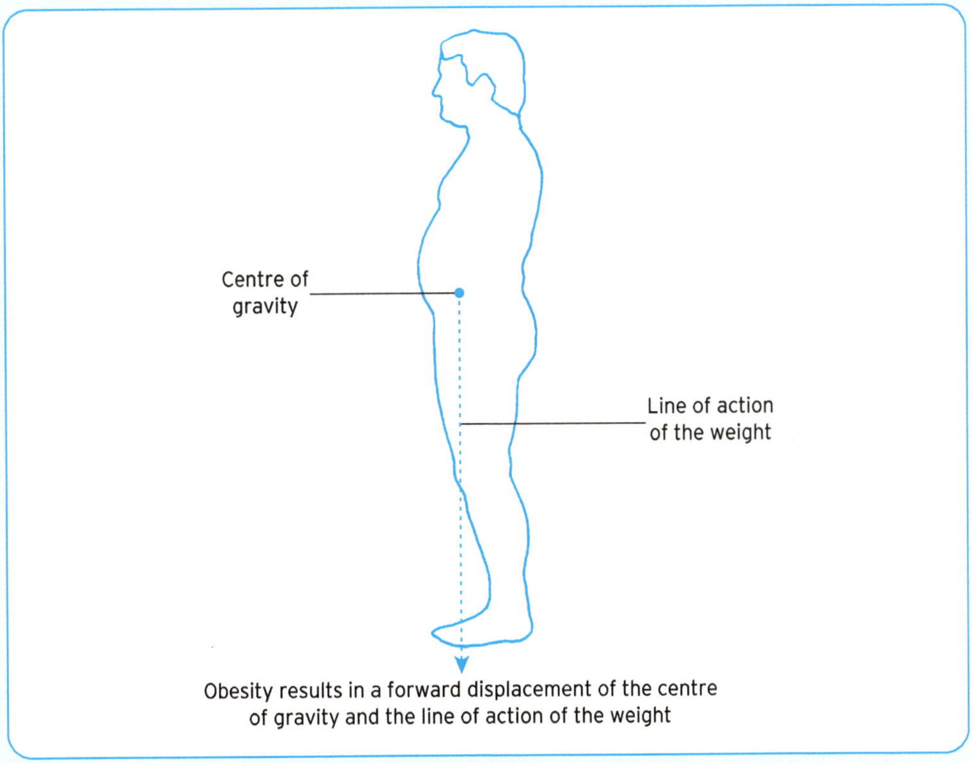

Figure 10.8
The forward displacement of the centre of gravity in obesity.

Stability

We have noted the meaning of the term 'centre of gravity'. Now we turn to the topic of stability. When we think about stability, it is helpful to imagine a vertical line passing through the centre of gravity. Consider Figure 10.9 for a moment.

- ***Which of the four shapes is in a stable equilibrium, and which will fall over?***

You are right if you have noted that a is in a stable equilibrium and will not fall over and that c is not in equilibrium and will fall over. The reason for this is that the line of action of its weight falls outside the base.

- ***What about b?***

In this case, the line of action of its weight falls on the edge of the base. The object will not fall over - it is in equilibrium, but it is an **unstable** equilibrium. Only a little force will cause it to fall over.

- ***What about d? Will d fall over?***

The answer is no, since although d looks similar to c, d has an extended base, and the line of action of the weight remains within this base. So the key to stability is the size of the base. The relevance of this is seen when we think about someone who is mildly intoxicated and finding it difficult to keep their balance.

- ***How does the person increase their stability?***

Perhaps you have realised that walking with the feet further apart, and thus widening the base, is an automatic attempt to increase stability.

- ***Can we make use of this principle in patients who are unstable? What artificial means are there of increasing the size of the base?***

You will have no difficulty realising that walking sticks, crutches and walking frames are all attempts to increase stability by widening the base, as Figure 10.10 shows. The important thing to note here is that all of these aids have to be fitted for the individual and their use

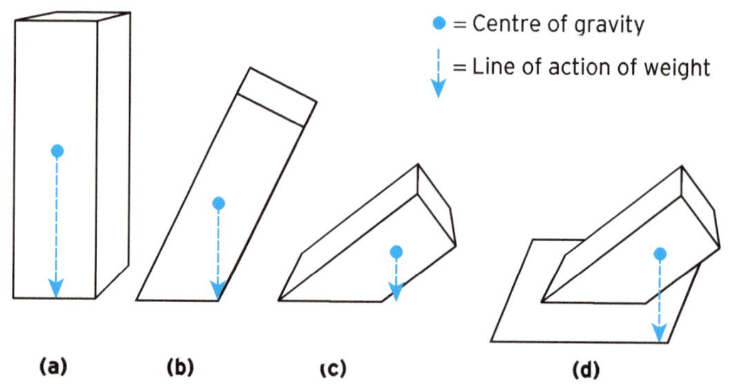

Figure 10.9
The stability of four shapes.

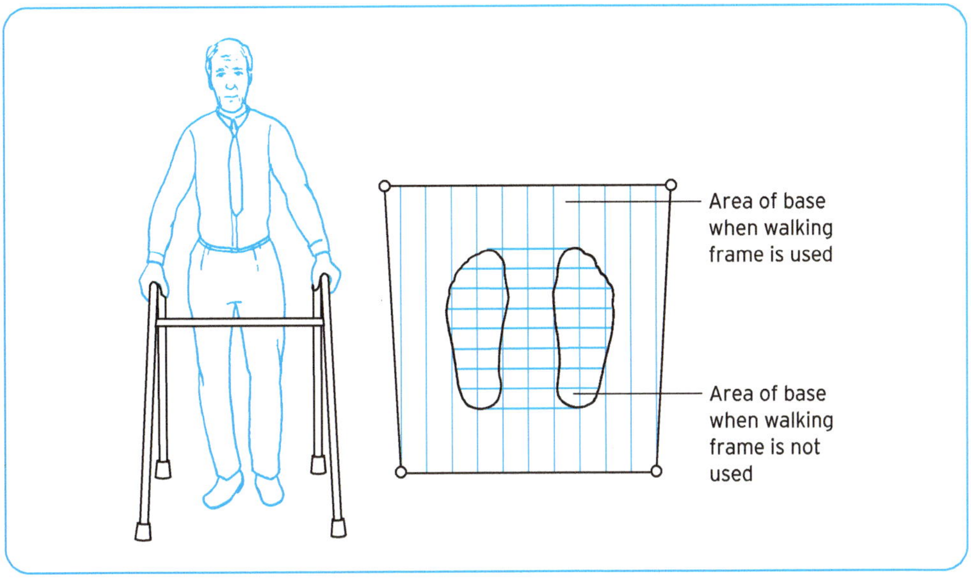

Figure 10.10
A walking frame increases the size of the base.

taught. For example, if crutches are to be effective, they have to be the right length for the patient. In addition, if the crutches are held vertically downwards, there is little effect on the size of the base – they have to be held at an angle away from the body.

Levers

A **lever** consists of a bar or a plank arranged so that it can pivot about a point referred to as the fulcrum (F). The plank used previously to illustrate the principle of the centre of gravity is one example of a lever. Levers also involve two forces – an effort force (*E*) and a resistance force (*R*). The latter is sometimes referred to as the **load**. Three types of lever are distinguished on the basis of the relationship between the fulcrum, the effort and the resistance. These three types of lever are referred to as first-order, second-order and third-order levers. Consider the three illustrations in Figure 10.11.

- ***What is the relationship between the fulcrum, the effort and the resistance in each of the types of lever?***

In a first-order lever, the fulcrum is between the two forces; in a second-order lever, the resistance is between the fulcrum and the effort; and in a third-order

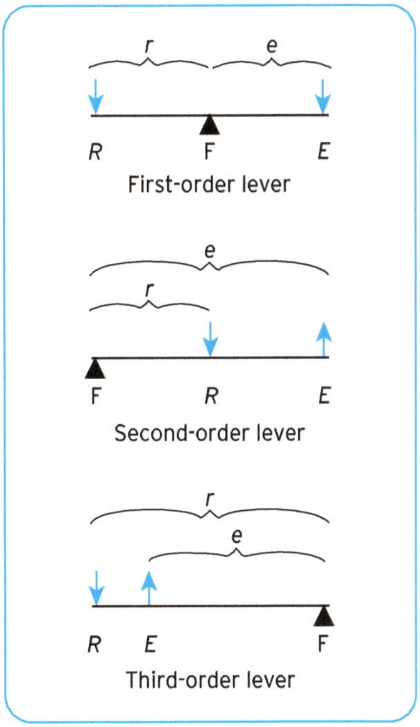

Figure 10.11
The three orders of levers.

lever, the effort is between the fulcrum and the resistance. Note too that the perpendicular (at right-angles) distance between the fulcrum and the line of action of the effort force is called the effort arm (*e*) and the perpendicular distance between the fulcrum and the line of action of the resistance force is called the resistance arm (*r*).

You will also be able to see that in second-order levers the effort arm is always longer than the resistance arm, while in third-order levers the resistance arm is always longer than the effort arm. In first-order levers, either arm may be longer or both may be the same length. Read that last sentence again. Now consider Figure 10.12.

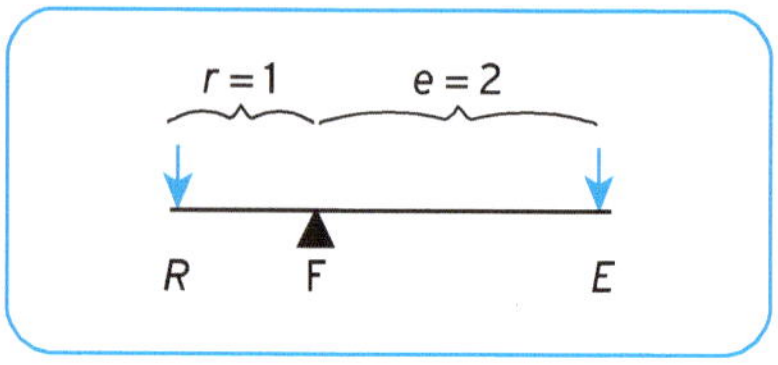

Figure 10.12
A first-order lever in equilibrium.

No doubt you had no trouble recognising that Figure 10.12 is a first-order lever, but note that in this case the effort arm is twice as long as the resistance arm. You might think 'So what?' After all, we did say that this could be the case. But imagine that our first-order lever is in a stable equilibrium - that is, it is balanced.

- ***Is the effort force (E) greater than, less than or equal to the resistance force (R)?***

Perhaps you have figured out that the effort force is less than the resistance force, since the effort force has a longer lever arm. In fact, the following equation is true:

$$Ee = Rr$$

Consequently, we can work out that in this case the value of the effort force (*E*) must be exactly half that of the resistance force (*R*), since the effort arm (*e*) is twice the length of the resistance arm (*r*). In fact, that is the whole point about first-order lever arrangements such as this - they enable us to oppose a resistance force with a lesser effort force by using a longer lever arm. In essence, we have just explained the use of a crowbar.

- ***Are levers important in the body?***

They are, indeed. Actually, bones act as levers, as we shall see in Practice point 10.5.

Practice point 10.5

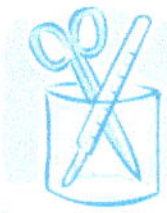

Levers and the body

If you remember the three types of lever, you will be able to recognise them when you see examples in the body. Three are shown in Figure 10.13.

An example of a first-order lever is flexion and extension of the neck, such as occurs when we nod the head. Standing on the toes, as one might to look over an obstacle, is an example of a second-order lever. Contraction of the biceps muscle of the upper arm is an example of a third-order lever. When the biceps muscle contracts, it becomes shorter and wider, and we can feel this increase in girth as it bulges in the upper arm. In this case, the biceps shortens to a relatively small extent compared with the distance through which the hand moves. Remember that in third-order levers, the effort arm is always shorter than the resistance arm. Consequently, the effort force must be greater than the resistance force, since this acts through a longer lever. Thus, in

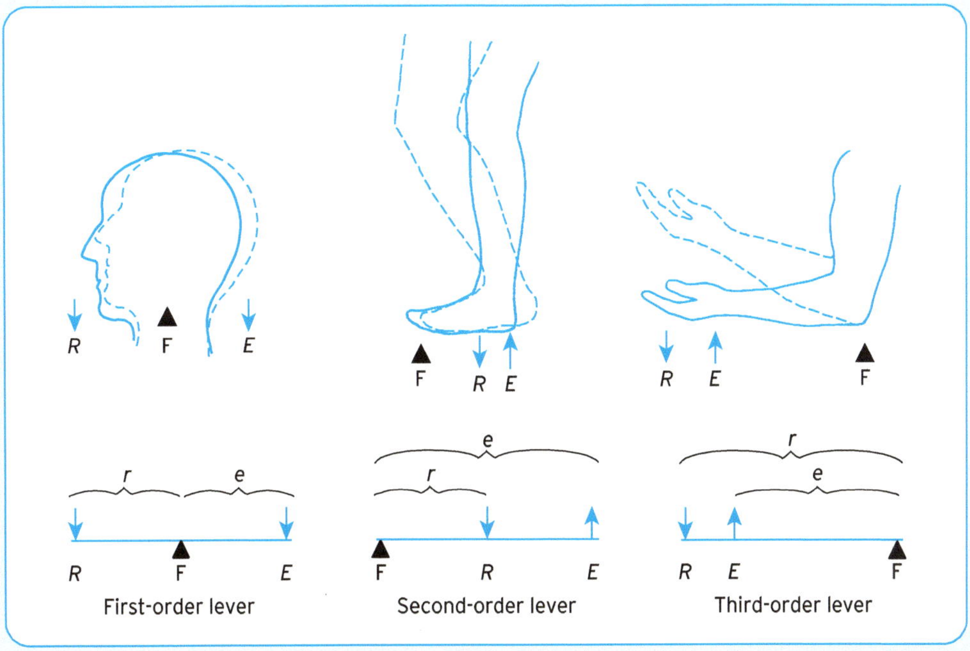

Figure 10.13
Three examples of levers in the body.

third-order levers, the resistance force is moved through a greater distance than the effort force, but the cost is that a greater effort force is required.

Levers and lifting

Figure 10.14 illustrates someone attempting to lift a sack. The first-order lever system involved is superimposed upon the image.

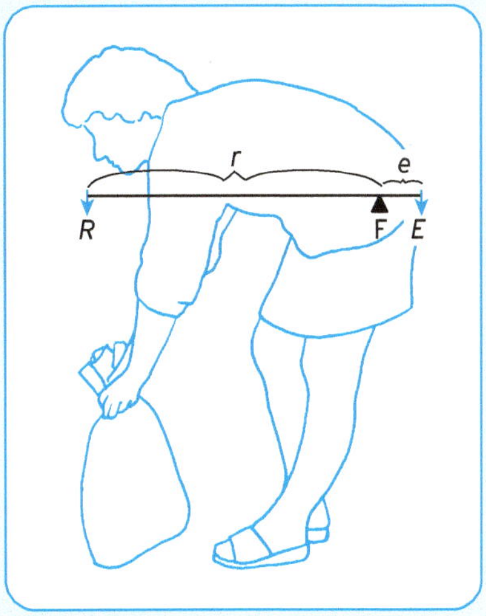

Figure 10.14
The lever system involved in lifting.

Once again the effort force is indicated by *E*, the effort arm by e, the resistance force by *R*, the resistance arm by *r* and the fulcrum by F. In this diagram, it is clear that the sack and the upper body provide the resistance force.

- ***What is providing the effort force?***

It is provided by the contraction of the muscles of the back. The point to note here is that because the fulcrum is close to the back, the effort force must be considerably larger than the resistance force, since the resistance force acts through the longer lever arm. The application of this understanding to practice is to note that the posture adopted by the individual in this diagram is much more likely to result in back injury than a posture in which the resistance arm is reduced in length.

- ***How could the resistance arm be reduced in length?***

Quite simply by bringing the resistance force (the sack) closer to the body. In addition, flexing of the spine should be avoided and the sack lifted by straightening the knees. The reason for this is explained in the next section. Finally, spreading the feet apart will improve stability by widening the base.

Levers and back injury

● ***How are back injuries sustained?***

As you might expect, there are many forms of back injury. One injury that you might have heard about is commonly called a slipped disc. The disc being referred to is an **intervertebral disc**. Intervertebral discs are located, as their name implies, between adjacent vertebrae (bones) of the spine. Each disc consists of an inner semi-fluid **nucleus pulposus**, which confers elasticity and compressibility. External to this is a strong outer ring of cartilage called the **annulus fibrosus**, which contains the nucleus pulposus and limits its expansion. This structure makes the discs highly suitable for their role in cushioning the force transmitted up the spine when walking, running and jumping. In addition, the discs allow the spine to flex (bend forwards) and to a lesser extent to bend from side to side.

In the case of a slipped disc, the nucleus pulposus protrudes through a rupture in the annulus fibrosus.

● ***Can you work out what the effects of this might be and how the condition might be treated?***

The effects result from compression of the spinal cord or a spinal nerve by the herniated disc, and this produces pain and sometimes numbness. Initial treatment includes **analgesics** (pain-relieving drugs), but surgical removal of a damaged disc is sometimes indicated.

● ***So how are slipped discs caused?***

Bending forwards to lift a heavy object, as described previously, is the cause. The effect of this on the disc is illustrated in Figure 10.1 5.

In this diagram, the forces applied to a disc while bending forwards and lifting a heavy object are shown. Note that this compression of the disc is not uniform along the whole breadth of the disc. The anterior portion is compressed, while posteriorly the disc is stretched; here, the annulus fibrosus is thinned and ruptured.

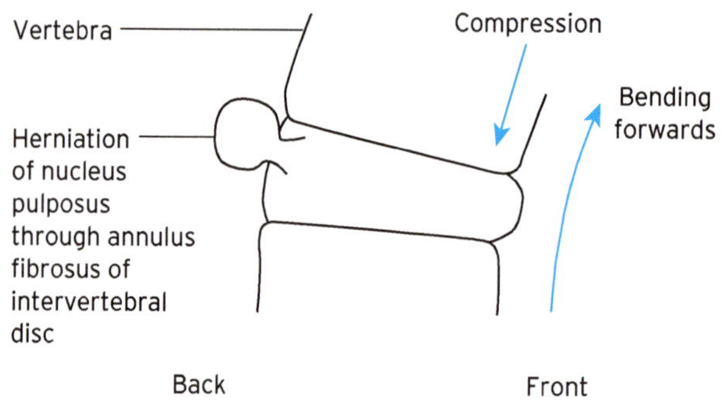

Figure 10.15
A slipped disc.

Pulleys

A pulley is a wheel with a groove around the rim that accepts a rope in the manner shown in Figure 10.16. If the pulley wheel rotates about a fixed axle - that is, the axle does not move up or down - it is referred to as a **fixed pulley**. Figure 10.16 is an example of a fixed pulley.

- ***What is the purpose of a fixed pulley?***

Fixed pulleys are used to change the direction of a force, but they do not produce any mechanical advantage - that is, an effort force of 100 N must be exerted to raise a resistance force (load) of the same value. There are also pulley systems (**moveable pulleys**) that produce a mechanical advantage, as shown in Figure 10.17. A moveable pulley is one whose axle is not fixed and that can, therefore, move up and down as well as rotate.

In the case of a single moveable pulley system, a load of 100 N requires an effort of only 50 N to lift it. More complicated pulley systems, such as a block and tackle, produce greater mechanical advantages.

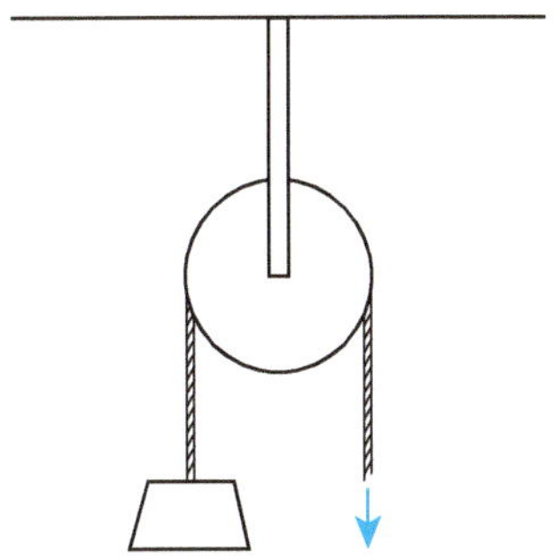

Figure 10.16
A fixed pulley.

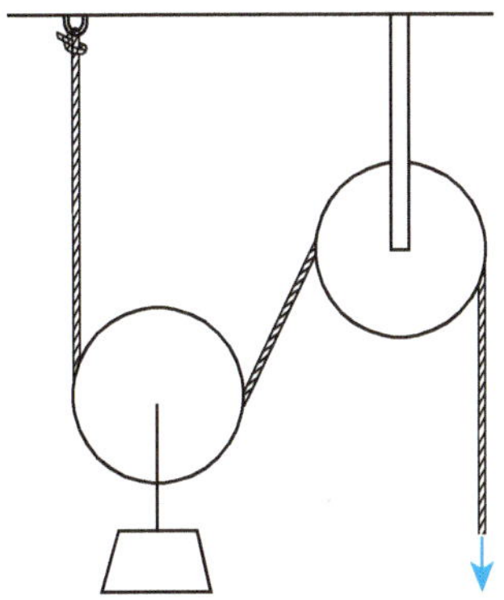

Figure 10.17
A single moveable pulley system.

Vectors

Remember that vector quantities are those that possess both size and direction. A force is one example of a vector quantity.

- ***What happens if an object is subject to two forces simultaneously? What are the net force and the direction of its action?***

To work out the answer to this question, we have to add together the two vectors in order to discover a single vector, called the resultant, which would have the same result. We can do this by drawing a vector diagram on a piece of graph paper. Consider Figure 10.18 as an example.

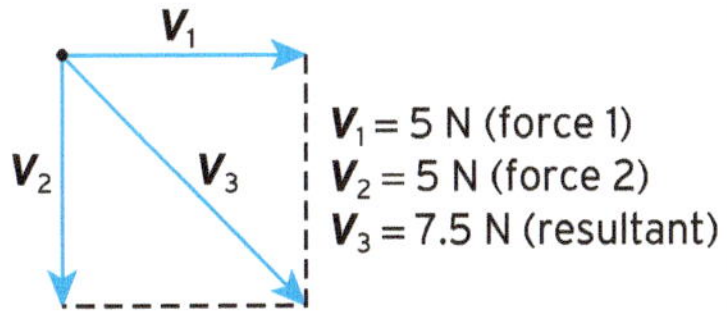

Figure 10.18
A vector diagram.

In this diagram, an object, represented simply by a dot, is subject to two forces acting simultaneously and at right-angles to each other. Lines, the length of which is proportional to the magnitude of the force, represent these forces. In this case, both forces are 5 N, and so both lines are of equal length. Note that the two lines form part of a parallelogram (a shape with parallel sides). If we now complete the shape, we can resolve the direction of the resultant by drawing a line from the object to the opposite corner of the parallelogram. The magnitude of the resultant can be calculated simply by measuring this line. The above discussion sounds rather theoretical - we need to relate it to practice. This is done in Practice point 10.6, in which vectors are related to orthopaedic traction.

Practice point 10.6

Pulleys, vectors and orthopaedic traction

Traction simply refers to a pulling force, and so the term 'orthopaedic traction' means the application of a pulling force to the bones. Orthopaedic traction is sometimes used to immobilise broken bones and to keep the broken ends in alignment, especially where muscle contraction tends to cause the broken ends to override each other, thus shortening the limb. Traction may be applied directly to the skeleton through pins inserted through a bone (skeletal traction) or indirectly through the skin using bandages (skin traction). Figure 10.19 shows one type of traction. Note that both fixed and moveable pulleys are used.

- ***Which of the pulleys are fixed, and which is moveable?***

Pulleys a, b and d are fixed, but pulley c is moveable. The presence of pulleys means that the force (weight) acts in a number of directions and that the leg is subject to two vectors. To work out the resultant, we have to draw a vector diagram - in fact, this is already done for you.

- ***So what is the direction of the resultant?***

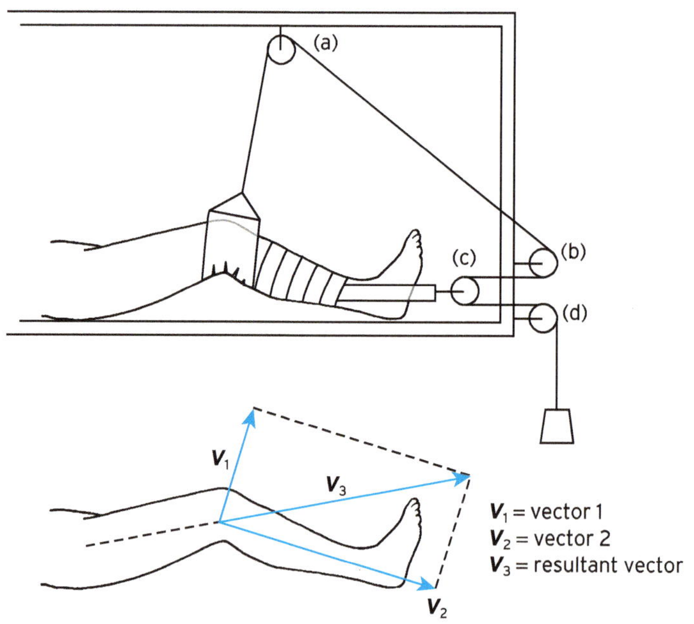

Figure 10.19
An example of orthopaedic traction.

It is in line with the shaft of the femur - the broken bone, in this case.

It is especially important to note that because a single moveable pulley is involved, the force applied to the leg is actually twice that of the weight applied to the rope. Clearly, if a mistake was made and too great a weight attached to the leg, the resultant traction on the leg would be considerable due to this mechanical advantage.

It is possible to see examples of traction in both paediatric and adult orthopaedic units. If you are involved in the care of a patient in traction, make an effort to find out more about the system involved and the nursing care of the patient. It is worth pointing out that developments in internal and external fixation techniques mean that the use of traction has declined in recent years.

In-text review

- ✔ Fainting caused by the pooling of blood in the legs is one example of the effect of gravity on the body.
- ✔ The centre of gravity of the body is normally within the pelvis, but it varies with position and obesity.
- ✔ An object does not fall over if the line of action of its weight passes through the base. This is an important consideration in the use of sticks, crutches and walking frames, which effectively widen the base.
- ✔ Levers are described as first-, second- or third-order, depending upon the relative positions of the fulcrum, resistance force and effort force.
- ✔ A first-order lever diagram can be used to examine the forces involved when lifting.
- ✔ Appropriate lifting techniques involve avoiding heavier weights than recommended, holding the weight close to the body and avoiding flexing of the spine.
- ✔ Pulleys are devices used for changing the direction of a force; some pulley systems also produce a mechanical advantage.
- ✔ The effect of two forces upon an object can be resolved using a vector diagram and the parallelogram method.

Summary

Aspects of science covered in this chapter such as the difference between vector and scalar quantities and Newton's laws of motion could be found in general science and physics textbooks. However, here they have been applied to health care. For example, Newton's first law was used to explain whiplash and the crash position. Nonetheless possibly the most important aspects dealt with are levers and moving and handling. During preparation to be a registered nurse you will no doubt have plenty of opportunity to learn more about the moving and handling of patients. A basic understanding of the science of levers will enable you to ensure patient safety and prevent back injury.

Summary points

- Scalar quantities, such as mass and speed, have only size, while vector quantities, such as weight, velocity, acceleration and force, have both size and direction.
- The behaviour of objects in motion is described in Newton's three laws.
- Fainting caused by the pooling of blood in the legs is one example of the effect of gravity on the body.
- The centre of gravity of the body varies with position and obesity.
- An object does not fall over if the line of action of its weight passes through the base.
- Levers are described as first-, second- or third-order, depending upon the relative positions of the fulcrum, resistance force and effort force.
- A first-order lever diagram can be used to examine the forces involved when lifting.
- Appropriate lifting techniques involve avoiding heavier weights than recommended, holding the weight close to the body and avoiding flexing of the spine.
- Pulleys are devices used for changing the direction of a force; some pulley systems also produce a mechanical advantage.
- The effect of two forces upon an object can be resolved using a vector diagram and the parallelogram method.

Self-test questions

1 Which one of the following measurements is a vector quantity?
(a) Length.
(b) Mass.
(c) Speed.
(d) Weight.

2 Which of the following statements are true?
(a) Velocity is an example of a vector quantity.
(b) An electron orbiting the nucleus of an atom is constantly accelerating.
(c) Force is an example of a vector quantity.
(d) Momentum is the product of mass and velocity.

3 Which of the following statements are true?
(a) When a person is sitting, the centre of gravity lies within the pelvis.
(b) When an individual is supine, the centre of gravity lies within the pelvis.
(c) Obesity causes an anterior displacement of the centre of gravity.
(d) The centre of gravity of a child lies outside the pelvis.

4 Which of the following statements are true?
(a) Whiplash injury can be explained by reference to Newton's second law.

(b) The statement 'to every action there is an equal and opposite reaction' is an expression of Newton's third law.
(c) Newton's first law is sometimes referred to as the law of inertia.
(d) Force = mass × acceleration.

5 Which of the following statements are true?
(a) Speed = distance/time.
(b) Acceleration = velocity/time.
(c) The acceleration of a fixed mass is proportional to the force applied to it.
(d) When two vehicles are stationary, the one with the greatest momentum is that with the greatest mass.

6 Which of the following statements are true?
(a) A seesaw is an example of a first-order lever.
(b) Flexing the elbow is an example of a third-order lever.
(c) Flexing the neck is an example of a third-order lever.
(d) Standing on the toes is an example of a second-order lever.

7 In the case of a first-order lever in equilibrium in which the resistance force is 10 N, the resistance arm 3 m and the effort arm 1 m, which one of the following is the value of the effort force?
(a) 120 N.
(b) 60 N.
(c) 30 N.
(d) 15 N.

8 In the case of a first-order lever in equilibrium in which the resistance force is 50 N, the resistance arm 1 m and the effort arm 10 m, which one of the following is the value of the effort force?
(a) 500 N.
(b) 250 N.
(c) 50 N.
(d) 5 N.

9 In the case of a fixed pulley, which one of the following is the minimum force that could be used to lift a load of 50 N?
(a) 100 N.
(b) 50 N.
(c) 25 N.
(d) 15 N.

10 In the case of a single moveable pulley, which one of the following is the minimum force that could be used to lift a load of 50 N?
(a) 100 N.
(b) 50 N.
(c) 25 N.
(d) 15 N.

Further study/exercises

1 **When you next visit a clinical area in which patients need help to move and position themselves, identify the moving and handling aids available and find out how to use them.**

2 **Suppose an immobile patient needs to be moved from a hospital trolley to a bed. How should this be done? What should you do to ensure the safety of the patient and the staff involved?**

Royal College of Nursing (2003). *Safer Staff, Better Care: RCN Manual Handling Training Guide and Competencies*. London: Royal College of Nursing.

Smith J. (ed.) (2005). *The Guide to the Handling of People*, 5th edn. Teddington: BackCare.

Steed R. and Tracey C. (2000). Equipment for moving and handling: hoists and slings. *British Journal of Therapy and Rehabilitation*, 7(10), 430-35.

Steed R. and Tracey C. (2000). Assisting independence and eliminating tasks for moving and handling. *British Journal of Therapy and Rehabilitation*, 7(12), 503-7.

Wilson C. (2001). Safer handling practice for nurses: a review of the literature. *British Journal of Nursing*, 10(2), 108-14.

11

Electricity, magnetism and medical equipment

Learning outcomes

After reading the following chapter and undertaking personal study, you should be able to:

1. Describe magnetism and distinguish between permanent magnets and electromagnets.
2. Give examples of the use of magnets in health care.
3. Distinguish between static and dynamic (current) electricity.
4. Explain the terms 'potential difference', 'current', 'resistance' and 'power' and identify the units used to measure each.
5. Briefly describe the effects of electrocution and distinguish between macroshock and microshock.
6. Identify important aspects of electrical safety.
7. Describe the action potential and relate this to nerve cells and the conduction system of the heart.
8. Briefly describe important medical uses of electricity, including the ECG monitor, the defibrillator, diathermy and the artificial pacemaker.

Introduction

It is probably not until a power cut that we come to realise how heavily dependent we are upon electricity - and not only for light. An average home in the West contains a large number of items of electrical equipment, including cookers, heaters, televisions and sound systems. It is probably not surprising, then, to discover that modern health care also shares this dependency upon electricity. In the course of your career, you will encounter medical equipment of many different kinds, some of which we describe in this chapter. Included are **electrocardiography** (ECG) machines, **artificial pacemakers**, and various scanners, such as **computerised tomography** (CT) and **magnetic resonance imaging** (MRI) machines. In this chapter, you will also learn about the importance of electricity in the proper functioning of the body, such as the electrical impulses transmitted in nerves. First, however, we spend some time thinking about a related phenomenon - magnetism.

Magnetism

Of all the phenomena described in this book, magnetism must be one of the most familiar.

- ***Think about the occasions when you have used a magnet.***

Most of us have owned a **magnet** and we may have used the magnetic pointer of a compass to help us find our way. Magnetism is not a newly observed phenomenon. The ancient Greeks noticed that certain stones attracted objects made of iron, and the description of these rocks as magnetic is derived from the name of the city of their discovery - Magnesia. Magnets can be divided into two types - **permanent magnets** and **electromagnets**.

Permanent magnets

The description of a magnet as permanent is probably self-explanatory, but this expression is used to identify magnets in which the magnetic field is not dependent on the flow of an electric current. Rubbing ferrous (iron-containing) metals with magnetic rock created the earliest permanent magnets. Subsequently, when small permanent magnets in the shape of a bar were floated on water, it was noticed that one end (pole) always pointed north, and so the ends of bar magnets came to be described as the north and south poles. Of course, this observation led to the development of the compass, in which the magnetic bar is shaped like a pointer. Such devices were in use by the Middle Ages. The need to float the pointer on water was subsequently eliminated by balancing the pointer on a pivot.

- ***What observations can we make when we bring together the poles of two bar magnets?***

Like poles repel; unlike poles attract. If you have ever owned a train-set with magnetic couplings, you may have worked this out long ago. You may also have performed an experiment at school in which iron filings are sprinkled upon a sheet of paper held above a bar magnet.

- ***When this is done, what do we observe?***

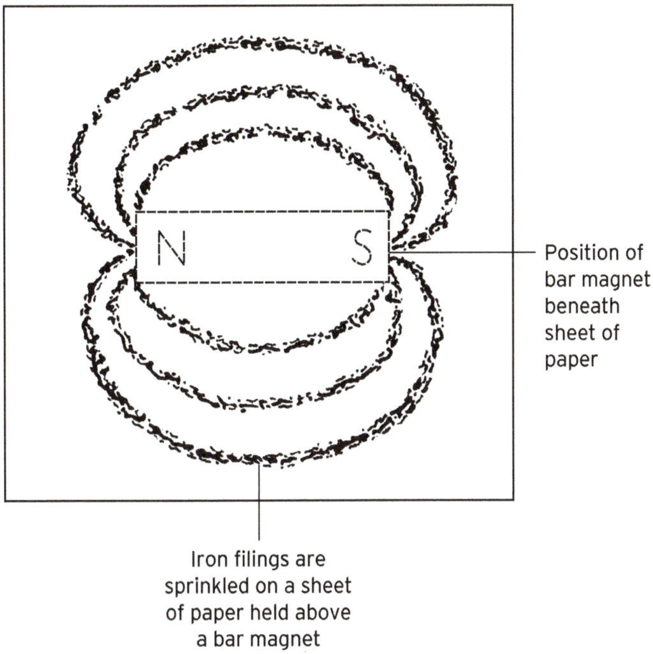

Figure 11.1
The effect of sprinkling iron filings on a piece of paper held above a bar magnet.

The iron filings do not remain scattered in a diffuse pattern, but instead they fall in a regular arrangement corresponding to magnetic lines of force, as shown in Figure 11.1.

These lines of force are collectively referred to as the **magnetic field**, which is the region in which magnetic force can be demonstrated. If we take a small compass, we could also demonstrate these lines of force by the movement of the needle. This is shown in Figure 11.2.

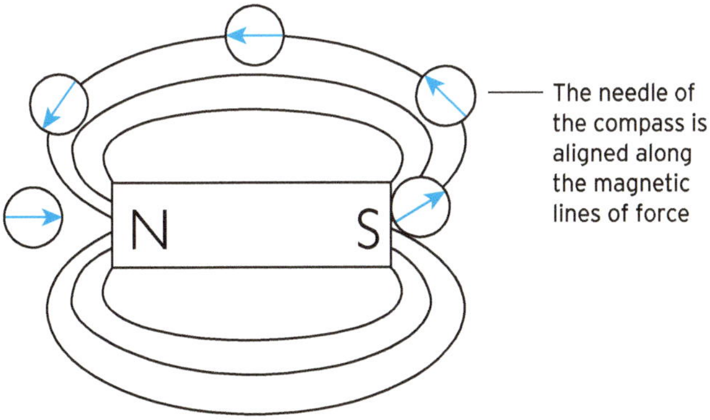

Figure 11.2
Using a compass to demonstrate magnetic lines of force.

Electromagnets

A connection between electricity and magnetism was confirmed when, in the early nineteenth century, it was shown that a magnetic field is present around a wire in which current is flowing. As soon as the current is turned off, the magnetic field disappears. This effect is shown in Figure 11.3.

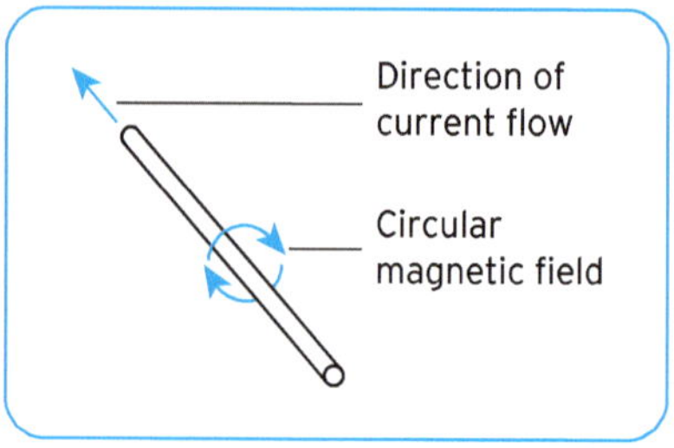

Figure 11.3
The magnetic field around a wire in which a current is flowing.

If the wire is formed into a coil that surrounds a cylinder, a magnetic field similar to that of the bar magnet is formed, and the device is called an **electromagnet**. This is illustrated in Figure 11.4. One use of large electromagnets is in cranes used to lift cars in scrap yards.

Are there medical uses of electromagnets?

Yes, there are. For example, you may witness an electromagnet being used to remove small metal objects that have penetrated the eye. Whether or not magnetic fields have wider implications for health is uncertain, as Practice point 11.1 explains.

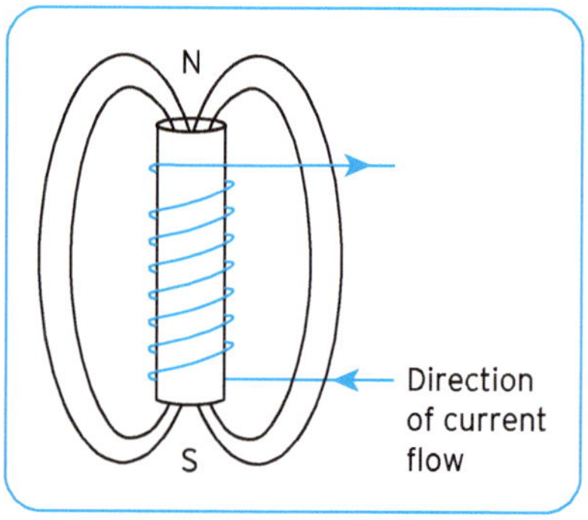

Figure 11.4
An electromagnet.

The solenoid

The magnetic field of an electromagnet is stronger if it contains an iron core; but if the core is not fixed when the current is flowing, the core will move forwards, to the north pole of the electromagnet. This effect is the basis of the **solenoid** or electrical switch. This is the kind of switch used in security doors fitted to apartments, since the solenoid can be operated from a distance. It also finds use in items of medical equipment, such as **artificial ventilators**.

Practice point 11.1

Magnetic fields and the body

At present, the beneficial or harmful effects of magnetic fields upon the body remain largely unconfirmed. Some people believe that magnetic fields may be used to alleviate inflammation and improve blood supply to injured areas. Magnetic bracelets can be bought from manufacturers who claim benefits in various conditions, such as joint disease. Others allege that magnetic fields associated with high-voltage power supplies may, in some way, contribute to illness. It will be interesting to see what research in this field reveals. It is certainly the case, however, that **artificial pacemakers** may be inhibited by magnetic fields; for this reason, patients who have such devices implanted should not lean over car engines that are running, since the ignition system develops strong magnetic fields.

Electricity

Like magnetism, electricity is a commonly experienced phenomenon, but one that is poorly understood. We commonly distinguish between two forms of electricity - static electricity and dynamic electricity.

Static electricity

Once again, the origins of this aspect of science go back to the ancient Greeks, who noticed that the semi-precious stone amber (fossilised tree sap) could be made to attract filaments of a cloth with which it was rubbed. In a similar way, you may have noticed that hair is attracted to a comb following vigorous combing. As a child, you may have torn up small pieces of paper in order to watch them 'jump' on to the comb as it was brought near to them. Centuries after the Greeks, any material with which this phenomenon could be demonstrated became known as an *electric*, a name derived from the Greek *elektron* (meaning amber), and the mysterious power of attraction came to be called electricity. We now know that the transfer of **electrons** (negatively charged subatomic particles) from one material to another causes the phenomenon of static electricity. In the above cases, this is achieved by rubbing. Electrons are described in more detail in Chapter 3.

Remember that only two types of charge exist - positive and negative. When electrons are transferred from one object to another, the recipient object becomes negatively charged and the object that has lost electrons becomes positively charged.

- ***What do we know about the behaviour of charged objects when they are brought together?***

Like charges attract, and unlike charges repel. Thus, static electricity is the phenomenon of a build-up of electrons. Since the electrons are not moving, the use of the description 'static' is quite appropriate.

- ***Does the build-up of electrons remain forever?***

No - eventually, something will happen to enable the electrons to be discharged. For example, they may leak away slowly through the atmosphere. This is especially so in humid conditions. Alternatively, they may be suddenly discharged by contact with a conductor. You may find this occurring when you make a hospital bed. These have wheels with rubber tyres, and so a build-up of charge is dissipated only when someone who is earthed touches the bed.

- ***Is static electricity dangerous?***

Not normally, although there are occasions when static electricity is potentially dangerous. For example, flammable gases may be ignited by the heat of a spark caused by the discharge of static electricity. During a storm, charged regions may develop in the atmosphere and the discharge of electrons from one region to another results in a very large spark, which we call lightning. The danger presented here is when a discharge is made to earth.

Insulators and conductors

Since we have already used the term **conductor**, it is probably a good idea to define it and compare conductors with **insulators**. Note that some materials do not allow the movement of electrons, and so when rubbing transfers electrons to them the charge is not lost. Such materials are called insulators or poor conductors. Examples are amber, plastic and rubber. Once again, you may have made use of this as a child. Rub an inflated rubber balloon against your jumper (the balloon and jumper are both good insulators). The balloon becomes charged and can be made to stick against the wall. Eventually, the charge leaks away and is the basis of the game to see who can get their balloon to stick the longest. Other materials, such as metals, are referred to as conductors, since electrons pass through them readily. Distinguishing between conductors and insulators is important when we move on to consider dynamic electricity.

Dynamic electricity

If static electricity involves the build-up of electrons in one place, then dynamic electricity involves the flow of electrons. One example of dynamic electricity in the body that we shall consider later on is the **electrocardiograph** (ECG - a trace of the heart rhythm). A consultant heart specialist once told me that he found it difficult to explain the ECG to healthcare staff who did not understand electricity. He had a point - it is much easier to explain electricity in the body or the operation of an item of medical equipment if the student has some knowledge of dynamic electricity. That is why we look at it here. A number of concepts have to be introduced if dynamic electricity is to be understood. We can introduce them by using a simple illustration - that of a water tank and tap, as shown in Figure 11.5.

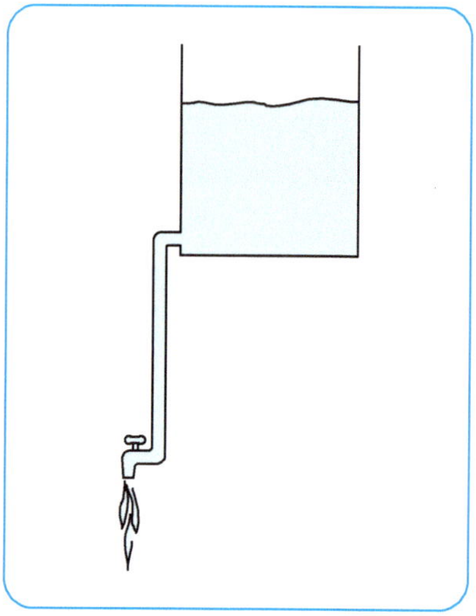

Figure 11.5
Illustrating dynamic electricity by using a water tank and tap.

You may wonder what a water tank and tap have to do with electricity, but stick with this illustration for a moment.

- ***What will happen if the tap is opened?***

Water will flow out of the tap. We could measure this flow in litres per minute (l/min).

- ***But why does the water flow?***

Once again, the answer is fairly obvious. It is because the tank is high up, perhaps in the loft, and the tap is low down, perhaps in the kitchen. In consequence, there is a pressure difference between the two points, and it is this pressure difference that causes the water to flow.

- ***And if the water in the tank was not replaced, what would happen to the flow rate as the volume in the tank became depleted?***

As the volume of water in the tank became depleted, the pressure difference between the tank and the tap would become reduced and the flow rate would fall.

- ***Could any other factor affect the flow rate?***

Yes - the diameter of the pipes could. Provided the pressure does not change, a greater flow rate could be maintained through a wider pipe.

- ***So, what has this illustration got to do with electricity?***

First, note that electrons also flow 'downhill' from a point of high concentration to a point of low concentration - that is, dynamic electricity consists of a flow of electrons from negative to positive. Actually, when electrons are flowing in this way, we say that there is a **current** of electricity, so perhaps the illustration of the tank of water and tap is not such a strange one after all. Incidentally, for this reason we also speak of dynamic electricity as current electricity.

- ***Can we measure electrical current just as we measure the flow of water?***

Yes we can, although we do not use l/min. The SI unit of current is the **ampere** (or amp), named after the scientist André Ampère. There is a current of one amp when one **coulomb** of charge is flowing each second:

Electrical current (amps) = number of coulombs/second

- ***What's that – a coulomb of charge?***

The charge of a single electron is far too small to be of practical use in the measurement of electrical current. Consequently, the SI unit of charge, the coulomb (named after Charles Coulomb), is used, which is much larger. In fact, one coulomb is equal to the charge of 1.6×10^{19} electrons.

- ***What pushes these electrons along? Is there an electrical equivalent of the pressure difference between the tank and the tap?***

Yes, there is. The term 'electrical potential' is the amount of energy per coulomb that a charge possesses. It is measured in joules per coulomb - a unit renamed the **volt** after the scientist Allessandro Volta. The difference in the electrical potential difference between two points is called the **potential difference**, and this too is measured in volts. Current flows between two points only when there is an electrical potential difference between them.

- ***Does the diameter of the wire through which a current is passing affect the current in the same way that the diameter of a pipe affects the flow of water?***

Once again, the answer is yes. Just as only the widest pipes can carry the greatest flow of water, so only the thickest wires can carry the greatest currents. You might have learned as much from experience. For example, a low current is conveyed from a transformer to the track of a toy train-set by thin wires, but the greater current that is carried to the transformer from the mains requires thicker wires.

The concept being introduced here is that of **resistance** - a property that impedes the flow of current through a conductor. Thicker wires offer less resistance. Resistance is dependent not only upon the diameter of the wire but also upon the material from which the wire is made, the least resistance being offered by the best conductors. The length of a wire also influences resistance – that is, resistance increases with length. The SI unit of resistance is the **ohm** (Ω), named after Georg Ohm. The relationship between current, electrical potential difference and resistance is given by the following equation (Ohm's law):

$$I \text{ (amps)} = V \text{ (volts)}/R \text{ (ohms)}$$

This means that when an electrical potential difference of 1 volt drives a current of 1 amp, the resistance is 1 ohm.

- ***What would happen if too great a current was passed through a wire?***

The answer is that some of the energy would be lost as heat and light. If the current is great enough, the heat generated will melt the wire, and we might say that the wire has 'burned out'. In order to avoid this, very thick wires supply X-ray machines, which require a potential difference of several thousand volts. Sometimes, however, the emission of heat and light is actually desired – in electric heaters and lightbulbs for example. In these cases, the diameter of the wire is chosen carefully so that the desired effect is produced without the wire melting. We might also select a wire of a certain thickness so that if too great a current is drawn through, it melts and the flow of current ceases.

- ***Have you worked out that this is a fuse?***

The problem with fuses is that, even with a low-current-rating 3-amp fuse, the current required to burn out the fuse is much greater than that required to kill. Consequently, electrical devices should be used with earth-leakage circuit breakers (see later).

Current flow

Although the illustration of the tank of water and tap works quite well, it does have one deficiency. It illustrates best the flow of current in one direction. For much of the time, however, we have to deal with current flow that changes direction.

Direct current

When electrons flow in one direction through a circuit, the current is described as **direct current** (d.c.). This is the type of current flow produced by batteries. Batteries may be of a number of types, but all make use of the fact that the atoms of certain metals dissociate (break up) when placed in an **electrolyte** solution (a solution of ions). For example, if a rod of zinc is partially immersed in a dilute solution of sulphuric acid (H_2SO_4), the zinc atoms dissociate into zinc ions (Zn^{2+}), which enter solution, and electrons, which remain in the rod. The dissociation of zinc is much more rapid than that of copper. Consequently, if a similar copper rod is inserted into the same solution, a potential difference will exist between the two rods. If a wire to form a circuit now joins the two rods, electrons will flow from the zinc rod to the copper rod – that is, there is a flow of current. Batteries that employ electrolyte solutions like this are referred to as wet cells. A car battery is an obvious example. Other batteries are called dry cells, since the electrolyte is in the form of a paste. Dry-cell batteries power electrical devices such as torches, toys and radios as well as artificial heart pacemakers that are implanted into the body.

Alternating current

In **alternating current** (a.c.), electrons flow first in one direction and then in the other direction. The domestic power supply is alternating current; in this case, the electrons flow 50 times in each direction every second, and we say that the current has a frequency of 50 hertz (Hz).

- ***Does a.c. have advantages over d.c.?***

It has some advantages. The energy losses in the power cables of electricity-generating companies are less when a.c. is used, and transformers can be used with a.c. (A transformer is a device that is used to change one voltage into another.)

- ***But if a.c. simply involves the rapid movement of electrons, what do we mean when we speak about using electricity?***

Electrons themselves are not being consumed; instead, energy is transferred by their oscillation, although the information that is really useful to have about electrical devices is the rate at which they consume energy - that is, power. Power is measured in the amount of energy used per second - joules per second (J/s). This is a further unit that has been renamed - this time after James Watt. The **watt** (W) is used to measure the power consumption of small electrical devices such as lightbulbs and we use this information when we make such choices as whether to buy a 60- or 100-watt bulb. We would probably choose a 60-watt bulb for a bedside lamp but a 100-watt bulb where greater brightness is required. The power used, however, does not tell us exactly how bright the bulb will be. A modern energy-saving bulb uses much less power than an old-fashioned bulb, and yet it is as bright. This is because it is more efficient and less energy is wasted as heat. Large items of electrical equipment, such as X-ray tubes, use so much power that the kilowatt (kW) is used instead of the watt (W). One kilowatt (kW) is equal to 1000 watts.

Electrocution

In this section, we are going to consider what happens in accidents when an electric current is applied unintentionally to the body and one occasion when we apply a large current on purpose.

- ***What two things are required for current to flow?***

An electrical potential difference is required to drive the current, and a circuit is needed through which the current can flow. It is important to keep these two factors in mind, since an understanding of them informs many aspects of electrical safety, some of which are given in Practice point 11.2. This is followed by an outline of first aid measures in the event of electric shock (Practice point 11.3).

Practice point 11.2

Electrical safety

In a textbook such as this, the advice given about electrical safety must be of a rather general nature. In addition, the hospital setting is sometimes treated differently from your own home. For example, in the home, an electrician would not usually be called to replace a lightbulb. In the hospital, however, there will be suitably qualified staff to carry out such tasks. A hospital will have a health-and-safety policy that covers electrical safety. You should familiarise yourself with the policies of the institutions in which you gain experience and, of course, you should follow them. Each department will also have a health-and-safety officer who can offer advice when required. Nonetheless, the following are some general points worth noting:

- Plugs should be fitted properly. In European Community (EC) countries, new items of electrical equipment already have plugs fitted.
- Each plug should be fitted with a fuse of the correct current rating for the piece of equipment to which it is attached.
- Hospitals will have a policy about the testing and checking of electrical equipment, and it should be adhered to. Testing is usually performed annually; the date of the test should be recorded on a sticker placed on the equipment.
- All equipment should be operated in accordance with the manufacturer's instructions.
- Objects containing fluids should not be placed on top of items of electrical equipment. This is a rather obvious point, but check out how cluttered a patient's bedside locker can become when personal items and a portable ECG machine compete for space.
- Do not operate electrical equipment with wet hands. Once again, this is a rather obvious point, but you may be rushing and anxious in an emergency. Consider the case of the patient who has suffered a cardiac arrest in the bathroom, where there is water on the floor. It may then be dangerous to operate electrical equipment such as the defibrillator.
- Equipment should be checked for signs of obvious damage, such as broken plugs and frayed flex. Damaged equipment should not be used – it should be labelled as damaged and be removed for repair by suitably qualified staff.
- Avoiding the creation of a circuit involving the patient should prevent microshock. For example, do not touch the patient at the same time as you touch an item of electrical equipment.

Why is electrocution potentially dangerous?

There are a number of reasons. An electric current may produce painful muscular contractions, and affected individuals may not be able to release themselves from the source of the current. Affected respiratory muscles experience sustained contraction, and the individual may not be able to breathe. Electrocution may also induce **cardiac arrest** – that is, the heart ceases to pump effectively. This does not necessarily mean that the heart is still. For example, the **arrhythmia** (abnormal rhythm) called **ventricular fibrillation** (VF) is characterised by rapid uncoordinated contractions. The appearance of the heart in this state

Practice point 11.3

First aid in electric shock

For a full description of what to do in electric shock, you should consult a first-aid manual. The following are some points for general guidance:

- Shout for help.
- Do not touch someone who is being electrocuted; tell others to keep away too.
- Do not make contact with the person via any conducting object.
- The current should be turned off at the mains.
- Once you have ensured that it is safe to do so, check that the patient is breathing and that there is a heartbeat.
- If breathing has ceased and a heartbeat is absent, commence cardiopulmonary resuscitation (mouth-to-mouth breathing and closed chest cardiac compression).
- Burns should be given attention only once breathing and a heartbeat have been restored.

has been likened to a bag of worms – a description that does at least convey the impression of a quivering but ineffective rhythm. Electrocution sometimes turns the heart's normal rhythm into VF.

- ***How is this treated?***

Perhaps you have heard of **defibrillation**? This means 'stopping fibrillation'; the device that achieves this is called a **defibrillator**. We consider this a little later.

Finally, in electrocution, burns may be produced at the site of entry of the current to the body and at its site of exit. These burns range from minor to very severe. Skin grafting may be required to repair damaged tissue; in the case of a severely burned limb, amputation may be performed.

- ***Is it possible, when accidents involving electricity take place, to predict the kind of effects that electrocution will produce in a particular case?***

There are many variables that affect the severity of the damage caused by an electric current passing through the body; some are described below.

Duration of current

This is perhaps the most obvious variable. The longer the duration, the worse the effects. Consequently, earth-leakage circuit breakers are designed to interrupt the current in a fraction of a second. These devices compare the current flowing in the two wires forming the circuit of the electrical device. These wires are called the live and neutral wires. Under perfect conditions, the current in each should be identical. If not, it means that some of the current is leaking away – perhaps to an individual who is being electrocuted. When this occurs, we say that the device is 'tripped' and the current flow is stopped.

Amount of current

The amount of current flowing is the most significant factor in determining the effects of electrocution. Currents of 1–5 mA (1–5 milliamps) will produce a definite shock, while death becomes possible at currents above about 10 mA.

- ***What factors determine the amount of current flowing?***

Remember Ohm's law ($I = V/R$)? Both potential difference and resistance influence the amount of current flowing.

Potential difference

Although electrical safety warnings often provide information about the electrical potential difference in volts, it is not the potential difference per se that is important but the current that it can drive. From Ohm's law, we can see that, provided the resistance remains unaltered, a greater potential difference will drive a greater current. The normal domestic electricity supply in the UK has a potential difference of 240 volts. This is certainly dangerous, but it is not as dangerous as overhead power cables, which carry thousands of volts. Each year, children are injured or killed as a consequence of playing around high-voltage supplies.

Resistance

Electrocution by the domestic supply of 240 V sometimes proves fatal, but other times it does not.

- ***Why is this?***

There are a number of reasons, but one is concerned with resistance. For example, the resistance offered by dry skin is many times greater than that of wet skin, and so the current driven by the same potential difference through wet skin will be higher than that through dry skin. Thus far, we have assumed that the current has to pass through the skin and other soft tissues in order to reach the heart. This is, of course, usually the case.

- ***Under what circumstances could a current be passed directly to the heart?***

One example is when a transvenous pacing wire is in place. In this case, a pacemaker wire is passed through the venous circulation (veins) to the right ventricle of the heart while the other end remains outside the body and is attached to an external impulse generator (pacemaker box). In a case such as this, even a very low current inadvertently passed down the wire to the heart may induce ventricular fibrillation (a form of cardiac arrest), since the high resistance of the skin and other body tissues has been bypassed. Indeed, the current required might even be below the level of perception of the individual through whom it is conveyed to the patient. Consequently, this form of electrocution is termed **microshock**, in order to distinguish it from the more common form, which we call **macroshock**.

Frequency

The heart is more susceptible to some frequencies of alternating current than others. For example, it is susceptible to the frequency of the domestic supply (50 Hz), while the very high frequency of **diathermy** (see later) causes burns without inducing muscle contraction or ventricular fibrillation.

In-text review

- ✔ Electricity involves the transfer of electrons.
- ✔ A build-up of electrons that are not flowing is referred to as static electricity.
- ✔ Dynamic (current) electricity involves the flow of electrons.
- ✔ Direct current involves the flow of electrons in one direction, while in alternating current the direction of current flow changes back and forth.
- ✔ The relationship between potential difference, current and resistance is given in Ohm's law.
- ✔ Power is the amount of energy consumed in one second and is measured in watts (joules/second).
- ✔ Electrocution occurs when there is a flow of current through the body, the effect of which is determined by the magnitude of the current, its frequency and duration.

Electricity in the body

The importance of electricity is probably demonstrated most clearly by the nervous system and in the generation of **action potentials**. Before we look at this, we ought to explain the function of the nervous system.

The nervous system

In Chapter 2 we considered the principle of feedback, as illustrated in Figure 11.6.

All feedback mechanisms involve three components - **receptors** (detectors), a **control centre** and **effectors** (structures that produce an effect/response). We have already noted that receptors monitor a **controlled condition** (e.g. body temperature) and provide information about it (input) to the control centre (e.g. the brain). The control centre generates instructions (output), which determine the response made by effectors. Inputs and output are messages about the operation of the body that are sent from one structure to another. Sometimes these messages take a chemical form (**hormones**), and sometimes they are nervous impulses (**action potentials**).

How is the nervous system organised?

People often say that the nervous system is complex. Indeed, if you are training to be a neurosurgeon, you would have to understand something of its complexity. For our purposes, however, you can begin to understand the nervous system first by noting that it has two main divisions - the **central nervous system** (CNS) and the **peripheral nervous system** (PNS).

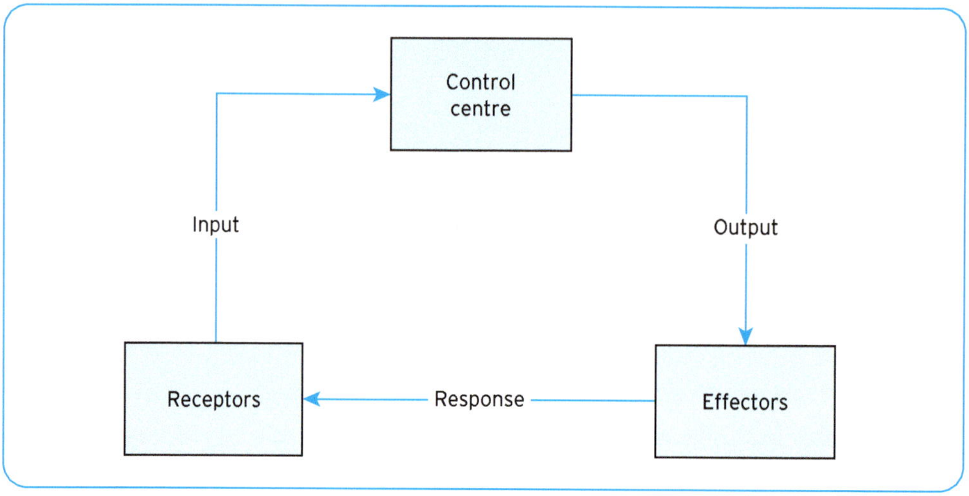

Figure 11.6
The principle of feedback.

It is in the CNS that we find many of the body's control centres; the job of conveying information to and from the CNS is done by the PNS. The CNS and PNS can each be subdivided further into two. The CNS consists of the brain and the spinal cord, while the PNS consists of the **sensory** and **motor** divisions. This is illustrated in Figure 11.7.

- ***To what do sensory and motor refer?***

The sensory division is the input to the CNS - it carries information about all that the body senses. The motor division is the output of the CNS. Much of this output is sent to muscles, which produce movement, but the description 'motor' also includes impulses sent to glands. The motor division can be subdivided further into the **somatomotor division** and the **autonomic division**.

In order to understand the role played by these two divisions, perform a simple exercise:

- ***Raise your arm.***

You can put it down again now. The point is that moving your arm was a conscious act. If you simply read on and decided not to perform the exercise, that too was a conscious act. You are illustrating the role of the somatomotor division. Here is another exercise:

- ***Dilate the blood vessels in your skin and turn red.***

In this case you have no choice: Flushing is an automatic response to being hot or embarrassed rather than a conscious act. Such automatic activities are under the control of the autonomic division. Finally, the autonomic division can be divided into two - the **sympathetic division** and **parasympathetic division**.

These are **antagonistic** - they have opposite effects.

- ***So which stimulates and which suppresses?***

It is not quite as clear-cut as that. For example, the sympathetic division raises the heart rate and the parasympathetic division slows it down. In contrast, concerning digestion, the

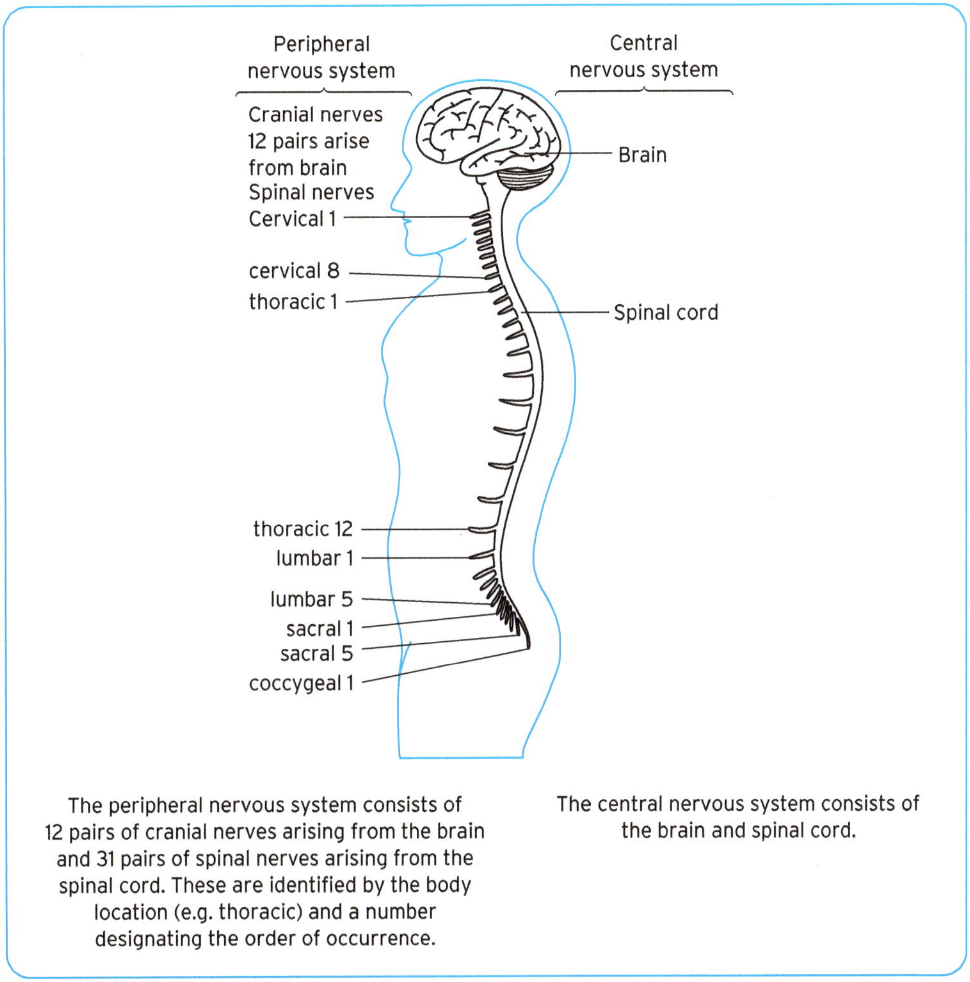

Figure 11.7
The central nervous system and the peripheral nervous system.

parasympathetic division stimulates the secretion of enzymes and the sympathetic division is suppressive. We might say that the sympathetic division stimulates active functions (such as the raising of the heart rate and other attempts of the body to get ready for vigorous exercise that we call the 'fight or flight response') and the parasympathetic division stimulates 'vegetative' functions (such as digestion). There are parts of the body, however, when this 'rule' does not apply. For example, both sympathetic and parasympathetic divisions stimulate salivary secretion (although each affects the composition of saliva differently), and the parasympathetic division mediates sexual arousal.

- ***In what structures do the nervous impulses travel?***

Nervous impulses travel in nerve cells (**neurons** - sometimes spelled neurones or referred to as nerve fibres). Like other cells of the body, neurons are microscopic, but they are organised into visible structures such as the brain, spinal cord and nerves. When we talk about nervous impulses, we are referring to an event called an **action potential**, explained below.

The action potential

Neurons (nerve cells) function as communication pathways because of their ability to transmit electrical impulses. This, in turn, depends on two features:

- A resting membrane potential – there is a potential difference (electrical gradient) across the cell membrane.
- Ion channels – pores that allow the movement of ions in or out of the cell. The channels may be open or closed, and they are, therefore, described as being gated. These are illustrated in Figure 11.8.

The neuron actively pumps sodium ions (Na^+) out of the cell in exchange for potassium ions (K^+). This means that the concentration of Na^+ is greatest immediately outside the cell, while the concentration of K^+ is greatest immediately inside the cell. We might describe this effect by saying that there is an ion concentration gradient across the cell membrane. The mechanism by which this is achieved is called the **sodium pump**. The ions are not exchanged one for one. Instead, two K^+ are exchanged for three Na^+. This results in an electrical potential difference across the cell membrane. This is important because it is a change in this potential difference that leads to the flow of current in the neuron. This potential difference can be measured.

What is the SI unit of electrical potential difference?

It is the volt (V), although this is too large a unit to use here. Instead, we use the millivolt (mV). (Remember that one volt equals 1000 millivolts.) The potential difference across the membrane of a nerve cell in which an impulse is not being conducted is referred to as the resting membrane potential, and its value is in the range of $^{-40}$ to $^{-90}$ mV. This means that the inside of the cell (**axoplasm**) is charged negatively compared with the outside. We describe the cell in this state as being polarised. This expression refers to having 'poles' or opposites – the inside is charged negatively compared with the outside.

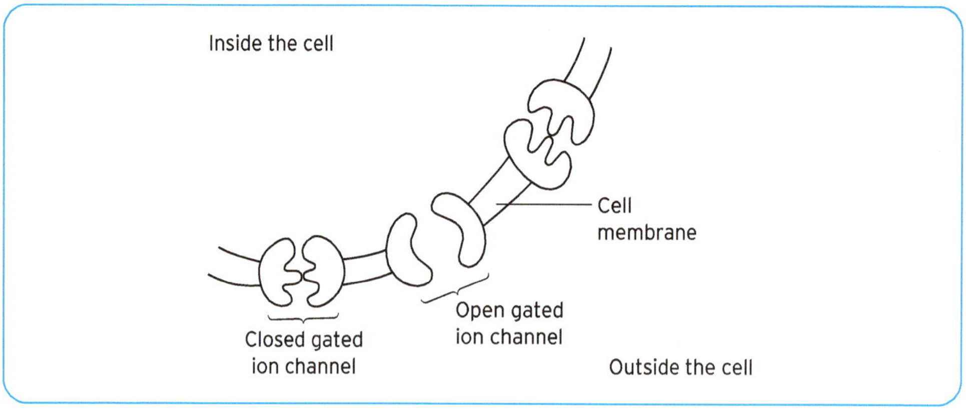

Figure 11.8
Ion channels.

● *So what happens for an impulse to be generated?*

The first point to note is that sodium channels open, and these allow Na^+ to diffuse through the cell membrane. This process is illustrated in Figure 11.9 - you might wish to refer to it as you work through this section.

● *In which direction does Na^+ move?*

You may have been able to work out that Na^+ diffuses into the cell. This is because the concentration of Na^+ is greater outside than inside the cell. Diffusion is the movement of a substance form a region of high concentration to a region of low concentration; it is explained more fully in Chapter 4.

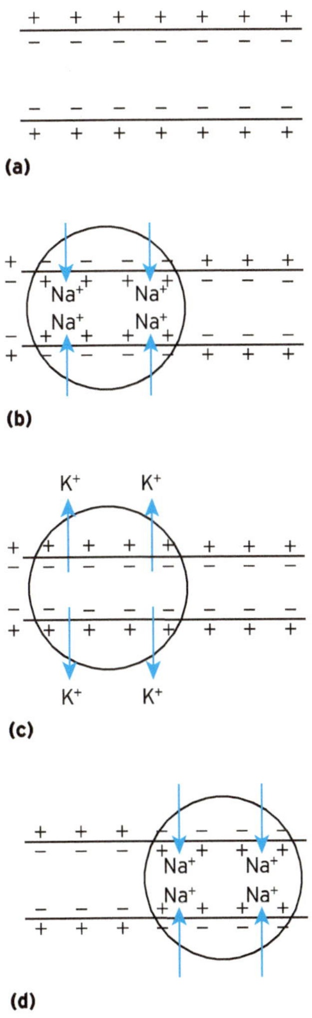

Resting state: the cell is polarised - that is, the inside is charged negatively compared with the outside.

Depolarisation: sodium channels open and Na^+ ions rush into the cell. At this point, the inside of the cell is charged positively compared with the outside.

Repolarisation: potassium channels open and K^+ ions diffuse out of the cell. At this point, the inside of the cell becomes charged negatively compared with the outside.

Depolarisation: an adjacent area of the neuron becomes depolarised.

Figure 11.9
The action potential.

- ***And what effect does this influx of Na^+ have on the membrane potential?***

Perhaps you have worked out that the axoplasm (contents of the nerve cell) becomes more positive. When this occurs, we say that the cell has depolarised. This expression means that it has lost its polarity, but it would be more accurate to say that its polarity has been reversed - the membrane potential may now be in the region of $^{+30}$ mV. Following the entry of Na^+, the sodium channels close and potassium channels open.

- ***In which direction does K^+ diffuse?***

It diffuses out of the cell, and the axoplasm (contents of the nerve cell) becomes negative again. Consequently, we say that the cell is repolarised - meaning that the call has 'regained' its polarity. Following repolarisation, the resting membrane potential is restored, but the cellular contents of Na^+ and K^+ are different. The cell still has a higher-than-normal Na^+ and a lower-than-normal K^+ content. The normal intracellular ion concentration is now restored by the action of the sodium pump. Note also that the changes described above bring about the same sequence of events in adjacent areas of the neuron, and this is repeated along its length. Consequently, an action potential consists of a wave of depolarisation and repolarisation, which passes down the length of the neuron. All nervous impulses are brought about in this manner, and so an understanding of this aspect of science is fundamental to an understanding of the nervous system as a whole. Without it, we cannot understand important conditions such as paralysis or how drugs such as **local anaesthetics** (drugs that remove sensation) work.

The conduction system of the heart

The heart is a hollow muscular pump with four chambers. The two upper chambers are called **atria** and the two lower chambers are called **ventricles**. The one-way flow of blood through the heart is ensured by the presence of valves. Actually, you might say that there are two blood circulations in the body - the right side of the heart pumps blood to the lungs (pulmonary circulation), while the left side of the heart pumps blood to the rest of the body (systemic circulation). Figure 11.10 is a schematic representation of the circulation, and Figure 11.11 shows the conduction system of the heart.

Clearly, if the heart is to be effective, then its contractions must be coordinated. To this end, the heart possess a conduction system through which the action potential, which brings about contraction, passes. The conduction system of the heart is comprised not of neurons, however, but of modified heart muscle cells. These cells are organised in one of two ways. They either form small masses called **nodes** or they form extended structures called **bundles** or **fibres**.

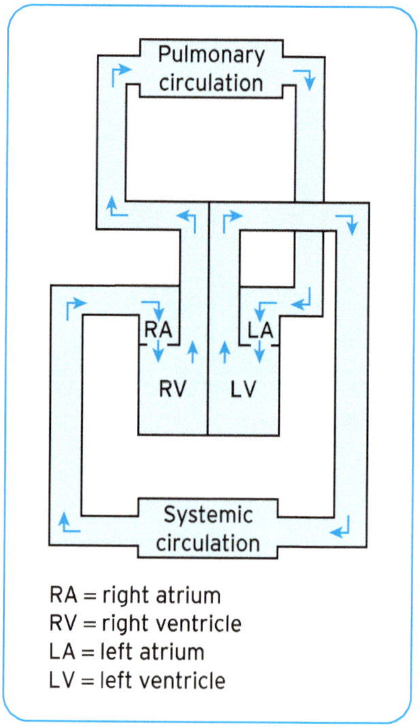

Figure 11.10
Schematic representation of the circulation.

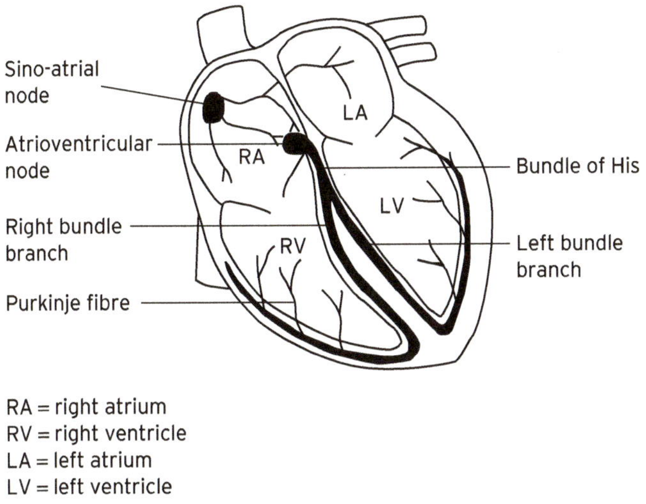

Figure 11.11
The conduction system of the heart.

The rate of contraction of the heart is determined by a small mass of tissue called the **sino-atrial node**, which is located in the wall of the right atrium. Consequently, this node is referred to as the **pacemaker**. The wave of depolarisation initiated by the sino-atrial node passes over the atria in a downward direction. As a consequence, the atria contract in a downward direction and so empty into the ventricles. Next, the wave of depolarisation is slowed down as it passes through a second node – the **atrioventricular node**.

- ***What purpose does the slowing of the impulse serve?***

This slowing of the impulse allows time for blood to flow into the ventricles. The wave of depolarisation now passes quickly to the apex ('tip') of the heart through bundles of fibres – first the **bundle of His** and then the two bundle branches. At the apex, each bundle branch gives rise to spreading fibres called **Purkinje fibres**.

- ***In which direction is the wave of depolarisation now passing?***

It passes upwards; as a consequence, the ventricles contract upwards and blood is pumped into the body's two main arteries – from the right ventricle into the **pulmonary artery** and from the left ventricle into the **aorta**.

At this point, it is probably worth pointing out that when medical images are taken (the simplest is the X-ray), the result is a visual representation of the structure of the body. Such images do not show how the body is 'working'.

- ***Can visual representations of the working of the body, such as the passage of an action potential through the heart, also be produced?***

In this case, a visual representation of the passage of electrical impulses through the heart can be created – it is called an **electrocardiograph** (electrocardiogram or ECG).

Important items of medical equipment

The ECG monitor

The electrocardiograph is sometimes described as a 'trace' (a line made by a recording instrument) of the rhythm of the heart. In order to explain how this is achieved, we introduce a rather old-fashioned term – 'cathode rays'. Cathode rays are streams of electrons produced by a heated filament that forms the negative **electrode** (**cathode**) of a device called the cathode ray tube. Since the cathode ray tube is the basis of the **oscilloscope** (hospital monitor), and of televisions too, it is important that we say something about how it works. The oscilloscope is illustrated in Figure 11.12.

The electrons produced at the cathode are accelerated towards the **anode** (positive electrode) because of the large potential difference between the two electrodes. After passing through a hole in the anode, the stream of electrons strikes a display screen that glows.

- ***So what would an observer see on the screen?***

An observer would see a glowing spot corresponding to the point at which the stream of electrons strikes the screen. Note, however, that before striking the screen, the beam has passed between two pairs of plates that are oriented at right-angles to each other and across which a potential difference can be applied. This means the beam can be deflected vertically or horizontally. In addition, the potential difference applied to the horizontally deflecting plates (x plates) increases steadily before suddenly changing polarity and steadily increasing once again.

- ***What effect does this have?***

To an observer, the fluorescent spot moves horizontally from the left of the screen to the right as the potential difference increases. The spot is then deflected to the left by the sudden change in polarity, but this happens too quickly to be seen. What the observer actually sees is what appears to be another spot moving from left to right. The process continues for as long as the power is switched on.

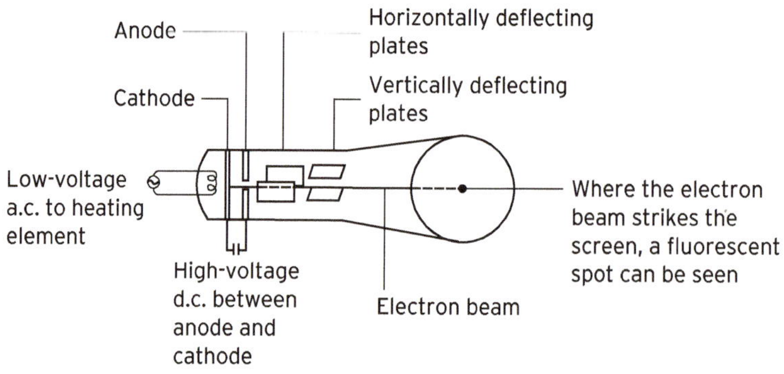

Figure 11.12
An oscilloscope.

What are the vertically deflecting plates (y plates) used for?

This question is best answered by considering the ECG monitor. In this case, electrodes are applied to the patient's chest and detect the small currents generated by the heart. These currents are then amplified and applied to the plates in order to produce a vertical deflection of the electron beam. The resultant wave pattern would be quite difficult to interpret were it not for the fact that the fluorescence of the screen persists for long enough for the eye to see the path taken by the spot.

What does a typical ECG trace look like?

We consider this in Practice point 11.4.

Practice point 11.4

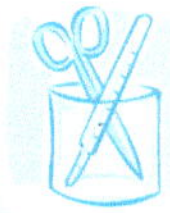

The normal ECG

Figure 11.13 shows what a normal ECG trace looks like.

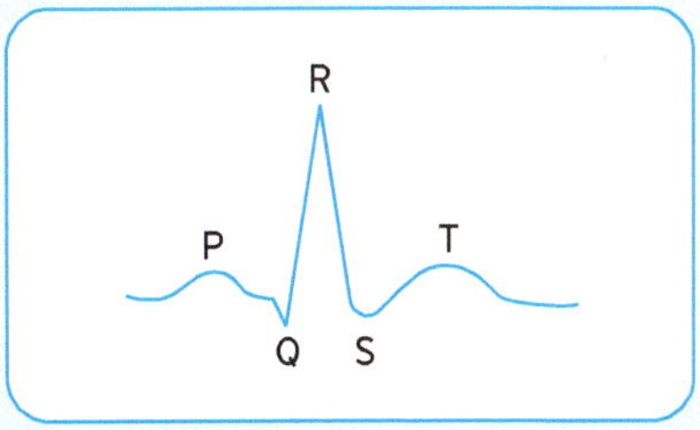

Figure 11.13
The normal ECG.

Note that several features are labelled. The first positive (upwards) deflection is labelled a P wave. This results from atrial depolarisation. Following this, there is a complex of waves called the QRS complex, which results from ventricular depolarisation. The T wave results from ventricular repolarisation. This normal pattern is referred to as **sinus rhythm**, because the wave of depolarisation originates in the sino-atrial node. Abnormalities of rhythm are referred to as **arrhythmias**, and you will learn about these during clinical studies. Although it is quite normal for the heart rate to speed up and slow down according to the needs of the body, arrythmias may produce an abnormal slowing (**bradycardia**) or an abnormal quickening (**tachycardia**) of the heart rate. When you are next involved in the care of a patient who is attached to an ECG monitor, have a look at the trace and see if you can identify the waves. Ask the staff to explain to you any arrhythmia.

Note too that the ECG machine is similar to the monitor, but instead of producing an image on a screen the trace is created by the deflection of a pen over the surface of a moving chart recorder. This paper trace can then be added to the patient's notes.

The defibrillator

Heart disease is the leading cause of death, particularly in developed countries. Sudden death due to heart disease is usually the result of an abnormal heart rhythm called **ventricular fibrillation**. This sometimes follows a **myocardial infarction** (heart attack), a condition in which part of the heart muscle dies when a clot occludes a **coronary artery** (artery supplying the heart muscle with blood). The termination of ventricular fibrillation by the administration of a strong electric shock is called **defibrillation** and the electrical device that generates the current is called a **defibrillator**.

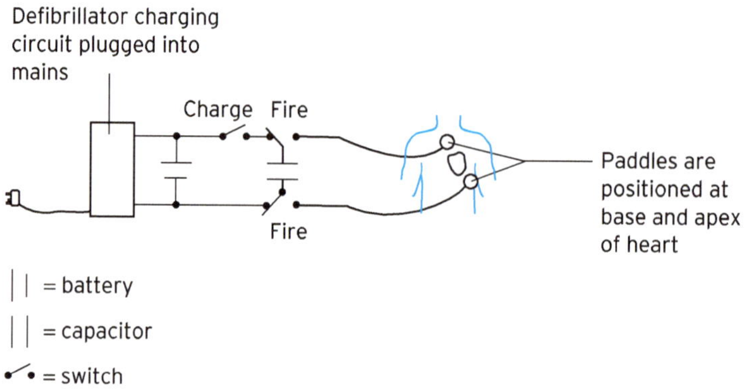

Figure 11.14
Simplified diagram of a defibrillator.

Have you seen a defibrillator?

You may not yet have seen a defibrillator in use, but if you have undertaken a practice placement in a hospital you should know where the nearest one is kept – you might be asked to get it urgently. Defibrillators may be operated from the mains electricity, but they also contain rechargeable batteries and can be operated when an external source of current is unavailable. This is only the case when the batteries are charged, and so when not in use, defibrillators should still be plugged in. The electrical component common to all defibrillators is the **capacitor** – a device responsible for storing charge. The capacitor may be charged either from the mains or from the internal batteries. This is done immediately before using the defibrillator when the charge button is pressed. The amount of energy to be used can be regulated and is administered to the patient via two electrodes placed on the chest (external defibrillation). Both electrodes have 'fire' buttons, both of which must be pressed if a charge is to be delivered. This feature reduces the likelihood of accidental discharge. A simplified circuit diagram for a defibrillator is given in Figure 11.14.

If the chest has been surgically opened, as is the case during a heart operation, sterile electrodes may be applied directly to the heart (internal defibrillation). It should be noted, however, that much less energy is required for internal defibrillation than for external defibrillation. Defibrillators are potentially dangerous pieces of equipment, and the proper procedure for their use must be followed. Some general advice about defibrillator safety is given in Practice point 11.5.

Diathermy

Diathermy involves the use of high-frequency alternating current for the purpose of cutting tissue (**electrosurgery**) and sealing blood vessels (**electrocautery**). The frequency of the current is indeed very high – 400 kHz to 3 MHz (up to 3 million Hz).

Practice point 11.5

Defibrillator safety

- Only staff members who have undergone training in the procedure to be followed should operate defibrillators. Having said this, automatic defibrillators are now appearing in public places, and these are designed to be used by untrained people. The device prompts the operator on the procedure to be followed.
- Defibrillators should be used only in accordance with the relevant hospital policy and the manufacturer's instructions.
- The capacitor should be charged to the correct energy level before defibrillation.
- Good contact with the skin is ensured by jelly pads, which serve as electrodes through which the current is delivered.
- Before defibrillation, the operator should give a warning in a clear voice and allow time for the resuscitation team time to stand back from the patient's bed.
- During defibrillation, the resuscitation team should not touch the patient, the bed or any conductive object in contact with the patient.
- During defibrillation, the patient's body must not be in contact with any conducting object through which the current may pass to earth.

Is diathermy not dangerous for the patient?

You might think so, and certain precautions do need to be taken, but remember that nerves and muscles are most sensitive to low frequencies, such as that of the domestic electricity supply (50 Hz); thus, they are unaffected by the high frequencies of diathermy. Note, too, that in monopolar diathermy, the current enters the body through the narrow diathermy probe - the active electrode, which is held by the surgeon - but leaves the body through a large electrode placed beneath the patient's buttocks or thigh (indifferent electrode). This arrangement is shown in Figure 11.15. The resistance to current flow offered by the tissues

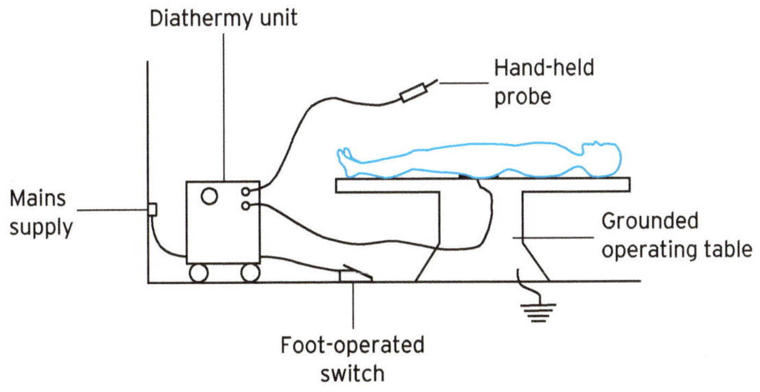

Figure 11.15
Monopolar diathermy.

of the body results in heating, but the current density is very much greater at the active electrode than at the larger indifferent electrode. Consequently, the temperature at the tip of the active electrode rises to several hundred degrees Celsius.

In electrocautery (sealing bleeding blood vessels), a bleeding vessel is gripped with artery forceps (a surgical instrument resembling scissors but used for grasping, not cutting), and these are touched with the active electrode. The heating effect dries out the cells of the vessel wall, and the cells shrink. This causes the vessel to contract and a clot forms within it. In this way, bleeding is arrested. In electrosurgery, a temperature of up to 1000 °C is created immediately beneath a narrow active electrode, and the cells disintegrate instantly. In bipolar diathermy, both electrodes are located within the probe held by the surgeon.

The artificial pacemaker

Heart disease may involve the conduction system as well as the heart muscle itself. The result is a disorder of conduction called a conduction defect. Conduction defects result in a slowed pulse rate (**bradycardia**). The pulse may be too slow to maintain cerebral (brain) perfusion and the patient loses consciousness (**Stokes-Adams attack**). **Sick sinus syndrome** and **atrioventricular block** are two examples of conduction defects. These may both be caused by an impaired blood supply to the heart caused by **atherosclerosis** (accumulation of fats and other substances in the walls of arteries). In sick sinus syndrome, there is a slowing of the rate of depolarisation of the sino-atrial node. Impulses are not blocked, however, as they travel through the conduction system, and therefore each ECG trace consists of a P wave, a QRS complex and a T wave. Consequently, we describe this as sinus bradycardia. In atrioventricular block, some of the impulses originating from the sino-atrial node are not transmitted by the atrioventricular node, and this is seen on the ECG as P waves that are not followed by QRS complexes.

Patients with a conduction defect can be helped by the fitting of an artificial pacemaker, which consists of a pulse generator that produces pulses of current to stimulate the heart to contract. As a temporary measure, the pulse generator may be external, but subsequently an implantable form is used. These are 'buried' in the fat somewhere around the chest - below the collarbone or the armpit. The current reaches the heart through a wire passed transvenously (through the venous circulation) to the right ventricle, as illustrated in Figure 11.16.

Transcutaneous electrical nerve stimulation (TENS)

Transcutaneous electrical nerve stimulation (**TENS**) is an electrical method of providing relief from pain. You might witness its use by women to alleviate the pain of early labour. As its name implies, TENS involves applying an electrical stimulus to the skin. Unpleasant effects such as muscle contraction can occur, but these are avoided by using high frequencies. The TENS apparatus is portable, which enables users to continue with their daily activities while wearing it.

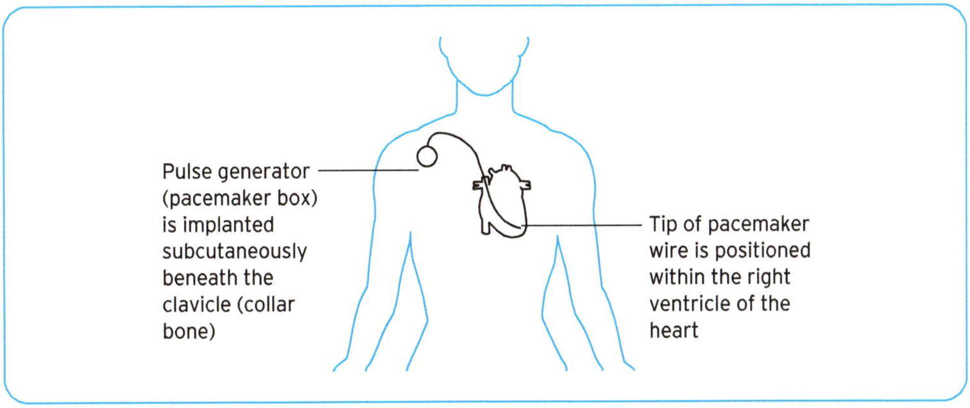

Figure 11.16
An implantable artificial pacemaker.

How does TENS work?

This is not an easy question to answer. It may be that the action potentials in sensory nerves stimulated by TENS act to block other sensory information that the brain would interpret as pain. It appears that part of the spinal cord acts like a gate, and the stimulation provided by TENS serves to 'close the gate' to other impulses. The gate-control theory of pain is commonly described in physiology and nursing textbooks, and you might like to find out more about it.

In-text review

- ✔ The nervous system is divided into the sensory and motor divisions.
- ✔ The motor division of the nervous system is divided into the somatomotor and autonomic divisions.
- ✔ The autonomic division of the nervous system is divided into the sympathetic and parasympathetic divisions.
- ✔ The action potential in nerve cells is one example of electrical current in the body.
- ✔ The movement of ions in and out of a cell creates an action potential.
- ✔ The conduction system of the heart is made up of modified heart muscle cells, not nerve cells.
- ✔ In the electrocardiograph (ECG), electrodes placed on the chest pick up the small currents created by the heart. These are then amplified and used to deflect the beam of a monitor or the pen of a moving chart recorder (ECG machine).
- ✔ Other important medical uses of electricity include the defibrillator, diathermy, the artificial pacemaker and transcutaneous electrical nerve stimulation (TENS).

Summary

We began this chapter by thinking about the number of electrical devices we have in our homes before going on to consider the science of magnetism and electricity. You will find this information in any introductory science textbook, but here we have applied it to the body, including the function of nerves and the regulation of the heartbeat. Finally, we returned to electrical equipment – this time to the devices, such as the ECG machine, found in the health-care setting.

Summary points

- → **Electricity involves the transfer of electrons.**
- → **A build-up of electrons that are not flowing is referred to as static electricity.**
- → **Dynamic (current) electricity involves the flow of electrons.**
- → **Direct current involves the flow of electrons in one direction, while in alternating current the direction of current flow changes in a cyclical manner.**
- → **The relationship between potential difference, current and resistance is given in Ohm's law.**
- → **Power is the amount of energy consumed in one second and is measured in watts (joules/second).**
- → **The action potential is one example of electricity in the body.**
- → **Important medical uses of electricity include the electrocardiogram (ECG), the defibrillator, diathermy, the artificial pacemaker and transcutaneous electrical nerve stimulation (TENS).**

Self-test questions

1 Which of the following statements is true?
   (a) Magnets in which magnetic force is dependent on the flow of an electric current are described as permanent.
   (b) The region in which magnetic force can be demonstrated is referred to as the magnetic field.
   (c) Like poles of bar magnets attract.
   (d) The magnetic lines of force that surround a wire through which a current is passing lie parallel to the wire.

2 Which of the following statements are true?
   (a) When objects become charged by rubbing, we find that opposite charges attract.
   (b) A build-up of electrons is referred to as static electricity.
   (c) Static electricity is also known as current electricity.
   (d) Objects through which electrons readily pass are known as insulators.

3 Which of the following statements are true?

(a) The current produced by a battery flows in one direction.

(b) Batteries may be constructed by placing two rods of the same metal in an electrolyte solution.

(c) The household electrical supply is an example of direct current.

(d) It is more economical to transmit alternating current over long distances.

4 Which of the following statements are true?

(a) Resistance increases with the length of a wire.

(b) Resistance increases with the diameter of a wire.

(c) The best conductors offer the greatest resistance.

(d) The resistance offered by dry skin is greater than that offered by wet skin.

5 Which of the following statements are true?

(a) The amount of current flowing is the most significant factor in determining the effects of electrocution.

(b) The heart is relatively insensitive to alternating current at 50 Hz.

(c) Direct currents cannot produce a fatal electric shock.

(d) The action of an earth leakage circuit breaker is to rapidly interrupt the flow of current.

6 According to Ohm's law, what would be the current flowing, in amps, when the potential difference is 5 volts and the resistance is 2 ohms?

(a) 10.

(b) 5.

(c) 2.5.

(d) 2.

7 Which of the following statements is true?

(a) The resting membrane potential of a neuron is approximately $^{-90}$ mV.

(b) The resting membrane potential arises because Na^+ is pumped into the cell.

(c) The sodium pump exchanges two K^+ for each Na^+.

(d) At rest, the inside of the cell membrane of a neuron is charged positively compared with the outside.

8 Which of the following statements are true?

(a) Depolarisation is brought about by an influx of Na^+.

(b) The membrane potential becomes more positive during depolarisation.

(c) Repolarisation is brought about by an influx of K^+.

(d) The membrane potential becomes more negative during repolarisation.

9 Concerning the ECG, which one of the following events results in a P wave?

(a) Ventricular depolarisation.

(b) Atrial depolarisation.

(c) Atrial repolarisation.

(d) Ventricular repolarisation.

10 Which one of the following statements correctly describes why diathermy does not result in ventricular fibrillation?

(a) The current used is too small.

(b) The resistance of the soft tissues is too high.

(c) The heart is insensitive to high frequencies.

(d) The potential difference used is too small.

Further study/exercises

1 We have mentioned the ECG and ventricular fibrillation, but what other common arrhythmia are there? Find out about the following:

- **Atrial fibrillation.**
- **Heart block (there are a number of different types).**
- **Ventricular tachycardia.**

Hampton J. R. (2003). *The ECG Made Easy*, 6th edn. Edinburgh: Churchill Livingstone.
Hampton J. R. (2003). *The ECG in Practice*, 4th edn. Edinburgh: Churchill Livingstone.

2 In addition to the ECG, a number of other electrical tests may be performed in hospital, including electroencephalography (EEG). Find out what the EEG involves from the Epilepsy Action website: www.epilepsy.org.uk/info/eeg.html

12

Light and vision

Learning outcomes

After reading the following chapter and undertaking personal study, you should be able to:

1 Describe transverse waves.

2 Describe light as an electromagnetic wave and identify it as part of the electromagnetic spectrum.

3 Explain what the term 'white light' means.

4 Describe the following properties of light: reflection, refraction, interference and polarisation.

5 Describe the effects of concave and convex lenses on parallel rays of light.

6 Using the explanations given in point 5, explain how lenses are used to correct the two vision defects hyperopia and myopia.

7 Describe the mechanism of vision and how we see.

8 Use the explanation given in point 7 to explain the different forms of blindness and, where appropriate, outline possible treatment options.

9 Briefly describe the mechanism of operation of the microscope and the fibre-optic endoscope.

10 Outline what is meant by the term 'laser' and give examples of the use of lasers in clinical practice.

11 Distinguish between the three bands of ultraviolet light and identify sources of each.

12 Using the explanation given in point 11, explain the effects of ultraviolet light on tanning, vitamin D synthesis and the development of skin cancer.

13 Using the explanation given in point 12, describe appropriate health-promotion advice regarding exposure to sunlight and the prevention of sunburn and skin cancer.

Introduction

When describing the life of his disabled daughter, Christopher Robin Milne pointed out that among the things we like to do, many are from the point of a spectator rather than as a participant. For example, many people who go to watch a football match would not have the stamina to play a game themselves and, under such circumstances, physical disability might have little effect on the person's ability to enjoy a match. In contrast, blindness may be contemplated fearfully, since it impairs the ability of a person to be a spectator. Of course, the blind football fan might very well listen to a game on radio, but what about someone who has been blind from birth? How does that person appreciate what is taking place? Even in our use of words to describe our understanding of something, we often use terms related to vision. We say 'I see' when we mean 'I understand' or ask someone to 'visualise' something when we mean 'imagine' it. Clearly, vision is very important - but what is vision?

Ask a photographer what photography is about and they will say something about composing interesting images or capturing a moment in time. Photographers often talk about the importance of light and describe getting up early in the morning or waiting for hours just to get the 'right light'. This serves to illustrate a point: We cannot consider seeing without 'looking at' light. In this chapter, we do just this before going on to consider light and the process of vision. We also consider optical instruments, such as the endoscope, and deal with some forms of light that we cannot actually see.

- ***So, then, what exactly is light, and how do we see?***

Theories about this have been put forward throughout history. One belief in the time of the ancient Greeks was that vision was the result of something being emitted from the eye itself - an idea that now sounds quite absurd. In the more recent past, Newton thought of light in terms of a stream of particles, while for some considerable time the behaviour of light as a wave has been accepted. Some of the properties of light, however, cannot be explained adequately by wave theory, and the notion of light as particles has re-emerged. Clearly, light is a complex phenomenon. For our purposes, much of what we observe of light, such as the way it changes direction when passing through the lens of our eye, can be explained on the basis of wave theory, and so this is where we begin.

Transverse waves

Imagine we have a tank of water in which a cork is floating. Dipping a hand in the water and moving it forwards and back, we then create a wave on the surface.

- ***What happens to the cork?***

The cork moves up and down when the wave passes, but note that the cork is not pushed forwards by the wave. The wave in our tank is an example of a **transverse** wave. Transverse waves are those in which a particle (the cork) move up and down at right-angles to the direction of the wave. The nature of a transverse wave is shown in Figure 12.1.

A number of measurements can be made of transverse waves, and some of these (wavelength, frequency, velocity) are described below.

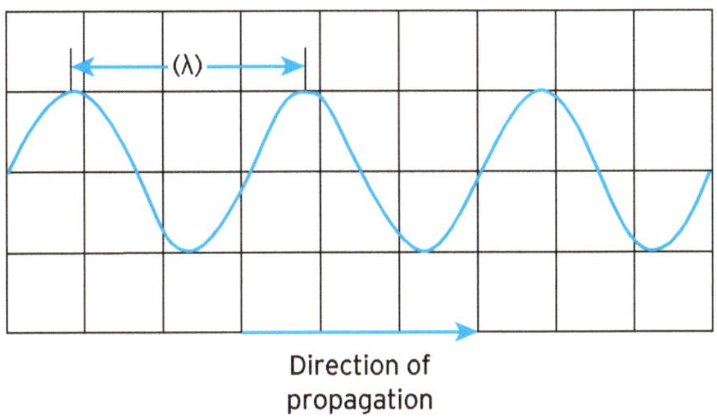

Figure 12.1
A transverse wave.

Wavelength (λ)

The wavelength of a transverse wave is the distance between two crests or two dips on successive waves.

Frequency

Frequency is the number of complete waves that pass a particular point in one second. You might hear frequency described in terms of cycles per second, but the proper name for this unit is the hertz (Hz).

Velocity

The velocity of a wave is how fast the wave is moving forwards. It is not a constant quantity but depends upon the medium through which the wave is passing. For example, light travels faster in air than it does in glass.

The electromagnetic spectrum

We have taken time to describe transverse waves because light may be thought of as the transfer of energy in the form of such waves. There is a problem here, however. In addition to being described as transverse, waves in a tank of water may also be described as **mechanical** - a reference to the fact that they require a material medium through which to pass.

- ***What about light? Does it require a material medium through which to pass?***

We know that it does not, since it crosses the vacuum of space.

- ***So, in the case of light, just what is it that is oscillating like our cork in the water tank?***

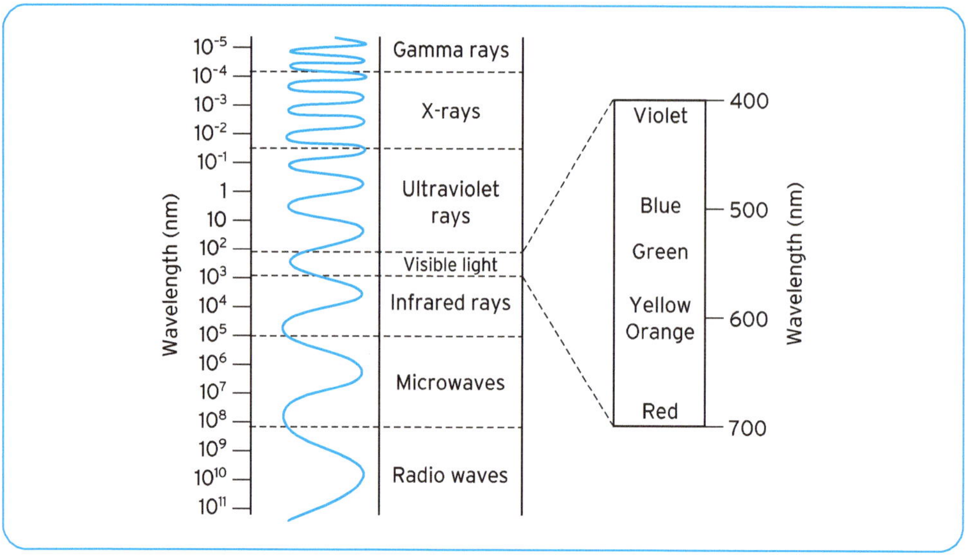

Figure 12.2
The electromagnetic spectrum.

The answer to this question is that light is an electromagnetic wave and that the properties that are undergoing movement are the direction of magnetic and electric fields. Electromagnetic waves are difficult to visualise because, unlike the water in our tank, these fields cannot be seen. Light is not an isolated electromagnetic phenomenon. Rather, it forms a small part of a spectrum of waves called the **electromagnetic spectrum**. This spectrum is illustrated in Figure 12.2. Have a look at this diagram for a moment. The electromagnetic spectrum includes **radio waves**, **microwaves**, **infrared rays**, **ultraviolet rays**, **X-rays** and **gamma rays**. Each form of electromagnetic radiation differs from the others by having a different wavelength and frequency. For example, radio waves have a longer wavelength and lower frequency than gamma rays. In this chapter, we concentrate on visible light, but we shall also mention ultraviolet light. Other forms of electromagnetic radiation, such as X-rays and gamma rays, are dealt with in Chapter 14. It is important, however, to realise that electromagnetic radiation forms a continuous spectrum of waves and that the wavelength at which the name given to a particular form of radiation changes is somewhat arbitrary. For example, there is no rigid boundary between ultraviolet rays and X-rays.

White light

In view of what we have noted above regarding the continuous nature of the electromagnetic spectrum, you may not be surprised to learn that visible light is not comprised of waves of a single wavelength. Instead, it is formed from a spectrum of visible wavelengths of between 400 and 700 nm (nanometres – of which there are 1000 million in a metre), each of which we perceive as a different colour. These colours become separated in a prism. We shall say more about this later; what is important to know now is that the result of adding these separate wavelengths together is the mixture of wavelengths that we call **white light**. This is discussed below.

The properties of light

● ***What happens to light when it hits an object?***

This depends upon the substance from which the object is made. For example, the object may transmit the light - that is, light passes through it. In this case, the substance is described as being transparent. Air, glass and pure water are examples of transparent substances. You might also add to this list clear solutions, such as sodium chloride/NaCl and glucose used in intravenous (i.v.) solutions (drips). Indeed, looking for this transparency is one of the important checks that nurses do on such solutions. If the solution is not clear or it has sediment, it should not be used and other samples from the same batch should be checked for contamination. Other substances transmit light, but in doing so scatter the light, so that objects viewed through the substance cannot be seen clearly. In this case, the substance is described as being translucent; frosted glass is an obvious example, but some intravenous solutions (e.g. **plasma**) are also translucent. Clearly it will help to know which solutions are meant to be transparent and which are translucent, so that contamination can be identified readily. Still other substances do not transmit light at all and are described as being opaque. Examples include wood and metal.

Reflection

● ***If light is not transmitted, what happens to the light?***

It might be absorbed, as is the case with dark objects, which when placed adjacent to each other can be difficult to distinguish. Alternatively, the light may bounce off some substances, and then we say that it has been **reflected**. Shiny opaque substances such as polished metals are good at reflecting light, but even transparent substances reflect some light. One example is glass, which is transparent and yet capable of producing glare due to reflection.

● ***Does a substance reflect all the wavelengths of light equally?***

Think about this for a moment and then answer a further question.

● ***Why does a red traffic light appear red?***

It appears red because it has a red filter - that is, only red light is able to pass through it.

● ***And what about other objects? Why does a red shirt, for example, appear red?***

An object appears red because it reflects only red light, while other frequencies are transmitted or absorbed. In pure blue light, there is no red to be reflected, and so the object appears black. If you have ever been to an event where coloured lights are used to produce a particular ambience, you will have observed this effect.

Refraction

We have already noted that light passes readily through transparent substances, but now we are going to deal with what happens when it passes from one transparent substance to another.

(i) Light ray enters glass at an angle to surface.
(ii) This is the path the light would take if it was not refracted on entering the glass.
(iii) Actual path of light through glass.
(iv) This is the path the light would take if it was not refracted on leaving the glass.
(v) Actual path of light on leaving the glass.

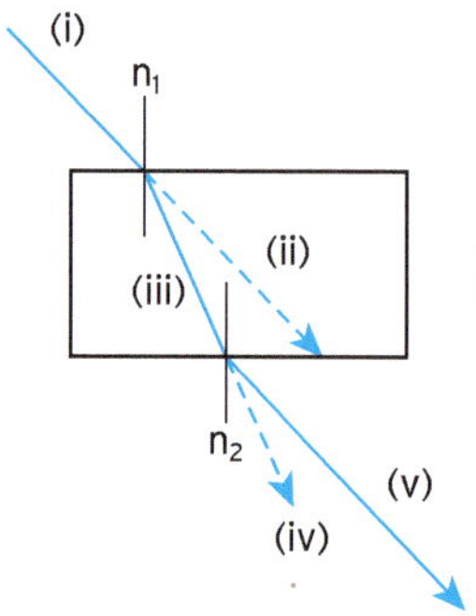

n_1 Normal at point of entry into glass.
n_2 Normal at point of leaving glass.

Figure 12.3
Refraction of light.

● ***Do you remember what we said about the velocity of light in glass and air?***

Perhaps you recall that light travels more slowly in glass than in air – in fact, the denser the substance, the slower light travels through it. Thus, light passing from air to glass slows down, and as it does so it bends. The light bends towards a line drawn at right-angles to the surface of the glass at the point at which the light strikes the glass. This line is called the **normal**. The bending of light in this way is called **refraction**. In contrast, when light leaves the glass and re-enters the air, it speeds up again and bends away from the normal. This process is illustrated in Figure 12.3.

● ***Do we experience the effects of refraction in everyday life?***

We do. One example is the distortion of the position of objects in water. Any child who has tried to catch fish using only a net knows that it is not as easy as it might first seem – this is not only because fish can be very quick. Have a look at Figure 12.4 for a moment.

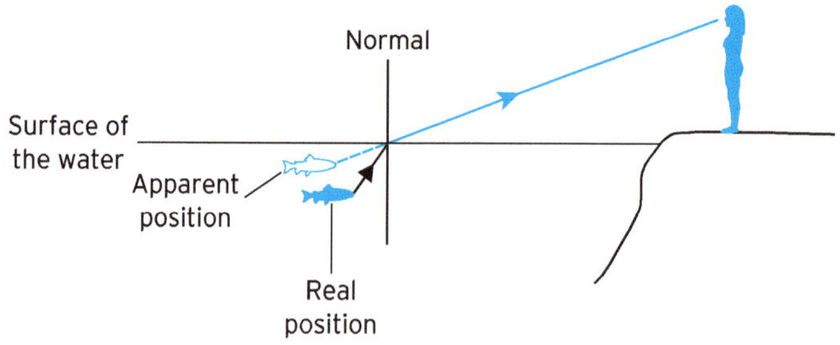

Figure 12.4
Refraction of light in water.

● *What happens to a ray of light reflected off the body of the fish as it leaves the water?*

You should remember that as light moves to a less dense medium, it accelerates and bends away from the normal. This creates a problem in the interpretation of the visual image for the brain of an observer, since the brain is used to light travelling in straight lines. Consequently, the apparent position of the fish is closer to the surface of the water than the actual position. People often say 'seeing is believing', but here is one example when our perception is not consistent with reality. There is clearly an important point here - especially if you are involved in caring for children: Bodies of water always appear shallower than they really are. Consequently, parents who warn their children 'it's deeper than you think' are, perhaps unwittingly, displaying knowledge of refraction.

Refraction also accounts for the splitting of white light into its separate wavelengths when it enters a prism, as shown in Figure 12.5. This separation of colours is due to the fact that the different wavelengths of visible light are refracted at different angles. This effect is clearly observed in natural prisms such as raindrops. When sunlight shines through water droplets, refraction causes the formation of a rainbow. Once you have understood refraction, you will find it much easier to comprehend the mechanism of vision, since the operation of the eye depends very much on its ability to refract light. In addition, refraction is the basis of the behaviour of lenses used to correct visual defects, as we shall see later in this chapter.

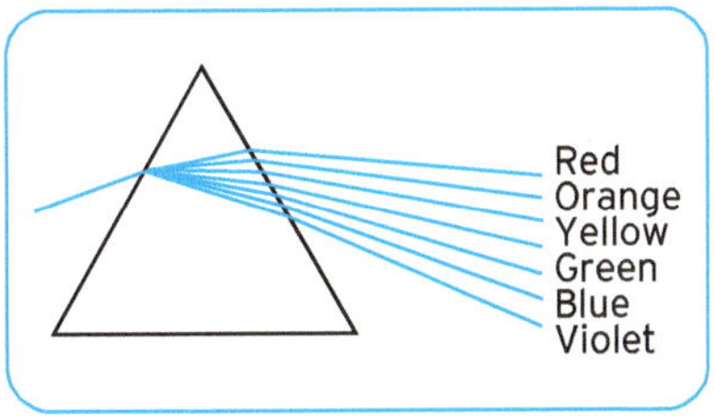

Figure 12.5
Refraction of light in a prism

Polarisation

Unpolarised light contains waves that oscillate (move up and down) in all possible planes at right-angles to the direction of propagation. This is illustrated in Figure 12.6. In contrast, polarised light consists of waves that oscillate in one plane only. This is also illustrated in Figure 12.6. The fact that light can be polarised is one piece of evidence that it exists as waves, since streams of particles could not be polarised.

● *How do we make use of this?*

Polarising filters may be used in sunglasses. In this case, the filter transmits only vertically polarised light. Since sunlight is unpolarised, polarising filters transmit only half of the direct sunlight incident upon them. But polarising lenses have an advantage over simple tinted lenses. We experience glare when sunlight is reflected from a flat surface such as a lake or a wet road surface, which has some degree of polarising effect in the horizontal plane. Polarising

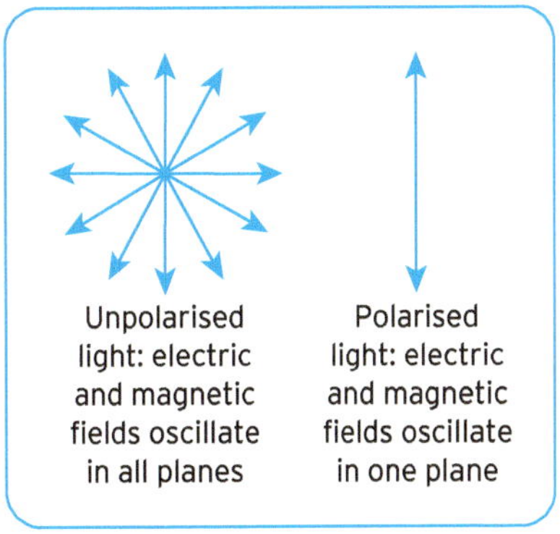

Figure 12.6
Unpolarised and polarised light

sunglasses do not simply cut down the transmission of light oscillating in all planes, as do ordinary tinted sunglasses; instead, polarising sunglasses eliminate light that is not oscillating in a vertical plane, and this has the greatest effect upon reflected light (glare). Many of us use tinted sunglasses or wear tinted spectacles on sunny days. We might even have specified a polarising (antiglare) coating. But high-quality sunglasses are especially important for people who suffer a degree of visual impairment, such as **cataract** (opacity of the lens of the eye). Later in this chapter we shall also explain how glasses with a ultraviolet (UV) filter can also give protection against cataract development.

In-text review

- ✔ Light is part of the electromagnetic spectrum.
- ✔ White light is formed from visible waves with a wavelength of between 400 and 700 nm (nanometres).
- ✔ When light strikes an object, the light may be absorbed, reflected or transmitted.
- ✔ The bending of light as it passes from one transparent substance to another is called refraction.
- ✔ The mechanism of operation of the eye depends on its ability to refract light.
- ✔ Lenses used to correct visual defects also work by refraction.
- ✔ Polarised light consists of waves that oscillate in one plane. Polarising spectacles reduce glare and the total light passing through them.

Lenses

Lenses are found in many forms of optical device, including microscopes, endoscopes (see later) and of course spectacles. Lenses are also found in the eyes of every creature that has vision, although they vary somewhat in structure. The purpose of all lenses, whether natural or synthetic, is to focus light at a particular point. But what exactly is a lens? A lens is a transparent object with a curved surface, such as is shown in Figure 12.7.

- ***What happens to light when it enters a lens?***

We consider this question in the following section.

Convex lenses

Figure 12.8 shows an example of a symmetrical double **convex** lens – that is, both sides of the lens are equally convex (thicker in the middle than at the edges). Such lenses are the simplest to consider. Note that in such diagrams, a line represents a beam of light. A segment of the lens is enlarged in order to show what happens when a beam of light (i) enters the lens. Note the position of the normal (line drawn at right-angles to the surface of the

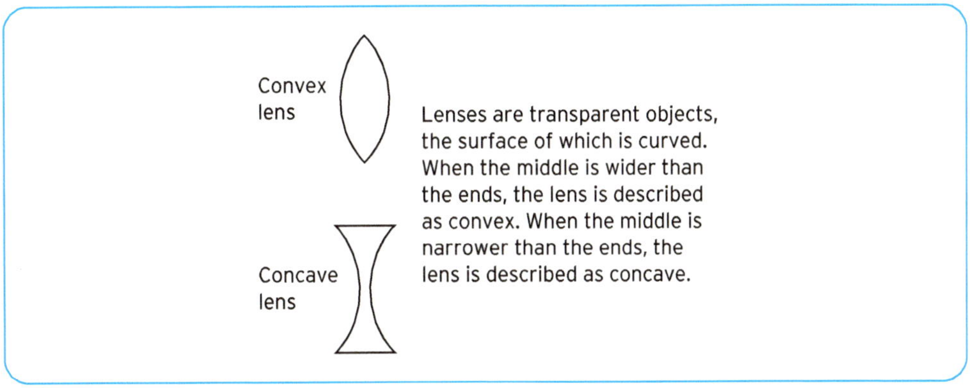

Figure 12.7
Lenses.

lens) to the surface of the lens that the light strikes (n_1) and the direction of the refracted ray as it passes through the lens (ii). Now note the position of the normal to the surface of the lens from which the light exits (n_2) and the direction of the ray as it re-enters the air (iii). Since the lens concerned is symmetrical, we can simplify the diagram and imagine the light ray being refracted only once from a vertical line, referred to as the principal axis, which is drawn through the centre of the lens. This is also shown in Figure 12.8.

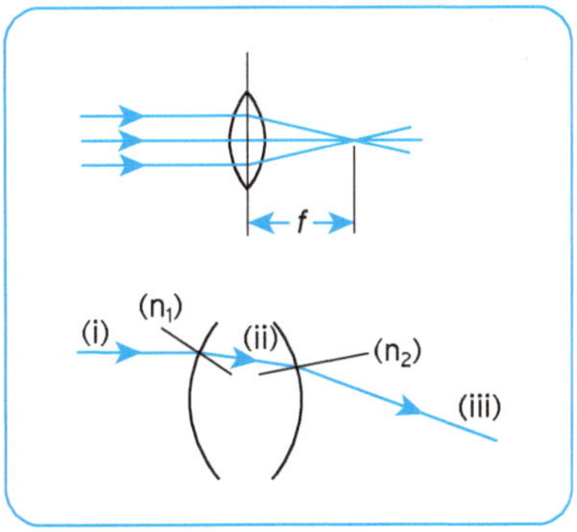

Figure 12.8
The effect of a convex lens on parallel rays of light.

- ***What is the effect of convex lenses on parallel rays of light?***

The light rays converge. Consequently, convex lenses may also be referred to as **converging lenses**. The shortest distance between the lens and the point at which light rays converge is called the **focal length**, and the point of convergence is the focal point or principal focus. Note that in the case of a convex lens, the focal point is behind the lens. If a piece of paper is held at this point, parallel rays of light from a distant object pass through the lens and are brought to a focus on the paper. This is a simple experiment that most children who have owned a magnifying glass have performed on a sunny day. When the magnifying glass is held facing the sun and the paper is held at the focal point, a yellow dot comes into focus on the paper. This is actually an image of the sun. Such an image is described as being real, since it can be projected on to a surface and viewed. In addition, the image in this case is also diminished (smaller than the object) and inverted (upside-down). This simple experiment is illustrated in Figure 12.9. Convex lenses are also used in the correction of certain vision defects. This is explained in Practice point 12.1.

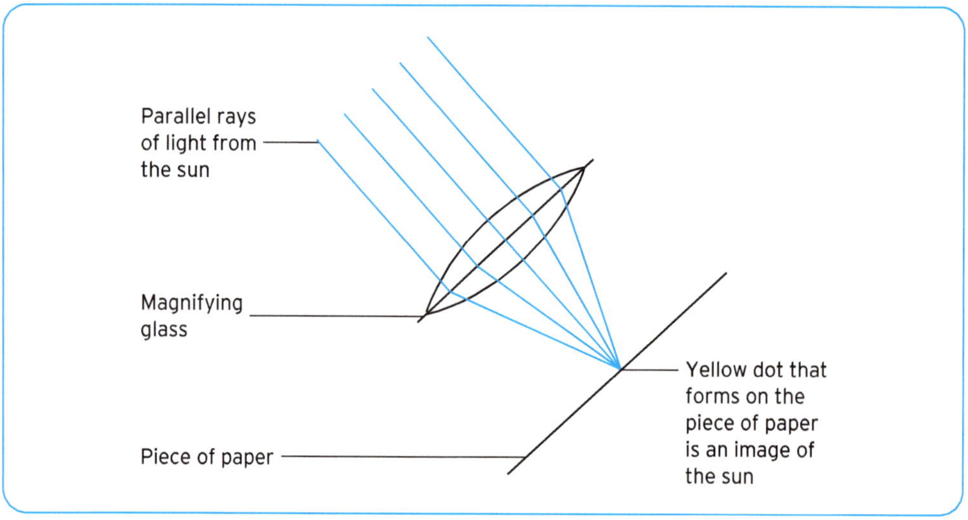

Figure 12.9
Using a convex lens to produce an image of the sun.

Practice point 12.1

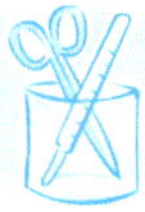

Convex lenses and the eye

Figure 12.10 is a cross-sectional diagram of the eye. The eye is a hollow spherical structure, the outer part of which is formed from three coats. The outermost is the tough sclera; interior to this is the vascular choroid. The innermost layer is the light-sensitive retina. At the front of the eye, the sclera becomes transparent, and this is known as the cornea. A thin transparent membrane called the conjunctiva covers the cornea, and this also forms the inner surface of the eyelids.

When we look at the eye from the front, we can see through the cornea to a pigmented doughnut-shaped muscle that is part of the choroid.

- ***What is this pigmented muscle called?***

This is the iris. It is the iris to which we refer when we describe the colour of someone's eyes. The hole at the centre of the iris is called the pupil. The pupil becomes constricted (decreased in size) with the contraction of muscle cells in the iris, which are arranged in a circular manner. In contrast, the contraction of muscle cells that radiate out from the pupil cause it to dilate (enlarge). By this means, the amount of light entering the eye under conditions of varying light intensity can be regulated.

Behind the iris, the choroid forms a ring of muscle called the ciliary muscle (ciliary body), and to this the lens is attached by inelastic suspensory ligaments. The space behind the cornea but in front of the lens (anterior chamber) is filled with a watery fluid called the aqueous humour, while the space behind the lens (posterior chamber) is filled with a more viscous substance called the vitreous humour.

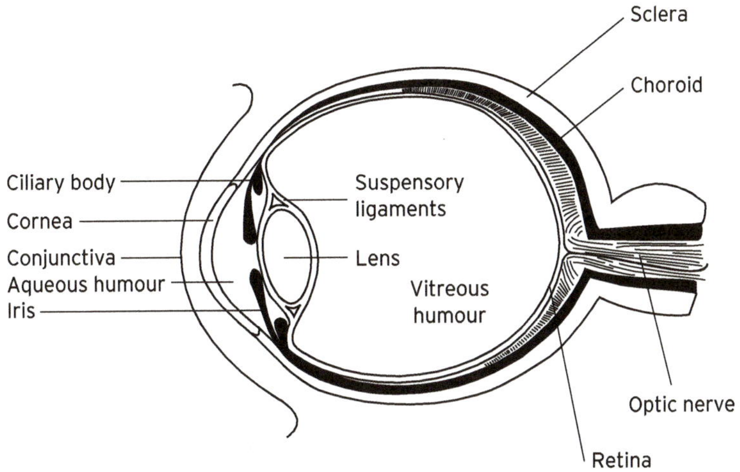

Figure 12.10
Cross-sectional diagram of the eye.

Figure 12.11 demonstrates how a real but inverted and diminished image of an object is formed on the retina. It is important to note here that although the eye contains a double convex structure called the lens, the cornea also acts like a lens. In fact, the cornea refracts light to a greater degree than does the lens itself.

● *Why have a lens at all?*

The answer to this question is that the lens performs the important role of accommodation. When parallel rays from a distant object enter the eye, they are focused on the retina by a relatively

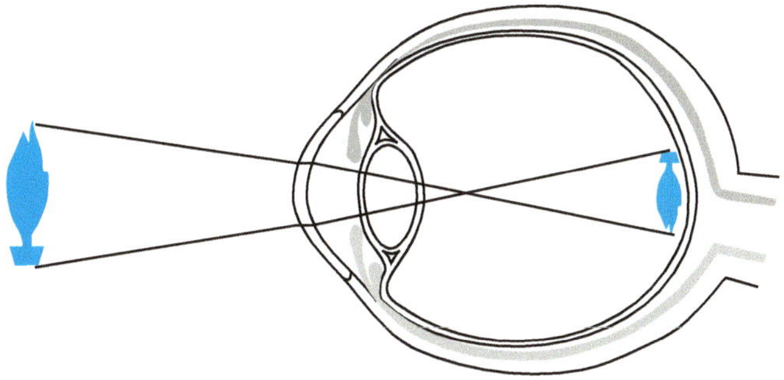

Figure 12.11
The formation of a real but inverted and diminished image on the retina.

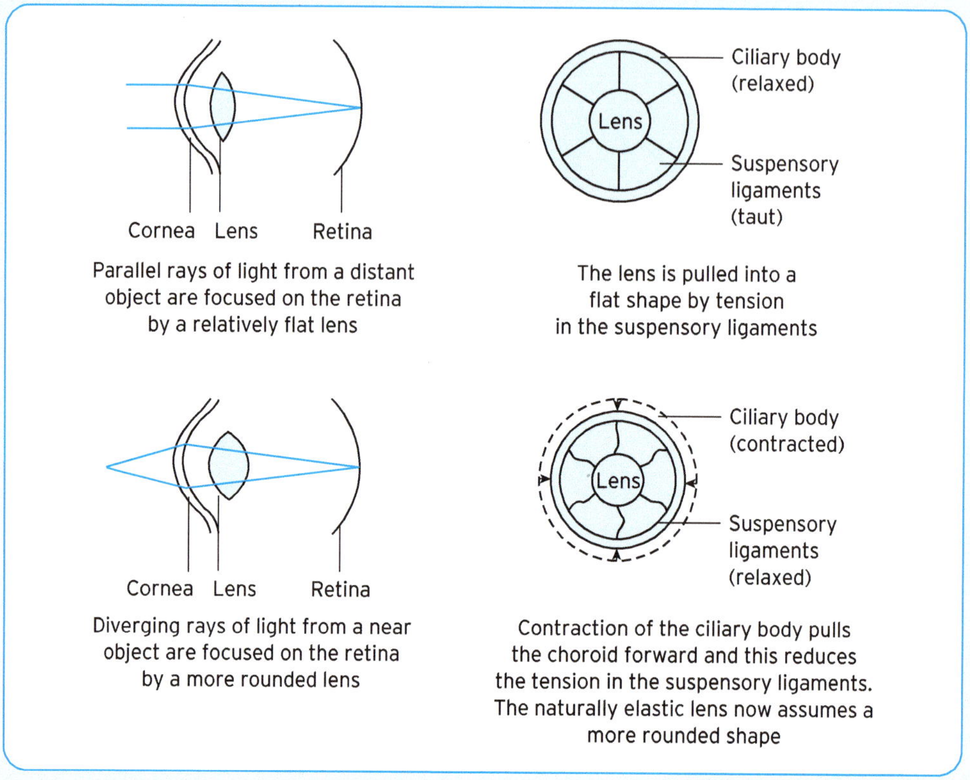

Figure 12.12
Accommodation.

flat lens. This is shown in Figure 12.12. The lens is made flat by the relaxation of ciliary muscles. In contrast, diverging rays from a near object require a stronger lens, and contraction of the ciliary muscles results in a more rounded lens. This is also shown in Figure 12.12. By this means, the eye is able to accommodate both near and distant objects.

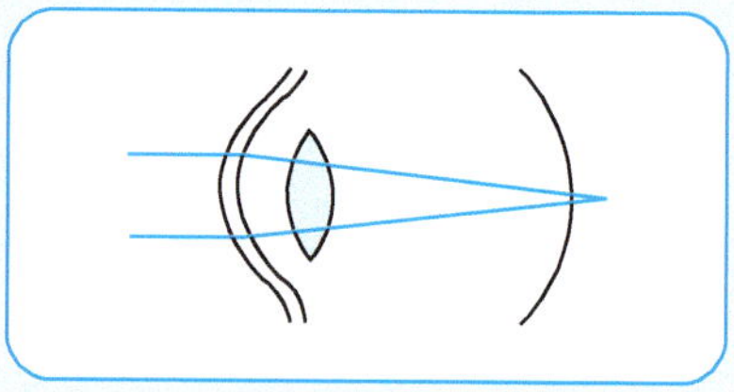

Figure 12.13
Hyperopia.

Convex lenses are also used in some spectacles. Consider Figure 12.13 for a moment.

- ***What is wrong with this eye?***

Light from the image is focused beyond the retina. This condition is called hyperopia (long-sightedness). What is required is an additional convex lens to correct the defect, and this is shown in Figure 12.14.

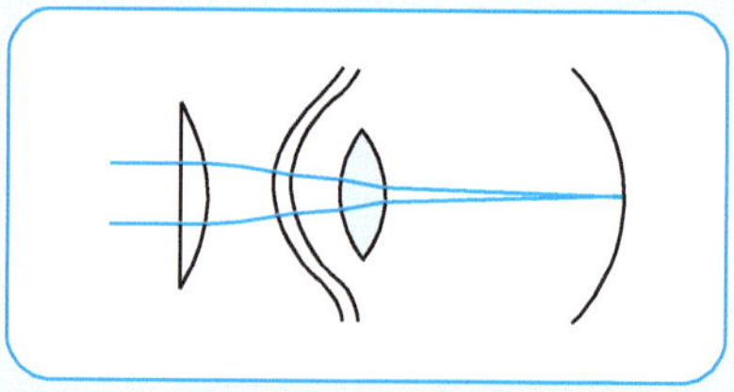

Figure 12.14
Correction of hyperopia.

Concave lenses

Figure 12.15 illustrates the effect of a double symmetrical concave lens on parallel rays of light. Note that, once again, refraction can be regarded as having taken place at the principal axis.

- ***What happens to the rays of light in this case?***

They diverge. Consequently, concave lenses are referred to as diverging.

- ***Where is the focal point in this case?***

To work out where the focal point is, we have to trace back the diverging rays to discover that it is in front of the lens. This is also shown in Figure 12.15.

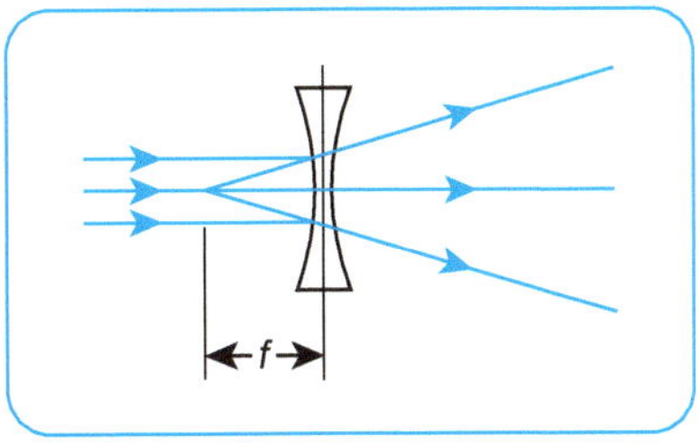

Figure 12.15
The effect of a concave lens on parallel rays of light.

- ***Can the image formed by a concave lens be seen?***

No. Since the focal point is actually in front of the lens, a screen placed there would block the entry of light into the lens. In this case, the image is described as being virtual. Concave lenses always produce virtual images. The use of concave lenses in correcting certain vision defects is described in Practice point 12.2.

Practice point 12.2

Concave lenses and vision

- ***Consider Figure 12.16 and decide what the problem is.***

In this case, light from the image is actually focused in front of the retina - a condition called myopia (short-sightedness).

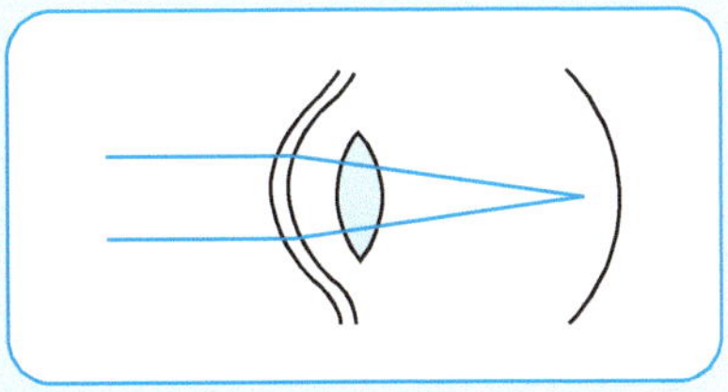

Figure 12.16
Myopia.

- ***What could be done about this?***

From what has been said already, you may realise that this problem can be corrected using a concave lens, as shown in Figure 12.17.

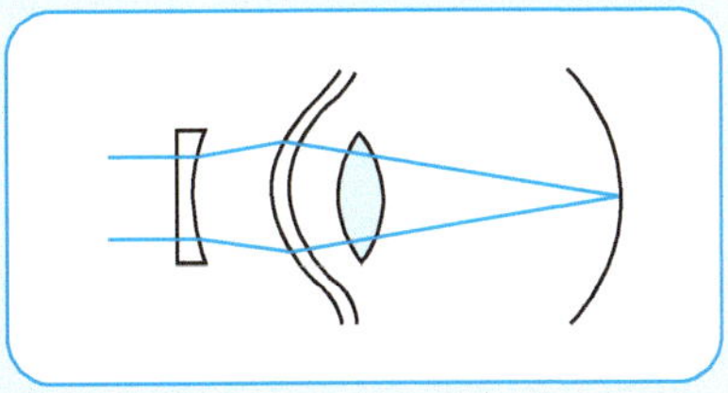

Figure 12.17
Correction of myopia.

In-text review

- ✔ A lens is a transparent object with a curved surface.
- ✔ When parallel rays of light pass through a convex lens, they converge.
- ✔ The cornea and lens of the eye are examples of convex lenses.
- ✔ Convex lenses produce real but inverted images - in the case of the eye, the image is produce on the retina.
- ✔ Convex lenses are used to correct hyperopia (long-sightedness), a condition in which an image is focused beyond the retina.
- ✔ When parallel rays of light pass through a concave lens, they diverge.
- ✔ Concave lenses produce virtual images.
- ✔ Concave lenses are used to correct myopia, a condition in which an image is focused in front of the retina.
- ✔ Accommodation refers to the changing of the shape of the lens of the eye from relatively flat to a more rounded (convex) shape. This enables both parallel and diverging light - from distant and near objects, respectively - to be focused on the retina.

How do we see?

Let us first of all think about our senses in general - touch, taste, hearing and smell as well as vision. These are all very different in nature, but the mechanisms of the senses involve two principal elements - detection and interpretation. The role of interpretation is undertaken by the nervous system (particularly the brain), the signals of which are electrical impulses in nerves. Organs of detection respond to physical phenomenon, such as light, by generating electrical signals, which the brain then interprets.

- ***In what part of the eye are light detectors located?***

Thus far, the structures of the eye that we have described have been concerned with focusing light on the retina at the back of the eye. Only the retina is sensitive to light. The retina contains millions of light-sensitive cells called rods and cones. These cells are so called because they resemble the shapes after which they are named. Collectively, they are described as photoreceptors - meaning light receptors or light detectors. They are illustrated in Figure 12.18. When light strikes photoreceptors, they generate electrical signals, which leave the eye via the optic nerve and eventually pass to the visual cortex in the occipital lobe of the brain (located at the back of the brain). It is here that the signals are interpreted as the visual images that we recognise.

- ***Why do we have two types of photoreceptor – rods and cones?***

Rods are responsible for black-and-white vision and are important in allowing us to see in low light levels. Cones allow us to discriminate colours under bright conditions.

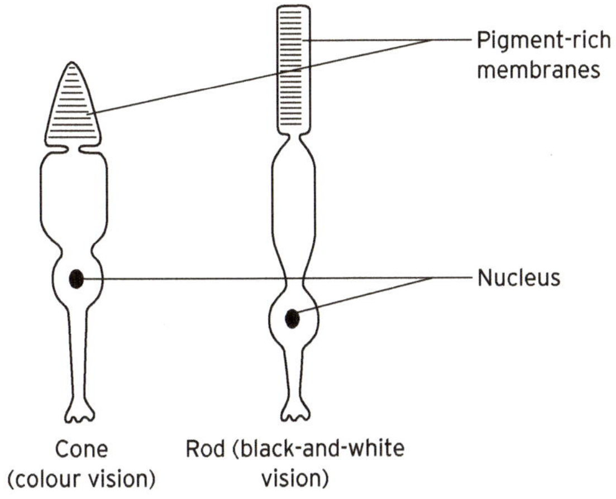

Figure 12.18
Photoreceptors of the retina.

How do rods and cones operate?

Remember that the job of the photoreceptors is to generate electrical currents. How this is achieved is best illustrated using rods, since these have been investigated most thoroughly. Rods make a purple pigment called rhodopsin from a yellow-coloured derivative of vitamin A called retinal and a protein called opsin. When light strikes rhodopsin, this pigment is broken down into retinal and opsin. Because this involves a colour change, it is often said that rhodopsin is bleached. It is this reaction that triggers the electrical currents that travel to the brain. Cones are believed to operate in a similar way, but the pigments they contain are less well understood than rhodopsin.

So is blindness caused by malfunction of photoreceptors? The answer to this question is that while there may be problems affecting photoreceptors, blindness can have many different causes, as Practice point 12.3 explains.

Practice point 12.3

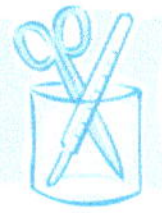

Blindness

Blindness refers to a partial or complete inability to see, but it is not a single condition. In fact, many disease processes can cause blindness. In order to understand them, consider what must happen for vision to occur. First, light must enter the eye and strike the retina. Next, visual pigments must be bleached and electrical signals generated. Finally, these signals must be conveyed to the brain, where they are interpreted.

So what might go wrong?

Take each of the above steps in turn. Light might not enter the eye. Damage to the eye can result in scarring, but one of the most common causes of the failure of light to reach the retina is opacity of the lens – a condition called cataract. The lens becomes progressively less transparent with age, but it is also affected by ultraviolet (UV) light (see later). Next, there might be a problem with the retina itself. The retina can become 'unstuck' from the layers beneath it, a condition called retina detachment. This develops when a retinal defect allows fluid to seep underneath, thus weakening its attachment. The illustration of wallpaper peeling off a damp wall is sometimes used to explain this condition. Another retinal problem is rod dysfunction, caused by a lack of vitamin A, which leads to the condition of night blindness. Finally, there may be an inability of the brain's visual cortex to interpret the electrical signals it is receiving. One case of this occurred in a lorry driver, who slipped off the back of his truck and struck his head. Unfortunately, he hit the back of his skull and damaged the occipital lobe beneath. It is in this lobe that the visual cortex is located; since all visual interpretation occurs here, the man lost his sight completely.

Can blindness be cured?

As you might expect, the answer to this question is 'it depends'. For example, cataract can be treated by surgical removal of the lens and night blindness can be treated with vitamin A supplements. There is no way, however, to restore damage to the brain or optic nerve.

In-text review

- ✔ Vision requires the operation of photoreceptors (light-sensitive cells) in the retina, nerve pathways to the brain and the visual cortex in the occipital lobe of the brain.
- ✔ Photoreceptors generate electrical signals when light strikes them. These signals are transmitted by the optic nerves to the visual cortex of the brain, where they are interpreted.
- ✔ There are two types of photoreceptor – rods and cones.
- ✔ Rods are responsible for black-and-white vision in low light levels and cones for colour vision under bright conditions.
- ✔ Rods make a pigment called rhodopsin, which is broken down when light strikes it. It is this reaction that triggers the generation of electrical signals.
- ✔ Blindness may result from conditions affecting the lens (e.g. cataract), the retina (e.g. retinal detachment) or the brain itself (e.g. brain injury).

Optical instruments

The slide projector

When introducing convex lenses, we explained how a real but diminished image of the sun could be formed. Now we show how a convex lens may be used to form an enlarged image of an object, in the manner shown in Figure 12.19. In order to illustrate how this is achieved,

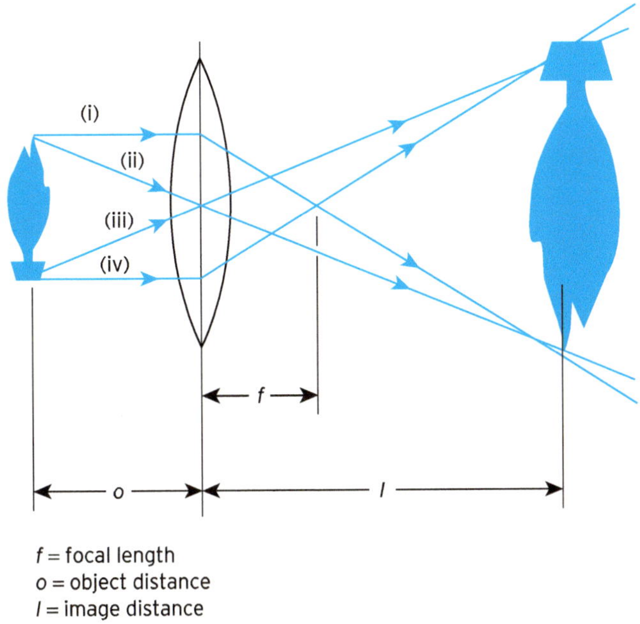

Figure 12.19
The operation of a slide projector.

four rays of light (i–iv) are shown. Rays i and iv are parallel and originate from the top and bottom of the object, respectively. In this case, the object is a slide of a tree. Note how these rays pass through the focal point. Unlike previous illustrations, their continuing path is also shown. Rays ii and iii both pass through the centre of the lens. The point of intersection of i and ii gives the top of the image, while the point of intersection of iii and iv gives the bottom of the image. Note that the image is both enlarged and inverted - perhaps you now understand why slides are inserted upside down into the projector. Convex lenses produce such real, enlarged, inverted images when the object is placed a distance from the lens that is close to its focal length.

The magnifying glass

Suppose we want to examine an object closely in order to take a detailed look at it.

- ***What would you do to achieve this?***

This is not a trick question. You would obviously hold the object close to the eye. But have a go at this - choose a small object and try to examine the detail of it.

- ***Any problems?***

Not initially. The closer the object is held to the eye, the bigger the image formed on the retina, and the easier it is to see the detail. If the object is brought very close, however, it

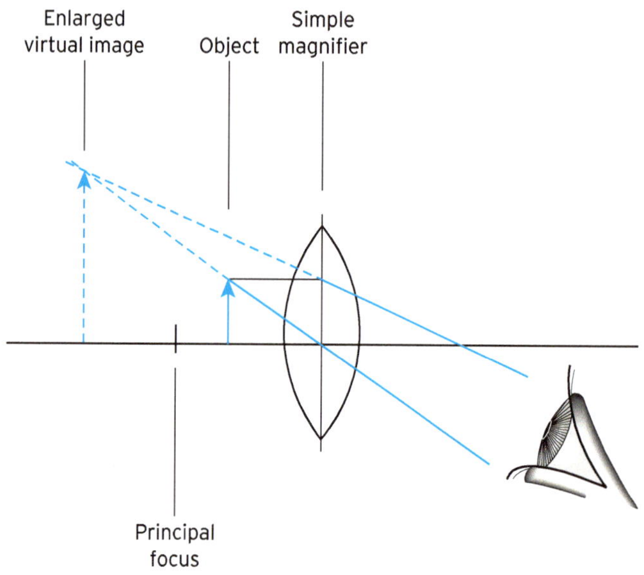

Figure 12.20
The use of a magnifying glass.

becomes out of focus and you can feel the eye strain. In a young person with healthy eyesight, an object may be brought as close as 10 cm and remain in focus.

- ***So how could we examine the object more closely?***

The answer is to use a magnifying glass. This is the simplest of all optical instruments and consists of a single convex lens. It is held close to the eye and the object positioned within its focal length such that a virtual image is formed in the manner shown in Figure 12.20. Note that this is the first time that we have encountered a virtual image produced by a convex lens, and so it is worth emphasising the arrangement once again. Note that the object is positioned within the focal length on one side of the lens, while the observer looks through the other side. It is also worth stressing that virtual images can be seen but they are referred to as 'virtual' because they cannot be projected on to a screen. One clinical use of the magnifying glass is in the examination of skin lesions, such as might be undertaken in the dermatology (skin) clinic.

The microscope

The microscope is a more complex optical instrument than the magnifying glass, since it contains two convex lenses. Its magnifying power is such that it can be used to examine objects that are not visible with the naked eye – cells, for example. Once these cells are prepared and presented on a glass slide, they form the object. The lens nearest the object is called the objective, and this always has a short focal length. It is positioned so that the object distance is just a little longer than the focal length of the objective. In this way, a

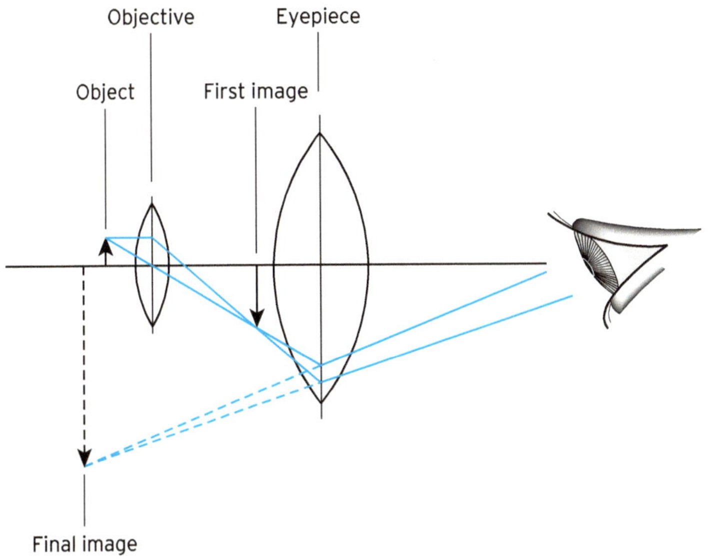

Figure 12.21
The operation of a microscope.

real and magnified image is produced within the body of the microscope. This is shown in Figure 12.21. The lens through which the observer looks is called the eyepiece lens, and this operates like a simple magnifying glass, using the real image generated by the objective to produce a very much magnified virtual image.

How do we work out the magnification produced by the microscope?

Usually, a microscope has three objectives mounted on a block, which rotates so that they are readily interchangeable. A single eyepiece is used, although this may be removed from the barrel of the microscope and changed if desired. To calculate the magnification produced, simply multiply the magnification produced by the eyepiece by that produced by the particular objective in use. A typical eyepiece magnification might be 10×; if used with a 20× objective, the resultant magnification is 200×.

Microscopes are useful in the examination of cells or samples of tissue taken from the body. These samples may be obtained through a needle, at the time of surgery or using a further optical device called an endoscope, as explained in Practice point 12.4.

Lasers

The word 'laser' is an acronym for light amplification by the stimulated emission of radiation. The creation of laser light is not described in this book, but it is helpful to know something about its nature. First, recall that white light consists of waves of different wavelengths - for this reason, it is sometimes referred to as 'incoherent'. Now imagine that light

Practice point 12.4

Endoscopy

An endoscope is simply a tubular device that is inserted into a body orifice or surgical wound for the purpose of examining the appearance of an internal structure - an ulcer of the stomach perhaps. Samples of exfoliated (shed) cells may be taken with a brush inserted through the endoscope, or the device may be used to obtain a tissue sample (biopsy). The simplest endoscopes are rigid metal tubes, but their diameter and inflexibility limits their use. Flexible fibre-optic endoscopes have more widespread application. These consist of parallel bundles of flexible glass fibres. Light is passed down the outer fibres so that an object within the body is illuminated. Light reflected from the structure being observed then passes up each fibre by being reflected many times within it. Finally, light emerges at the end of the fibre outside the body. Provided the relative positions of the fibres remain fixed, the image presented to the observer consists of many pieces of visual information equal in number to the number of glass fibres. We might describe the image as a kind of mosaic - not of tiles but of light. The operation of an endoscope is illustrated in Figure 12.22.

Endoscopes are available for different purposes and are named after the structure they are designed to visualise. The procedure of examination is described in a similar way. For example, gastroscopes are used to examine the stomach - a procedure called gastroscopy. You might like to read about the nursing care required before, during and after endoscopy.

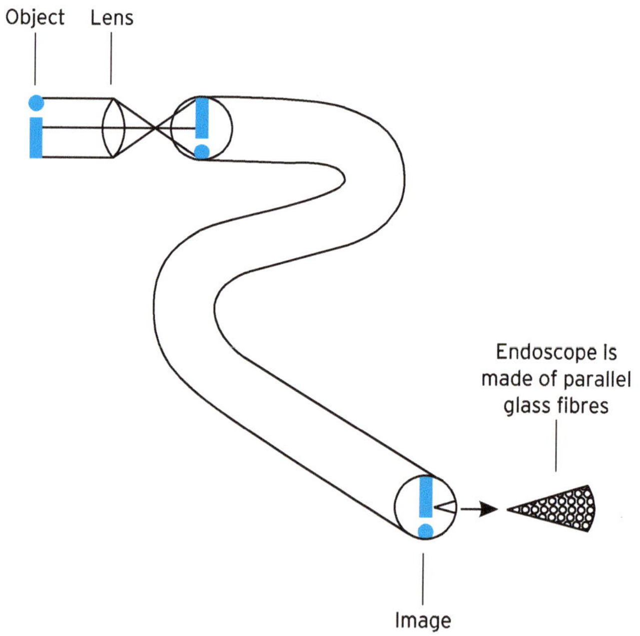

Figure 12.22
The operation of a fibre-optic endoscope.

of a single wavelength is produced. Such light may be described as monochromatic, but it remains incoherent since the waves are not in phase. In contrast, laser light consists of monochromatic light in which all the waves are in phase, and the expression 'coherent light' is used. The light produced may form part of the visible spectrum or may be infrared or ultraviolet.

- ***What medical use can be made of laser light?***

The medical use of lasers is based upon a number of effects of laser light, including photoblation and photocoagulation. Photoblation is the destruction of tissue by a beam of laser light. The beam may be used for cutting tissue in a similar manner to a scalpel or for more widespread destruction, for example of tumours. Photocoagulation is the coagulation of blood that occurs as a consequence of the heat produced by the laser light. Consequently, laser surgery is relatively bloodless.

Ultraviolet radiation

Ultraviolet (UV) radiation comprises electromagnetic waves within a range of wavelengths of 100-400 nm. It is generally the case in most of the electromagnetic spectrum that the shorter the wavelength, the greater the penetrating ability of the waves. In the case of ultraviolet light, however, the longer wavelengths penetrate deeper into the body. Three bands of ultraviolet radiation are described:

- Ultraviolet A (UVA): 315-400 nm.
- Ultraviolet B (UVB): 280-315 nm.
- Ultraviolet C (UVC): 100-280 nm.

Ultraviolet C

This band has the shortest wavelength and is least penetrating. It has a high frequency, however, and carries greater energy than do UVA or UVB.

- ***Are considerations of penetrating power and energy important?***

Yes. Since UVC penetrates no deeper than the skin and yet carries greatest energy, it has the greatest capacity to cause burns. Fortunately, UVC in sunlight is filtered out by the atmosphere's ozone layer.

- ***How do environmental pollutants affect the ozone layer?***

You have probably heard about ozone depletion, and this clearly has important implications in terms of the amount of ultraviolet radiation that is incident upon our bodies.

Despite the potentially damaging effects of UVC, we make good use of this band of UV light when germicidal lamps produce it artificially. As their name implies, germicidal lamps are used to kill microorganisms (bacteria and fungi) and are employed as a means of sterilisation - for example, of the inside of inoculation cabinets used in the microbiology laboratory.

Ultraviolet A

UVA is the band of UV light with the longest wavelength and greatest penetrating power. It is able to penetrate the epidermis to reach the dermis. It has a low frequency, however, and therefore carries the least energy. UVA is a poor initiator of tumour development, but it does damage the enzyme systems responsible for repairing genetic material (deoxyribonucleic acid, DNA) and so increases the carcinogenic effects of UVB. Because of the deeper penetration of UVA, it damages the extracellular matrix of the dermis, causing the skin to become inelastic and wrinkled - an effect sometimes described as premature ageing.

UVA is present in sunlight, even in winter; sunbeds, therapeutic lamps and fluorescent tubes also produce UVA. UVA does not trigger tanning as strongly as does UVB, and this fact should be borne in mind by people who use sunbeds excessively, especially in view of the potential harm caused by UVA. UVA is used therapeutically in the treatment of some skin conditions. Psoralen UVA (PUVA) is a form of photochemotherapy in which the patient takes an oral dose of the light-sensitising drug psoralen before exposure to UVA. PUVA is used in the treatment of psoriasis.

Ultraviolet B

UVB is sometimes described as the most active component of sunlight.

- ***What does this term actually refer to?***

It is a reference to the fact that UVB in sunlight has the greatest impact on our bodies.

- ***Why is this?***

Remember that UVC carries the most energy and so potentially is the most damaging band. UVC, however, is filtered out by the ozone layer. On the other hand, UVA is highly penetrating but carries less energy. In between these bands is UVB, which is of sufficient energy and penetrating power to cause harm. Figure 12.23 shows the penetration of UVA and UVB and Practice point 12.5 explains the effects of UV light on the body.

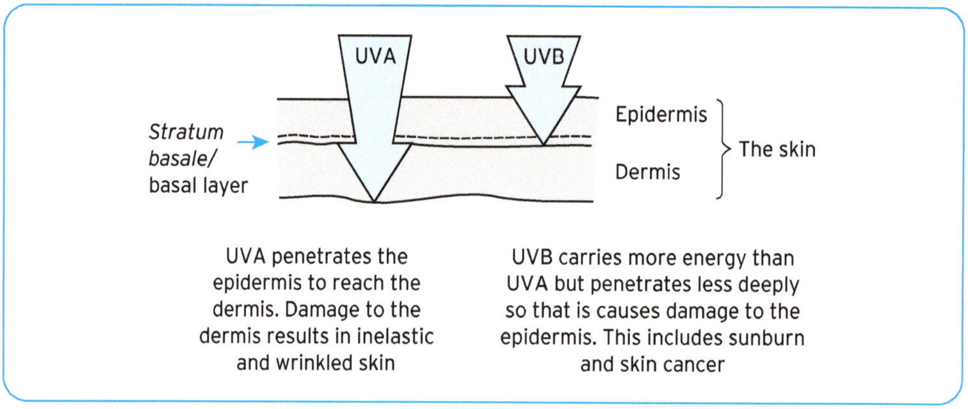

Figure 12.23
The penetration of UVA and UVB.

Practice point 12.5

The effects of UV light on the body

Ultraviolet light has a number of effects on the body. Several of these are detrimental, but there are some positive effects too.

Vitamin D synthesis

UVB is responsible for the conversion in the dermis of the skin of the substance 7-dehydrocholecalciferol to cholecalciferol - one form of vitamin D (D_3). Vitamin D synthesis by the body also involves stages in the liver and kidney. The important point to note here is that we are not entirely dependent upon a dietary intake of vitamin D and that vitamin D synthesis is one positive benefit of UVB. You can find out more about vitamin D and the effects of deficiency in Chapter 7.

Tanning and sunburn

The colour of the skin of an individual depends upon a number of factors, including the presence of pigments. The most important of these is melanin. Melanin is produced in the basal layer of the epidermis by cells called melanocytes.

- ***Does the number of melanocytes differ in people of different races?***

You might think so, but in fact this is not the case. The number of melanocytes does not vary with race, age or sex. The amount of melanin produced, however, does vary with race and also with exposure to sunlight. In addition, the distribution of melanocytes is not uniform. There are relatively few melanocytes on the trunk, but there are more in the penis, scrotum and areola of the nipple.

Melanocytes have processes that project upwards between the superficial keratinocytes (skin cells). Melanin is contained in membrane-bound structures called melanosomes. Under the stimulation of UV light, melanosomes pass along these processes and are taken up by the keratinocytes.

The rate of production of melanin increases with increasing exposure to UV light, and it is the accumulation of melanin in the skin that is responsible for tanning. Melanin serves to protect cells from damage caused by UV light. DNA contained in the nucleus is particularly susceptible. Perhaps it is not surprising that melanosomes are not distributed randomly within the keratinocytes but instead are concentrated above the nucleus, thus affording the greatest protection. Despite the protective effects of melanin, the development of a tan takes a considerable number of days, and people who do not regulate their exposure to the sun experience the inflammation and erythema (redness) that characterises sunburn.

Skin cancer

The incidence of skin cancer in Britain has risen rapidly in the past two decades, making it the second most common form of cancer.

- ***Who gets skin cancer? Is it difficult to treat?***

Skin cancer is an unusual condition, since it is more common in affluent than poor people and reflects the extent of exposure to sunlight. Skin cancer is not a single disease - there are three forms. The most dangerous form is malignant melanoma, which accounts for 10% of cases. Malignant melanomas spread rapidly, and this is one of the reasons why they are so dangerous. Malignant melanomas are more common in younger people and can be linked to periods of sunburn and overexposure. This means that health-promotion advice about exposure of young people to sunlight is currently very important.

Basal cell carcinoma and squamous cell carcinoma are more common and account for 90% of cases of skin cancer. These are rarely fatal if treated early. It is thought that they result from cumulative exposure to the sun rather than to acute episodes of overexposure. Consequently, they tend to appear on the more exposed parts of the body in later life, especially in individuals who have worked outdoors a lot.

- ***Who provides health-promotion advice about the effects of the sun?***

Advice may be sought from general practitioners, practice nurses and pharmacists, but any nurse may have the opportunity to pass on information about avoiding the damaging effects of the sun. In addition, most sunscreen containers provide some information, perhaps in the form of a leaflet. Some sources differ in the information given; for example, some classify skin types into four groups, while others use six groups. There is general agreement about some of the advice, however, and this appears in Practice point 12.6.

Practice point 12.6

Sun protection

- Select a waterproof sunscreen with an adequate sun protection factor (SPF). The SPF is a way of denoting the extent of protection afforded by different sunscreens. For example, an SPF of 15 multiplies the period of time it takes to burn by 15. Everyone should use a sunscreen with an SPF of at least 15; people with paler skin should use a sunscreen with a higher SPF rating. The sunscreen chosen should be hypoallergenic and perfume-free and should screen out both UVA and UVB.
- Apply the sunscreen 15–30 minutes before going out in the sun, and rub it in well. Repeat the application approximately every 2 hours throughout the day and additionally after swimming. Remember to use an SPF15 lip balm too.
- Avoid excessive exposure of the skin to the sun. Wear light-coloured, closely woven, loose-fitting clothing. Light colours reflect heat while dark colours absorb it, so light-coloured, loose-fitting clothing will help you to feel cooler. Lightweight clothing provides little protection against UV light, which will instead simply pass through lightweight clothing. Consequently, garments should be closely woven. Wearing a wide-brimmed hat protects the head and neck.
- Avoid the sun between 11:00 and 15:00, especially in countries near the Equator. At other times, limit your time spent in the sun. Weather forecasts may indicate how long it is likely to take to burn, but clearly this is only a guide and does not take into account individual factors.
- Wear sunglasses that conform to BS2724:1987, since prolonged exposure to ultraviolet may cause the lens to become opaque – a condition known as a cataract. Cataracts are the most common cause of blindness, although sight may be restored by removal of the lens.
- Avoid wearing cosmetics in the sun, since these may increase your skin's sensitivity to the sun.
- Babies under 6 months of age should be kept out of the sun altogether, while an SPF50 preparation should be applied to children. In addition, children should always wear T-shirts and hats in the sun.
- UV light can be reflected by water, snow and buildings, so it is important to apply sunscreen, even if you are sitting in the shade. UV light also penetrates cloud, so it is still possible to burn on an overcast day.

In-text review

- ✔ An endoscope is a tubular device inserted into the body for the purpose of visual inspection.
- ✔ Lasers produce monochromatic light, all the waves of which are in phase. Laser light can be used to destroy damaged tissue and tumours.
- ✔ Ultraviolet (UV) light comprises electromagnetic waves with wavelengths in the range 100–400 nm.
- ✔ UV light is responsible for one step in the skin in the manufacture of vitamin D.
- ✔ UV light triggers the production of melanin by melanocytes of the skin (tanning).
- ✔ UV light is implicated in causing skin cancer.

Summary

Light has been described as a visible part of the electromagnetic spectrum. The action of lenses upon light has been described, and this has been related to vision and the correction of simple sight defects. The mechanism of vision has been explained and the operation of important optical devices such as microscopes, endoscopes and lasers has been examined. Finally, the benefits and dangers of ultraviolet (UV) light have been discussed and related to protecting the skin from sunburn and cancer.

Summary points

- → **Transverse waves are those in which particles oscillate in a direction that is perpendicular to the direction of propagation of the wave.**
- → **Light is an example of an electromagnetic wave and forms part of the electromagnetic spectrum.**
- → **Visible light has a wavelength of between 400 and 700 nm.**
- → **Different wavelengths of light are seen as different colours.**
- → **Refraction is the bending of light as it travels through transparent materials of different densities.**
- → **Lenses are transparent objects with curved surfaces, which may be described as being either concave or convex.**
- → **Hyperopia is the condition in which an image is brought to a focus beyond the retina. It is corrected with a convex lens.**
- → **Myopia is the condition in which an image is brought to focus in front of the retina. It is corrected with a concave lens.**
- → **Ultraviolet (UV) light is made up of electromagnetic waves within the wavelength range 100–400 nm.**
- → **UVB is responsible for tanning and the synthesis of vitamin D, but it is also implicated in the development of skin cancer.**

Self-test questions

1 Which of the following statements are true?
(a) Frequency is measured in hertz (Hz).
(b) Wavelength is the maximum displacement of a particle from its rest position,
(c) Frequency is the number of complete waves that pass a particular point in one second.
(d) The wavelength is the number of complete waves that pass a particular point in one second.

2 Which of the following statements are true?
(a) Ultraviolet waves have a shorter wavelength than visible light.
(b) Electromagnetic waves are mechanical waves.
(c) Mechanical waves do not require a material medium through which to pass.
(d) Infrared waves have a shorter wavelength than ultraviolet.

3 Which of the following statements are true?
(a) When light enters a more dense medium it speeds up.
(b) When light enters a more dense medium, it bends towards the normal.
(c) When light enters a less dense, medium it speeds up.
(d) When light enters a less dense medium, it bends away from the normal.

4 Which of the following statements are true?
(a) Refraction accounts for the splitting of white light into its separate wavelengths when it enters a prism.
(b) Rainbows are caused by reflection.
(c) White light is formed from a spectrum of visible wavelengths of between 400 and 700 nm.
(d) Substances that transmit light, but in doing so scatter it, are described as translucent.

5 Which of the following statements are true?
(a) Concave lenses always produce real images.
(b) A magnifying glass is an example of a convex lens.
(c) A convex lens may be used to produce a real and magnified image.
(d) In a microscope, the objective produces a real, magnified image.

6 Which of the following statements are true?
(a) In hyperopia, the image is focused in front of the retina.
(b) In myopia, the image is focused in front of the retina.
(c) Hyperopia is corrected using a convex lens.
(d) Myopia is corrected using a concave lens.

7 Which of the following statements are true?
(a) Myopia is sometimes referred to as short-sightedness.
(b) Hyperopia is sometimes referred to as long-sightedness.
(c) Parallel rays of light from a distant object are focused on the retina by a relatively flat lens.
(d) Diverging rays of light from a near object are focused on the retina by a rounded lens.

8 Which of the following statements are true?
(a) UVC carries more energy than UVB.
(b) UVB is more penetrating than UVA.
(c) UVA is more penetrating than UVC.
(d) UVB carries more energy than UVA.

9 Which of the following statements are true?
(a) UVA is used as a means of sterilisation.
(b) UVB does not penetrate the ozone layer.
(c) UVB has been implicated in skin cancer.
(d) UVA is produced by sunbeds.

10 Which of the following statements are true?
(a) Everyone should use a sunscreen with an SPF of at least 15.
(b) Those with the palest of complexions should use a sunscreen with an SPF of 50.
(c) Melanosomes are cells that produce melanin.
(d) Increased exposure to sunlight results in increased melanin production.

Further study/exercises

1 Myopia and hyperopia have been described, but what are the following vision defects:

- **Astigmatism.**
- **Glaucoma.**
- **Presbyopia.**

2 What resources are available to help someone who is loosing their vision?

Royal National Institute for the Blind (RNIB) website: www.rnib.org.uk

13

Sound and hearing

Learning outcomes

After reading the following chapter and undertaking personal study, you should be able to:

1. Identify sound waves as mechanical waves.
2. Describe the characteristics of longitudinal waves.
3. Outline the decibel scale for measuring the perceived loudness of sound.
4. State the importance of wearing hearing protection in noisy environments.
5. Describe the mechanism of hearing.
6. Briefly describe the two main forms of deafness.
7. List some of the important aspects of communicating with someone who has a hearing impairment.
8. Outline the piezoelectric effect and briefly describe the medical use of ultrasound.
9. Describe the Doppler effect and outline the medical use of Doppler ultrasound.

Introduction

Have you ever wondered how important sound is to us? Hearing a person's voice is important for communication, and much of our enjoyment in life involves hearing. How would you feel about not being able to enjoy music, for example? In contrast, loss of hearing makes communication difficult and affects our enjoyment of life. Perhaps most significantly, hearing loss may isolate deaf people from others. Deaf people have to make a great effort to communicate and maintain relationships with others. As an example, someone once described that, as a little girl, her grandfather regularly took her to the cinema. This is not an unusual thing to do, but in this case the girl's grandfather had become deaf following an explosion in the trenches of the First World War. If we reflect on this for a moment, we soon realise what an effort the grandfather was making. Although he heard nothing of the movies, he took his granddaughter to see them in order to maintain a relationship with her. So, then, hearing is very important; but before we consider the mechanism of hearing and how it may be lost, we shall investigate sound.

Sound

Sound is a form of wave but, unlike light waves, sound waves are mechanical in nature - that is, they require a material medium through which to pass, and they cannot cross the vacuum of space. When we think of sound, we usually think of waves passing through air, but sound can be transmitted through different kinds of substance - even our bodies, as we shall see later.

Sound waves are **longitudinal waves** in which particles of the medium in which the wave is passing (e.g. air or water) move back and forth in the direction in which the wave is moving. Sound waves are produced by vibration - for example, vibration of the tuning fork illustrated in Figure 13.1. When the tuning fork is struck, the prongs vibrate - that is, they move in and

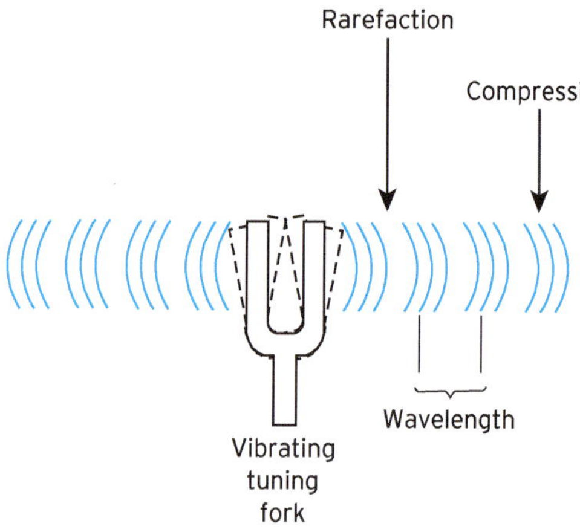

Figure 13.1
The vibration of a tuning fork.

out. When the prongs move outwards, the adjacent air is compressed; when the prongs move inwards again, the air pressure between the prong and the compression falls; this is referred to as a **rarefaction**. This process is repeated, and the series of compressions and rarefactions that results is referred to as a longitudinal wave. Longitudinal waves contrast with **transverse waves** (see Chapter 12), where the direction of oscillation is at right-angles to the direction in which the wave is moving. The production of sound by the vibration of the tuning fork is not dissimilar to the way in which the vocal cords vibrate in speech production (see Practice point 13.1).

Practice point 13.1

Speech

If you run your fingers down the anterior surface of your neck you should feel the rigid structure commonly referred to as the voice box or, more correctly, the **larynx** (Figure 13.2). The larynx is a hollow structure made of cartilage that is continuous with the **pharynx** (the common passage way for food and air) above and the **trachea** (windpipe) below. The larynx contains two strong elastic structures, called the **vocal cords**, which are separated by a space called the **glottis**. Sound is produced by the vibration of these cords, which in turn causes the air passing through the glottis to vibrate.

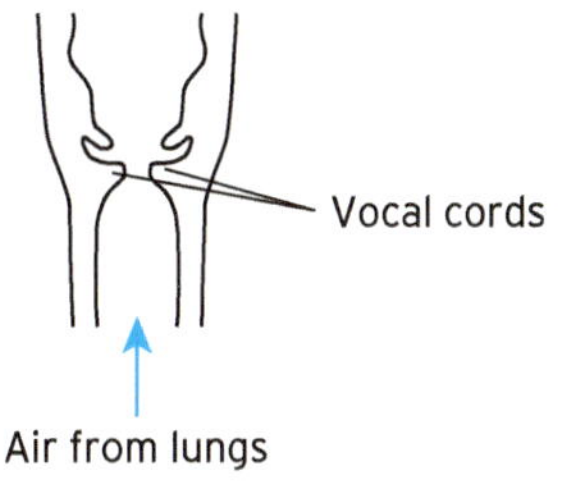

Figure 13.2
The larynx and vocal cords.

Sound is normally generated only during expiration (breathing out); inspiration occurs silently. Consequently, inspiratory sounds may be important indicators of some form of pathology. For example, **stridor** is a high-pitched inspiratory sound associated with spasm of the vocal cords (**laryngospasm**), which may occur during an allergic reaction or in the presence of inflammation of the larynx (**laryngitis**). In contrast, the presence of growths (tumours, e.g. cancer) on the vocal cords may impair their vibration and produce hoarseness.

A number of properties of longitudinal waves can be described, including wavelength, frequency, amplitude, intensity and loudness.

Wavelength

In longitudinal waves, the **wavelength** is the distance between two adjacent compressions or two adjacent rarefactions.

Frequency

The **frequency** of longitudinal waves is defined in the same way as for transverse waves - it is the number of complete waves that pass a particular point in one second. In everyday language, we often refer to pitch rather than frequency. We describe high-frequency sound waves as being high-pitched and low-frequency sound as low-pitched.

Is pitch the same as frequency?

Not quite. Frequency is a measurable quantity, while pitch refers to the individual's perception of the sound. Human ears can detect sound within the frequency range 20–20 000 Hz (oscillations per second), although this varies somewhat between individuals.

Although you may be familiar with the fact that ageing often results in some degree of reduction of sensitivity to sound, did you know that the range of frequencies that can be heard becomes narrower with age? There is in fact a selective loss of hearing, which affects the higher frequencies. In order to obtain some idea of what it is like to experience this, perform the following simple experiment. Turn on the radio and adjust the volume to a little below the comfortable listening level. This simulates a reduction of overall sensitivity. Now adjust the tone to full bass. This simulates a reduction of sensitivity to higher frequencies. You will still be able to hear what is being transmitted, but you will find yourself having to concentrate quite hard to understand the spoken words. There is a practical point here. What do we do when trying to communicate with someone who is partially deaf? We try to speak more loudly, but in doing so our voices become higher-pitched, and the patient with reduced sensitivity to higher frequencies may understand this less easily.

So what determines the frequency at which an object will vibrate?

Perhaps the most obvious determinant is the length of the vibrating medium. The longer the medium, the lower the frequency produced. The term 'medium' sounds a little vague, but it is used here to encapsulate vibration in all kinds of substance, including the metal prongs of a tuning fork, the strings of a stringed instrument and the column of air in a wind instrument. In the case of a tuning fork, the longer the prongs, the lower the frequency of the note produced. Some stringed instruments, such as the piano, contain a large number of strings of different lengths, and simply striking different strings produces sound of different frequencies. In other stringed instruments, such as the guitar and violin, holding down the string changes the frequency of the note produced, and this has the effect of varying the length of the vibrating section. In wind instruments, the length of the vibrating column of air may be changed using a system of valves or, in the simple case of a recorder, by covering a different number of holes in the body of the instrument.

The tension in the medium also affects frequency – the greater the tension, the higher the frequency. This principle is also used in stringed instruments, which are tuned by adjusting the tension in each of the strings so that each vibrates at a specific frequency. Different frequencies are also produced by the vocal cords through the mechanism of varying the tension within them. The vocal cords are stretched in order to produce higher frequencies and relaxed to produce lower frequencies.

One of the important properties we might want to know about sound is its loudness. For example, we might want to know how loud a hospital is at night. (If you have ever been a hospital patient, you will know that hospitals are very noisy.)

In the next section, we look at a number of properties of sound, including amplitude, intensity and loudness.

Amplitude

The amplitude is the maximum displacement of a particle from the rest position. The amount of energy carried by the wave and the loudness of the sound are both related to amplitude.

Intensity and loudness

Intensity is an expression of the amount of energy carried by a wave - it is also proportional to the square of the amplitude.

- ***What is the relationship between intensity and loudness?***

Let us imagine a sound of pure frequency - say, 5000 Hz. As the intensity increases, so does the perceived loudness.

- ***So can we equate intensity with loudness?***

We cannot precisely equate these two, since intensity is a measurable quantity, while loudness is a subjective perception. In fact, the human ear is not equally sensitive to all frequencies that are audible, and so two different frequencies, each with the same intensity (that is, carrying the same amount of energy), may be perceived as having different degrees of loudness. What is needed is a scale that enables us to compare the perceived loudness of different sounds - the **decibel** scale.

Table 13.1 lists some different sounds and their approximate rating on the decibel scale, along with a figure for the multiple threshold of intensity - that is, how many more times the sound is louder than the threshold of hearing (the quietest sound that can be heard). Note that the decibel scale is a logarithmic scale. This is a scale based on powers of ten - remember

Table 13.1 **The decibel rating and multiple threshold of intensity for various sounds.**

Sound	Decibel level (dB)	Multiple of threshold intensity
Threshold of hearing	0	1
Rustling leaves	10	10
Quiet room	20	10^2
Empty street	30	10^3
Room in house - no-one talking	40	10^4
Quiet conversation	50	10^5
Normal conversation	60	10^6
Loud conversation	70	10^7
Lecture	80	10^8
(N.B. Danger of hearing damage with prolonged exposure beyond this level)		
Loudest parts of orchestral music, factory machinery	90-100	10^9-10^{10}
Loud indoor music	110	10^{11}
Pain threshold	120	10^{12}

from Chapter 1 that we can express a large number as a power of 10, so that 100 (10×10) becomes 10^2. To understand the implications of this, consider the decibel level of rustling leaves (10 dB) and a quiet room (20 dB).

- ***Does this mean that an empty room is twice as noisy as rustling leaves?***

No - look at the multiple of the threshold of intensity. The sound of a quiet room is 100 times (10^2) more intense than the threshold (1), while the sound of rustling leaves is only 10 times louder than the threshold. This means that a quiet room is 10 times as loud as rustling leaves.

The measurement of the intensity of sound becomes important at high intensity, and potentially damaging, levels. In this context, hearing protection is discussed in Practice point 13.2.

Practice point 13.2

Hearing protection

Since noise may induce hearing loss (see later), protecting the ears from excessive noise is important. Employers are required to follow strict standards of noise control and provide ear protection for their employees. Many factories have high noise levels due to the operation of machinery. Some obvious examples of noisy environments include printing works and bottling plants. Clearly, employees in such environments should be encouraged to take responsibility for their own health and wear the ear protectors provided; occupational health nurses may have a role in encouraging this. Practices such as using radio headphones beneath ear protectors should be discouraged, since the noise level produced by playing music under such circumstances can be excessive. Self-inflicted hearing damage caused by the playing of loud music and visiting clubs and raves cannot be legislated against easily, but in Britain local authorities are able to take action against persistent 'noise polluters'.

Resonance

An object may be caused to vibrate at a range of different frequencies, but it will vibrate maximally at a particular frequency: This is the **resonant frequency**. If a sound wave with the same frequency as the resonant frequency of the object is produced, the object will begin to vibrate in time with the wave. This effect is demonstrated easily using two identical tuning forks with the same resonant frequency. One is struck and the note produced can be heard; in addition, the prongs can be seen to be vibrating. When this fork is held near the second fork, this too begins to vibrate, and we say that it is resonating.

Resonance is an everyday experience. For example, you might be driving a car and note that at a particular speed, a part of the dashboard or an object within the car starts to vibrate and make a sound. This is because at a particular speed, the vibration produced by the car engine matches the resonant frequency of a component in the dashboard or an object within the car, and these begin to vibrate maximally in time with the engine vibration. Go a little slower or a little faster and the sound disappears, since the engine vibration no longer matches the resonant frequency of the object.

- ***Is resonance important within the body?***

Resonance of air in the mouth, nose, pharynx and nasal sinuses is responsible for the characteristics of the voice produced. In addition, the **basilar membrane** of the inner ear (see later in this chapter) contains fibres of different lengths, and these resonate maximally at different frequencies. They thus form the basis of hearing different frequencies. The mechanism of hearing itself is more fully explained in Practice point 13.3.

In-text review

- ✔ Sound waves are longitudinal mechanical waves.
- ✔ The tension and length of a vibrating object determine the frequency of sound produced.
- ✔ The intensity of sound is measurable, but loudness is a subjective perception.
- ✔ The decibel scale is logarithmic, and so the intensity of a normal conversation (60 dB) is ten times that of a quiet conversation (50 dB).
- ✔ The frequency at which an object vibrates maximally is called the resonant frequency.
- ✔ If a sound wave is produced with the same frequency as the resonant frequency of an object, the object will begin to vibrate in time with the wave.
- ✔ Resonance occurs in the basilar membrane of the inner ear and is an important component of the mechanism of hearing.

Practice point 13.3

The mechanism of hearing

The mechanism of hearing involves the outer ear, the middle ear, the inner ear and the brain. The brain undertakes the interpretation of nervous impulses conveyed to it via the cochlear division of the vestibulocochlear nerve; this is not discussed here. Instead, we shall describe the structures involved in the detection of sound.

The outer ear

The outer ear consists of the **pinna**, the **external auditory canal** and the **tympanic membrane** (eardrum). Locate these structures on the diagram in Figure 13.3. The pinna is the external structure that we commonly refer to as the ear in everyday language. It is not as prominent in humans as in some other animals, but its role is to direct sound waves into the external auditory canal. This is a tubular structure that works like a funnel. It is open to the atmosphere at its external end, but the internal end is closed by the tympanic membrane.

- ***The external auditory canal contains* ceruminous glands *that* secrete cerumen. *What purpose does this secretion have?***

Cerumen is referred to more commonly as earwax. Together with outward-pointing hairs, cerumen discourages insects from entering the ear and helps to trap dust. The end of the

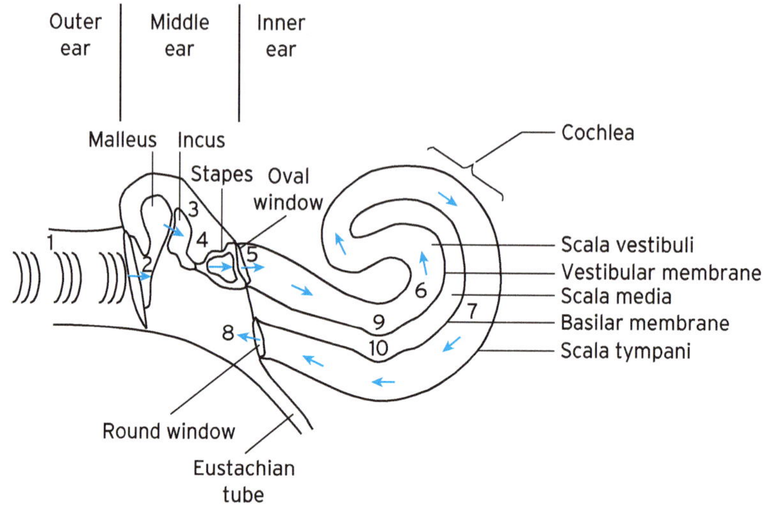

Figure 13.3

The outer ear, middle ear and inner ear.

(1) A sound wave passes along the external auditory canal. (2) A compression causes the tympanic membrane to bulge inwards; as a consequence, it pushes against the malleus. (3) The malleus pushes against the incus. (4) The incus pushes against the stapes. (5) The stapes pushes against the oval window and causes it to bulge inwards. (6) The sound wave is transmitted through the perilymph of the scala vestibuli. (7) The wave continues through the perilymph of the scala tympani. (8) A compression causes the round window to bulge outwards, into the middle ear. (9) The vestibular membrane vibrates in time with the sound wave. (10) The basilar membrane vibrates in time with the vestibular membrane.

external auditory canal inside the skull is covered by the tympanic membrane. The effect of sound waves upon the tympanic membrane is to cause the membrane to vibrate.

The middle ear

The middle ear is a small chamber inside the skull that contains three small bones referred to as the **ossicles**. These bones are named the **malleus**, the **incus** and the **stapes**. The literal meaning of these names is the hammer, the anvil and the stirrup, respectively, and they look a little like the objects after which they are named. The malleus is in contact with the tympanic membrane and, as a consequence, the two vibrate in time with each other. The malleus in turn moves the incus, which in turn moves the stapes. Finally, the stapes pushes against a covered opening called the oval window.

- ***What exactly do these bones achieve?***

They may be likened to a set of levers that serve to increase the amplitude of vibration by as much as by 20 times. This is important, because the wave that passes down the air-filled tympanic membrane ultimately will be transmitted in the fluid of the inner ear, and a greater force is required to set fluid in motion than air. Before we move on to consider the inner ear, we should note that a second membrane-covered opening exists below the oval window; this is the round

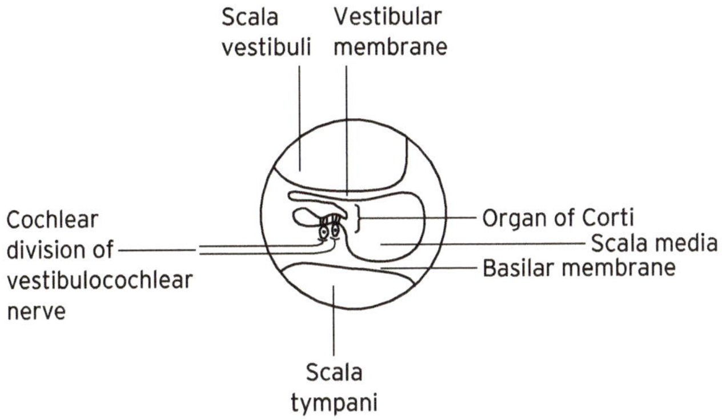

Figure 13.4
The cochlea.

window. Its role will become clear a little later. Note too that the middle ear is not a closed space - a tube called the **eustachian tube** vents the middle ear. This tube connects the middle ear with the pharynx and allows pressure differences on either side of the tympanic membrane to be equalised. You can find out more about this in Chapter 6.

The inner ear

The inner ear is formed by a number of structures, some of which are concerned with balance rather than with hearing. The part of the inner ear that is concerned with hearing is the cochlea, which is illustrated in Figure 13.4. The cochlea is a spiral-shaped chamber that contains three fluid-filled channels - the **scala vestibuli**, the **scala media** and the **scala tympani**. The scala vestibuli begins on the side of the oval window opposite to the stapes, spirals up to the apex of the cochlea and leads to the scala tympani, which spirals down the cochlea to the round window. The fluid that fills these two channels is called **perilymph**. Note that the movement of the stapes back and forth causes the oval window to vibrate, and this sets up a longitudinal wave in the perilymph, which eventually is transmitted to the round window. As a consequence, the oval and round windows move synchronously but in opposite directions.

Now let us consider the remaining chamber - the scala media. This too is filled with fluid, but in this case the fluid is called **endolymph**. Note that the scala media is, in effect, sandwiched between the two other membranes. Because of this, the floor of the scala vestibuli (**vestibular membrane/Reissner's membrane**) forms the roof of the scala media, and the floor of the scala media (basilar membrane) forms the roof of the scala tympani. Make sure that you can locate these structures on the diagram in Figure 13.4 before we proceed.

The apparatus of sound detection is called the organ of Corti, and this is located in the scala media. It is illustrated in Figure 13.5. The organ of Corti contains auditory receptor cells that have microscopic hair-like projections called cilia. For this reason, they are often referred to as hair cells. The cilia are attached to the tectorial membrane, which floats in the endolymph above the hair cells. In the basilar membrane, the hair cells are connected to sensory nerve cells (neurons) that collectively form the cochlear division of the vestibulocochlear nerve.

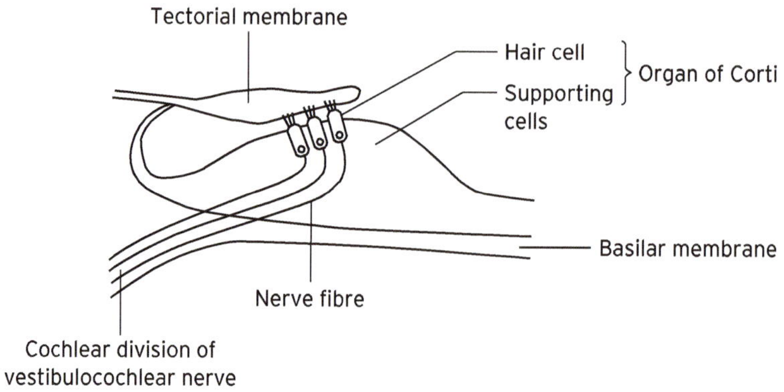

Figure 13.5
The organ of Corti.

● *How does this arrangement enable us to hear?*

We have already noted how vibrations are set up in the perilymph by the movement of the oval window. These vibrations are transmitted readily across the vestibular membrane, which is very thin. This means that the endolymph also vibrates in sympathy with the oval window. Vibrations of the endolymph then cause the basilar membrane to vibrate. Although the entire length of the basilar membrane is capable of vibration, it vibrates maximally at a specific point determined by the frequency of vibration of the endolymph. This is an example of resonance.

The basilar membrane contains fibres, called stiff fibres, of different lengths, all of which begin at the base of the cochlea. Many pass part way along the basilar membrane, while the longest pass all the way up to the apex of the cochlea. In the case of low-frequency sounds, the basilar membrane vibrates maximally at its apex, while in the case of high-frequency sounds the basilar membrane vibrates maximally at its base. At the point of maximum movement of the basilar membrane, the motion of **cilia** (hair-like projections) of cells referred to as hair cells initiates nervous impulses that are conveyed to a specific region of the auditory cortex of the brain. (This is the part of the brain where the interpretation of sound takes place.) Of course, most sounds are complex mixtures of frequencies, which result in the stimulation of a number of regions of the organ of Corti and finally to patterns of nervous impulses, which the brain has to interpret. More frequent impulses result from sound waves with greater amplitude (loud) than from those with lower amplitude (quiet). In this way, the brain receives information about both the intensity and the frequency of sound.

Nurses study physiology, such as the mechanism of hearing, with a specific purpose – to understand illness and how to help the patient. With this in mind, deafness is discussed in Practice point 13.4.

Practice point 13.4

Deafness and its forms

Loss of hearing may be partial or complete. Some forms of deafness occur in children, while others are associated with ageing.

- ***When deafness is suspected, how is hearing assessed?***

The simplest form of hearing test is conducted on babies by health visitors as part of developmental assessments. An attempt is made to distract the baby using a rattle in order to confirm that the infant can hear. In older children and adults, an **audiometric test** is used. This involves listening to sounds of different frequency and intensity through headphones and reporting when a sound can be heard, for example by pressing a signalling button.

The causes of deafness can be placed in one of two groups - **conductive deafness** and **sensorineural deafness**.

Conductive deafness

This form of deafness results from an impaired conduction of sound to the cochlea and results from a problem affecting the outer ear or middle ear. Possible causes include the occlusion of the external auditory canal by wax, the accumulation of tenacious secretions in a middle ear infection (**otitis media** - sometimes called glue ear) and damage to the ossicles. As a general rule, conductive deafness is easier to treat than sensorineural deafness. Some treatments are simple; for example, accumulated wax is softened by the daily instillation of olive oil into the external auditory canal over a period of about five days followed by ear syringing. Although this is a simple procedure commonly performed by practice nurses and other nurses, there is a risk of causing damage to the tympanic membrane, and so only properly trained staff should carry out this procedure. Otitis media is not uncommon in children and initially may be treated with antibiotics. If otitis media is persistent, however, the tympanic membrane may be perforated surgically and a grommet (a simple valve) inserted in order to allow the fluid in the middle ear to be discharged. Another mechanical problem is the age-related degeneration of the ossicles, which results in their failure to magnify the amplitude of vibration. This form of deafness is usually managed by electronic amplification - that is, the affected individual wears a hearing aid.

Sensorineural deafness

Damage to the cochlea or its associated nervous pathways results in sensorineural deafness. In this form of deafness, sounds are perceived as being quieter and may also be distorted; **tinnitus** (the subjective experience of noise in the absence of an external stimulus) may also be present. As a consequence, a hearing aid may be of little value to a person with this form of deafness. Sensorineural deafness may occur as part of the ageing process (**presbycusis**), may be induced by drugs (e.g. the antibiotic gentamicin), may follow some infections (e.g. measles, mumps, chickenpox, rubella) or may be induced by noise.

Having considered the forms of deafness, you may wonder how best to communicate with someone who has a hearing impairment. This is discussed in Practice point 13.5.

Practice point 13.5

Communicating and hearing impairment

When communicating with someone who has a hearing impairment, it is useful to bear in mind the following points:

- Position yourself directly in front of the person and do not turn around while still talking to the person.
- Do not speak until you have the person's attention.
- Find out whether the person can lip-read or normally uses a hearing aid. This information should be recorded in the patient's nursing notes.
- If a hearing aid is normally used, it should be fitted and working.
- Do not use exaggerated lip movements.
- Speak slowly, raising your voice only a little.
- Confirm that the patient has understood what you have said before continuing a conversation.
- Rephrase sentences if the patient experiences difficulty.
- Be patient - do not give up and abandon any attempt to communicate.
- Try other means of communicating, such as with gestures. You may have to learn some sign language in order to communicate with people who use this.

Thus far, we have considered sound and hearing. Clearly the two are related, but just as there are sounds so quiet that we cannot hear them, so there are frequencies to which we are not sensitive - particularly very high frequencies. Just because we cannot hear a sound does not mean to say that such frequencies are unimportant - we put high-frequency sound to medical use, as you will see in the next section.

Ultrasound and the piezoelectric effect

In this section, we look at an effect that links crystals, submarines and modern medical scanning techniques. Science is never boring, but sometimes we have to stick with unusual topics before we understand a point related to clinical practice.

When a force deforms certain crystals, such as quartz, a small voltage is created across the crystals. This is termed the **piezoelectric effect**, and crystals that demonstrate it are called **piezoelectric crystals**. If a small voltage is applied across such crystals, they demonstrate a deformation. This is called the **reverse piezoelectric effect**. Alternating current produces intermittent deformations - that is, the crystal vibrates. These vibrations generate sound, the frequency of which is higher than that which can be heard by human ears - we call it **ultrasound**. Piezoelectric crystals are not recent discoveries - the piezoelectric effect was first observed in the late 1800s, and in the First World War ultrasound detection of submarines was developed (sonar - **so**und **n**avigation **a**nd **r**anging). Ultrasound is also employed to create images of the body, as explained in Practice point 13.6.

Practice point 13.6

Ultrasound and the body

Ultrasound may be used to produce an image of internal structures of the body. This involves placing an ultrasound **transducer** against the body surface and directing the ultrasound waves towards the structure to be imaged. You may recall that a transducer is a device for converting one form of energy into another. The ultrasound transducer uses the reverse piezoelectric effect to generate ultrasound and the piezoelectric effect to detect ultrasound echoes (reflections) bounced back from internal structures. Such reflections occur at any interface between tissues of different densities - for example, between healthy tissue and a tumour. These reflections are then used to produce a visual image of the structure that has been scanned. Ultrasound has certain advantages over other scanning techniques: ultrasound scanners are portable and less expensive than many other imaging devices; an ultrasound scan is not invasive and involves little discomfort for the patient; and ultrasound is without the risks associated with ionising radiation (see Chapter 14).

- ***Do you know of some of the uses of ultrasound?***

Since ultrasound is believed to be a safe method of scanning, it finds use in obstetrics in the imaging of the foetus. Ultrasound scans can be used to determine the age of the foetus and to detect foetal abnormalities such as **spina bifida** (a spinal defect). Until recently, little could be done to treat deformities of the developing child, except to educate the parents. More recently, surgeons have begun to develop techniques for operating on a child while it is still developing in the uterus. More conventionally, abdominal organs such as the liver may also be scanned using ultrasound; the detection of **neoplasms** (new growths such as a cancer) is one obvious use.

Finally, short-duration high-intensity ultrasound waves may be used to break up kidney stones - a procedure called **lithotripsy**. An alternative method is surgical removal of the stones.

The Doppler effect

Have you noticed that the pitch of the sound of a speeding motorcycle increases as it gets nearer but decreases as it moves away? This is known as the **Doppler effect**.

- ***Would you notice the same change in pitch if you were riding the motorcycle?***

No. Provided that the motorcycle is travelling at constant speed, the engine note remains the same.

- ***Why is it that an observer notices a change in pitch?***

In order to answer this question, remember that pitch is related to frequency - we perceive high-frequency sounds as being high-pitched. Remember, too, that frequency is the number of waves that pass a particular point in one second. The motorcycle engine emits a sound wave of a certain frequency (true frequency), but as it travels towards us, we receive a greater number of waves per second - that is, the received frequency is greater. In contrast, as the motorcycle travels away from us, the received frequency is less than the true frequency. The difference between the true frequency and the received frequency is described as a Doppler shift.

- ***So does the Doppler effect have any medical uses?***

It does, as Practice point 13.7 makes clear.

Practice point 13.7

The Doppler effect and the body

First, let us note that the Doppler effect can be demonstrated with all frequencies of sound, including ultrasound.

- ***What would happen if we directed an ultrasound wave at flowing blood?***

We would be able to detect a Doppler shift in the frequency of the reflected wave. If the blood is flowing towards the transducer, the reflected wave will have a higher frequency than that of the original wave; but if the blood is flowing away from the transducer, the reflected wave will have a lower frequency than that of the original wave.

- ***What if we directed the ultrasound wave to a narrowed part of the vessel?***

The velocity of blood in narrowed vessels is increased. (If you are unsure about this, check out Chapter 6.) For now, it is sufficient to note that the Doppler effect can be used to detect changes in blood flow, such as might occur in disease processes such as **atherosclerosis** (narrowing of the arteries due to the accumulation of fat and other substances in the artery wall).

In-text review

- ✔ The outer ear consists of the pinna, the external auditory canal and the tympanic membrane.
- ✔ The middle ear contains the ossicles.
- ✔ The inner ear contains the spiral-shaped cochlea.
- ✔ The cochlea contains three fluid-filled channels - the scala vestibuli, the scala media and the scala tympani.
- ✔ The scala vestibuli begins at the oval window and spirals to the apex of the cochea.
- ✔ The scala tympani spirals down from the apex of the cochlea to the round window.
- ✔ The scala media is found between the scala vestibuli and the scala typani and contains the apparatus of sound detection - the organ of Corti.
- ✔ Sound waves cause vibrations in hair cells found in the organ of Corti. This results in nervous impulses, which are conveyed to the auditory cortex of the brain, where they are interpreted as sound.
- ✔ Deafness may be conductive or sensorineural.
- ✔ Ultrasound consists of waves with a frequency higher than that which can be heard by humans.
- ✔ Ultrasound can be used to generate visual images of body structures.
- ✔ The Doppler effect can be used with ultrasound to detect narrowing of blood vessels.

Summary

We began this chapter began with an illustration of how important hearing is to communication and our ability to socialise with other people, before going on to describe sound as a mechanical longitudinal wave. We also explained the measurement of the intensity of sound using the decibel scale, and important aspects of hearing protection were given. Most importantly, the mechanism of hearing was described and some possible causes of deafness were given. Finally, the use of ultrasound in the production of visual images of the body was explained.

Summary points

- Sound waves are mechanical longitudinal waves.
- The perceived intensity of sound is measured on the decibel scale.
- The mechanism of hearing involves the conduction of sound waves through air in the outer ear, through the bones of the middle ear and through the fluid of the inner ear.
- Deafness may be classified as either conductive or sensorineural.
- Sensorineural deafness may result from noise exposure; thus, wearing hearing protectors in noisy environments is important.
- Internal structures may be scanned using ultrasound waves produced by the reverse piezoelectric effect and detected using the piezoelectric effect.
- Short-duration high-intensity ultrasound waves may be used to break up kidney stones (lithotripsy).
- The Doppler effect may be used to detect narrowing of blood vessels.

Self-test questions

1 Which of the following statements are true?
(a) Sound waves are electromagnetic.
(b) Sound waves are longitudinal.
(c) Sound waves are mechanical.
(d) Sound waves are transverse.

2 Which of the following statements are true?
(a) One wavelength is the distance between adjacent rarefactions.
(b) One wavelength is the distance between adjacent compressions.
(c) One wavelength is the distance between a compression and an adjacent rarefaction.
(d) One wavelength is the number of waves that pass a point in one second.

3 Which of the following statements are true?

(a) The longer the vibrating medium, the lower the frequency of sound produced.

(b) The shorter the vibrating medium, the higher the frequency of sound produced.

(c) The greater the tension in the vibrating medium, the lower the frequency of sound produced.

(d) The greater the tension in the vibrating medium, the higher the frequency of sound produced.

4 Which of the following statements are true?

(a) Sound is conducted through the outer ear in air.

(b) Sound is conducted through the middle ear in fluid.

(c) Sound is conducted through the inner ear in fluid.

(d) The inner ear is vented by the eustachian tube.

5 Which of the following statements are true?

(a) The amplitude is the maximum displacement of a particle from the rest position.

(b) Loudness is a subjective perception.

(c) Intensity is not measureable.

(d) Two waves with different frequencies but with the same intensity may be perceived as having different degrees of loudness.

6 If an empty street is rated at 30 dB and normal conversation at 60 dB, how much louder is normal conversation than an empty street?

(a) Twice as loud.

(b) Half as loud.

(c) One hundred times as loud.

(d) One thousand times as loud.

7 Match the structures on the left with the appropriate locations on the right.

(a) Organ of Corti	(i) Outer ear
(b) Ossicles	(ii) Brain
(c) Ceruminous glands	(iii) Middle ear
(d) Auditory cortex	(iv) Inner ear

8 Match the structures on the left with the appropriate description on the right.

(a) Basilar membrane	(i) Roof of scala tympani
(b) Vestibular membrane	(ii) Located within the scala media
(c) Tympanic membrane	(iii) Outside the cochlea
(d) Tectorial membrane	(iv) Roof of scala media

9 Which one of the following structures does not form part of the middle ear?

(a) Malleus

(b) Eustachian tube

(c) Stapes

(d) Hair cell

10 Which one of the following is a form of sensorineural deafness?

(a) Accumulated wax in the external auditory canal.
(b) Presbycusis.
(c) Tenacious fluid in the middle ear.
(d) Degeneration of the ossicles.

Further study/exercises

1 Recently, a good deal of attention has been given to cochlear implants. What are they, and who benefits from them?

The Ear Foundation: www.earfoundation.org.uk/search

Royal National Institute For The Deaf (RNID) website: www.rnid.org.uk/

Cochlear implants factsheet: www.rnid.org.uk/information_resources/factsheets/medical/factsheets_leaflets/cochlear_implants.htm

National Deaf Children's Society website: www.ndcs.org.uk

Deaf children and cochlear implants: www.ndcs.org.uk/information/childhood_deafness/cochlear_implants/

2 It is well known that hospitals can be noisy places. The next time you are in a care setting where patients need to rest, identify possible sources of noise and suggest ways in which the noise level could be reduced. This exercise might be particularly important at night. Can you find any nursing research on this subject?

Biley F. (1994). Effects of noise in hospitals. *British Journal of Nursing*, 3(3), 110-11.

Cabrera I. N. and Lee M. H. M. (2000). Reducing noise pollution in the hospital setting by establishing a department of sound: a survey of recent research on the effects of noise and music in health care. *Preventive Medicine*, 30(4), 339-45.

Hilton B. A. (1986). Noise: who says hospitals are quiet places? *Canadian Nurse*, 82(5), 24-8.

14

Radiation in diagnosis and treatment

Learning outcomes

After reading the following chapter and undertaking personal study, you should be able to:

1. Distinguish between ionising radiation and non-ionising radiation and relate this distinction to radiation safety in clinical practice.
2. Describe four forms of ionising radiation and compare their penetrating ability and relate this to their usefulness in clinical practice.
3. Explain what is meant by the term 'radioactive decay' and describe alpha decay and beta decay.
4. Explain the concept of half-life.
5. Explain how X-rays are produced and relate this to the investigation of illness.
6. Outline the biological effects of ionising radiation and relate this to radiation safety in clinical practice and to patients receiving radiotherapy.
7. Describe important aspects of radiation protection for health-care workers.
8. Briefly describe the following imaging techniques: simple X-ray, cine radiography, computerised tomography (CT) and radionuclide scans.
9. Describe the use of ionising radiation in the treatment of cancer.

Introduction

You may have watched police-chase television programmes in which a thief abandons a stolen car and makes his escape on foot, only to be followed by a helicopter with night-vision equipment. This is a good illustration that being 'seen' does not always depend upon visible light. In fact, visible light is only a small part of a spectrum of waves that we call the **electromagnetic spectrum**. We introduced this spectrum in Chapter 12, noting that electromagnetic waves radiate from their point of origin and that the word '**radiation**' may be used to describe such waves. When used in this way, the term 'radiation' simply refers to something being emitted. Electromagnetic waves are often referred to as radiation, but the term may also be applied to particles, some of which are described later. Furthermore, although mention of radiation can conjure up thoughts of danger, no such meaning is implied in the word itself. In the example above, night-vision equipment detects infrared radiation emitted by hot objects such as bodies; this example probably does not cause you anxious thoughts. On the other hand, many people do not like the thought of nuclear power stations on their doorstep. When we express a fear of radiation, we are, in fact, referring to **ionising radiation**, which consists of electromagnetic waves or particles, which, when striking matter, cause the production of ions. Since ionising radiation (e.g. X-rays) is used medically to produce images of the body and to destroy cancers, we consider it in this chapter.

The nature of ionising radiation

Ionising radiation includes high-frequency electromagnetic rays such as **X-rays** and **gamma rays**, as well as particles such as **alpha particles** and **beta particles**. We look at each of these in turn and subsequently relate their relevance to clinical practice.

Alpha particles (helium nuclei)

Alpha particles are helium nuclei - that is, helium atoms from which two electrons have been lost. Helium nuclei may be represented in the following way: ${}^{4}_{2}He$

- ***To what do the figures refer?***

The lower figure is the atomic number (number of protons in the nucleus) and the upper figure is the mass number (sum of the number of protons and neutrons). In a helium nucleus, there are two protons and two neutrons, so the atomic number is 2 and the mass number is 4. Alpha particles have a relatively poor penetrating power, as Figure 14.1 shows. A sheet of paper may stop alpha particles, and they certainly do not penetrate deeper than the skin.

Beta particles (electrons)

Beta particles are actually electrons. They have poor penetrating power, although it is greater than that of alpha particles. Beta particles penetrate living tissue to a depth of about 1 cm and may be stopped by a thin sheet of metal foil.

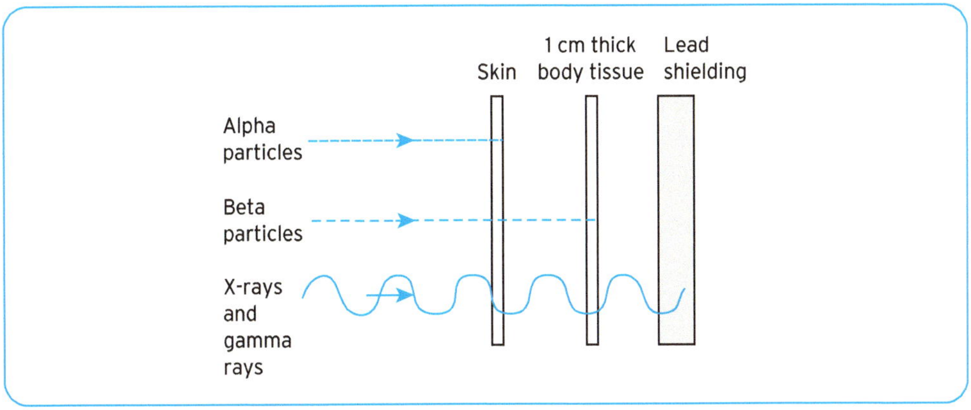

Figure 14.1
The penetrating ability of different types of ionising radiation.

Gamma rays and X-rays

These are both highly penetrating forms of electromagnetic radiation. Both readily penetrate the body and are stopped only by lead shielding several centimetres thick. This makes them potentially very dangerous, as well as potentially useful. Penetrating ionising radiation can be used to produce images of internal structures of the body and to treat cancerous growths within the body. Although gamma rays and X-rays have a similar nature, they are produced differently. Gamma rays are emitted by the unstable nuclei of certain elements; a few of these elements are naturally occurring, but most are produced in nuclear reactors. In contrast, X-rays are produced electrically in an **X-ray tube** or a **linear accelerator**.

Radioactivity and radioactive decay

The nuclei of isotopes of certain elements are unstable and break up. (Isotopes are atoms with the same atomic number but different mass numbers – that is, the same number of protons in the nucleus, but different numbers of neutrons.) In the process of breaking up, such isotopes spontaneously emit gamma rays or particles, and as a consequence they are referred to as **radioisotopes**. The spontaneous particulate or electromagnetic emissions are referred to as **radioactivity**, and the breakup of the nuclei that leads to these emissions is called **radioactive decay**. From what we have noted above about the nature of radiation, you will no doubt have realised that there are three forms of radioactive decay: alpha decay, beta decay and gamma decay.

Alpha decay

One example of an alpha emitter is uranium-238 (^{238}U). This is chosen as an example because you may very well have heard of uranium, even if you have not studied science before.

- ***To what does the number after the name of this element refer?***

It is not the atomic number of uranium, since all isotopes of uranium have an atomic number of 92. It is, in fact, the mass number of a particular isotope of uranium. When thinking about radioactive isotopes, the mass number is always given along with the name of the element, so that different isotopes are readily distinguished.

- ***What happens when an atom of uranium-238 emits an alpha particle?***

To answer this question, examine the incomplete equation below:

$$^{238}_{92}\text{U} \rightarrow {}^{4}_{2}\text{He} + ?$$

Note that when a helium nucleus is emitted from an atom, the mass number is reduced by four and the atomic number is reduced by two. The resultant element, therefore, has a mass of 234 and an atomic number of 90. Note that since the atomic number is no longer 92, this is not simply another isotope of uranium - an atom of a new element has been formed. The name of the element with the atomic number 90 is thorium. You could check this by looking at the periodic table in the appendix at the back of this book. We are now in a position to complete the equation for the radioactive decay of uranium-238:

$$^{238}_{92}\text{U} \rightarrow {}^{4}_{2}\text{He} + {}^{234}_{90}\text{Th}$$

Actually, ^{234}Th is also an unstable isotope and decays. The decay that begins with ^{238}U involves a number of unstable isotopes and, as a consequence, continues for many years. The process of radioactive decay comes to an end only when stable isotope is formed - in this case, it is an isotope of lead.

Beta decay

Beta rays consist of streams of electrons. The key to understanding beta decay is to note that these electrons originate not from the electron shells surrounding the nucleus of an atom but from the nucleus itself. You may wonder how this can be, as the nucleus is comprised only of protons and neutrons. The answer is that in some isotopes, the neutron is capable of breaking up to form a proton and an electron. The proton is retained in the nucleus and the electron is emitted.

- ***What happens to the mass number and the atomic number of an isotope that decays in this manner?***

First, note that the mass number does not change: Although a neutron has broken up, a proton has been produced, and protons and neutrons have identical masses. Second, note that the atomic number actually increases by one. Remember that the atomic number is the number of protons within the nucleus and, as we have already noted, an additional proton has been created by the breakup of a neutron. So let us look at an example. We shall consider iodine-131 (^{131}I), an isotope with medical significance - it is used to produce images of the thyroid gland in the neck and also to treat thyroid cancer, as we shall see later.

$$^{131}_{53}I \rightarrow ^{131}_{54}Xe + e^-$$

^{131}I decays by beta emission to an element that also has an atomic mass of 131 - remember that the atomic mass does not change. The atomic number increases to 54; the element with an atomic number of 54 is xenon.

Gamma decay

The emission of high-frequency electromagnetic rays referred to as gamma rays does not involve the loss of subatomic particles, and so there is no change in either the atomic number or the atomic mass. One gamma emitter of medical importance is cobalt-60 (^{60}Co). We shall say more about this isotope a little later in this chapter.

The concept of half-life

Each radioisotope has a specific rate of decay. Some isotopes decay quickly, while others decay very slowly indeed. The important thing to note is that the fraction of the total number of nuclei of a particular isotope that decay in a given period of time is constant. Consequently, it makes little sense to attempt to define the total life of an isotope. Instead, the concept of **half-life** is used. There are three ideas here: physical half-life, biological half-life and effective half-life. The **physical half-life** of an isotope is the length of time it takes for half of the existing nuclei to decay. Table 14.1 lists some isotopes along with their mode of decay, physical half-life and, for some, the biological half-life too. This latter concept is explained shortly, but for now you will be able to see that the range of values is very wide indeed.

- ***If we take a 1-g sample of $^{60}_{27}CO$, which has a half-life of approximately 5 years, how much of it would remain after 5 years?***

Only half would remain - 0.5 g. It is worth pointing out that the mass of matter in our sample would not have fallen to 0.5 g. Instead, our sample would consist of 0.5 g of the original isotope plus its decay products.

Table 14.1 Half-lives of some important isotopes.

Isotope	Type of decay	Physical half-life	Biological half-life
$^{14}_{6}C$	Beta	5730 years	35 days
$^{24}_{11}Na$	Beta	15.02 hours	29 days
$^{42}_{19}K$	Beta	12.36 hours	43 days
$^{60}_{27}Co$	Beta	5.27 years	-
$^{131}_{53}I$	Beta	8.04 days	180 days
$^{235}_{92}U$	Alpha	7.04×10^8 years	-
$^{238}_{92}U$	Alpha	4.47×10^9 years	-

- ***Will our sample be only half as radioactive after 5 years?***

The answer is no – the radioactivity will not decrease by half, since many of the decay products are themselves radioactive.

Half-life, as we have described it above, is referred more correctly to as physical half-life in order to distinguish it from biological half-life. **Biological half-life** is the time taken for the amount of a specific radioisotope that has entered the body to be reduced by half as a consequence of natural biological processes, regardless of whether the isotope has decayed. For example, the isotope may be eliminated in the urine. In clinical practice, when isotopes have been administered to a patient, both the physical half-life and the biological half-life are important, and so a further concept – effective half-life – is used. **Effective half-life** refers to the time required for an amount of a specific isotope to fall to half its original value as a result of both its radioactive decay and its biological elimination. Understanding these concepts is of help when caring for patients to whom isotopes have been administered. Practice point 14.1 deals with the problem of the elimination of isotopes in body fluids.

Practice point 14.1

Isotopes and body fluids

In view of what we have noted above about the difference between physical and biological half-lives, you will no doubt have realised that if an isotope that has been administered to a patient is eliminated before it has decayed, then the body fluids in which it is present will be radioactive and will require careful handling. If you work in an environment where such patients are cared for, there will be a hospital policy describing the safe disposal of urine, faeces and vomitus, which you should of course follow.

In-text review

- ✔ Ionising radiation includes streams of particles (alpha particles/helium nuclei and beta particles/electrons) and electromagnetic waves (X-rays and gamma rays).
- ✔ Alpha particles and beta particles result from the decay of unstable nuclei of radioisotopes, while other radioisotopes emit gamma rays.
- ✔ X-rays are produced electrically.
- ✔ The skin stops alpha particles; beta particles penetrate soft tissue to a depth of about 1 cm; and only thick lead shielding stops X-rays and gamma rays.
- ✔ The length of time it takes for half of the original number of nuclei of an unstable isotope to decay is referred to as the physical half-life.
- ✔ Biological half-life is the time taken for the amount of a specific radioisotope that has entered the body to be reduced by half as a consequence of biological processes.
- ✔ Effective half-life refers to the time required for an amount of a specific isotope to fall to half its original value as a result of both radioactive decay and biological elimination.

One of the forms of ionising radiation with which we are most familiar is X-rays. The designation 'X' was first given to signify that, at the time of their discovery, their nature was unknown. The use of X-rays as a medical device to show the internal structure of the body became so common that the name 'X-ray' was used to refer to the medical imaging technique as well as the rays themselves. In Practice point 14.2, we explain how X-rays are used.

Practice point 14.2

X-rays

We have described X-rays as electrically produced electromagnetic waves. The most common use of X-rays is in the production of visual images of the internal structures of the body. This is such a common procedure that the term 'X-ray' is used in reference to the procedure as well as to the rays themselves. During the procedure, X-rays are directed towards the patient, who lies above or stands in front of an X-ray-sensitive film. This film is the X-ray equivalent of the light-sensitive film in the back of a conventional camera. The X-rays that meet a less dense area of the body are able to pass through it, strike the film and expose it, while other rays are stopped by denser tissue of the body. The image that is formed may be likened to a shadow. It is, however, a shadow cast by X-rays rather than by light; because of the penetrating power of the rays, it is a shadow of internal structures. Note, too, that once the film has been developed, the unexposed areas appear white and the exposed areas appear black. Figure 14.2 shows what an X-ray looks like.

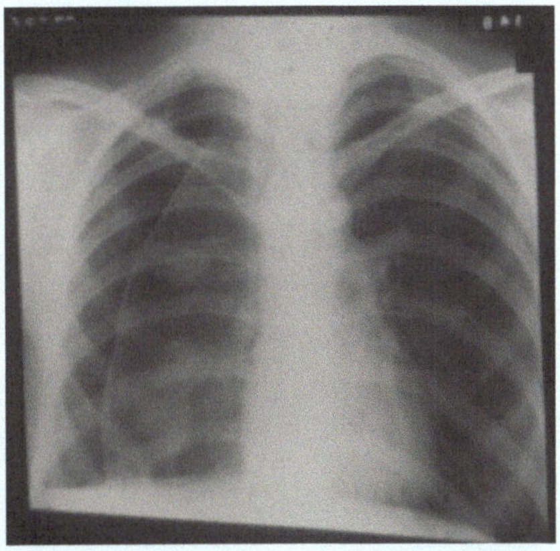

Figure 14.2
A chest X-ray.

You may wonder how X-rays are produced. They are generated when a stream of electrons strikes a metal target. In a simple X-ray tube, the electrons are generated by a heated element and then attracted to the target by an electrical potential difference (see Chapter 11) of several hundred thousand volts. Such apparatus is suitable for generating X-rays with sufficient energy to form an image of the body (that is, to take an X-ray).

The high-energy X-rays required to treat cancers require a linear accelerator. This piece of equipment uses a different method to generate a stream of very high-energy electrons. Nonetheless, the X-rays themselves are still produced when these electrons strike a metal target.

- ***Are there limitations to the usefulness of an X-ray?***

Every procedure has its limitations, and the simple X-ray is no exception. First, note that the image produced is two-dimensional, and one body structure may be partially obscured by another in front of it in the same way that an individual may be obscured by another in a group photograph. Of course, if someone takes a second photograph, this time from a different angle, then it may be possible to see the person who was previously obscured. This is exactly what is done in the case of X-rays – they are taken from different angles. For example, you may see the expressions

'A-P' and 'lateral' written on X-ray request cards. A-P stands for anterior-posterior, meaning an image taken with the X-ray tube in front and the film behind of the patient. The term 'lateral' means a view taken from the side; left or right should be specified.

A second limitation of the simple X-ray is that the density of the body's soft tissues is approximately the same as that of water, and so the boundary between one soft-tissue structure and another is indistinct. This can be overcome in some situations - take the stomach as an example.

- ***How could the structure of this hollow organ be made more visible?***

The description of the stomach as hollow is a clue to the answer to this question. We could ask the patient to drink a **radio-opaque** medium. Radio-opaque means opaque to X-rays - that is, X-rays do not readily penetrate it. The medium may or may not be opaque to light. Having swallowed such a medium, the patient is tilted so that the medium coats the interior of the stomach. When an X-ray is taken, the wall of the stomach is then contrasted against the medium. For this reason, such a radio-opaque medium is also referred to as a **contrast medium**. In this example, the contrast medium consists of an emulsion containing barium sulphate; the procedure is termed a **barium meal**. This procedure may be used in order to confirm the presence of a lesion within the stomach. If a gastric (stomach) ulcer is present, a crater filled with barium can be seen. A small quantity of barium within the crater may even be observed for some time after the stomach has emptied. If a **neoplasm** (new growth/tumour) is present, however, the outline of the stomach will be irregular. You might like to find out more about contrast radiography, for which a variety of contrast media are available. Some of these are suitable for injection into the bloodstream.

The effects of ionising radiation

We have described ionising radiation as radiation that is capable of producing ions. A number of mechanisms are involved in the process of ionisation, including the ejection of electrons from their orbit when an atom is struck by the radiation. Some of the ions produced are oxidising agents and some are reducing agents (see Chapter 3), or in some other way they may be toxic to cells. Sometimes cells are able to repair the damage produced, but if the intensity of the radiation is too great or the period of repair between exposures is too short, then cells may die. Even if a cell does survive, damage to its genetic material (deoxyribonucleic acid, DNA) may impair its function. Such a genetically damaged cell may be described as 'mutant'. When such a cell reproduces, the altered genetic material will be replicated, and subsequently a malignant tumour (cancer) may develop. If the mutated cell is a gamete (sex cell - oocyte or spermatocyte), then the embryo that results from the fusion of this sex cell with another may possess a genetic defect. Without a fuller description of the effects of ionising radiation, it becomes obvious that unnecessary radiation exposure should be avoided.

So, then, we have good reason to treat radiation with caution. On the other hand, if electromagnetic radiation is damaging, it can also be used to damage unwanted or diseased cells. For this reason, health-care workers who are exposed to ionising radiation need protection. This is explained in Practice point 14.3. There is a paradox here: Radiation both causes cancer and is used to treat cancer. We look at this later on in the chapter.

Practice point 14.3

Radiation protection for health-care workers

In an introductory science textbook such as this, any advice given about radiation protection must be of a general nature. When any procedure involving ionising radiation is performed, however, you should follow the relevant hospital policy. In addition, in the UK, all X-ray and radiotherapy departments are required to have a radiation protection supervisor who can be contacted for advice. Having noted the above, probably the most important thing to understand about radiation is that the intensity varies inversely with the square of the distance from the source. This is referred to as the **inverse square law**. This means that the intensity varies inversely with distance - the greater the distance from the source, the lower the intensity. Second, note that intensity is not reduced in direct proportion to the distance but as a square of the distance.

- ***If you were to double the distance between yourself and a source of radiation, by how much would the intensity be reduced?***

The intensity would be reduced by a factor of four (2^2) - that is, when the distance to the source is doubled, the intensity is reduced to a quarter. This is illustrated in Figure 14.3. Therefore, if you are present in a ward when portable X-ray equipment is being used, stand away from the patient and do not stand directly in front of an X-ray beam: It makes more sense to stand behind the X-ray machine than in front of it!

What we have noted about the inverse square law is true when there is no barrier between the individual and the source, but another method of reducing radiation exposure is to use some form of shielding. In the X-ray department, the radiographer will stand behind a partition while taking the X-ray and observe the patient safely through a window of lead glass.

- ***What if the patient is anxious about the procedure or in danger of falling?***

It is rarely necessary for a nurse to remain with a patient during an X-ray. If the patient is anxious, give reassurance before the procedure and then step behind the partition while the X-ray is being taken. If you are concerned about the patient's physical safety, then use pillows and bean-bags to help the patient maintain position and side rails to ensure the patient's safety.

Some procedures require staff to be present. In such cases, the staff exposed to radiation wear lead rubber aprons. These aprons need to be cared for carefully. They are always hung from

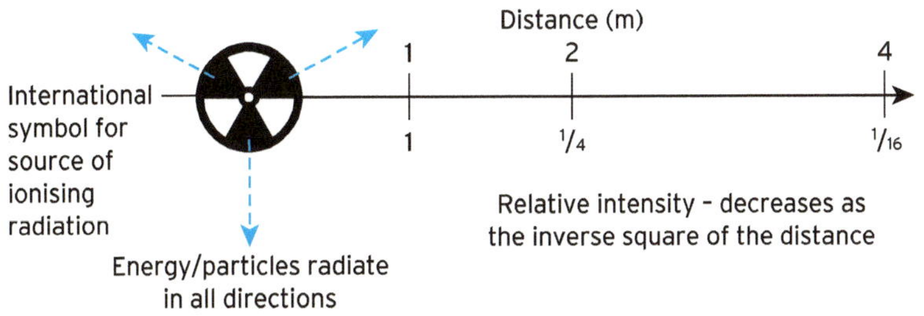

Figure 14.3
The inverse square law.

strong hangers when not in use; they should never be folded over the back of a chair or left crumpled on the floor. If this is allowed to happen, cracks may appear in the apron, which will act like a funnel through which radiation can pass.

Some patients have radioisotopes implanted in their bodies as part of the treatment of cancer. You need to restrict the time you spend with such individuals. Staff who are exposed to radiation frequently, such as radiographers and nurses working in radiotherapy wards, wear badges containing radiographic film. Different regions of the badge have different thicknesses of shielding, so the film is exposed to different degrees according to the amount of radiation exposure. This provides a way of determining how much radiation has been received in a fixed time period. If the maximum permitted exposure were reached, the continued exposure to radiation would not be permitted and, for a period of time, the health-care worker would have to be deployed in duties that did not involve radiation exposure.

Finally, we can summarise radiation protection under three headings - distance, shielding and time.

The measurement of radiation

You may see radioactivity expressed in a number of different units. Units are currently in use include the **becquerel** (Bq), the **gray** (Gy) and the **sievert** (Sv). The becquerel measures the radioactivity of a source of radiation in terms of the number of disintegrations per unit of time. One becquerel equals one nuclear disintegration per second. Although this unit is important for scientists, it is not so useful for health-care workers. What is needed in health care is a unit that measures the amount of energy absorbed by the body; such a unit is the gray. One gray is equivalent to the absorption of one joule of energy per kilogram of body tissue. The gray also has limited use, however, because different forms of radiation produce different effects, even when the absorbed dose in grays is the same - that is, even when the same amount of energy has been absorbed. The sievert takes into account the biological effects of the different forms of radiation; and this unit is used in clinical practice.

In-text review

- ✔ The term 'X-ray' is used not only of a type of electromagnetic radiation but also of the imaging procedure in which such radiation is used.
- ✔ X-ray images are shadow images of internal body structures produced when an X-ray-sensitive film is placed behind the subject and penetrating X-rays are directed through the body.
- ✔ The production of ions in biological tissue, some of which may be toxic, accounts for some of the damaging effects of ionising radiation.
- ✔ Ionising radiation may produce cell death or damage the genetic information of cells.
- ✔ Distance from source, time of exposure and shielding are the factors that should be considered in connection with radiation exposure.

When a patient undergoes investigation for an illness, medical staff have, in addition to X-rays, many more imaging techniques available to them. Some of these are explained in Practice point 14.4.

Practice point 14.4

Other important radiological diagnostic procedures

In addition to the simple X-ray, there are a number of other important radiological diagnostic procedures, including cine radiography, fluoroscopy and computerised tomography.

Cine radiography

When a simple X-ray is taken, the X-ray film serves the same purpose as a photographic film, and we might describe the result as an X-ray 'still'. Cine radiography involves the use of cine X-ray film, and a moving X-ray image is obtained. This is, therefore, analogous to the cine camera. The cine camera has been replaced by video and digital imaging, and so the term may sound rather old-fashioned. Cine radiography is especially useful when a dynamic process is to be imaged - blood flow, for example. Suppose a patient is suspected of having a narrowed blood vessel. This may be investigated by injecting into the bloodstream a contrast medium, which then circulates through the vessel under investigation. The procedure is referred to as **angiography**; a common form is **coronary angiography** - imaging the **coronary arteries** (the arteries that supply the heart with blood). In this case, a catheter (tube) is inserted through the **aorta** (the main artery of the body) via the **brachial artery** of the arm or via the **femoral artery** of the leg. As the catheter approaches the heart, its tip is directed towards one of the coronary **ostia** (opening of a main coronary artery). The contrast medium is injected through the catheter under force, and at the same time the cine X-ray image is filmed. By this means, an image of the coronary arteries is obtained as the contrast medium flows through them. This enables medical staff to locate a narrowed or occluded portion and to plan surgery to bypass it.

Fluoroscopy

When certain substances are struck by ionising radiation, they emit visible light (**fluoresce**). Fluorescence can be used to produce an image of the body by positioning the patient between an X-ray tube and a fluorescent screen in a procedure called **fluoroscopy**. Note that an image is present only for as long as X-rays strike the fluorescent screen. If a permanent record is required, then a radiograph or cine X-ray has to be taken. X-ray fluoroscopy is often combined with other investigations, especially those in which a device has to be positioned within the body. For example, in coronary angiography, the doctor views a fluoroscopic image of the chest as a radiopaque catheter is directed through the aorta to the heart.

Computerised tomography (CT)

In recent years the number of scanning techniques available to doctors has increased greatly. Even if you are not involved closely in these procedures, it is helpful to patients if you can explain what they should expect. The size of some scanners can be intimidating, especially when heavy motorised parts move close to the body. You should have no difficulty understanding what computerised tomography is, however, if you remember that the Greek word '*tomos*' means slice. In the case of a simple X-ray, a body structure in front of an organ may obscure it from view. Clearly it is helpful if we can view an image of the body just as though it had been 'sliced up', and that is exactly what CT images look like – a series of transverse (horizontal) slices through the body.

During a CT scan, the patient lies still as a thin beam of X-rays is passed through the body to a detector. As the CT scanner rotates, the X-rays are directed through the patient from every angle. A computer is used to build up the slice-by-slice image of the patient's body based upon the intensity of the X-rays generated and the intensity of the X-rays that reach the detector.

In the procedures explained in Practice point 14.4, ionising radiation is produced outside the body and directed towards the body in order to produce an image. Other imaging techniques involve the administration to the patient of a radioisotope and the build-up of an image from the radiation emitted from the patient's body. This is explained in Practice point 14.5.

Practice point 14.5

Radioisotope scans

Although it sounds somewhat frightening, the administration of radioisotopes to patients as part of diagnostic testing is not at all uncommon. Such tests depend upon the body dealing with the radioisotope in the same way as it deals with non-radioisotopes of the same element. The use of radioisotopes in diagnosis may be illustrated using the example of the **thyroid gland**. This endocrine gland is located in the neck and produces the hormone **thyroxine**, which is important in carbohydrate metabolism. The mineral iodine is essential for the manufacture of thyroxine and a radioisotope of iodine (^{131}I) can be used to investigate thyroid dysfunction in two ways:

Urinary excretion of ^{131}I

In this test, the patient is given a measured dose of ^{131}I. The patient's urine is collected for 48 hours and the amount of isotope excreted is measured. In **thyrotoxicosis** (overactive gland), a greater-than-normal amount of ^{131}I is concentrated in the thyroid gland and less is excreted, while in **myxoedema** (underactive gland) the reverse is true.

Thyroid scan

If the urinary excretion of ^{131}I is abnormal, the patient may have a thyroid scan. In this test ^{131}I, ^{125}I or ^{123}I is administered to the patient. The radiation emitted by the isotope is then detected by a gamma camera, which builds up an image from the emissions from the gland. The radioactive iodine is most concentrated in overactive regions of the gland, and emissions from these regions are correspondingly greater, giving rise to so-called 'hot areas'. In contrast, underactive regions take up less iodine than normal and give rise to correspondingly reduced emissions and 'cold areas'; such an area may be suggestive of thyroid cancer.

Although we have placed some emphasis on the dangerous nature of ionising radiation, its ability to destroy the body tissue is put to good use in the destruction of cancers, as explained in Practice points 14.6 and 14.7.

Practice point 14.6

Radiation in the treatment of cancer

The damaging effects of ionising radiation upon cells have already been described, but in this practice point we turn to the use of radiation to kill cancerous cells - a treatment referred to as **radiotherapy**.

Rapidly dividing cells are commonly more sensitive to radiation than are cells that divide at a slow rate. Since cancer cells usually divide rapidly, radiation has a greater effect upon them than upon normal tissue. Nonetheless, the sensitivity of malignant tumours (cancers) to radiation varies. Some tumours are highly **radiosensitive** but others are much less so. The degree of radiosensitivity is an important factor in determining the suitability of radiotherapy as a treatment in a particular case. It is also important to note that some of the normal cells of the body, particularly epithelial cells, also divide rapidly; these include cells of the bone marrow, intestinal epithelium and hair follicles. Consequently, radiotherapy produces some unpleasant side effects through its action upon these tissues, including anaemia (reduced number of **erythrocytes** (red blood cells), which are produced in the bone marrow), diarrhoea and hair loss. There are other effects, too; you might like to find out what they are.

- ***Can the effects of radiotherapy upon normal healthy tissue be limited?***

Yes, since healthy tissue normally recovers more quickly from radiation exposure than does cancerous tissue. Consequently, the radiation dose may be divided between numbers of treatments, each treatment providing a fraction of the dose required. The time period between treatments enables the healthy tissue to recover. In addition, beams of radiation may be directed at a malignant tumour at different angles through the skin in a technique called **multiple-field therapy**. This means that the healthy tissue receives only a part of the dose that reaches the cancer.

Practice point 14.7

Types of radiotherapy

In **external-beam radiotherapy**, a beam of X-rays or gamma rays is directed at the body from an external source. This technique is also called **tele-radiotherapy** - a term derived from a Greek word meaning 'far'. X-rays of sufficient energy for use in radiotherapy are produced from the rapid deceleration of high-energy electrons in a linear accelerator, while gamma rays are emitted by the nuclei of the atoms of certain radioisotopes, such as ^{60}Co (cobalt-60). The ability of the linear accelerator to produce a beam of deeply penetrating high-energy X-rays that can be focused precisely upon a tumour means that X-ray radiotherapy is much more common than gamma-ray radiotherapy. Although high doses of radiation are administered during radiotherapy, the dose is focused upon the tumour and the exposure localised. Once the treatment is complete, it is perfectly safe to be with and touch the patient. It is important to stay out of the treatment room when radiotherapy is being administered, although staff can observe patients via closed-circuit television and communicate via an intercom.

External-beam radiotherapy is not the only form of radiotherapy. In **internal radiotherapy**, a radioisotope is implanted within the body. For this reason, the treatment is sometimes referred to as **brachy therapy**, from a Greek word meaning 'near'. There are three forms of internal radiotherapy. In **intracavity implantation**, the isotope is contained in some form of receptacle that is implanted in the body cavity in order to irradiate adjacent structures. For example, ^{137}Cs (caesium-137) may be used to treat carcinoma of the cervix or vagina. In **interstitial implantation**, the isotope is surgically implanted directly into a malignant tumour in the form of beads, needles or wires: This method ensures that the tumour receives the greatest dose of radiation. One example of interstitial radiotherapy is the insertion of ^{192}Ir (iridium-192) needles into a tumour of the tongue. Finally, radioisotopes may also be administered systemically. Perhaps the most notable is the oral administration of ^{131}I in the treatment of cancer of the thyroid gland. The use of this isotope in the diagnosis of thyroid dysfunction has already been described, but in higher doses the beta radiation emitted will actually kill malignant cells.

- ***Is the rest of the body irradiated as well?***

Remember that the body metabolises radioisotopes in the same way as non-radioisotopes and that the thyroid gland concentrates iodine within it. Consequently, although the thyroid tumour cells are killed, the rest of the body receives only a very small radiation dose. Nonetheless, staff must protect themselves from radiation emitted by patients who have radioisotopes implanted within their bodies. Patients receiving internal radiotherapy are cared for in single rooms, and the length of time spent with each patient is strictly controlled. The exposure of staff can be limited still further by the technique of **afterloading**. In this form of treatment, an empty tube that will eventually contain the isotope is implanted into the relevant body cavity. Subsequently, the isotope is loaded into the tube remotely, but it may be removed again when staff need to enter the room.

In-text review

- ✔ In addition to simple X-rays, other important investigations include cine X-rays, fluoroscopy and computerised tomography (CT) scans.
- ✔ Radioisotope scans involve the administration to the patient of a radioisotope. The radiation emitted from the patient is then used to build up an image of the body.
- ✔ Radiotherapy makes use of the damaging effects of radiation to destroy cancerous cells.
- ✔ External-beam radiotherapy and internal radiotherapy (including intracavity and interstitial radiotherapy) are the different forms of radiotherapy.

Summary

In this chapter, we have dealt with some important scientific topics, such as radioisotopes and radioactive decay. In the 'nuclear age', perhaps everyone should have a degree of understanding of these topics. The purpose of this chapter, however, is not simply to increase the general knowledge of the reader. Instead, the material has been related specifically to clinical practice by reference to imaging techniques and treatments such as radiotherapy. As a health-care worker, you may encounter radiation more frequently than a member of the general public. Consequently, the section in this chapter dealing with radiation protection is especially important.

Summary points

- Ionising radiation includes both streams of particles, such as alpha particles (helium nuclei) and beta particles (electrons), and electromagnetic waves, such as X-rays and gamma rays.
- Alpha particles and beta particles result from the decay of unstable nuclei.
- X-rays are produced electrically, while some radioisotopes emit gamma rays.
- The skin stops alpha particles; beta particles penetrate soft tissue to a depth of about 1 cm; but only thick lead shielding stops X-rays and gamma rays.
- The length of time it takes for half of the original number of nuclei of an unstable isotope to decay is referred to as the half-life.
- The production of ions in biological tissue, some of which may be toxic, accounts for some of the damaging effects of ionising radiation.
- Distance from source, time of exposure and shielding are the factors that should be considered in connection with radiation exposure.
- Important imaging techniques in which ionising radiation is employed include the simple X-ray, cine radiography, computerised tomography (CT) scans and radionuclide scans.
- Ionising radiation may also be used to destroy malignant cells, and therefore it plays an important role in the treatment of cancer.

Self-test questions

1 Which one of the following is an accurate definition of isotopes?
(a) Atoms with the same number of electrons but with a different number of protons.
(b) Atoms with the same number of neutrons and electrons.
(c) Atoms with the same number of neutrons but with a different number of protons.
(d) Atoms with the same number of protons but with a different number of neutrons.

2 Which of the following statements are true?
(a) Alpha particles are more penetrating than beta particles.
(b) Beta particles are more penetrating than X-rays.
(c) X-rays are more penetrating than alpha particles.
(d) Gamma rays are more penetrating than alpha particles.

3 Match the forms of radiation on the left with the descriptions on the right.

(a) Alpha particle	(i) Electromagnetic radiation emitted by an isotope
(b) Gamma ray	(ii) Helium nucleus
(c) Beta particle	(iii) Electromagnetic radiation produced electrically
(d) X-ray	(iv) Electron

4 Suppose a radioisotope has a physical half-life of 5 years. How much of an original mass of 16 g will remain after 20 years?

(a) 8 g.
(b) 4 g.
(c) 2 g.
(d) 1 g.

5 Suppose that you are standing 2 m away from a source of radiation and you then move to a position 4 m away. By how much will the intensity of the radiation have fallen?

(a) 1/2.
(b) 1/4.
(c) 1/8.
(d) 1/16.

6 Which form of ionising radiation is emitted in the following reaction $^{60}_{27}Co \rightarrow ^{60}_{27}Co + ?$

(a) Alpha particles.
(b) X-rays.
(c) Gamma rays.
(d) Beta particles.

7 When a $^{238}_{92}U$ atom emits an alpha particle, it decays to which of the following?

(a) $^{59}_{27}Co$.
(b) $^{239}_{94}Pu$.
(c) $^{235}_{92}U$.
(d) $^{234}_{90}Th$.

8 Identify the missing element in the following equation: $^{131}_{53}I \rightarrow ? + e^-$

(a) $^{131}_{54}Xe$.
(b) $^{131}_{53}Xe$.
(c) $^{130}_{53}Xe$.
(d) $^{126}_{51}Xe$.

9 Match the investigations on the left with the descriptions on the right.

(a) Radionuclide scan	(i) A technique that results in images of transverse slices through the body
(b) CT scan	(ii) An image of a contrast medium passing through a blood vessel
(c) Angiography	(iii) A technique that involves the administration of a radioisotope
(d) Simple X-ray	(iv) A still, two-dimensional image of the internal structures of the body

10 Which one of the following currently describes the reason why it is possible to trace the metabolic pathways of the body using isotopes of the naturally occurring elements of the body?

(a) They are used in such small amounts that they do no harm.
(b) They have very short half-lives and so do no harm.
(c) They emit only gamma rays.
(d) They are metabolised in the same way as non-radioactive isotopes.

Further study/exercises

1 **Patients who are undergoing radiotherapy often experience unpleasant side effects. What are the important aspects of nursing care when these effects are present?**

Cancer BACUP website: www.cancerbacup.org.uk/Home
General information on radiotherapy: www.cancerbacup.org.uk/Treatments/Radiotherapy/Generalinformation
Cancer Research UK website: www.cancerhelp.org.uk/default.asp
Radiotherapy: www.cancerhelp.org.uk/help/default.asp?page=166

2 **Other diagnostic procedures include positron-emission tomography (PET) and nuclear magnetic resonance imaging (MRI). What do these procedures involve?**

Cancer Research UK website: www.cancerhelp.org.uk/default.asp
PET scan: www.cancerhelp.org.uk/help/default.asp?page=152
MRI scan: www.cancerhelp.org.uk/help/default.asp?page=149
NHS Direct: www.nhsdirect.nhs.uk/index.asp
Online encyclopaedia PET scan: www.nhsdirect.nhs.uk/en.aspx?articleID=427
Online encyclopaedia MRI scan: www.nhsdirect.nhs.uk/en.aspx?articleID=556

15

Genetics in health and illness

Learning outcomes

After reading the following chapter and undertaking personal study, you should be able to:

1. Describe the structure of a nucleic acid.
2. Describe the structure of deoxyribonucleic acid (DNA) and compare it with that of ribonucleic acid (RNA).
3. Define the terms 'chromatin', 'chromosome', 'diploid', 'haploid' and 'gene' and relate these definitions to normal healthy cells.
4. In connection with the replication of normal healthy cells, describe the following:
   - DNA replication.
   - The cell cycle and mitosis.
   - How meiosis differs from mitosis.
5. Describe briefly the three types of RNA – messenger RNA (mRNA), ribosomal RNA (rRNA) and transfer RNA (tRNA).
6. Differentiate between a codon and an anticodon.
7. Describe transcription and translation.
8. Explain the terms 'locus', 'allele', 'genotype', 'phenotype', 'homologous', 'homozygous' and 'heterozygous' and relate the explanations to genetic disease.
9. Identify normal traits that you might see in people that you meet each day and that are examples of simple autosomal inheritance (dominant and recessive), incomplete dominance (co-dominance), multiple alleles and polygenic inheritance.
10. Use a Punnett square in order to show the possible combination of alleles that may be inherited from parents and relate this to patients in clinical practice.
11. Give examples of the following patterns of genetic disease – simple autosomal inheritance (dominant and recessive), incomplete dominance (co-dominance) and sex-linked disorders – and give examples from clinical practice.
12. Describe briefly what is meant by a chromosomal aberration and give an example.

Introduction

When looking at photographs of people, have you ever noted similarities in the appearance of family members over several generations? If so, you were making an observation about **genetics**. The word 'genetics' is derived from '*genesis*' meaning creation, but really it is the study of **heredity**. Heredity is the transmission of physical characteristics (e.g. eye colour) from parents to children; it is also the study of diseases that have a genetic basis, e.g. **cystic fibrosis**. '*Genesis*' is also the origin of the word '**gene**', which is the name given to sections of **deoxyribonucleic acid (DNA)**. DNA is a large molecule that carries **genetic information** about such diverse things as eye colour, hair texture and which enzymes are made in the body. DNA is located in the **nucleus** of the cells of the body, and this is where we begin our study.

The nucleus of the cell

The cell (Figure 15.1) is the smallest living structure of an organism. The entire substance of a cell is referred to collectively as **protoplasm**, and it is separated from the outside environment by a membrane called the **cell membrane**. Most cells have an oval or spherical structure called the **nucleus** located within the protoplasm. The substance of the nucleus is collectively referred to as **nucleoplasm**, while the rest of the cell substance is called **cytoplasm**. Nucleoplasm is separated from cytoplasm by a membrane that forms the boundary of the nucleus; this membrane is called the **nuclear membrane**. This membrane contains pores (channels) through which molecules may enter or leave the nucleus.

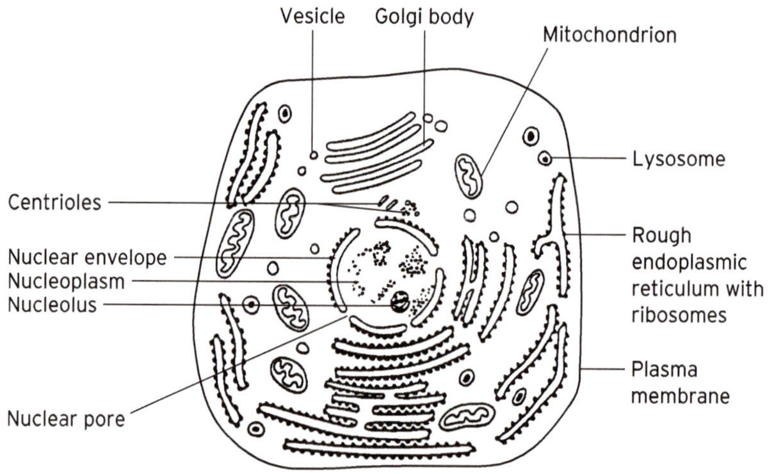

Figure 15.1
A typical animal cell. (From Cornwell A. and Miller R. (1997) *Longman Study Guides. A-Level and AS-Level Biology*. Harlow: Longman.)

Within the nucleus, **chromosomes** are found. These are important genetic structures made of DNA. Chromosomes can be seen with a light microscope, but they are visible only when the cell is actively dividing (reproducing).

- ***How many chromosomes do human cells possess?***

To answer this question, it is important to explain that the body's cells form two groups - **gametes** and **somatic cells**. Gametes are the sex cells - **ova** (eggs) in females and **spermatozoa** (sperm) in males. All other cells are described as somatic. In somatic cells there are 23 pairs of chromosomes - the so-called **diploid number**. (The prefix 'diplo' means double, but here 'diploid' refers to the full number of chromosomes.)

- ***Why do we say '23 pairs' and not simply '46'?***

Chromosomes are arranged in pairs according to their size and shape. Such pairs are referred to as **homologous chromosomes/homologous pairs**. One member of each homologous pair is derived from the mother and the other is from the father. One pair of chromosomes carries information about sex, and these are the **sex chromosomes**. The remaining 22 pairs do not carry information about sex and are called **autosomes**.

- ***How many pairs of chromosomes do gametes possess?***

Gametes possess only 23 chromosomes - the so-called **haploid number**. (The prefix 'haplo' means single, but here 'haploid' refers to the reduced number of chromosomes.) Twenty-two of these chromosomes are autosomes, and one is a sex chromosome.

There are two types of sex chromosome; they are given the designation X and Y. Female somatic cells (non-sex cells) possess two X chromosomes, while ova (the female gamete/sex cell) possess a single X chromosome. (Remember somatic cells are diploid and gametes are haploid.) Male somatic cells possess one X chromosome and one Y chromosome; spermatozoa contain either one X chromosome or one Y chromosome. A new individual is formed when haploid gametes fuse in a process called **fertilisation**. This is the process that takes place after sexual intercourse, in which one of millions of male spermatozoa deposited in the reproductive system of the female penetrates a single ovum. The sex of the new individual is determined by which sex chromosome (X or Y) the spermatozoon is carrying, since the ova always carry an X chromosome. If the spermatozoon is carrying an X chromosome, then the new individual will be female (XX); if the spermatozoon is carrying a Y chromosome, then the new individual will be male (XY).

Chromosomes consist of deoxyribonucleic acid (DNA) and its associated proteins. Before cell division, DNA forms a mass of threads called **chromatin**. Electron micrographs (photographs taken with an electron microscope) show that chromatin resembles beads on a string. Each bead-like structure is called a **nucleosome** and consists of DNA wrapped twice around a core of eight proteins called **histones**. During the early stages of cell division, DNA is replicated (copied) and the chromatin coils to form the discrete structures that we call chromosomes. At this stage, it can be seen that each chromosome consists of two parts called **chromatids** joined by a structure called a **centromere** (Figure 15.2). Each pair of chromatids carries the same genetic information.

What is DNA made of?

Francis Crick and James Watson first described the structure of DNA in 1956. DNA is made of subunits (building blocks) called **nucleotides**. Each nucleotide has three components:

- a five-carbon atom sugar molecule
- a phosphate group
- An organic compound referred to as a **base** (the word 'base' refers here to 'foundation' and is used in reference to a major component of a molecule).

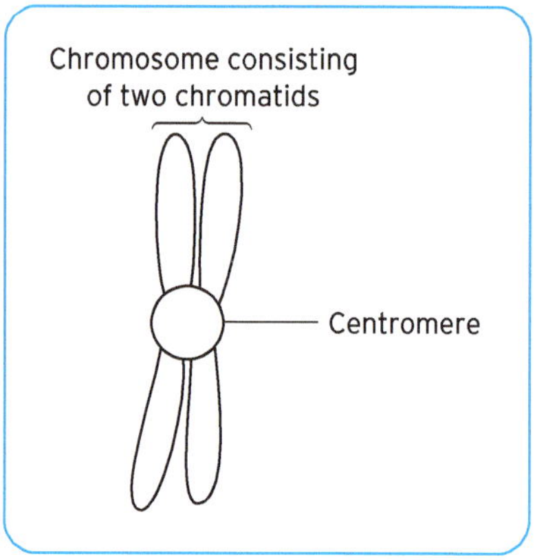

Figure 15.2
The structure of a chromosome.

The structure of a nucleotide is shown in Figure 15.3. Nucleotides that form DNA have the sugar **deoxyribose** and one of four bases - **adenine**, **thymine**, **guanine** or **cytosine**.

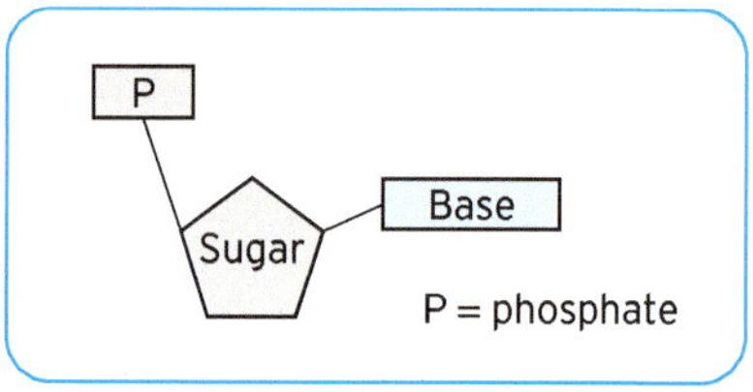

Figure 15.3
The structure of a nucleotide. (From Miller C. and Barber M. (1997) *Longman Study Guides. GCSE Biology*. Harlow: Longman.)

DNA possesses two chains that are formed from the bonding of the sugar of one nucleotide with the phosphate group of another. Consequently, these chains are sometimes referred to as **sugar-phosphate backbones**. Bonds formed between the bases then join these two chains. Adenine always bonds with thymine and guanine always bonds with cytosine. On first examination, this arrangement looks rather like a ladder, but actually the two sugar-phosphate chains spiral around each other. In fact, that is how the structure of DNA is described - as a double helix (Figure 15.4).

DNA is not the only nucleic acid - there is another called **ribonucleic acid** (**RNA**). RNA differs from DNA in three important ways:

- RNA consists of only a single strand of nucleotides.
- In the nucleotides that form RNA, the sugar is **ribose**, not deoxyribose.
- The base **uracil** is found instead of thymine.

DNA: the genetic code

DNA is often described as the body's genetic code. This is because DNA acts as the instructions for which proteins the body should make, and how the body should function.

How can a chemical act as a code?

To answer this question, let us think about codes in general. Codes are systems of characters (letters, numbers or symbols) that are used to represent words. Codes look mysterious

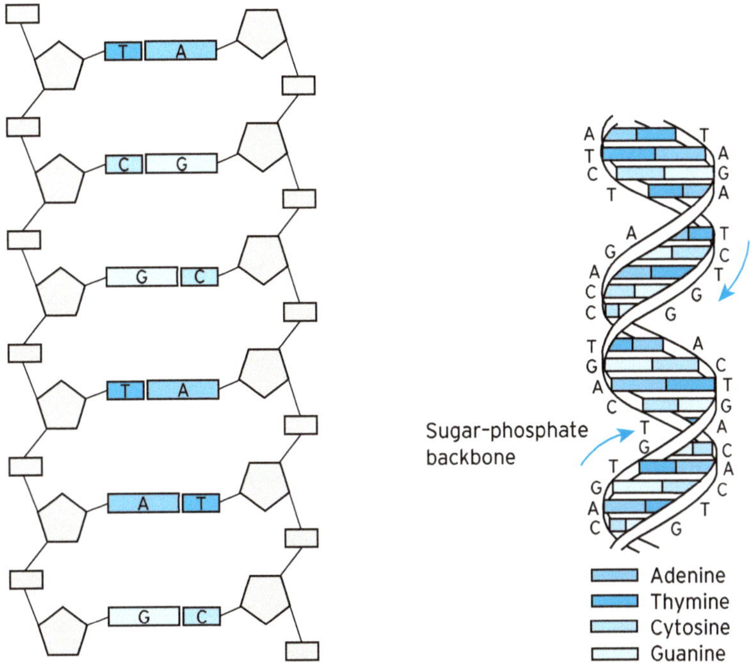

Figure 15.4
The structure of DNA. (From Miller C. and Barber M. (1997) *Longman Study Guides. GCSE Biology*. Harlow: Longman.)

until you know that the meaning of a word is determined by the sequence of characters in the code. It is similar with the genetic code - it appeared mysterious until it was discovered that its meaning is in the sequences of bases in DNA. These are arranged in triplets (groups of three), which are referred to as **codons**. Each codon acts as a code for a specific **amino acid** - there are 20 amino acids in nature.

- ***How many codons would you expect?***

You might think that there should be 20 codons, but in fact there are 64. Some amino acids are specified by more than one codon - a condition referred to as **redundancy**. In addition, some codons have functions other than coding for specific amino acids. Some codons indicate the point at which a code for a particular protein begins; these are referred to as **start codons**. Other codons indicate the point at which the code for a particular protein ends and are referred to as **stop codons**.

At this point, it is probably worth returning to a term introduced earlier - **genes**. These are segments of DNA that code for a specific protein. Genes form a section of a strand of DNA located between a start codon and a stop codon. There are thousands of genes in human DNA. Later in this chapter, we shall explain how the body uses the genetic code, but before we do this we need to consider how DNA is replicated.

DNA replication

If a cell is to divide (reproduce), it must replicate its DNA so that 23 pairs of chromosomes can be passed on to each of the resulting new cells. New cells are always called **daughter cells**. The first process in DNA replication is the unwinding of the double helix, as shown in Figure 15.5. Next, newly synthesised bases pair with the bases of the two original strands. In this way, two DNA molecules result. Each DNA molecule consists of a strand of the original molecule and a new strand. Consequently, DNA replication is said to be semi-conservative, as it conserves one old strand as part of each new strand.

Once DNA has been replicated, the cell is able to divide to produce two new cells. This is what we consider next.

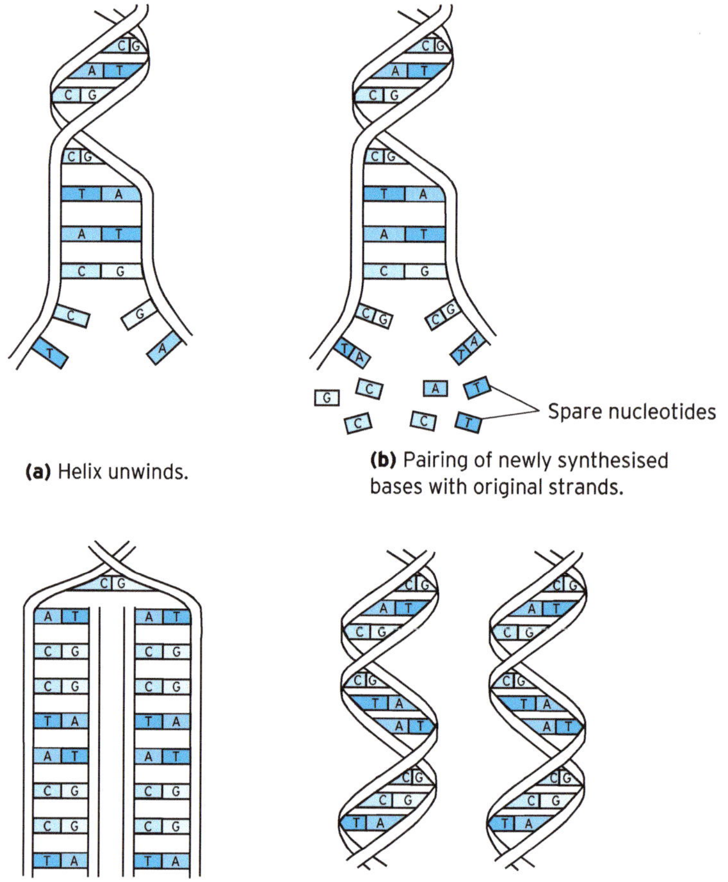

(a) Helix unwinds.

(b) Pairing of newly synthesised bases with original strands.

(c) Two strands begin to form.

(d) Two complete strands.

Figure 15.5
DNA replication. (From Miller C. and Barber M. (1997) *Longman Study Guides. GCSE Biology*. Harlow: Longman.)

Mitosis and the cell cycle

Cells need to reproduce so that damaged cells are replaced and growth takes place. Some cells, such as those of the basal layer of the skin, divide rapidly throughout life, while others, such as neurons in the brain, do not divide at all after birth. Figure 15.6 is a diagrammatic representation of the lifecycle of a somatic cell.

The cell cycle can be divided into two parts - **interphase** and **mitosis** (cell division). We consider each stage in turn.

Interphase

When a cell is not actively dividing, it is said to be in interphase. Interphase can itself be divided into distinct phases, which are represented in Figure 15.6. S stands for synthesis and refers to DNA synthesis (DNA replication); G_1 and G_2 are periods of growth, while G_0 is a period of rest. In G_0, the cell is actively metabolising but not growing or synthesising DNA.

Mitosis (cell division)

Cell division in somatic cells is referred to as **mitosis**, although strictly speaking this term refers only to the manner in which chromosomes are distributed between two newly forming cells (daughter cells). The division of the parent cell into two daughter cells is called **cytokinesis** (cytoplasmic division). Mitosis is divided into four stages called **prophase**, **metaphase**, **anaphase** and **telophase** (Figure 15.7). These are followed by cytokinesis. Each stage is described below.

Prophase: in this first stage of mitosis, chromosomes become visible and it can be seen that each is made of two chromatids. At the end of prophase, the nuclear membrane breaks down

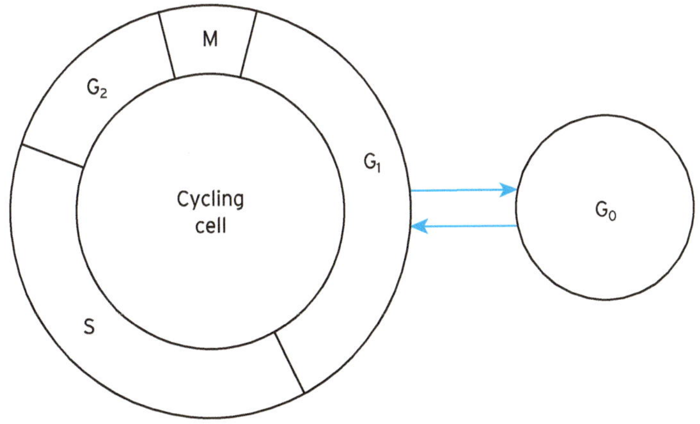

Figure 15.6
The cell cycle.

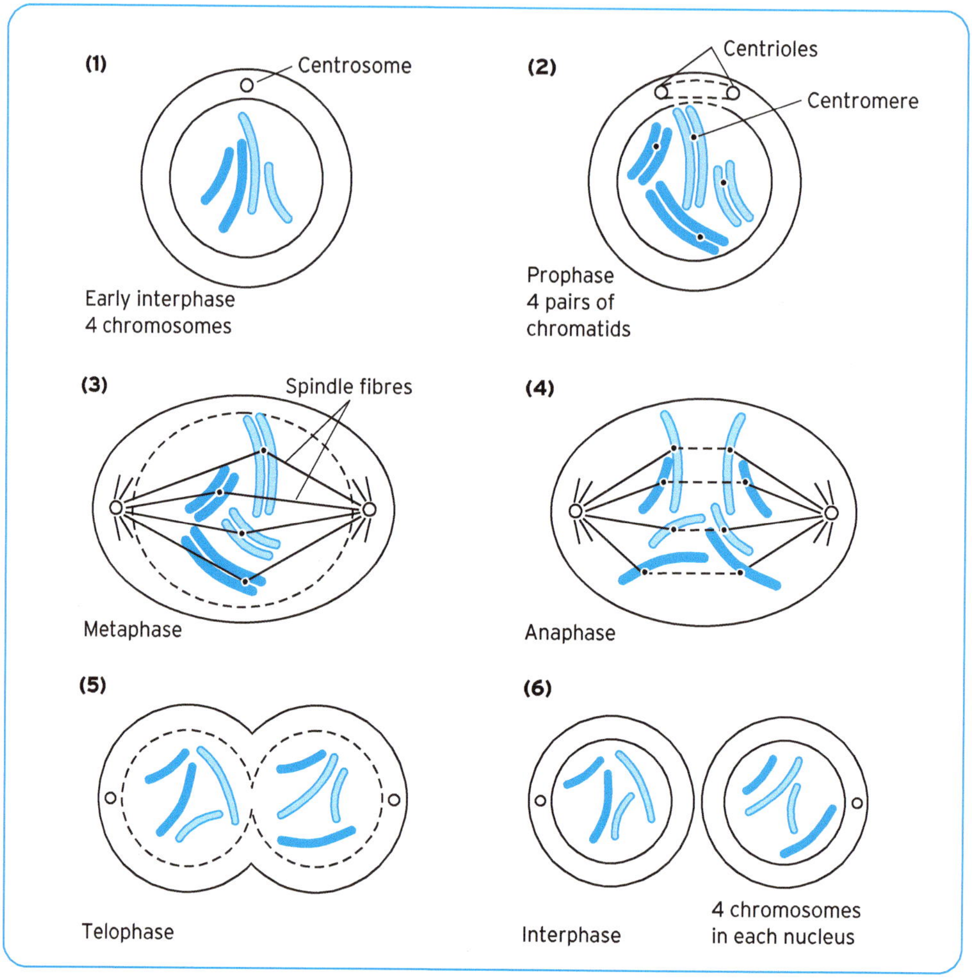

Figure 15.7
Mitosis. (From Sheeler P. (1996) *Essentials of Human Physiology*, 2nd edn. Dubuque: Wm. C. Brown.)

and fibres form between structures called **centrioles**. Centrioles are normally found adjacent to the nucleus in a region called the **centrosome**, but in prophase the centrioles move to opposite poles of the cell. The fibres that form between them are referred to as **spindle fibres**.

Metaphase: during this stage, chromosomes become attached along the centre of the spindle fibres at a position called the equatorial plate.

Anaphase: this stage is characterised by splitting of the centrosomes so that 'sister' chromatids separate and begin to move to opposite ends of the parent cell. From this point, each chromatid is regarded as a separate chromosome.

Telophase: in this stage, the DNA of both sets of chromosomes begins to uncoil and form thread-like chromatin again. The mitotic spindle disappears and a nuclear membrane forms around both sets of chromosomes.

Cytokinesis: cell division is completed when the cytoplasm of the parent cell is divided between the two newly forming cells.

In view of this sequence of events, we can summarise mitosis as the process of cell division that occurs in somatic cells and that leads to the production of two diploid daughter cells. Two important points about mitosis are that it is a controlled process and that only the right number of cells is produced for normal growth or replacement of dead cells. Sometimes, however, the process does not proceed normally, as Practice point 15.1 makes clear.

Practice point 15.1

Cancer

Cell division is normally a well-regulated process, so that the rate of production of new cells is adequate for the purposes of growth and repair. Sometimes, however, cells escape the normal controlling mechanisms, and a **neoplasm** (new growth) results. Neoplasms can produce unpleasant effects through a number of mechanisms, including the compression of vital structures such as nerves and blood vessels. Such effects are referred to as **space-occupying lesion effects**. Neoplasms are sometimes referred to as tumours, and they are of two kinds.

Benign neoplasms consist of cells that resemble those from which they arise, while the cells of **malignant neoplasms** are highly abnormal. As well as space-occupying lesion effects, malignant tumours spread out and invade adjacent structures in a way that resembles the spreading of a crab's legs. For this reason, malignant tumours are often referred to as **cancers**. You may wish to find out more about the difference between benign and malignant neoplasms.

We have seen that mitosis is the process of cell division that takes place in somatic cells. Gametes (sex cells) are produced in the gonads (reproductive organs) by a different process, which is explained below.

Meiosis

Cell division in the **gonads** (reproductive organs) takes place by **meiosis** - a different process from mitosis in somatic cells.

- ***What is the reason for this difference?***

To answer this question, recall that gametes differ from somatic cells in having only 23 chromosomes rather than 23 pairs of chromosomes. Meiosis is a process whereby only one of each homologous pair is distributed to each gamete. For this reason, meiosis is said to be a reduction division. In fact, meiosis involves two divisions. Before the first division, DNA replication takes place in a similar way to mitosis. The first meiotic division results, therefore, in two diploid cells. The second meiotic division takes place without additional DNA replication, and so the final result is four haploid cells. Meiosis is clearly a more complicated process than mitosis, but each stage is given the same name as in mitosis; a Roman numeral is added in order to indicate whether the first or second division is being referred to (prophase I, prophase II, etc.). The details of meiotic division are not given here, but the key events that take place in prophase I are explained.

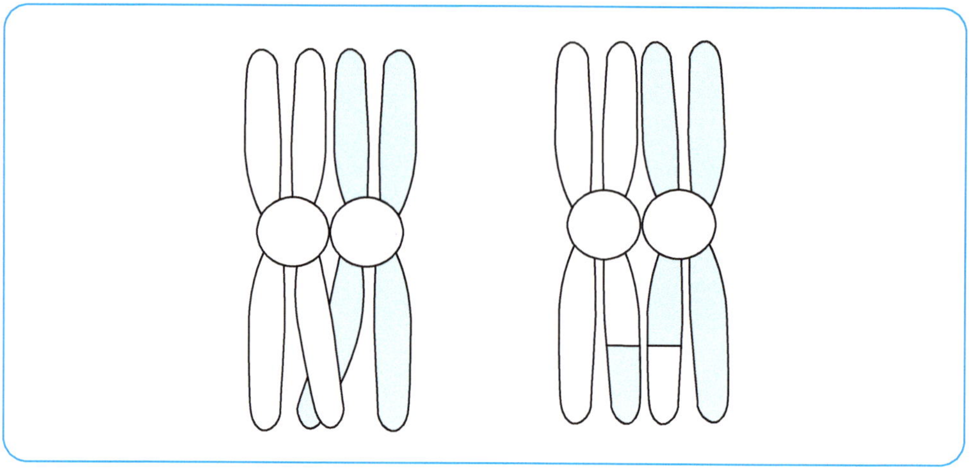

Figure 15.8
Crossing over.

Key events in prophase I

Certain events occur in prophase I that do not occur in prophase of mitosis. In prophase I, chromosomes thicken and shorten. They then arrange themselves in homologous pairs, each individual chromosome consisting of two chromatids. For this reason, when a homologous pair joins together, the structure that is formed is referred to as a **tetrad** (meaning four). It is worth remembering that one member of a homologous pair is derived from the mother and the other from the father. Following tetrad formation, pieces of DNA are exchanged between homologous pairs in a process referred to as crossing over (Figure 15.8).

- ***What is the significance of crossing over?***

Remember that gametes possess only 23 chromosomes rather than 23 pairs. Crossing over ensures genetic variability by ensuring that each gamete receives chromosomes that contain a combination of maternal and paternal genetic information.

In-text review

- ✔ Genetics is the study of heredity.
- ✔ The genetic information of a cell is contained within its nucleus.
- ✔ Chromosomes are structures that are present in the nucleus and formed from tightly coiled deoxyribonucleic acid (DNA).
- ✔ The bases in DNA are arranged in triplets (codons) that form a code for protein synthesis.
- ✔ There are 23 pairs of chromosomes in human somatic cells and 23 chromosomes in human gametes.
- ✔ Somatic cells divide by mitosis, a process that leads to the formation of two diploid daughter cells.
- ✔ Gametes are the result of a meiotic division, a process that results in the formation of four haploid daughter cells.

Protein synthesis

No matter what job a protein does, all proteins are made up of chains of simple molecules called **amino acids** joined together by chemical bonds called **peptide bonds**. We have already noted that DNA is a code for protein synthesis, but you may wonder why this is important. Proteins form essential components of our body. Some proteins, such as **collagen**, are of structural importance; **actin** and **myosin** are the contractile proteins of muscle; and other proteins are referred to as functional and perform the roles of **enzymes**, **hormones** and **antibodies**. In essence, the way in which our bodies function is due to proteins of one kind or another. Consequently, whatever controls protein synthesis ultimately determines our physical characteristics and body function.

So, then, the code for protein synthesis is located within the nucleus; we consider next how it is employed to make protein. First, we return to RNA - in fact to three forms of this nucleic acid: ribosomal RNA (rRNA), messenger RNA (mRNA) and transfer RNA (tRNA).

Ribosomal RNA (rRNA)

Proteins are synthesised in cytoplasmic organelles called **ribosomes**. Ribosomes are made of **rRNA**, which is synthesised in the nucleus and enters the cytoplasm via nuclear pores. Ribosomes are made of two subunits (a large subunit and a small subunit), and these join together before protein synthesis takes place.

Messenger RNA (mRNA)

In essence, **mRNA** is a copy of a DNA gene that is made in the nucleus in a process referred to as **transcription** (literally, 'copying'). mRNA then leaves the nucleus via a nuclear pore and enters the cytoplasm. This copy of the genetic code forms the instruction for protein synthesis that is read by a ribosome. You probably now understand why this form of RNA is described as a 'messenger'. In effect, mRNA acts as a messenger from the nucleus to the ribosome.

Transfer RNA (tRNA)

tRNA molecules consist of three nucleotides, the base sequence of which is referred to as an anticodon. Each tRNA molecule picks up a specific amino acid and functions as a means of transferring it to a ribosome, where protein synthesis takes place in a process called **translation**.

In describing the three types of RNA, the processes of transcription and translation have been mentioned. We now move on to explain these processes in more detail.

Transcription

Remember that transcription is the process by which mRNA is synthesised in the nucleus. The first stage of this process is the separation of DNA base pairs so that the double helix unwinds, just as it does before replication. Only one of the strands of DNA is involved in mRNA synthesis, however, and this is referred to as the **sense strand**. The other strand is referred to as the **antisense strand**. As the DNA double helix unwinds, the bases of mRNA nucleotides pair with the corresponding DNA nucleotides in the manner shown in Figure 15.9. In this way, a single strand of mRNA is assembled alongside the sense strand.

The process does not begin and end at random. Remember that certain DNA codons perform the role of identifying the point at which a gene begins (start codons) and others the point at which it ends (stop codons). Consequently, mRNA synthesis begins with a start codon and ends with a stop codon. In addition, recall that although the bases adenine, guanine and cytosine are common to both DNA and RNA, DNA alone has thymine and RNA alone has uracil.

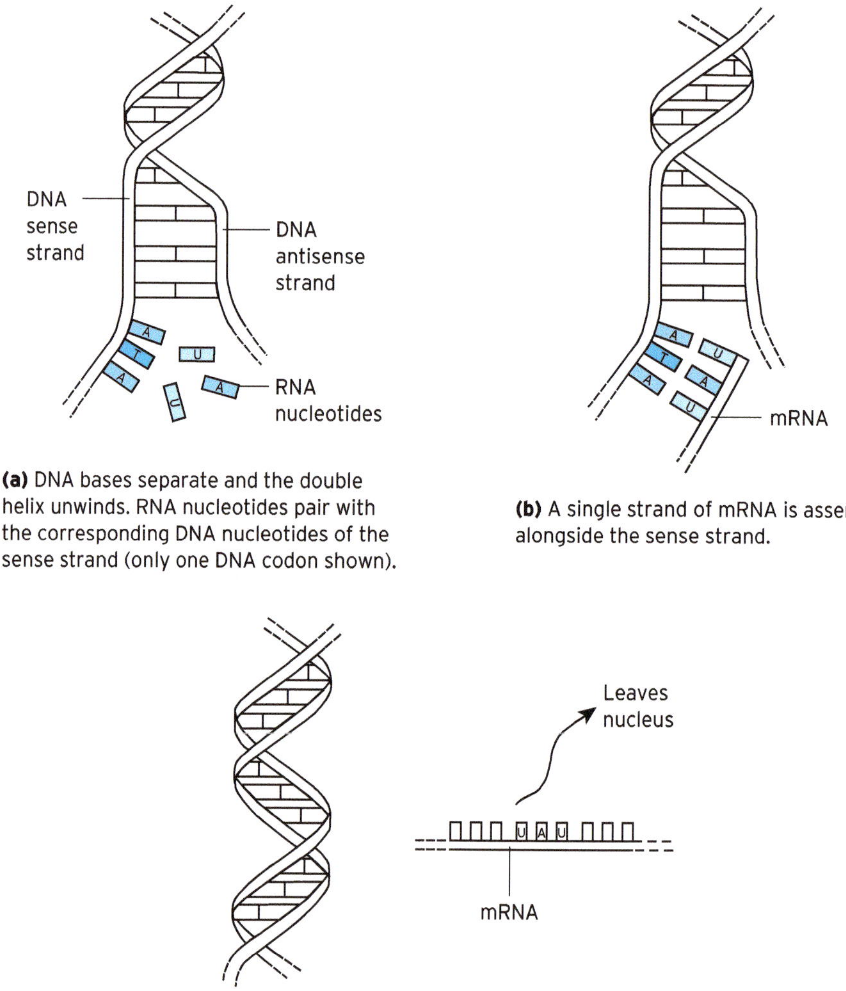

(a) DNA bases separate and the double helix unwinds. RNA nucleotides pair with the corresponding DNA nucleotides of the sense strand (only one DNA codon shown).

(b) A single strand of mRNA is assembled alongside the sense strand.

(c) An mRNA strand is completed and leaves the nucleus via a nuclear pore. The double helix of DNA is restored.

Figure 15.9
Transcription.

- ***If a DNA codon contained the bases ATA, what would be the corresponding mRNA codon?***

The correct answer is UAU.

- ***What now happens to the mRNA strand?***

Once an mRNA strand has been completed, it leaves the nucleus via a nuclear pore and enters the cytoplasm.

Translation

In the cytoplasm, a ribosome becomes attached to an mRNA strand at a start codon and the process of translation begins. We might summarise this process by saying that the code in the form of a sequence of bases in mRNA is translated into a sequence of amino acids in a protein chain. During translation, the ribosome moves along the length of the mRNA molecule from the start codon to the stop codon. This process is shown in Figure 15.10.

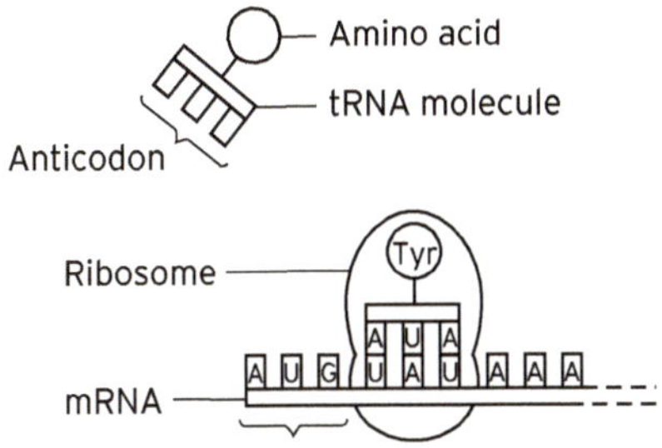

(a) The ribosome has reached the first codon after the start codon (UAU). A tRNA molecule with a corresponding anticodon (AUA) becomes attached. This tRNA molecule carries the amino acid tyrosine (Tyr).

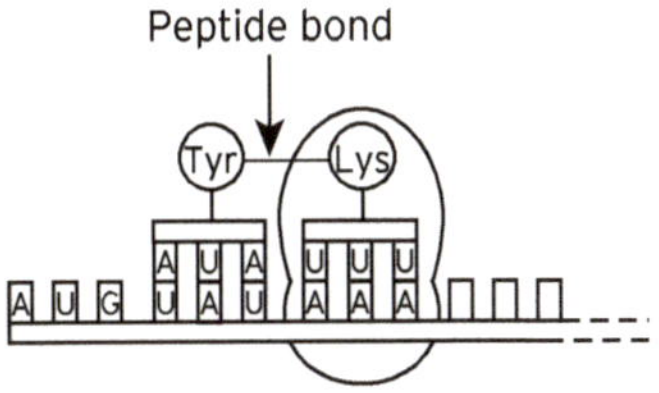

(b) The ribosome moves along to the next codon (AAA). A tRNA molecule with a corresponding anticodon (UUU) becomes attached. This tRNA molecule carries the amino acid lysine (Lys). Tyrosine and lysine become joined by a peptide bond.

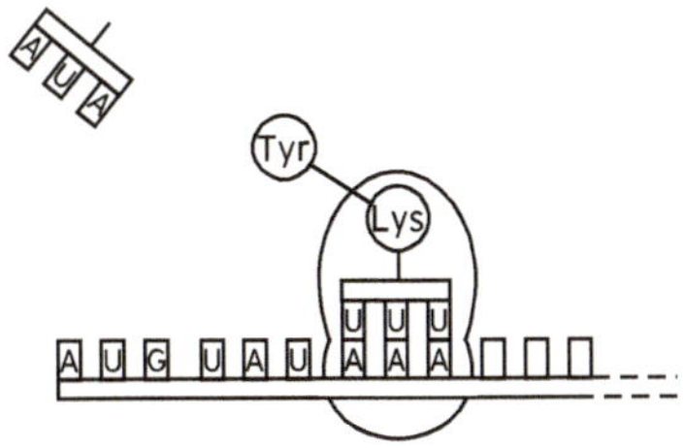

(c) The first tRNA molecule leaves the ribosome and becomes free to pick up another tyrosine molecule. The ribosome will now move on to the next codon.

Figure 15.10
Translation.

Let us imagine that the ribosome has reached the first codon after the start codon - UAU in Figure 15.10. At this point, a tRNA molecule with the corresponding anticodon (AUA) becomes attached to the mRNA molecule. Remember that each tRNA molecule carries a specific amino acid. The tRNA molecule with the anticodon AUA carries the amino acid tyrosine. The ribosome now moves along the mRNA strand and a second tRNA molecule becomes attached. At this point, the amino acids of the first and second tRNA molecules are joined by a peptide bond. The first tRNA molecule then leaves the ribosome and becomes free to pick up another amino acid, while the ribosome moves on to the third codon, where the process is repeated. In this way, the code for the synthesis of a specific amino acid is read by the ribosome until a stop codon is reached. At this point, the manufacture of the new protein is complete.

Thus far, we have been dealing with what might be termed the building blocks of genetics - nucleic acids. We have also examined processes such as translation that occur in the cell. We now move on to consider the impact of these processes on people - that is, inheritance.

Genetic inheritance

The nature of genetics is such that much of its study seems scientific and rather distanced from people. The reality is quite different, as you will see as we consider inheritance. Initially we do this using examples unrelated to illness, before proceeding to consider some common genetic diseases.

The position that a gene occupies on a chromosome is referred to as a **locus** (plural **loci** - the English word 'location' comes from the same origin). Genes that occupy the same loci on homologous chromosomes are said to be **alleles** or allelic genes. Alleles code for the same trait, such as eye colour; however, they do not necessarily code for the same expression of that trait. For example, one allele may code for blue eyes and the second allele for brown eyes. When both alleles code for the same expression of a trait, the individual is said to be **homozygous** for that trait. If alleles code for different expressions of a trait, then the individual is said to be **heterozygous**. The genetic makeup of an individual - that is, which genes are possessed - is termed the **genotype**, while the expression of the genes is termed the **phenotype**.

- ***In the case of the heterozygous individual, which of the two alleles is expressed?***

When one allele is expressed fully over another, that allele is said to be **dominant**, while the allele that is not expressed at all is said to be **recessive**. Characteristics that are expressed by dominant genes can be observed in both the homozygous dominant state (possessing two dominant alleles) and the heterozygous state (possessing one dominant allele and one recessive allele), while characteristics that are expressed by recessive genes can be observed only when an individual is homozygous recessive (possessing two recessive alleles). When referring to genotypes, it is customary to identify each gene using a single letter. This is given as a capital letter in the case of a dominant gene and as a lower-case letter for a recessive gene. The simplest cases are those in which a characteristic is determined by only two alleles of a single gene present on an autosome (non-sex chromosome) - that is, simple autosomal inheritance.

Simple autosomal inheritance

Consider the example of dimples in cheeks, the presence of which is determined by a dominant gene. Let D stand for the dominant (dimples) gene and d the recessive (absence of dimples) gene. Table 15.1 gives the possible genotypes and phenotypes in this case.

Table 15.1 The simple autosomal inheritance of the dimples in cheeks gene.

Genotype	Phenotype
DD (homozygous dominant)	Dimples present
Dd (heterozygous)	Dimples present
dd (homozygous recessive)	Dimples absent

Recessive genes express certain traits - flat feet are an example. Let D stand for the dominant (normal arches) gene and d stand for the recessive (flat feet) gene.

- ***What are the possible genotypes and phenotypes in this case?***

Check your answer against Table 15.2.

Table 15.2 The simple autosomal inheritance of flat feet.

Genotype	Phenotype
DD (homozygous dominant)	Normal arches
Dd (heterozygous)	Normal arches
dd (homozygous recessive)	Flat feet

In Table 15.3, a number of normal human traits and genetic diseases are listed according to whether the gene concerned is dominant or recessive.

The punnet square

If we had to work out which genes a child might inherit from two parents of known genotype, it would be rather easy to mix up in our minds the possible letter combinations. It is much easier if we write down the genotypes of the parents, but we can make matters simpler still

Table 15.3 Phenotypes expressed by dominant and recessive genes.

Phenotype due to the expression of dominant genes (DD or Dd)	Phenotype due to the expression of recessive genes (dd)
Normal skin pigment	Albinism
Freckles	Absence of freckles
Ability to roll tongue into a U shape	Inability to roll tongue into a U shape
Normal arches	Flat feet
Dimples in cheeks	Absence of dimples
Unattached earlobes	Attached earlobes

by using the Punnet square. This is a simple device consisting of a square divided into four boxes. The possible alleles derived from the father are placed to the left of the square and the possible alleles derived from the mother are placed above the square. In order to work out the possible genotypes of the parents' children, the alleles of the parents are combined in turn. Suppose we take the case of parents of whom both are heterozygous for the dimples gene (Dd). Remember that this gene is dominant, and so both parents have dimples. The use of the Punnet square in this case is demonstrated below:

	D	d
D	DD	Dd
d	Dd	dd

- ***What are the possible genotypes and phenotypes of the children?***

They are DD (dimples present), Dd (dimples present) and dd (dimples absent).

- ***What is the probability of the parents in the above example having a child with dimples?***

It is three out of four, or 75%. The probability of having a child without dimples is thus 25%.

Incomplete dominance

Incomplete dominance is the condition that exists when both alleles are expressed in the heterozygous state. The inheritance of hair texture is a good example. In this case, the individual who is homozygous for the curly hair gene has curly hair and the individual who is homozygous for the straight hair gene has straight hair.

- ***What is the phenotype of the heterozygous individual?***

The heterozygous individual has an intermediate hair texture - that is, wavy hair.

Multiple allele inheritance

Although only two alleles are inherited for each gene, that does not necessarily mean that only two alleles exist. In some cases, there are multiple alleles, such as the ABO blood group system. Early attempts at blood transfusion were sometimes successful, but at other times they were disastrous and the recipient of the blood died. It was not until the ABO blood group system was discovered that it became possible to select only blood from individuals whose **erythrocytes** (red blood cells) were compatible with the proposed recipient. Compatibility depends upon the **antigens** (chemical groups on the surface of the erythrocyte) that an individual possesses. There are only two antigens - the alpha antigen (α) and the beta antigen (β).

Table 15.4 Determination of ABO blood group.

Alleles possessed		Antigens possessed	ABO blood group designation
I^A	I^A	α	A
I^A	i	α	A
I^B	I^B	β	B
I^B	i	β	B
I^A	I^B	α and β	AB
i	i	None	O

- ***Is there an allele that codes for each of these antigens?***

Yes - one allele (I^A) codes for the alpha antigen and another allele (I^B) codes for the beta antigen. There is a third allele (i), however, that codes for 'no antigen'. The alleles I^A and I^B are co-dominant genes, while i is recessive.

- ***Are we now in a position to work out the different antigen combinations?***

Yes - but remember that each individual will possess only two alleles - one on each homologous chromosome. The possible antigen combinations and blood group designations are given in Table 15.4.

Let us now use a Punnett square to answer a question.

- ***What is the probability of a child of blood group O being born to heterozygous parents of blood group A?***

To answer this question, first note the genotypes of the parents. Since they are both heterozygous for the blood group A, they must have the genotype I^Ai. We can now use a Punnett square to work out the possible genotypes of the children, as shown below:

	I^A	i
I^A	I^AI^A	I^Ai
i	I^Ai	ii

There is a probability of one in four children (25%) born to the above parents having blood group O (ii).

Polygenic inheritance

When several genes control a trait, the term **polygenic inheritance** is used. Examples of polygenic inheritance traits include eye colour, hair colour and skin colour. In the case of skin colour, there are three separate genes involved, and each has two alleles: Aa, Bb and Cc. The genotype AA, BB, CC leads to a very dark-skinned phenotype and the genotype aa, bb, cc leads to a very light-skinned phenotype. Suppose two such individuals were to have children.

- ***What would be the possible phenotypes?***

Once again we need to draw a Punnet square.

	abc	abc
ABC	Aa, Bb, Cc	Aa, Bb, Cc
ABC	Aa, Bb, Cc	Aa, Bb, Cc

In this case, all the children would have a skin tone of intermediate darkness.

Inheritance of sex

We have already seen that all ova and 50% of spermatozoa carry an X chromosome, while the remaining 50% of spermatozoa carry a Y chromosome. We can illustrate the inheritance of sex using a Punnett square.

	X	X
X	XX	XX
Y	XY	XY

On this basis, 50% of children should be male and 50% female. It is important to point out, however, that chromosomes determine genetic sex. Initially, both male and female embryos develop identically until about seven weeks after fertilisation. After this time, genes present on the sex-determining region of the Y chromosome (SRY) are responsible for initiating male development. When the SRY is absent, the embryo continues to develop physiologically as a female despite possessing a Y chromosome.

Thus far, we have considered examples of the genetics of physical features, such as eye colour and blood group. We next consider diseases that have a genetic basis.

Genetic disease

Cystic fibrosis (simple autosomal recessive)

Cystic fibrosis is often used as an example of an autosomal recessive disorder since it is relatively common, affecting about one in 2000 live births. It is not necessary to know a great deal about a genetic disorder in order to understand how it is transmitted. You may be interested to learn, however, that the gene of importance in this case codes for protein that regulates the movement of chloride ions (Cl^-) across epithelial membranes that line airways, ducts and hollow organs. On initial examination, this appears to be a rather insignificant function, but when the defective gene is present the affected individual has serious health problems, some of which are outlined in Practice point 15.2. For the time being, let us consider the case of a child with cystic fibrosis being born to parents, neither of whom has the disease. Let D stand for the (dominant) normal gene and d for the (recessive) cystic fibrosis gene.

Practice point 15.2

Cystic fibrosis

The gene of importance in this case codes for a protein that regulates the movement of chloride ions across epithelial membranes. These are the membranes that line airways, ducts and hollow organs. Patients with the abnormal gene produce thick mucus; an effect of this early in life is bowel obstruction. In the respiratory system, the mucus has the effect of making sputum difficult to cough up; people with cystic fibrosis require daily chest physiotherapy. Even when this is performed, they are predisposed to serious lung infections. Over a period of years, the lungs become damaged and the patient may experience heart failure. For this reason, people with cystic fibrosis may ultimately undergo combined heart and lung transplantation.

- ***What are the genotypes of the parents?***

To answer this question, remember that since the defective gene is recessive, the disease is present only in homozygous recessive individuals (dd); the child in the above example must have inherited defective genes from both parents. Since neither parent has the disease, however, they must both be heterozygous (Dd).

- ***What term is used to describe individuals who possess a single recessive gene for a disease?***

They are referred to as carriers. They possess the defective gene, but since the gene is recessive the disease is not expressed in the heterozygous state. Carriers can, of course, pass the gene on to their children, as the above case shows. The Punnet square helps us to explain the above example more fully:

	D	d
D	DD	Dd
d	Dd	dd

Parents who have a child with cystic fibrosis often ask the question 'What is the chance of having another child with the disease?'

- ***What answer would you give?***

If you have checked the Punnett square, you should realise that it is 25%. There is the same probability of having a normal child and a 50% probability that a child will be a carrier.

Note that although cystic fibrosis is an autosomal recessive disease, it is relatively common. It is a common misconception that recessive traits are rare and dominant traits common, but this is not the case. In the section below, we briefly explain Huntington's disease as an example of an autosomal dominant disease. You might not have encountered this disease during your training - or even heard of it. There are two reasons for this. The disease is indeed uncommon, and most patients are encountered in the mental health context, since a major manifestation of Huntington's disease is dementia.

Huntington's disease (simple autosomal dominant)

This disease occurs even when a single defective gene is inherited - that is, it is an example of autosomal dominant inheritance. Huntington's disease involves a progressive degeneration of the nervous system, the symptoms of which include depression, chorea (involuntary dance-like movement) and dementia. Not all genetic diseases are evident at birth, and in the case of Huntington's disease the manifestations do not become evident until the third or fourth decade. You might like to imagine what you would feel like to discover that a loved one is developing dementia in his or her thirties or forties. What kind of support might the affected family require?

Having considered a recessive trait and a dominant trait, you have probably anticipated that the next section deals with a co-dominant trait - and indeed it does. Sickle cell anaemia is not included just to complete the picture, however. It has been chosen because it is a significant genetic disease affecting a particular ethnic group, and it is important in a study of genetics to reflect the multicultural nature of our society. You may be surprised to learn that up to 25% of Africans carry the sickling (abnormal) gene, but usually in the heterozygous (less serious) state.

Sickle cell anaemia (co-dominance)

Remember that co-dominance (incomplete dominance) is the condition that exists when both alleles are expressed in the heterozygous state. Sickle cell anaemia (sickle cell disease), which affects individuals of African and Caribbean descent, is a good example. This condition results from a gene defect that causes an abnormality of the red blood cell pigment **haemoglobin**. This molecule is important in oxygen transport, since oxygen binds to it to form **oxyhaemoglobin**. When the defective gene is present in the homozygous state, the abnormal haemoglobin produced precipitates within red blood cells, which, as a consequence, become sickle-shaped. Abnormally shaped red blood cells have a shorter lifespan than normal red blood cells, and **anaemia** (reduced number of red blood cells) results. In the heterozygous state, normal and abnormal haemoglobin is produced, and therefore the tendency for red blood cells to sickle is less. This leads to a milder form of the condition, referred to as **sickle cell trait**.

The normal gene is usually designated Hb and the sickling gene as Hb^S. Let us now consider the case of parents, both of whom have sickle cell trait and who are, therefore, heterozygous (Hb^AHb^S).

- ***What are the probabilities of the following children being born?***
  (a) Unaffected child.
  (b) Child with sickle cell trait.
  (c) Child with sickle cell disease.

In order to answer this question, you will need to draw a Punnet square. If you have done this correctly, you will see that the answers are (a) 25%, (b) 50% and (c) 25%. If you are unsure about this, check your Punnet square against the one given below:

	Hb^A	Hb^S
Hb^A	Hb^AHb^A	Hb^AHb^S
Hb^S	Hb^AHb^S	Hb^SHb^S

Of course, such genetic considerations can appear removed from nursing, until one begins to think how genetic problems affect health. The effects of sickle cell anaemia are explained in Practice point 15.3.

Practice point 15.3

Sickle cell anaemia

For much of the time, the patient with sickle cell disease is quite well. The disease is characterised, however, by episodes of severe illness called **sickling crises**, especially in childhood. These episodes may be brought on by physical stressors such as dehydration, exposure to cold and infection, but sometimes they occur for no obvious reason. When a sickling crisis occurs, possible manifestations are pain, pyrexia (elevated temperature), **anaemia** and **jaundice**.

Pain

Sickle-shaped blood cells clump together and get stuck in small blood vessels, preventing normal blood flow, which causes pain. This occurs in the hands, arms, legs, back and abdomen and should be treated with **analgesics** (pain-relieving drugs). It is best, although not always possible, to avoid conditions that bring on a crisis.

Pyrexia

Infections often produce pyrexia, and the patient's temperature should be measured (see Chapter 9). A person with sickle cell disease is at risk of developing severe infections, especially pneumococcal pneumonia. For this reason, penicillin is taken **prophylactically** (preventatively).

Anaemia

Sickle-shaped erythrocytes are fragile and have a shortened lifespan. For this reason, the patient may be anaemic (reduced erythrocyte numbers/reduced amount of haemoglobin in the blood). It is especially important for the patient to maintain an adequate intake of the B group vitamin folic acid, found in leafy vegetables, which is required for the manufacture of erythrocytes (see Chapter 7). In a severe crisis, it may be necessary for the patient to receive a blood transfusion in order to restore the normal numbers of erythrocytes.

Jaundice

When damaged erythrocytes are destroyed in the body, a pigment called **billirubin** is released. This is quite normal, but the early death and destruction of sickle-shaped cells means that there is an excess of billirubin in the body, and the skin and **sclera** (white) of the eye take on a yellow tinge; this is called jaundice. Eventually, the body processes the excess pigment, but looking for yellowing of the skin and the sclera is an important assessment measure.

Sex-linked disorders

Thus far, the traits and disorders that we have considered have been the result of genes carried on autosomes. These traits and disorders affect males and females equally. We now turn to sex-linked disorders, which affect males rather than females and in which a defective recessive gene is carried on an X chromosome.

Sex-linked disorders are probably best demonstrated by **haemophilia** A. The term 'haemophilia' literally means 'blood love', and it is applied to conditions in which blood coagulation is impaired and there is a tendency to bleed severely following injury (or even spontaneously). Haemophilia is caused by the absence of one of a number of chemical substances called **clotting factors**. In the case of haemophilia A, clotting factor VIII is missing. The defective gene responsible is carried on the X chromosome and this is usually designated X′ in order to distinguish it from a normal X chromosome. The genotype of haemophiliac males is, therefore, X′Y.

- ***Why, when the defective gene is recessive, do males with the genotype X′Y develop haemophilia?***

In order to answer this question, first note that X and Y chromosomes are not homologous in the true sense. The Y chromosome is only about a third of the size of the X chromosome and lacks some of the genes that are present on the X chromosome, including the gene for the production of factor VIII. Consequently, in the male with the X′Y genotype, the defective gene is not masked by a normal (dominant) gene on the Y chromosome. In contrast, females with the genotype X′X possess a normal (dominant) gene on the second X chromosome, and so the defective (recessive) gene is not expressed; such females are, however, able to pass on the defective gene and so are referred to as carriers.

- ***What about females with the genotype X′X′?***

The X′X′ genotype usually results in spontaneous abortion early in pregnancy, and so affected individuals are not encountered.

- ***Use a Punnett square to work out the possible genotypes and phenotypes of children born to parents of the genotypes XY and X′X.***

	X′	X
X	XX′	XX
Y	X′Y	XY

The possible genotypes and phenotypes are X′X (carrier female), XX (normal female), X′Y (haemophiliac male) and XY (normal male).

Chromosomal abnormalities

Thus far, we have considered abnormalities of specific genes. In contrast, chromosomal abnormalities (aberrations) affect the whole of a chromosome or a significant part of it. The most familiar is probably **Down's syndrome**, in which there are three copies of chromosome number 21 (**trisomy 21**). This defect results from either a failure of homologous chromosomes to separate in the first meiotic division or a failure of sister chromatids to separate in the second meiotic division. Such a failure is referred to as **non-disjunction** and results in a gamete that possesses both copies of chromosome number 21. The oocyte is most commonly affected. When fertilisation by a normal spermatozoon takes place, the child inherits three copies of the twenty-first chromosome. The characteristics of Down's syndrome include low IQ, poor muscle tone, short stature, protruding tongue and **epicanthal** folds (folds of skin over the inner junction of the eyelids).

In-text review

- ✔ Transcription is the synthesis of mRNA from the sense strand of DNA.
- ✔ Translation is the process by which proteins are synthesised.
- ✔ Translation occurs when anticodons of tRNA molecules pair with the codons of mRNA and amino acids carried by tRNA are joined together by peptide bonds.
- ✔ The patterns of genetic inheritance may be described as simple autosomal (dominant and recessive), co-dominance (incomplete dominance), multiple allele inheritance, polygenic inheritance and sex-linked inheritance. The following are examples:

Inheritance	Example
Simple autosomal (recessive)	Cystic fibrosis
Simple autosomal (dominant)	Huntington's disease
Co-dominance	Sickle cell anaemia
Multiple allele	ABO blood group
Polygenic	Colour of eyes, hair and skin
Sex linked	Haemophilia A

- ✔ The possible combinations of alleles inherited from parents of known genotype can be demonstrated using a Punnett square.

Summary

The early parts of this chapter dealt with the science of genetics, including the structure of the nucleic acids DNA and RNA. Covering such material is not an end in itself - the aim is to understand the genetic basis of disease. In a general science textbook such as this, only a few genetic conditions, such as cystic fibrosis, have been considered. Previously, these have been thought of as incurable and difficult to treat. In the working lives of you who use this book, however, there will be advances in the treatments available, particularly in genetic engineering (the science of altering the genotype of individuals). The gene responsible for cystic fibrosis was identified some years ago, and it is hoped that scientists will develop ways of incorporating normal genes into individuals with such genetic disease.

Summary points

- Chromosomes are structures that are present in the nucleus and formed from tightly coiled deoxyribonucleic acid (DNA).
- The bases in DNA are arranged in triplets (codons) that form a code for protein synthesis.
- There are 23 pairs of chromosomes in human somatic cells and 23 chromosomes in human gametes.
- Somatic cells divide by mitosis, a process that leads to the formation of two diploid daughter cells.
- Gametes are the result of a meiotic division, a process that results in the formation of four haploid daughter cells.
- The synthesis of mRNA from the sense strand of DNA is referred to as transcription.
- The synthesis of protein that occurs when the anticodons of tRNA molecules pair with the codons of mRNA is referred to as translation.
- The patterns of genetic inheritance may be described as simple autosomal (dominant and recessive), incomplete dominance (co-dominance), multiple allele inheritance, polygenic inheritance and sex-linked inheritance.
- The possible combinations of alleles inherited from parents of known genotype can be demonstrated using a Punnett square.

Self-test questions

1 Which of the following statements are true?
(a) Chromosomes are visible throughout the lifecycle of the cell.
(b) Chromatin is present within the cytoplasm of a cell.
(c) Chromosomes are formed from tightly coiled DNA.
(d) Histones are formed from DNA.

2 Which of the following statements are true?
(a) Gametes possess 23 pairs of chromosomes.
(b) Somatic cells possess 22 pairs of autosomes.
(c) Somatic cells possess one pair of sex chromosomes.
(d) Gametes possess one sex chromosome.

3 Which of the following statements are true?
(a) DNA consists of a single strand of nucleotides.
(b) RNA contains the base uracil.
(c) RNA consists of a single strand of nucleotides.
(d) DNA contains the base uracil.

4 Which of the following statements are true?
(a) Mitosis occurs in somatic cells.
(b) Meiosis leads to the formation of four haploid cells.
(c) Mitosis leads to the formation of two haploid cells.
(d) Tetrad formation occurs in prophase I of meiosis.

5 Which of the following statements are true?
(a) A triplet of DNA bases is referred to as a codon.
(b) A tRNA molecule contains three nucleotides.
(c) A triplet of mRNA bases is referred to as an anticodon.
(d) An mRNA molecule consists of three nucleotides.

6 Which of the following statements are true?
(a) Transcription is the process by which mRNA is synthesised.
(b) The DNA strand involved in mRNA synthesis is referred to as the antisense strand.
(c) The process that leads to the synthesis of protein is referred to as transformation.
(d) The nucleus is the site of protein synthesis.

7 Match the term on the left with the appropriate description on the right.

(a) Alleles	(i) Non-sex chromosomes
(b) Autosomes	(ii) Genes that code for the same trait
(c) Ribosomes	(iii) Proteins associated with DNA
(d) Histones	(iv) The sites of protein synthesis

8 What is the probability in simple autosomal recessive inheritance of the birth of a child with a trait when the parents are heterozygous for this trait?
(a) 25%.
(b) 50%.
(c) 75%.
(d) 100%.

9 What are the possible combinations of alleles of children born to parents with the blood groups AB and O? (Hint: use a Punnett square.)
(a) I^Ai, I^Ai, I^BI^B, I^BI^B.
(b) I^Ai, I^Ai, I^Bi, I^Bi.
(c) I^Ai, I^Ai, I^Ai, I^Ai.
(d) I^AI^A, I^BI^B, I^AI^B, ii.

10 Match the genetic diseases on the left with the appropriate descriptions on the right.

(a) Cystic fibrosis	(i) Simple autosomal dominant
(b) Haemophilia A	(ii) Simple autosomal recessive
(c) Huntington's disease	(iii) Incomplete dominance
(d) Sickle cell anaemia	(iv) Sex-linked

Further study/exercises

1 Describe the health problems experienced by individuals with cystic fibrosis and identify their nursing needs.

Madge S. (2002). Cystic fibrosis. *Professional Nurse*, 17(6), 343-4.
Ratjen F. and Doring G. (2003). Cystic fibrosis. *Lancet*, 361(9358), 681-9.
Cystic Fibrosis Trust website: www.cftrust.org.uk/index.jsp
NHS Direct: www.nhsdirect.nhs.uk/index.asp
Online Health Encyclopaedia Cystic Fibrosis: www.nhsdirect.nhs.uk/en.aspx?ArticleID=118

2 Outline the role of the genetic counsellor.

Crouch D. (2005). It's a bridge between science and people. *Nursing Times*, 101(7), 24-5.
Gulland A. (2001). Dealing with the facts of life. (Role of genetic counsellors.) *Nursing Times*, 97(36), 26-7.
Harrison S. (1995). Viewpoint. Practice tips: in the genes shop. *Nursing Standard*, 10(8), 50.
Visser A. and Bleiker E. (1997). Genetic education and counselling. *Patient Education and Counselling*, 32(1-2), 1-7.

16

Microbiology

Learning outcomes

After reading the following chapter and undertaking personal study, you should be able to:

1 Identify four types of microorganism and describe their characteristics.

2 Explain how bacteria are identified.

3 Describe various host-microorganism relationships and relate these to health and illness.

4 Identify the routes by which microorganisms enter the body and relate these to clinical practice.

5 Identify potential sources of infection and mechanisms of transmission of microorganisms with particular reference to clinical practice.

6 Describe how cross-infection can be prevented, especially in the health-care environment.

7 Describe the response of the body to infection.

8 Define immunity and distinguish between innate and acquired immune mechanisms.

9 Explain the process of immunisation and relate this to health.

10 Describe how in clinical practice samples of microorganisms are obtained for examination in the microbiology laboratory and outline the tests that are performed there.

11 Distinguish between cleaning, disinfection and sterilisation and describe the role played by each in the prevention of infection, with special reference to the hospital environment.

12 Describe how infections are managed and the role of antibiotics.

13 Explain antibiotic resistance and outline the ways in which it may be avoided.

Introduction

Microbiology is the study of organisms that are not visible to the naked eye (**microorganisms**) - that is, they can be examined only with the aid of a microscope or, in the case of the smallest microorganisms, with an electron microscope. When we think of microorganisms, we probably think of those that cause disease (**pathogens**). Indeed, as this chapter is being completed, the first UK bird death (a swan) caused by the H51N strain of bird flu has just been reported, and the British government has decided to continue culling badgers in an experiment to determine the effect of badgers on **tuberculosis** (TB) in cattle. Add to these examples the ongoing **AIDS** (acquired immune deficiency syndrome) **pandemic** (worldwide epidemic) and frequent reports of hospital superbugs, and one wonders whether there is space in the tabloids for any other news.

Many microorganisms, however, are not pathogens, and some microorganisms fulfil important roles in the environment. For example, many microorganisms live on dead and decaying matter (**saprophytes**) and fulfil an important recycling function in the environment; some soil bacteria produce nitrogen-containing compounds required by plants, while other microorganisms are involved in the production of foods such as cheese and yoghurt. Even our fight against pathogens depends upon microorganisms, since **antibiotics** are derived from them.

- ***So where should our study begin?***

Perhaps we should describe how microorganisms are named.

Naming microorganisms

In most cases, a convention is followed in the naming of microorganisms. Before this is explained, perhaps we should point out that all life on earth is divided into five kingdoms.

- ***Can you name any of the five kingdoms?***

You should have no difficulty naming the animal and plant kingdoms; you might also have given fungi too. The remaining two kingdoms are **monera** and **protista**. Each kingdom is subdivided into groups, until finally the name of the individual species is given. It is not necessary to learn the different subgroups, but it helps to understand the convention applied to the naming of species. This convention is referred to as **binomial nomenclature**, since two names are used to identify each organism. The names are given in Latin and understood by scientists the world over. For example, humans are *Homo sapiens* - which means 'wise man'. Whether the human race is wise is debatable - the point is that the names used in the binomial system do have a meaning that is an attempt to say something about the characteristics of the organism being referred to. Note that by convention, Latin is italicised and only the first name starts with a capital.

- ***Not so difficult, then - have a go at* Felis domesticus. *What species is this?***

Did you work out that it is the domestic cat? Microorganisms are given their names in a similar way, for example *Streptococcus faecalis*. In this case, the first name tells you something about the shape of the organism - we explain this later.

So what does faecalis tell us?

You should have no difficulty working out that it tells you that the organism is found in the faeces. This convention is followed in most but not all cases, as you will see later. In addition, the name is sometimes abbreviated, so that *Streptococcus faecalis* becomes *Strep. faecalis*. Although this is perfectly acceptable, in this introductory text abbreviated forms have been avoided in order not to be confusing. Having explained how microorganisms are named, we now introduce the four types of microorganism: **bacteria**, **viruses**, **fungi** and **protozoa**.

Bacteria

In Chapter 15, the structure of a typical animal cell was described. It was noted that the entire contents of the cell are collectively referred to as **protoplasm** and that this is separated from the outside by the **cell membrane**. Within the cell is located the **nucleus**, which contains the cell's genetic information. The contents of the nucleus (**nucleoplasm**) are separated from the rest of the cell contents (**cytoplasm**) by the **nuclear membrane**. Within the cytoplasm are a number of other structures that perform specific functions for the cell. For example, **mitochondria** generate energy and **ribosomes** make protein. These structures are referred to collectively as **organelles** - a term that means 'little organs'. We could say that just as organs such as the heart perform specific functions for the body, so organelles perform specific functions for the cell. This type of cell structure is described as **eukaryotic**.

So what about bacteria – are they similar?

Bacteria are single-celled microorganisms, some of which are similar in size to human cells. For example, the bacterium that causes **anthrax** (*Bacillus anthracis*) is about 6 µm (6 microns - there are 1000 microns in a millimetre) in diameter and the **erythrocyte** (red blood cell) is about 8 µm (8 microns) in diameter. That is where the similarity ends, however. Bacteria have a cell structure that is unlike that of any other organism.

What are the differences between bacterial cells and eukaryotic cells?

The cytoplasm of bacteria contains no compartments or distinct organelles, genetic material is not membrane-bound in a nucleus and the cell is bound by a special structure called the **cell wall**. This type of cell structure is described as **prokaryotic**. We are perhaps used to referring to the animal kingdom and the plant kingdom, but bacteria are so different that they have a kingdom of their own called monera - it means 'alone'.

Types of bacteria

So, bacteria are microscopic and difficult to see, but are they hard to find?

Actually, no. Bacteria cover the surfaces of our bodies and are present in the food we eat; some bacteria are present in the high temperatures of sulphur springs and others deep within the polar ice. It is almost impossible to find a place where there are no bacteria, although the special measures taken in hospital operating theatres do limit their numbers somewhat.

- ***If bacteria thrive in diverse environments, there must be different types.***

Yes, this is certainly true, and we divide bacteria into a number of groups. The first divisions are the **archaebacteria** and **eubacteria**. Archaebacteria are distinct from all other types of bacteria, in terms of both their structure and the chemical processes that take place within them. Archaebacteria are found in some of the most hostile environments on earth, but they are not of medical significance, so we shall not consider them further. All other bacteria are classified as eubacteria, or true bacteria. This division is divided further into three groups based upon the mode of nutrition - this classification sounds strange, but we do the same with people when we ask 'Are you vegetarian?' **Photoautotrophs** (light self-feeders) contain **chlorophyll** (the green pigment found in plants) and use energy in the form of light to produce nutrients. **Chemoautotrophs** (chemical self-feeders) derive the energy they need from inorganic molecules, such as ammonia (NH_4); for example, nitrifying bacteria are found in root nodules of some plants (e.g. peas and beans) and convert ammonia into nitrates - a form of nitrogen that can be used by other plants. Organic gardeners make use of this by planting peas or beans in the season before other vegetables that require a lot of nitrogen. Finally, there are the **heterotrophs** (other feeders), which obtain their nutrients from organic molecules.

- ***Is there a purpose to describing this classification?***

First, it is probably helpful to understand that monera is a kingdom of diverse organisms that play important roles in the health of our planet. Not all bacteria cause disease; in fact, only some heterotrophs do so. Incidentally, you have probably also realised that, just like the bacteria that cause disease, humans are heterotrophs.

Identifying bacteria

A number of characteristics are used to identify bacteria, including appearance, staining reactions, metabolism and ability to form spores.

Appearance

The appearance of individual organisms is used as a means of identifying species. Four morphological (shape) forms exist (Figure 16.1) - **cocci**, **bacilli**, **vibrio** and **spirochaetes**.

Individual cocci are round, but groups occur together. In **diplococci**, the organisms are arranged in pairs. An example is *Neisseria gonorrhoeae* - the organism that causes **gonorrhoea**. Clusters of cocci are called **staphylocci** - an example is *Staphyloccus aureus*. This organism is part of the normal skin flora (organisms that normally live on the skin and cause no harm). Some members of this group, however, do also cause wound infections. In **streptococci**, the organisms are arranged in chains. Streptococci cause a wide range of infections, including sore throats.

Bacilli are rod-shaped organisms - the rods appear singly or in chains. A number of bacilli, such as *Salmonella enteritidis* and *Escherichia coli*, cause food poisoning.

Vibrio are curved bacteria - an example is *Vibrio cholerae*, which causes **cholera**.

Spirochaetes are spiral-shaped and include *Treponema pallidum* - the organism that causes **syphilis**.

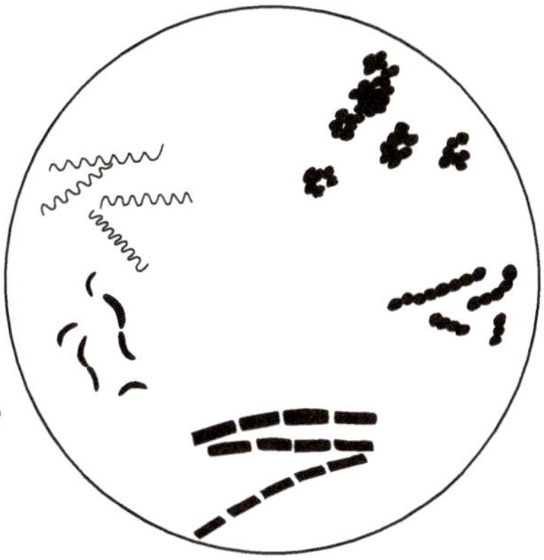

Figure 16.1
Four shapes of bacteria.

Staining reactions

The most important staining reaction is the **Gram stain**. A thin film of a specimen is smeared on to a glass microscope slide and stained with both violet and red dyes. Depending upon which dye is taken up, the organisms will appear purple (Gram-positive) or pink (Gram-negative). The difference in staining reactions reflects differences in the composition of the cell wall.

Metabolism

Like humans, some bacteria require the presence of oxygen in the environment. Such bacteria are called obligate **aerobes** - *Mycobacterium tuberculosis*, which causes tuberculosis (TB), is an example. Organisms that are unable to tolerate the presence of oxygen are called obligate **anaerobes** - *Clostridium tetani*, which causes **tetanus**, is an example. **Tetany** is a sustained muscular contraction that can have a number of causes. Since the toxins produced by *Clostridium tetani* cause tetany, the condition that results from infection by this organism is caused tetanus. If you have not heard of this condition, it is probably because immunisation against it is undertaken during childhood and it no longer causes the number of deaths that it once did.

Spore formation

Various Gram-positive species are able to form **spores**. In unfavourable conditions, the microorganism develops a protective capsule in which it lies in a dormant condition and is referred to as a **spore**. The spore is able to tolerate extremes of conditions, such as high temperatures, and is resistant to chemical disinfectants. The spore may remain dormant for many years, but when favourable conditions return it will 'germinate' and the organism will resume its active lifecycle. *Clostridium tetani* and *Bacillus anthracis* are examples of spore-forming organisms.

Reproduction of bacteria

The use of the term 'reproduction' here is a misnomer. Populations of bacteria increase when individual bacterial cells grow, duplicate their genetic material and divide into two in a process called **binary fission**.

- ***So if the first generation consists of only a single cell, the next will consist of two, the next four, the next eight, and so on?***

Exactly so, and provided that there is a continuous supply of nutrients, the rate of growth can be very rapid indeed. A new generation may be produced every 5 minutes, but more commonly every 30 minutes - 'slow coaches' may take several days. In the space of a few hours, a small number of bacteria could become many millions.

Viruses

Perhaps the first thing we should note about viruses is that they are too small to be seen with a light microscope. You might wonder how they could have been discovered at the end of the nineteenth century, long before the invention of the electron microscope. Scientists realised that viruses existed when they were able to show that some infectious agents passed through filters designed to trap bacteria. It also became clear that these agents could multiply only inside living cells and, therefore, scientists concluded that they must lack some of the apparatus required for reproduction. In part, we can say that they were right. In reality, however, viruses are not living organisms at all. Viruses do not have a cellular structure but consist instead of a core of **nucleic acid** (either DNA or RNA) and a protein coat or **capsid**. Because viruses cannot replicate themselves, they are dependent on the host to do this for them. Consequently, they are **obligate parasites** - they can exist only at the expense of another organism. Viruses are responsible for disease in both plants and animals; they also infect bacteria. A specific virus can infect only a specific species of organism; in a limited number of cases, more than one species may be infected. An obvious example is **human immunodeficiency virus** (HIV), which is thought to have been introduced to humans from African monkeys. Although HIV infection is extremely serious, many viral illnesses are minor and self-limiting, as explained in Practice point 16.1.

Practice point 16.1

Self-limiting viral infections

We have already noted that viruses are not living organisms. There is a very important point to be made about treating viral infections - if viruses are not alive, they cannot be killed. In fact, there are very few effective **antiviral agents** (drugs used to treat viral infections). It is just as well that many viral infections are minor and self-limiting - after a short period of illness, the body deals with the infection without any specific treatment. Perhaps you have visited the doctor with a sore throat but been given no treatment. This is because most sore throats are viral in nature and the prescription of antibiotics is not required.

- ***Couldn't the doctor prescribe antibiotics as a precaution?***

Since antibiotics do not shorten the length of a viral illness such as a sore throat, a cold or uncomplicated influenza (flu), it would serve no purpose to prescribe antibiotics. To do so would expose the patient to any complications that the antibiotics might cause. Excessive use of antibiotics may also lead to antibiotic resistance, as we discuss later.

- ***So how are self-limiting viral illness managed?***

Since the illness will resolve spontaneously, any treatment is given purely to alleviate symptoms. Think about a severe cold or influenza.

- ***What are the symptoms?***

Symptoms might include **pyrexia** (elevated temperature), discomfort such as headache or **myalgia** (muscle pain), lethargy, nasal congestion and cough.

- ***What would you advise the patient to do?***

Lethargy is easy to deal with - just rest. Pyrexia and discomfort can be alleviated by an **analgesic** (pain-relieving drug) that also lowers the temperature; **aspirin** and **paracetamol** are both good examples. (It is important to note, however, that although these drugs are readily available over the counter, there are restrictions on their use. A pharmacist will be able to give advice about the most suitable over-the-counter medicine, and the information leaflet enclosed with each drug should always be read before taking the first dose.) Cold remedies often include a decongestant to help with nasal congestion, although these drugs can also be bought separately; **pseudoephedrine** is a common example. **Pholcodine** is an example of an **antitussive** (suppresses cough), but such drugs should be used only if the cough is not productive (coughing up sputum).

- ***Think through why this is the case.***

If a patient is expectorating (coughing up sputum), the cough is serving a very important function - getting rid of the sputum. Suppressing the cough is clearly not a good idea in these circumstances - if sputum is not coughed up, then it may impair respiratory function, and congested respiratory passages are an environment in which bacteria can grow. Incidentally, secretions can be loosened and made easier to expectorate by old-fashioned steam inhalations.

- ***'I went to the doctor with a cough and a cold and he didn't prescribe any treatment. I didn't get better – in fact, I got worse. When I went back a week later, he gave me antibiotics, which cleared it up in a week. Why didn't he give me them to start with?'***

Does this sound familiar? It is unfortunately true that some viral infections resolve only slowly; perhaps the patient fails to rest and the illness worsens. A virus may cause the initial infection, but following this the patient also succumbs to a bacterial infection. It is to treat this that antibiotics are prescribed.

Viral replication

Viruses are the ultimate parasite, being completely dependent on their host in order to replicate. Think about this for a moment: A virus enters the cell of a susceptible organism, where the viral nucleic acid acts as a code for the host cell to make more viral nucleic acid and protein coats that are assembled into new viruses. These leave the cell and move on to infect other cells, perhaps being transmitted to a second individual, before the process begins once more. If this did the cell no damage, then it would probably be unnecessary to include it in this textbook, but unfortunately the host cells may die as a consequence of infection.

In addition, infection by a virus sometimes transforms a normal host cell into a cancer cell, and this is more serious than the viral infection itself. For example, the Epstein-Barr virus causes the illness **glandular fever**, which produces flu-like symptoms. In some cases, the illness is severe and the individual experiences a prolonged period of weakness. A small number of sufferers, however, subsequently develop a form of lymphatic cancer (**Burkitt's lymphoma**/syndrome).

Fungi

When we think of fungi, we probably think of the multicellular organisms we also call mushrooms. Fungi, however, are a kingdom of eukaryotic organisms, most of which feed on dead or decaying organic material (**saprophytes**) and play an important role as recyclers in our environment. Most fungi are multicellular, but some, such as yeasts, are unicellular. Some fungi are also parasites and feed on living organisms. Examples of the latter include **ringworm** (not a worm at all) and athlete's foot. Fungi are composed of slender filaments called **hyphae** (singular = **hypha**). A mass of hyphae is called a **mycelium**. Hyphae grow into a food source and secrete enzymes to break it down and release nutrients. Hyphae often form fluffy masses that we see on top of spoilt food, but some species also produce large reproductive structures that we recognise as mushrooms.

Most fungi reproduce both sexually and asexually. The kingdom is classified into four divisions. The first three divisions are based upon the characteristics of the sexual stages of reproduction. Although fungi in these three groups are important in the environment, they do not cause disease and so are not dealt with here. The fourth division includes all the species that are unable to reproduce sexually and are referred to as **imperfect fungi**. These reproduce by the production of spores and they include some important disease-producing fungi.

Protozoa

We now come to the final kingdom of organisms important in the study of human disease - the kingdom Protista. Protists are eukaryotic organisms; most are single-celled, but some are multicellular. The kingdom is divided into groups based upon which other organisms the protists resemble. **Algae** are plant-like protists, **slime moulds** are fungus-like protists and **protozoans** are animal-like protists. Members of the latter group interest us here, since they cause disease in humans. Protozoa are grouped into four phyla (groups), depending on how the organism moves. They are the **amoebas**, **flagellates**, **ciliates** and **sporozoans**.

Amoebas

In physiology, the movement of certain **leukocytes** (white blood cells) is referred to as **amoeboid** – meaning 'like an amoeba'. That's fine if you know what an amoeba is but not very clear if you don't. Amoebas are often described as shapeless single-celled organisms – but clearly every organism has a shape, so what is meant by this term? Amoebas are able to move by pushing out cytoplasm in one area and retracting it from another. As cytoplasm is pushed outwards it is thought to resemble a foot, but as the cytoplasm continues to stream forward the foot disappears. For this reason, the term **pseudopods** (meaning 'false feet') is used. Pseudopodia are important in both the nutrition and movement of amoebas. Amoebas engulf their prey by forming pseudopodia around the prey. The prey is then contained in a **vacuole** (fluid-filled sac) within the amoeba, whereupon enzymes digest the prey. The process is referred to as **phagocytosis** – a term that means 'cell eating' (Figure 16.2).

Amoebas are abundant in both fresh and salt water. Some cause disease, such as *Entamoeba histolytica*, which is responsible for amoebic **dysentery**. This disease occurs mainly in tropical and subtropical countries, where it causes diarrhoea. The infection may be acute or chronic and is transmitted to others by the ingestion of contaminated fruit, vegetables and water. The use of human faeces as a fertiliser is responsible for a high incidence in some regions. Dysentery is further explained in Practice point 16.2, which deals with travel health.

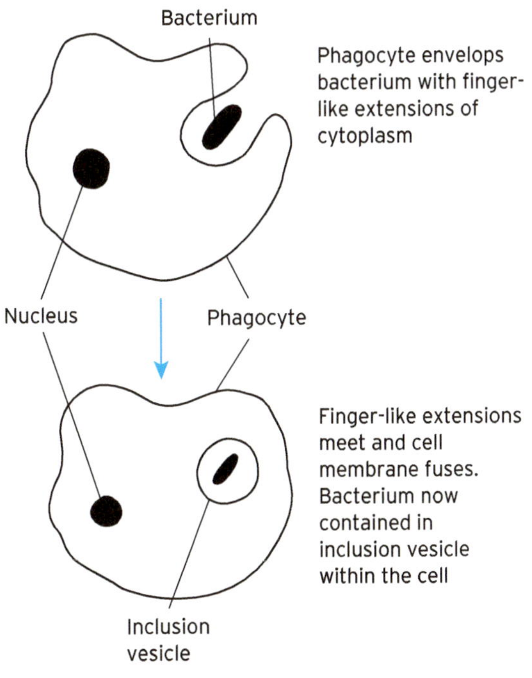

Figure 16.2
Phagocytosis.

Practice point 16.2

Travel health – dysentery

- ***Someone asks you for health advice regarding a holiday in the tropics. What would you say about dysentery?***

You might want to explain how dysentery is transmitted. In addition, many good travel health practices are common to a variety of illnesses, including drinking only boiled or bottled water.

- ***What about vegetables?***

You have probably worked out that you should avoid eating raw vegetables in the tropics, since they may have been grown in contaminated soil. You might think that fruit ought to be safe, but you cannot guarantee this. Fruit may have been washed in contaminated water, and there have even been cases of fruit being injected with water in order to make it look more appealing.

It would also be worth explaining what to do in the event of illness. The problem caused by diarrhoea is of fluid and electrolyte loss, and so the traveller should carry sachets of rehydration salts (available from a pharmacy).

Flagellates

This is a group of organisms characterised by the possession of at least one **flagellum** - a whip-like structure that is used for movement. The organism is propelled as the flagellum beats backwards and forwards. *Trypanosoma gambiense* and *Trypanosoma rhodesiense* are examples of flagellates that cause disease in humans - African **sleeping sickness**. The organism is transmitted by the tsetse fly after it has fed on the blood of an infected person. The symptoms caused by sleeping sickness include fever and skin eruptions, but in the longer term the blood-borne parasites may enter the **cerebrospinal fluid** of the brain, producing a chronic disease characterised by lethargy and drowsiness, hence its name. Eventually, sleeping sickness is fatal. Since insects transmit a number of tropical diseases, the use of insect repellents in tropical countries is important.

Ciliates

This group of protists gains its name from a Latin word meaning 'eyelash' - a reference to the hair-like **cilia** that cover the organism. Cilia beat in a coordinated way that enables movement. *Balantidium coli* is a ciliate that inhabits the intestinal tract of pigs and can cause dysentery in humans.

Sporozoans

Sporozoans are non-motile parasites with a complex lifecycle involving sexual and asexual phases and transmission from host to host by various species of insect. Of the diseases caused by sporozoans, **malaria** is the most important.

Malaria

Four members of the genus plasmodium cause malaria: *Plasmodium falciparum*, *Plasmodium vivax*, *Plasmodium malariae* and *Plasmodium ovale*. Malaria is characterised by intermittent pyrexia (raised temperature) with **anaemia** (reduced oxygen-carrying capacity of the blood) due to the destruction of erythrocytes (red blood cells). Symptoms can be diverse and severe, especially in malignant malaria (caused by *Plasmodium falciparum*), where capillaries can become obstructed by infected erythrocytes. Although the chances of dying from an attack of malaria are not large, the untreated disease is likely to take a chronic relapsing course. Malaria is a very widespread disease of the tropics, and as a consequence it accounts for the highest number of deaths worldwide of any single infectious disease.

The lifecycle of *Plasmodium*

Since malaria is so important worldwide, we spend some time describing the rather complicated lifecycle of the causative organism. In the first phase of infection (pre-erythrocytic phase - meaning that which occurs before erythrocytes are involved), the parasite is introduced into the blood through a bite by a female **Anopheles mosquito** (Figure 16.3). The sporozoans soon disappear from the blood, but they have not been killed. Instead, they have entered

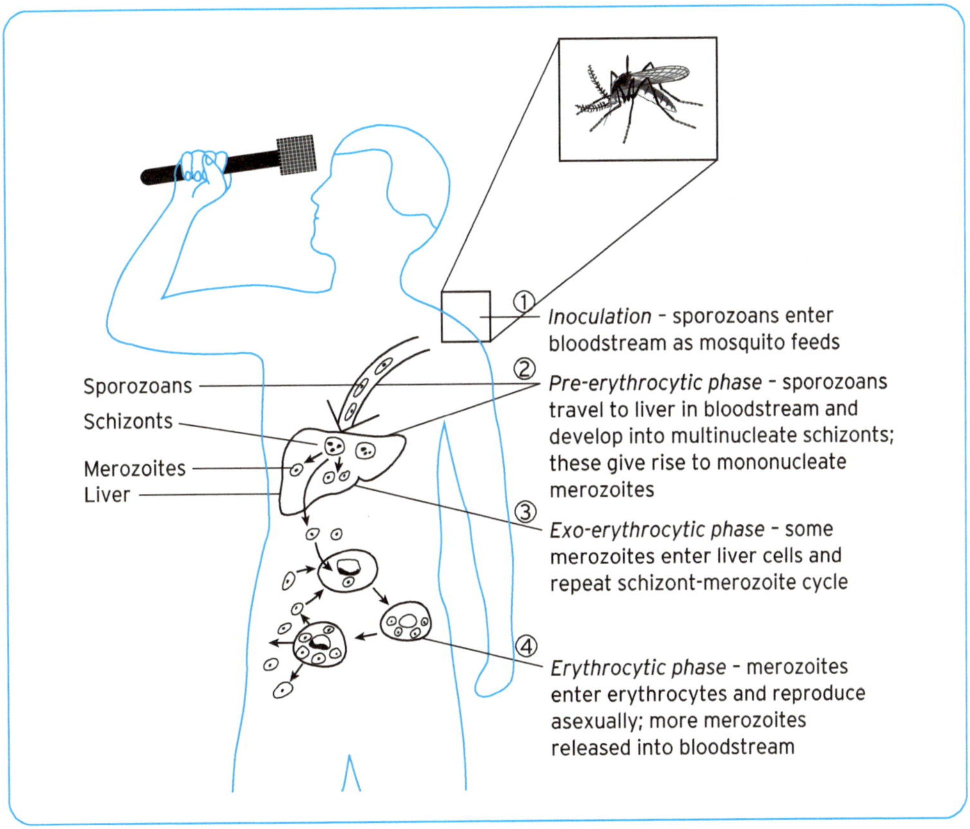

Figure 16.3
Lifecycle of the anopheles mosquito.

liver cells, where they develop into large multinucleate cells (cells with multiple nuclei) called **schizonts**, which give rise to small mononucleate (cells with a single nucleus) **merozoites**. In the next phase (exo-erythrocytic phase - meaning the phase that occurs outside erythrocytes), some merozoites enter other liver cells and repeat the schizont-merozoite cycle.

The main asexual phase is the erythrocytic phase, in which the merozoites enter erythrocytes and develop there. As you might expect, each stage of development through which the organism passes is given a further, difficult-to-pronounce name. It is sufficient to know, however, that the result of this development process is the release of even more merozoites into the blood, where they infect new cells.

- ***Is there a purpose to learning about these stages?***

The disappearance from the blood of the parasites in the first stage helps us to understand why the patient has no symptoms early on.

- ***So if someone has contracted malaria on holiday, when will they show symptoms?***

Unless the holiday is very long, the symptoms will probably not occur until they return home. A potential problem is that if health-care staff have not seen malaria before, a diagnosis may be delayed. For this reason, we have spent some time describing this disease.

- ***So what actually causes the sudden severe pyrexia?***

This occurs when merozoites are released into the blood in the erythrocytic phase. Incidentally, the exo-erythrocytic phase persists for a long time in *Plasmodium vivax* infection and accounts for relapses after the parasite has been eradicated from the blood.

- ***Why doesn't the body destroy the parasite?***

In its complex lifecycle, the parasite undergoes changes that enable it to repeatedly evade the immune system.

- ***So is that the whole of the lifecycle of the malaria parasite?***

Not quite. Some merozoites develop into sexual cells (**gametocytes**), but sexual reproduction does not take place in the human. The lifecycle is completed only when a female Anophyles mosquito feeds on the human's infected blood. In view of the significance of mosquitoes in spreading malaria, these small creatures feature strongly in malaria prevention measures outlined in Practice point 16.3.

Host–microorganism relationships

Before we consider infectious disease further, we ought to clarify some important terms. The term '**symbiosis**' refers to the close living association of two different species of organism. Symbiosis takes a number of forms. In **commensalism**, one species benefits from the association while the other neither benefits nor is harmed. The surface of our skin supports the growth of a range of bacteria, sometimes described as skin commensals or normal skin flora. Our skin forms an environment on which the organisms grow, but we experience neither harm nor benefit as a consequence. **Mutualism** refers to a close relationship in which both organisms

Practice point 16.3

Malaria prevention

Since Anophyles mosquitoes are the sole carriers of malaria to humans, prevention depends on effective anti-mosquito measures. These include the use of insecticides in houses and insecticide-impregnated mosquito nets over beds. Insect repellents may also be applied to the body. Mosquitoes require water to breed, and so the risk of being bitten is greater near rivers and lakes. At these places, it is best to cover up as much of the skin as possible. Having said this, it is not possible to avoid sites where mosquitoes can breed - they actually need very little water, and you may have seen native British mosquitoes emerging from small pools of water, such as rain butts and puddles.

The mainstay of prevention measures is drug treatment. There are three problems, however. The first is that drug resistance is common and different drug regimes are required, depending upon which country, or even which area within a country, is visited. In the UK, practice nurses usually give travel advice, and you may be interested in this role. In view of the seriousness of malaria, considerable responsibility is borne by the nurse when planning a course of drugs.

- ***Have you heard of any problems associated with malaria prophylaxis (prevention)?***

All drugs are capable of producing side effects, but some of the drugs used in malaria prophylaxis produce severe side effects. The side effects depend upon which drugs are used, but gastro-intestinal disturbance is common.

- ***What can be done about this?***

The worse thing that can happen is the patient stops taking the medication - after all, malaria is potentially fatal. Patients should be made aware of the side effects and of the importance of compliance with the regime. Gastrointestinal disturbance may be lessened if the drug is taken with food. If side effects are serious, it may be possible to take an alternative drug.

In order to be effective, malaria prophylaxis needs to be taken some weeks before and after the period spent in the high-risk area. Occasionally, patients leave the seeking of travel advice until late in their holiday plans, so that there is insufficient time to complete all the required preparation. Perhaps more often the patient returns home feeling well and then discontinues the prophylaxis prematurely.

benefit, but this kind of relationship does not exist in humans. The third type of relationship is **parasitism**, in which one organism benefits but the other is harmed. When the parasite is a microorganism, it is described as a pathogen and the harm done to the host is the disease.

It is probably worth pointing out that the above descriptions are not absolutely clear-cut. For example, the species *Staphylococcus aureus* is a skin commensal, but when a wound occurs *Staphlococcus aureus* may infect that wound. We could say that *Staphylococcus aureus* is taking the opportunity presented by the creation of the wound. In fact, that is the very expression used to describe what happens - we say that the organism is an **opportunist pathogen**. The important point here is that although *Staphylococcus aureus* is causing an illness (the wound infection), it does not need to do so in order to complete its lifecycle. It was already living and reproducing on the skin of the patient before the wound occurred, and at that point it was causing no harm. Compare this with a microorganism that cannot reproduce without causing disease; such organisms are called **obligate pathogens**. All viruses are obligate pathogens.

- ***So, then, does the presence of an organism not always mean that there is an infection?***

That is correct. An **infection** occurs when an organism is living and reproducing in or on the host's tissues and causing damage (disease). The host's body will respond to this in a number of ways, and we discuss this later. If the presence of an organism produces no response and causes no damage, we simply refer to **colonisation**.

- ***So colonisation is not a problem?***

Although colonisation may not be an immediate problem, it does result in a reservoir of microorganisms that may find their way to sites where they become opportunist pathogens. Consider a further example: Within our large intestines, we all carry *Escherichia coli*. At this location, it is a normal gut commensal, but *Escherichia coli* is capable of causing infection elsewhere. It may be transferred to the urinary tract and cause **cystitis** (infection of the bladder), or following ineffective handwashing it may be transferred to a wound or to food.

- ***So are all pathogens equally capable of causing disease?***

No - the ability of a pathogen to cause disease depends upon its **virulence**. Virulence varies between species and even between strains of the same species.

In-text review

- ✔ Microbiology is the study of organisms that are not visible to the naked eye (microorganisms).
- ✔ Life on earth is divided into five kingdoms: animals, plants, fungi, monera and protista.
- ✔ Organisms are named using binomial nomenclature - so called since two names are used to identify each organism.
- ✔ Animal cells are characterised by a eukaryotic cell structure whilst microorganisms may be prokaryotic or eukaryotic.
- ✔ Four types of microorganism are important in disease: bacteria, viruses, fungi and protozoa.
- ✔ Bacteria are identified on the basis of their appearance, staining reactions, metabolism and ability to form spores.
- ✔ The term 'symbiosis' refers to the close living association of two different species of organism.
- ✔ In commensalism, one species benefits from the association while the other neither benefits nor is harmed, e.g. the normal skin flora.
- ✔ In parasitism, one organism benefits from the association but the other is harmed. When the parasite is a microorganism, it is described as a pathogen and the harm done to the host is a disease.

The response to infection

Immunity is the body's ability to resist infectious disease; the system that controls immunity is called the **immune system**. The immune system is also involved in other functions, including the detection and destruction of cancer, but this is not dealt with here.

The immune system

Think for a moment about one of the systems of the body - the respiratory system, perhaps.

- ***What are its important structures?***

Your list probably includes the lungs and the upper and lower airways. It is not too difficult to think about the respiratory system, since the structures are large and easy to locate. The immune system is not so easy to picture. Its principal components are microscopic (e.g. cells in the blood) and it operates throughout the body - within structures of other systems, in fact. In order to explain how the body responds to an infection, some of the important components of the immune system are briefly described here.

Bone marrow

Blood-cell production (**haematopoiesis**) takes place in the red bone marrow of flat bones such as the sternum (breast bone). Among the cells produced are the **leukocytes** (white blood cells), which play an important role in immunity.

Leukocytes

Two groups of leukocyte exist: **Granulocytes** are so called because their cytoplasm has a granular appearance. The content of these granules determines the staining properties of three types of granulocyte. **Basophils** take up basic dyes ('phil' comes from '*philos*', meaning to love), **eosinophils** take up the acidic dye eosin and **neutrophils** show no dye preference.

Agranulocytes are leukocytes that do not possess granules. There are two types - **lymphocytes** and **monocytes**.

- ***What functions do the various leukocytes perform?***

Neutrophils are **phagocytes** that engulf microorganisms (phagocytosis) and destroy them with enzymes. Monocytes have the ability to be transformed into **macrophages** (literally, 'big eaters'), which have a considerable capacity for phagocytosis. There are a number of different types of lymphocytes, some of which are involved in the production of **antibodies** (**immunoglobulins** - an expression that means globular proteins of the immune system). Basophils produce **histamine** and eosinophils are involved in allergic reactions.

Thymus gland

The **thymus gland** develops beneath the sternum in foetal life and is involved in the development of a certain type of lymphocyte (**T lymphocyte** or T cell). Lymphocytes that are not processed in the thymus are referred to as **B lymphocytes** or B cells.

Immune mechanisms

Immune mechanisms are described as either **innate** or **acquired**.

Innate mechanims

The word 'innate' means 'inborn' or 'inbuilt', which is a very good description of a group of mechanisms that are the same in each member of a species. You might say that the body does not have to develop or 'learn' these defences. In addition, innate mechanisms do not adapt to the different microorganisms that the body encounters. For this reason, innate immunity is also referred to as non-adaptive. Innate immunity includes many different mechanisms - only some are described here, including physical barriers, chemical substances, **phagocytosis** and **inflammation**.

Physical barriers

The most obvious physical barrier is the skin on the outside of our body, which is several layers thick. The outer layer of skin is made up of tough dead cells, which are made waterproof by the substance **keratin**; this arrangement provides a barrier to the entry of microorganisms. After foetal life, we do not have to develop skin to protect us, and our skin does not change according to which microorganisms we encounter. The skin is then a good example of innate (non-adaptive) immunity.

Chemical substances

A number of chemical substances in the body help to prevent infection. One example is **hydrochloric acid** in the stomach - few microorganisms will survive this hostile environment. The skin is also acidic - **sebum**, which is secreted to keep the skin supple, contains **fatty acids**; the mildly acidic environment allows commensals to grow, but pathogens are inhibited. Not all protective chemicals are acidic, however - tears are protective of the eyes due to the presence of the enzyme **lysozyme**.

Phagocytosis

Neutrophils and macrophages are the body's phagocytes. The movement of these cells resembles that of an amoeba. When a microorganism is encountered, the cytoplasm is projected around it and the microorganism is engulfed (Figure 16.4). The microorganism is now contained within the phagocyte but surrounded by a section of the phagocyte cell membrane in a structure called a vacuole. Within the phagocyte cytoplasm are lysozomes that contain digestive enzymes. Lysozomes fuse with the vacuole and empty their contents into the vacuole. The microorganism within it is then digested before the vacuole moves to the edge of the cell and its contents are removed in a process called **exocytosis** (see Figure 16.4). Incidentally, pus is the accumulation of the end products of this microorganism-digesting process.

Inflammation

Think about what happens when a small wound occurs. Perhaps the wound is so small that you don't notice it at first. After a while, however, it starts to become more painful and the wound edges become red and swollen. If the wound is large enough, you might be able to feel that it is warmer than the undamaged tissue. We say that the wound is inflamed.

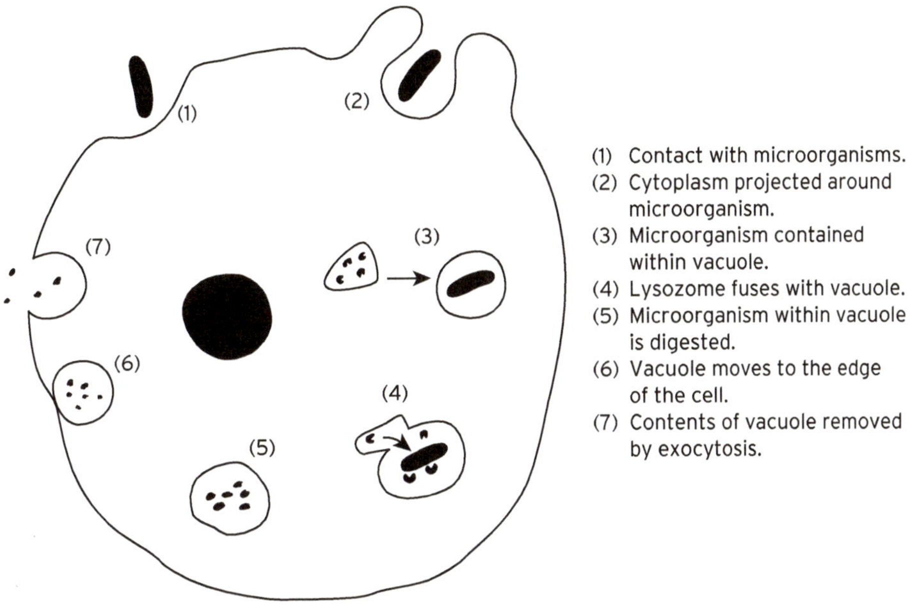

Figure 16.4
Stages of phagocytosis.

- ***So to begin with the wound is not very sore, but then something happens to increase the pain and to cause redness, swelling and warmth?***

Yes, that is correct - these changes are the body's response to injury rather than part of the injury itself.

- ***What purpose is served when the body's response to injury increases pain?***

One obvious effect is that the injured person starts to protect and guard the damaged tissue; if there was no pain, this would not occur. Inflammation is the response of the body to injury that serves to deliver important substances to the site of injury. When tissue is damaged, whether by a cut or damaged by a pathogen, substances are released from the affected cells. For example, **basophils** release **histamine**. These substances are **vasoactive**, meaning they have an effect on blood vessels - they cause the blood vessels to dilate.

- ***Presumably the dilation accounts for the redness and warmth of the wound edges?***

Exactly so - this redness is referred to as **erythema**. The smallest blood vessels (capillaries) become leaky, and fluid and cells are lost from the blood, causing swelling.

- ***Why is this important?***

It allows the phagocytes to appear in large numbers at the site of injury. In fact, phagocytes are attracted to move towards the chemical substances released at the site of injury in a process called **chemotaxis**.

Acquired immunity

- ***Have you suffered from chickenpox?***

This is an infectious disease that is usually contracted in childhood - most people will have had the disease before adult life.

- ***If you answered 'yes', do you worry about getting it again?***

The answer is almost certainly 'no'. You may have been so unconcerned that you have not thought to ask this question before. You are quite right to be unconcerned. The fact is that once people have had chickenpox, they become immune. This is clearly not because of some innate mechanism - after all, they did get the disease once. The immunity has been acquired - in fact, that is the name given to this type of immunity - **acquired immunity**.

- ***Does immunity to chickenpox extend to other infectious diseases?***

No - when people become immune to chickenpox, they do not at the same time become immune to other infectious diseases. For this reason, acquired immunity is also referred to as **specific** immunity.

There are two aspects of acquired immunity - **humoral** and **cell-mediated**. Cell-mediated immunity refers to the activity of specialist types of T lymphocyte, while humoral immunity refers to the production of **antibodies** (immunoglobulins). The word 'humour' refers to body fluids, such as blood, breast milk and saliva, but it is antibodies present in body fluids that account for acquired immunity. These two aspects of acquired immunity are interrelated, but in this basic text only the production of antibodies is explained. For further details, you are advised to consult a physiology textbook.

Before antibody production is described, the term '**antigen**' needs to be explained. Antigens are large chemical groups that appear on the surface of cells. They act as a kind of code that the immune system uses to distinguish between **self** and **non-self**. B lymphocytes bind to antigens on the surface of microorganisms, after which they begin to grow and multiply, resulting in two populations of identical cells or clones (Figure 16.5). One population called **plasma cells** produce antibodies (immunoglobulins) in great numbers, but after some time they die. Consequently, the antibody level also begins to fall.

- ***What do antibodies actually do?***

Antibodies inactivate antigens in a number of ways. For example, antibodies cause antigens to clump together to become more susceptible to phagocytosis.

- ***But if the antibody level declines after the first infection, how is the body protected against further infections?***

Remember that the multiplication of B lymphocytes creates two populations. The second population consists of **memory cells**. These do not produce antibodies straight away but are able to do so if the antigen in encountered a second time. You could say that the body 'remembers' the infection and how to produce antibodies to fight it. This explains why a person becomes immune to chickenpox after the first infection. Of course, the process is a little more complex than the simplified picture presented here. For example, different

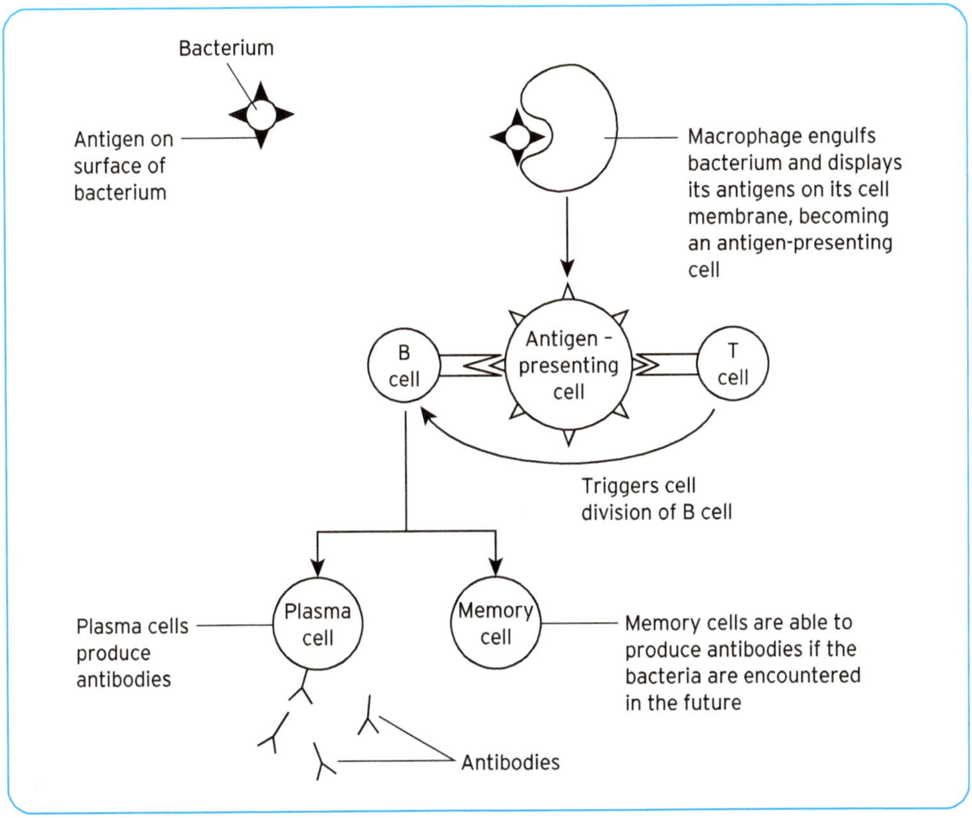

Figure 16.5
The production of antibodies.

types of T lymphocyte control the process. At this point in your studies, however, the above synopsis of acquired immunity will suffice.

● *Do health-care workers really need to know about acquired immunity?*

Perhaps we should ask some further questions. Recently, concerns about the safety of the MMR (measles, mumps and rubella) vaccination appeared in the media, with the result that many parents decided not to have their children immunised. Consequently, these children are exposed to the risks of some infectious diseases. You will not be able to answer questions about the safety concerns of MMR if scientists differ in their opinions, but could you explain what happens in the body following immunisation? In addition, on entering the health-care field, you were probably immunised against the serious blood-borne disease hepatitis B. Do you know what the risks of this disease are and why immunisation is effective? If not, how were you able to give consent to receive the immunisation? Whatever your answers to these questions, it is clearly important that all health-care workers have some level of understanding about acquired immunity for the reason that all are exposed to both the risks of infectious diseases and the immunisation against them. Immunisation is further explained in Practice point 16.4.

Practice point 16.4

Immunisation

In this section, we provide a brief explanation of immunisation so that you may have a basic understanding of how it is achieved. This understanding may help you to decide which immunisations you will consent to have yourself and give you the basis of a simple explanation for patients.

In the eighteenth century, people were highly anxious about contracting the infectious disease **smallpox**, since many people died from this. (The word 'pox' is the plural of 'pock', meaning pustule - a pus-filled skin lesion. Smallpox is a disease that produces small pustules - a descriptive name given at a time when the cause of infectious diseases was poorly understood.) Despite the fact that in the eighteenth century the cause of disease was not known, doctors did observe the effects of immunity - people who got smallpox and survived did not contract it again. Doctors made crude attempts at immunisation involving the inoculation of material taken from the skin lesions (pox) of sufferers. Here, the word 'inoculation' masks a rather unpleasant procedure - a knife deliberately contaminated with pus from a patient with smallpox was used to open a wound in the hitherto healthy subject. The obvious problem with this approach was that the inoculated person might very well contract smallpox and die.

If antigens of the causative organism of an infectious disease could be administered without the risk of the disease, then the recipient would develop immunity safely. You may be surprised to learn that some modern immunisations actually contain live organisms, but these have been cultured in such a way as to weaken them (**attenuated**). Other immunisations contain killed organisms or an altered form of the toxin produced by a microorganism called **toxiod** (tetanus).

Immunisations are usually administered by **intramuscular** (into muscle) or **intradermal** (into the dermis of the skin) injection. At some point, you might find it helpful to consult a nursing textbook to learn about correct injection techniques.

Virulence

Virulence is the name given to the characteristics of a microorganism that favour its survival in or on the host and its ability to cause disease. The factors that influence virulence include the ability to grow in or on the host, to evade host defences and to damage the host.

Ability to grow in or on the host

Nutrition

Some pathogens are able to synthesise certain nutrients, but to the greatest extent they obtain them from the tissues in which they live. The availability of nutrients may be one factor that determines whether an organism is able to live at a particular site. The **exudate** of a wound and an excess of pulmonary secretions both provide nutritious environments for bacterial growth.

Temperature

An organism is more likely to cause an infection if the host temperature is within its own optimal temperature range. Host susceptibility also varies with temperature. In everyday language, we recognise this by referring to upper respiratory tract infections as 'colds'.

pH

Most organisms grow within the pH range of the body's tissues. The slight acidity of the skin surface, however, deters some organisms, and the strongly acidic stomach contents offer some protection against swallowed organisms.

Other factors

There are a number of diverse examples that are not easy to fit into any classification. Consequently, a number of examples are given:

- Projections (**pili**) on the surface of *Neisseria gonorrhoea* enable the organism to adhere to the lining of the cervix and urethra.
- *Staphylococcus aureus* and *Streptococcus pyogenes* have receptors for **fibronectin**, a **glycoprotein** (molecule made up of a sugar and a protein) found on the surface of cells.
- *Staphylococcus epidermidis* produces a slime that enables it to stick to plastic such as intravenous **canulae** and giving sets.

Ability to evade host defences

The ability to evade host defences depends on many complex properties and so we deal with this only superficially. Some bacteria are able to resist phagocytosis (being engulfed by the body's defensive white blood cells), while others are engulfed but not subsequently destroyed. Resistance to phagocytosis is dependent upon the surface characteristics of the microorganism, such as the possession of a polysaccharide (type of carbohydrate) capsule.

Ability to damage the host

Occasionally, pathogens structurally damage the tissue that they infect. In most cases, however, damage is the result of the microorganism's biochemical activity - specifically, the production of toxins and enzymes. Toxins are bacterial products or constituents of the micro-organism itself that fall into one of two groups - **exotoxins** and **endotoxins**. Living bacteria (mainly Gram-positive organisms) produce exotoxins. Exotoxins diffuse into the surrounding tissue and are circulated in the bloodstream. They are highly toxic proteins that produce specific effects. Nonetheless, they are inactivated by heat and neutralised by specific antibodies. Endotoxins form part of the bacterial cell wall (typically of Gram-negative organisms) and are released only when the organism dies. They are non-specific in their action and are relatively heat-stable. Examples of toxin-producing organisms are given in Table 16.1. It should be borne in mind that some organisms that do not produce toxins nonetheless cause disease.

Table 16.1 Toxin-forming bacteria.

Exotoxin-forming organisms		Endotoxin-forming organisms	
Organism	Disease	Organism	Disease
Clostridium botulinum	Botulism	*Salmonella typhi*	Typhoid fever
Clostridium tetani	Tetanus	*Neisseria meningitidis*	Meningococcal meningitis
Corynebacterium diptheriae	Diptheria	*Shigella sonnei*	Dysentery

Table 16.2 Enzymes produced by bacteria.

Type of enzyme	Action	Example
Coagulase	Leads to formation of fibrin clot that protects organism from phagocytosis	*Staphylococcus aureus*
Fibrinolysin	Destruction of fibrin - assists in spread of microorganism	*Streptococcus pyogenes*
Hyaluronidase	Destroys hyaluronic acid that joins cells together - assists spread of microorganism	*Clostridium perfringens*
Collagenase	Breaks down collagen and destroys muscle	*Clostridium perfringens*
Lecithinase	Destroys lecithin, a component of cell membranes	*Clostridium perfringens*
Deoxyribonuclease	Breaks down DNA	*Clostridium perfringens, Streptococcus pyogenes*

Many pathogens produce disease by releasing enzymes that damage the body in some way. Table 16.2 gives some examples of enzyme-producing bacteria.

In-text review

- ✔ Immunity is the body's ability to resist infectious disease; the system that controls immunity is called the immune system.
- ✔ The immune system operates throughout the body within structures of other systems. Its principal components are microscopic (e.g. leukocytes/white cells in the blood).
- ✔ Immune mechanisms are described as either innate or acquired.
- ✔ Innate mechanisms are inbuilt and include physical barriers, chemical substances, phagocytosis and inflammation.
- ✔ Acquired mechanisms involve development of the ability to resist specific diseases following exposure to them.
- ✔ There are two aspects of acquired immunity - humoral and cell-mediated.
- ✔ Humoral immunity refers to the production of antibodies.

Sources of infection

Let us think back for a moment to the example of *Staphylococcus aureus*. Suppose a patient with this skin commensal is admitted to hospital after sustaining a serious wound - perhaps they have been in a road traffic accident. Subsequently, the wound becomes infected with *Staphylococcus aureus*. Let us now ask a rather obvious question.

- ***From where did the infecting organism come?***

It came from the patient's own skin - this is an example of **endogenous infection** (self-infection). Now imagine that the staff in the hospital ward wash their hands ineffectively and transfer the organism to another patient, who then develops a wound infection. This is an example of **exogenous infection**.

- *In everyday language, we use an alternative term for 'exogenous infection'. What is it?*

Perhaps you know that we normally speak of cross-infection. Sources of cross-infection can be objects in the environment, members of staff and other patients. For example, organisms may be spread by a bar of soap or on dust particles floating in the air. Incidentally, we also refer to hospital-acquired (**nosocomial**) infection.

Routes of entry

- *So how do organisms enter the body?*

Even if you have not studied science before, you should be able to come up with some good answers to this question. Depending on how you classify them, there are four routes of entry: inhalation, ingestion, inoculation and congenital transmission.

Inhalation

Perhaps it is not surprising that the organisms that enter the body via inhalation tend to cause illnesses of the respiratory tract - think about coughs and colds. **Tuberculosis** is another, much more serious respiratory disease. In addition, many childhood illnesses enter the body via inhalation, including measles.

- *So what is actually inhaled?*

If an individual exhales forcibly or coughs, they will release droplets of respiratory secretions into the air. We do not mean visible droplets - these are far too large to travel far or be inhaled. In addition, large droplets will be readily filtered in the nose and airways. Large droplets may fall to the ground, however, and the organism subsequently may be circulated in the air on small dust particles. In contrast, droplets less than about 5 μm (5 microns) in diameter can travel in the air and may reach the lower airways when inhaled.

- *So how might droplet inhalation be prevented?*

It is good practice to provide a patient with a respiratory tract infection with tissues and a disposal bag to place them in when used. The bag should be changed regularly. If a patient is expectorating (coughing up) sputum, then a sputum pot with a lid should be provided. This should be labelled with the patient's name and date - then it will not be given to another patient by mistake and can be replaced daily.

Ingestion

Organisms that cause infection of the gastrointestinal tract enter the body by being ingested in contaminated food or water. Examples include *Salmonella enteritidis*, which causes salmonella food poisoning. The common term 'food poisoning' is something of a misnomer, since 'poisoning' implies toxins but no toxin is involved in this case (a better term would be **salmonellosis**). *Salmonella enteritidis*, present in contaminated food, is ingested; the organisms multiply in the body, causing dairrhoea, vomiting and fever. Salmonellosis is an example of a **zoonotic infection** - zoonoses are diseases that are transmitted from animals to humans. *Salmonella enteritidis* is found in domestic livestock, although it often fails to give rise to any symptoms in its animal hosts. It may also be present in eggs.

- ***How could salmonellosis be prevented?***

Salmonella enteritidis grows readily at room temperature and will survive light cooking. Consequently, meat (especially chicken) and eggs should be cooked thoroughly. The organism survives freezing, although refrigerator temperatures will slow the growth rate. Cross-contamination is possible, and so cooked food and raw meat should be kept separately. Some people become asymptomatic carriers - that is, they carry the organism but they have no symptoms. The danger then is that inadequate handwashing during food preparation may result in the organism being transferred to previously uncontaminated food.

Inoculation

In this context, the term **inoculation** refers to transmission across a breech in the skin or mucous membranes. Sometimes, the term 'injection' is used instead, and indeed needles are often involved. Two examples are infection of an intravenous cannula site (drip site) by *Staphylococcus epidermidis* and transmission of hepatitis B virus through needle-sharing by drug addicts. A wound, including a surgical incision, is another example, as is inoculation by the mouth parts of biting insects. A mosquito transmits the plasmodium that causes malaria, while the trypanosome that causes African sleeping sickness is transmitted by the tsetse fly. Perhaps a less obvious example is anal intercourse and the transmission of human immunodeficiency virus (HIV); the recipient of secretions from an infected individual is at great risk because of trauma to the anal mucosa.

In the above cases, it is not possible to make general comments about prevention of infection - specific interventions are required. Hospital policies specify the frequency with which intravenous cannulae and giving sets should be changed, and staff should always wash their hands before attending to such therapies. Needle-exchange programmes, where drug addicts can replace used needles with sterile needles, are an attempt to reduce the incidence of blood-borne cross-infection in this group of people. The use of condoms helps to reduce the likelihood of transmission of HIV, and there are specific drug regimes for malaria prevention.

Congenital transmission

Although the placenta has features that help to prevent microorganisms from crossing it, some microorganisms are passed from mother to foetus. This type of transmission is sometimes referred to as 'vertical'. Examples include transmission of *Treponema pallidum*, the spirochaete that causes syphilis, and rubella virus, which causes German measles. Human immunodeficiency virus (HIV) may be contracted in this way, but transmission is more likely by contact between the foetus and maternal blood at birth.

Methods of transmission

Airborne spread

Inhalation has already been described as a possible route of entry for respiratory organisms that cause respiratory illness. Other organisms, however, are also airborne. Think about the following question:

- ***Why were nurses traditionally taught to make beds?***

It is certainly true that some patients spend a good deal of time in bed, and comfort measures such as clean and unwrinkled sheets are important. But when changing sheets, why were nurses taught to loosen a dirty sheet, fold it carefully and drop it into a linen skip without letting it touch the uniform or bed curtains?

- ***Why not pull it from the bed and carry it down the ward?***

Have you worked out that the purpose of the rather old-fashioned, formalised way of making a bed was to prevent shed skin cells from being shaken into the atmosphere or deposited on the uniform or bed curtains? Although these precautions were directed at airborne spread, they were not aimed at respiratory illness.

- ***So what organism were they directed against?***

The above precautions were meant to reduce the spread of skin commensals such as *Staphylococcus aureus*. Such traditional nursing tasks have rather gone out of fashion, but there is a sound rationale for them. The emergence of resistant strains of *Staphylococcus aureus* means that measures to prevent transmission should be emphasised once again.

Under the heading of airborne spread, we should mention the organism that causes Legionnaire's disease - *Legionella pneumophila*. This organism is a problem in contaminated water, but it is dealt with here since ingestion is not a problem. Look at the name of the organism.

- ***What does 'pneumophil' tell us?***

'Pneumo' refers to the lungs and 'phila' is derived from '*philos*', meaning to love. So *Legionella pneumophila* is an organism that loves the lungs - that is, it causes **pneumonia** (infection of the lung tissue). The organism enters the lungs via droplets of contaminated water - like those created by air-conditioning units and showers.

- ***How can infection be prevented?***

The key to the prevention of infection by any microorganism is to identify the kind of environment it likes and then change the environment so that it cannot grow or break the chain of its transmission. In this case, person-to-person transmission does not occur, but we do know that *Legionella pneumophila* likes stagnant water at a temperature of up to 45 °C.

- ***So the answer is simple – just keep water temperatures high.***

Exactly so, which is why we often see warnings about water temperatures above the taps in public buildings - the water is stored at a high temperature. Cold water comes direct from the water mains, and so organism growth in storage is not then a problem.

Contaminated food and water

We have previously considered ingestion as one means by which organisms enter the body, and we gave *Salmonella enteritidis* as an example. We now consider further cases of food and water contamination, while Practice point 16.5 deals with basic food hygiene.

Escherichia coli

This is a Gram-negative bacillus, of which a great many strains exist. Some of these strains are normal gut commensals, but others cause gastroenteritis in which diarrhoea and vomiting lead to dehydration. Laboratory tests are used to identify the different stains.

Escherichia coli 0157 has been responsible for a small number of very serious outbreaks. One of the most serious outbreaks took place in Lanarkshire in 1996. The outbreak was eventually traced to a single butcher's shop, but not until 20 people had died.

Listeria monocytogenes

This Gram-positive bacillus may cause serious illness such as **meningitis** (infection of the meninges - the membranes covering the brain). The ability of the organism to cross the placenta means that it is a particular problem during pregnancy. A pregnant woman who becomes infected with *Listeria monocytogenes* may have mild flu-like symptoms or be asymptomatic. Unfortunately, the consequences for the foetus are more serious and include spontaneous abortion. Infection has sometimes been attributed to unpasteurised milk and cheese made from it; consequently, pregnant women are advised to avoid these foods.

Contact

Contact with a source of infection is the main route by which organisms are spread. Sometimes a distinction is made between **direct** contact and **indirect** contact. Direct contact refers to contact between a person with an infection or carrying a microorganism and others who are not infected.

- ***Which microorganisms are involved in transmission by direct contact?***

You probably will not be surprised to learn that skin commensals (e.g. *Staphylococcus aureus*), organisms infecting intravenous infusion equipment (e.g. *Staphylococcus epidermidis*) and any organism infecting a wound are transmitted readily by direct contact. You may be more surprised, however, to learn that organisms causing upper respiratory tract infection are often spread in this way rather than by being airborne.

- ***What is the best way to prevent spread by direct contact?***

You might suggest that we need to break the contact, and you would be right. But think about this a little more. Let us take the example of a typical hospital ward - perhaps it has four bays, each with six patients.

- ***This doesn't seem to be a good idea – we take 24 sick people and put them all together.***

Yes, that is exactly what we do and you are right - it is not a very good idea. Worse still, the same nurses care for all the patients. You might describe this as a recipe for cross-infection. This is not the end, however: some health-care workers, e.g. doctors and physiotherapists, also have contact with patients in other wards and departments - there might be several hundred patients in a regional hospital in the UK, and the opportunities for cross-infection are great indeed.

- ***How, then, do we break the contact?***

The most significant practice that health-care workers can undertake to stop the spread of microorganisms is to wash their hands between touching each patient.

- ***So then the problem is solved?***

Not exactly - think about it for a moment. Imagine that you are working in a hospital ward and a patient in the toilet uses the call buzzer. The patient needs your help to clean himself

Practice point 16.5

Food hygiene

When nursing physically ill patients, it is important to monitor the nutritional state of the patients, and thus nurses often have to deal with patients' food. Nurses are rarely involved in actually preparing food, but they may be involved in helping patients to eat or simply in taking food to patients. The following lists some important points regarding basic food hygiene measures, but insufficient information is provided for formal training in food handling.

General points

- The kitchen should be clean.
- Hands should be washed before food is handled.
- In the home, kitchen towels should be changed regularly.
- In institutions, paper towels should be used instead of fabric towels.
- Refrigerator temperatures should be monitored.
- People with gastrointestinal symptoms should not prepare food.

Safe storage

- Food should be stored in a refrigerator.
- Raw meat and cooked foods should be kept separately - the raw food should be on the bottom shelf so that it does not drip on to cooked food.
- Food in damaged containers (e.g. bulging tins) should not be consumed.
- Sell-by dates should be observed - but note that it is still possible for food to spoil before the sell-by date.

Preparing food

- Hands should be washed before preparing food and after preparing raw meat and eggs.
- Wounds on the hand should be covered with an appropriate waterproof dressing.
- Utensils should be kept clean, and separate chopping boards should be used for raw meat and other food.
- Fruit and vegetables should be washed in running water.

Cooking food

- Allow adequate thawing times before frozen food is cooked. Once thawed, food should not be refrozen without cooking if first.
- Ensure that the oven is at the correct temperature before cooking begins.
- Ensure food is cooked thoroughly - if necessary, use a food thermometer.
- If there is a delay before serving, cooked food should be kept hot - do not allow it to remain warm for a prolonged period.
- If food is to be stored after cooking, it should be cooled rapidly and placed in the refrigerator. Once again, it should not be allowed to remain warm.

after having a bowel movement. You are certainly going to wash your hands after that. After helping the patient back to his bed, another patient asks you to check the intravenous infusion site (drip site) on the back of her hand because it has become painful. Before you do this, you need to wash your hands. Having dealt with this, a colleague asks for your help repositioning an immobile patient in the next bay.

- ***What do you need to do first?***

Yes, wash your hands. Are you starting to get the point? Washing your hands between direct contact with each patient is very inconvenient and time-consuming. It is never going to be easy to break the contact, but no matter how inconvenient or difficult, your hands must be washed between contact with each patient.

- ***Is there no alternative to handwashing?***

When handwashing is done properly, it is very effective, but when entering and leaving a ward or when moving from one person to another after normal social contact, an antiseptic hand rub may be used instead. Next time you undertake a clinical placement in a hospital, check out the handwashing policy and other requirements for prevention of cross-infection. In the meantime, read Practice point 16.6, which describes typical handwashing practice.

Practice point 16.6

Social handwashing technique

The following description explains important points that might form part of a typical hospital procedure for social handwashing - that is, before normal social contact with a patient. More thorough handwashing is required before invasive procedures.

Hands should be washed in the following circumstances:

- As soon as the hands are visibly soiled.
- Between contact with different patients.
- After handling any items that are soiled or contaminated. Note that certain items, such as a sputum pot, may not be visibly soiled but may well be contaminated with microorganisms.
- Before handling food or food-related items, such as cutlery.

Liquid soap is satisfactory for a normal social handwash. Antiseptic solutions must be used before undertaking clinical procedures, when a more lengthy handwash is required. Soap dispensers should be used until completely empty and then replenished. Bar soap should be avoided, since it can itself be contaminated.

Elbow-operated mixer taps should be used and the temperature of the water temperature adjusted so that it is quite warm but not hot enough to cause discomfort or scalding.

Adequate liquid soap is applied to the hands so that lather can be created. The hands are rubbed together for approximately 30 seconds in the following way (Figure 16.6):

1. Palm to palm.
2. Palm of one hand over back of other, then alternate.
3. Between fingers - fingers interlocked and rubbed back and forth.

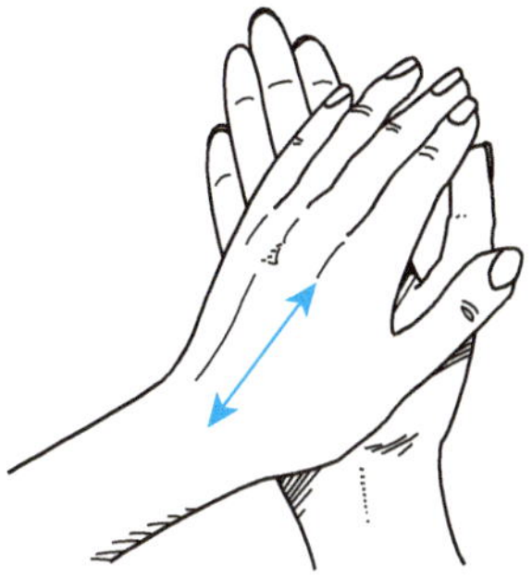

(1) Palm to palm.

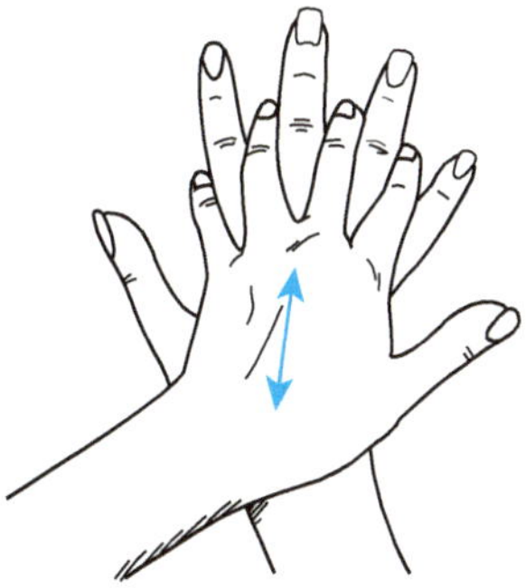

(2) Left palm over back of right hand, then reverse hands.

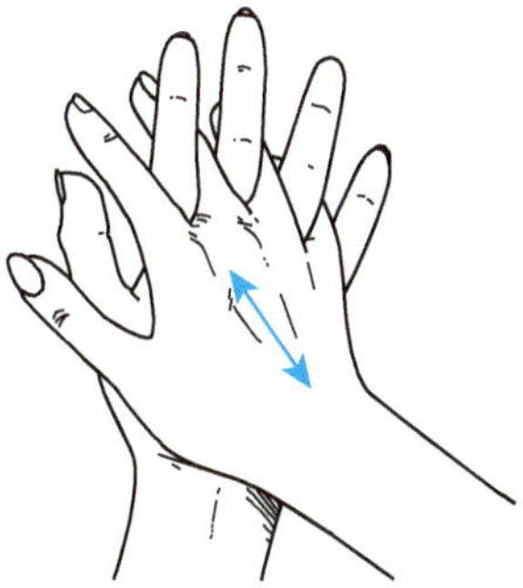

(3) Palm to palm with fingers in between each other.

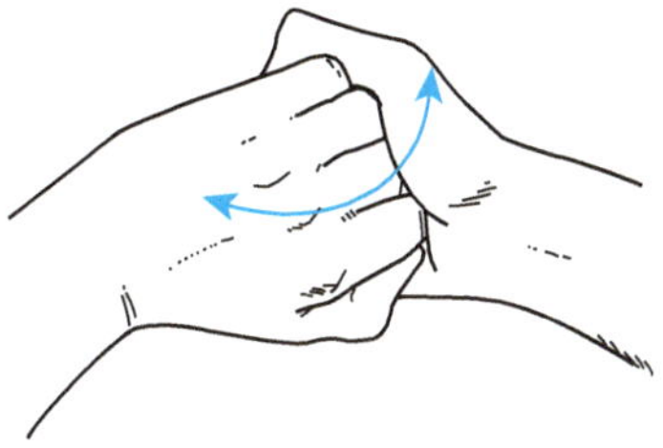

(4) Back of left fingers in palm of right hand, then reverse hands.

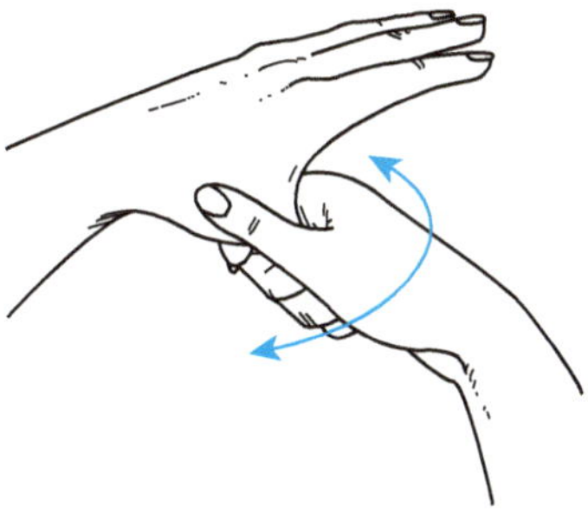

(5) Clasp left thumb in palm of right hand and rotate, then reverse hands.

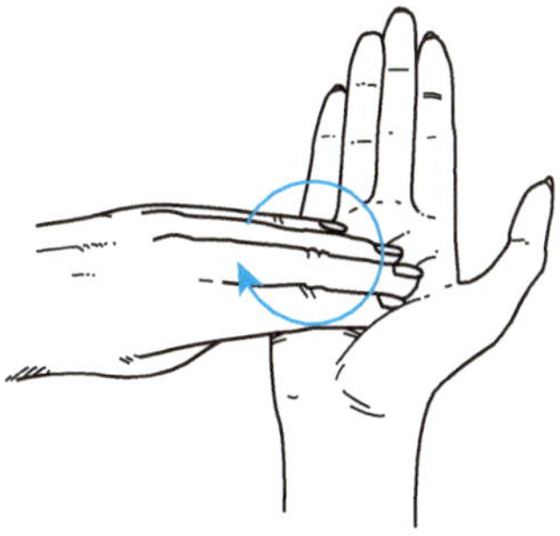

(6) Rotate fingers of left hand in palm of right hand, then reverse hands.

Figure 16.6
The procedure of handwashing.

4 Fingers of one hand to palm of other, then alternate.

5 One hand clasps thumb of the other and rotated back and forth, then alternate hand and thumb.

6 Fingers of one hand rubbed in palm of the other, then alternate.

7 One hand rubs wrists of the other arm, then alternate.

It is important to note that the physical action of rubbing removes soiling and transient microorganisms. Antiseptics have an additional chemical effect, but frequent use may cause irritation or soreness. This may lead to reluctance to wash the hands and cause small breaks in the skin, which can become a source of microorganisms. Consequently, it is preferable to reserve antiseptics for clinical procedures and to use liquid soap for normal social handwashing.

Cuts and abrasions should be covered with a waterproof dressing.

If hands are physically clean - that is, not soiled with dirt - then a hand rub may be used as an alternative to handwashing. Note that hand rubs do not contain detergents - the active component is alcohol. This means that they are ineffective at removing physical soiling of the hands. Hand rubs are ideal for use on entering a clinical area and between normal social contact with patients. Sufficient rub is applied to the hands so that the entire skin surface is covered. The hands are rubbed together until dry. The alcohol will not take long to evaporate, so if too little is applied the hands may have dried before all areas are covered.

- ***What, then, is indirect contact?***

This refers to the transmission of microorganisms from one person to another via an object of some kind. Such objects are sometimes described as **fomites**. The object may be moveable and used by more than one person; crockery and cutlery are obvious examples - and most of us would not wish to share such objects without them being washed thoroughly first.

- ***Can you think of objects that we sometimes share and that are actually involved in personal hygiene?***

Perhaps you have worked out that bars of soap and domestic towels are examples. For this reason, you should not see these used in hospitals, except for personal use by a single patient. For some years, the authors of this book conducted with student nurses experiments in handwashing. Bacteria would be taken from the unwashed and washed hands of students and grown in a hospital laboratory. Different types of soap and handwashing solution were used. Many students were surprised to see that after washing with used bar soap, the number of bacterial colonies grown actually increased. The used soap was acting as a fomite.

Other fomites are static and it is the people who move. For example, you might wash your hands very well after using the toilet and then unknowingly open the toilet door with a handle that has been touched by someone who did not wash their hands.

Insect vectors

The term 'vector' is derived from a Latin word meaning 'to carry' and is used here since insects do not function simply as a kind of fomite - they actually move about and carry microorganisms from one person to another. Indeed, the microorganism might complete part of its lifecycle within the insect - we have already mentioned malaria and African sleeping sickness in this context. In both these cases, the organism enters the body by inoculation - a bite. Insect vectors do not always function in this way, however. For example, flies transmit the Gram-negative bacillus *Shigella sonnei*, which causes bacillary dysentery, from faeces to food; the organism then enters the body by ingestion. Nonetheless, the number of cases caused by faecal contamination of the hands is probably very many times greater than that caused by flies.

In-text review

- ✔ The term 'endogenous infection' (self-infection) is used when an infection occurs because of the transfer of microorganisms from one part of a person's body, e.g. the skin, to another, e.g. a wound.
- ✔ The term 'exogenous infection' (cross-infection) is used when an infection occurs because of the transfer of microorganisms from one person to another.
- ✔ The term 'nosocomial' refers to hospital-acquired infection.
- ✔ There are four possible routes of entry of microorganisms into the body: inhalation, ingestion, inoculation and congenital transmission.
- ✔ There are four possible methods of transmission of microorganisms: airborne spread, contaminated water, contact (direct or indirect) and insect vectors.
- ✔ Removing a reservoir of microorganisms or preventing their transmission can prevent cross-infection.
- ✔ The single most effective means of preventing cross-infection in health care is effective handwashing.

Microbiology samples

Since microorganisms are not visible with the naked eye, laboratory tests are required for their identification.

- ***What is it that is actually tested?***

For a microbiological test to be performed, some kind of sample is required - of body fluid, for example. Certain body fluids, such as **cerebrospinal fluid** (CSF - a fluid that cushions the brain and spinal cord), can be obtained only during specialised procedures. Others, such as urine, are obtained easily, and it is these that we concentrate on here. Practice point 16.7 provides general advice concerning obtaining specimens for microbiological examination.

Urine specimens

A specimen of urine for microbiological examination is obtained when the patient has symptoms of **cystitis** (infection of the urinary bladder). Symptoms include **frequency** (passing urine frequently), **urgency** (urgent need to void) and, sometimes, pain on passing urine. In addition, infected urine often has an unpleasant smell. Nurses often perform a quick test for the presence of Gram-negative organism using nitrite urinalysis strips. The reagent strip is dipped into a specimen of urine and the presence of nitrites confirmed by a change in colour of the reagent pad.

Practice point 16.7

Obtaining specimens for microbiological examination

Important general points common to obtaining various types of specimen include identification, container, collection and transport.

Specimen identification

Identify the type of specimen required from the microbiology laboratory request card. Next, check the identity of the patient concerned. Ensure that the patient details are correct on both the card and the specimen container. Patients are identified by four items of information: full name, date of birth, address and hospital unit number.

Specimen container

Ensure that the specimen container is the correct type. For example, a simple urinalysis does not require a sterile container, but a urine specimen for microbiological examination does.

Specimen collection

Ensure that the specimen is collected with regard to proper sampling technique. For example, urine specimens need to be collected without contamination by skin commensals. Note that when specimens are being collected, there may be a threat of cross-infection, and so precautions are required. For example, when obtaining a stool specimen, disposable gloves and an apron should be worn.

Specimen transport

Specimen collection should be timed so that the specimen arrives quickly at the laboratory. Little purpose is served by obtaining a specimen at night if it is not examined until the following morning. A delay gives time for contaminating organisms to multiply and produce confusing results. All specimens of body fluids should be transported in containers with tightly fastened lids. They should then be placed upright in racks or sealed plastic bags.

- ***If a positive nitrite test confirms the presence of Gram-negative bacteria, why is a sample of urine required for the microbiology laboratory?***

Treatment could be commenced on the basis of the nitrite test alone. The specific organism causing the infection would not have been identified, however, and the antimicrobial drug to which the organism is sensitive would not be known. For this reason, it is preferable to obtain a urine specimen for the microbiology laboratory before any drug therapy is commenced.

- ***If the nitrite test is negative, is a urine specimen for the laboratory not required?***

Remember that a positive nitrite test only confirms the presence of a Gram-negative organism. If the test is negative, there might still be an infection caused by another type of organism. Consequently, a urine specimen for microbiological examination is obtained on the basis of the symptoms alone.

Can the same urine specimen be used for urinalysis and microbiological examination?

Certainly not – the sample that has had the reagent strip dipped into it has been contaminated. The problem with collecting urine samples is that it is far too easy to contaminate the sample. First, the correct sterile container needs to be obtained. Once the top has been removed, care must be taken to avoid touching the inside of the top or the container. The patient is then asked to urinate into the container. This is not as easy as it sounds, since skin commensals are easily washed into the sample as urination commences. This is particularly the case in women; to avoid contamination, the **labia** should be separated and the middle of the stream collected. It is a little easier in men, since the foreskin is usually easily retracted, although once again the middle of the stream is collected. Incidentally, if you see the abbreviation MSU (sometimes MSSU), this refers to a **mid-stream specimen of urine**.

Some patients who are unable to pass urine normally have a urinary **catheter** (a type of long tube) passed into the urinary bladder via the urethra (the tube that leads from the bladder to the outside). Urinary catheters are invariably problematic, for a number of reasons, including increased incidence of infection. One way to reduce the incidence of catheter-related cystitis is to avoid disconnecting the catheter from the drainage bag. Each time the tubing is disconnected, there is the opportunity for microorganisms to enter. Instead, the bag is emptied via a tap at its base.

If a specimen of urine is required, how is it obtained?

If you check along the length of the catheter, you will find a self-sealing sleeve. A sterile needle can be inserted here and a sample of urine withdrawn into a syringe.

Stool specimens

Stool (faecal) specimens are obtained easily using a container in which a spoon is incorporated into the lid. The patient is asked to pass a stool into a container (a card bedpan liner) without passing urine too. A scoop of faeces can then be placed in the container and the lid sealed.

Sputum specimens

Sputum is part of an important mechanism for trapping microorganisms before they reach the lowest airways. When an infection of the lungs or lower airways is present, it may be possible to identify the organism in the sputum.

How is a specimen of sputum obtained?

The patient is asked to spit into a sterile container, but there is a problem here. If you use the word 'spit', that is exactly what you will get – spit (saliva) rather than secretions from the lungs.

Could you ask the patient to cough instead?

Indeed, you could – try for a moment by giving a cough yourself.

- ***Where did the noise of the cough come from?***

From the throat - that is still not good enough - we need sputum from the lungs. One way to ensure that the secretions collected come from the lower airways and lungs is to begin by asking the patient to slowly and deeply breathe in and out three times. If there is an excess of pulmonary secretions, this simple exercise may trigger an episode of effective coughing, so have the specimen container ready. If not, at the end of the third inhalation encourage the patient to give a 'huff' - that is, to breathe out forcibly through the mouth (you might need to demonstrate this first). The aim of this exercise is not to create a noise from the throat but to forcibly exhale sputum from the lungs.

Wound specimens

A sample of microorganisms from a wound can be obtained using a sterile wound swab - this looks rather like a large cotton bud in a sealed container. The seal is broken and the swab removed without allowing it to become contaminated. The wound is wiped gently with the sterile end; the swab is then returned to its container. If a wound is exuding or pus is present, a specimen should be obtained on the swab. In large wounds, parts may show signs of healing but other areas may be infected: Ensure you do not drag pus from the infected area on to parts of the wound that are healing.

Blood cultures

Two important terms must be distinguished at this point. **Bacteraemia** is a transient condition in which bacteria are present in the blood but the host's defences then destroy them. This can occur after insertion of a urinary catheter or following wounding with a dirty object. When microorganisms are actively reproducing in the bloodstream, the patient becomes gravely ill and the term **septicaemia** is used. The patient urgently requires an intravenous (into a vein) course of antibiotics.

- ***Which antibiotics?***

In order to identify the causative bacteria and discover which antibiotics the organism is sensitive to, two samples of blood are required. From these, the organism can be cultured (grown). Strict aseptic technique is used to obtain the blood from a patient's vein.

- ***Can you work out why two samples are needed?***

One is used to grow aerobic bacteria and the other to grow anaerobic bacteria.

Other specimens

There are many other types of specimen for microbiological examination that are beyond the scope of a basic science book. Nonetheless, you might be interested to find out about them. Two examples are listed below:

- When bacterial meningitis is suspected, a sample of cerebrospinal fluid (CSF) is obtained during a procedure called **lumbar puncture** (a needle is passed between the lumbar vertebrae in order to aspirate CSF from around the spinal cord).
- Sexually transmitted diseases are increasing in prevalence in the UK. Swabs may be taken from the urethra in men and the vagina and cervix in women.

Microbiological tests

It is worth pointing out that once appropriate specimens have been obtained, laboratory tests are undertaken on the specimens rather than on the patient. Such tests are described as 'direct' – the tests are performed directly on the microorganisms.

- ***What, then, are 'indirect' test?***

In contrast to direct tests, indirect tests are not performed on the microorganisms but on the patient in an attempt to identify some form of response to infection. Two examples are given below:

Serological tests

The word '**serological**' is derived from the word '**serum**' and refers to the fluid components of blood (meaning not the cells). In the present context, serological tests are those performed on a sample of the patient's blood.

Venereal disease research laboratory test

This test is used to quantify antibodies to the organism *Treponema pallidum*, which causes the venereal disease syphilis. The test is used as a screening tool to confirm a diagnosis and also to monitor the progress of the patient under treatment.

Hypersensitivity tests

Heaf test

This test employs a **Heaf gun** – an injection device that delivers purified protein derivative (PPD) to multiple punctures of the dermis of the skin. PPD is a protein derivative of *Mycobacterium tuberculosis*, the organism that causes tuberculosis (TB). If the patient is suffering from tuberculosis, has had the disease or has been immunised against it, the patient will develop an allergic (hypersensitivity) reaction to PPD and the puncture sites will become red and inflamed.

- ***What use is this test of allergy?***

In developed countries, where immunisation against tuberculosis is routine, the Heaf test is used to confirm that a child has responded to immunisation and has become immune to the disease. Antibodies confer immunity; the presence of antibodies is confirmed by allergic reaction to PPD. You may remember having a Heaf test performed or the site being examined some time afterwards. If you look carefully on your upper arm, you might still be able to see the faint circular scar left by the test. In contrast, when tuberculosis immunisation has not taken place, the Heaf test can be used in the diagnosis of the disease.

The microbiology laboratory

This section provides a basic introduction to some of the tests performed in the microbiology laboratory. A detailed description is beyond the scope of this book, but the reader will gain an appreciation of some of the main techniques employed once a specimen has left the patient.

Cultivation of microorganisms

Unless you have studied microbiology before, the expression 'cultivation' probably sounds rather strange. After all, it refers to nurturing - the expression is often used of gardeners caring for prized plant specimens, but here we are talking about disease-causing organisms.

- ***Do we really mean that the organisms are nurtured in the microbiology laboratory?***

Yes, that is what occurs: Microorganisms present in a specimen are given ideal conditions in which to grow. If microorganisms are to be identified and various tests performed upon them, then the microbiologist requires a supply in pure culture - that means each species grown separately and not mixed up together.

Cultivation of bacteria

The classical way to grow bacteria is referred to as **plating out**, since the growth medium is contained in special shallow culture plates with overlapping lids. The plates are sometimes called **Petri dishes** after a German bacteriologist. A wire loop is sterilised by passing it through a flame and then allowed to cool.

- ***Why does the wire loop need to be sterilised?***

When obtaining a specimen, you will have taken care to prevent contamination - the intention is to grow the bacteria present in the specimen rather than bacteria from the nurse's hands or the environment. Contamination must also be avoided in the microbiology laboratory, and so the wire loop is sterilised each time before it is used. Next, a small quantity of the specimen (e.g. sputum, pus, etc.) is picked up and streaked across the culture medium. The wire loop is allowed to cool first after sterilisation in order to not kill the bacteria in the specimen.

- ***What would happen if bacteria were now simply allowed to grow in this dish?***

A great many microorganisms would grow very close together. Instead, the first streaks are confined to a segment of the Petri dish; then the wire loop is sterilised again and a second segment of the dish is streaked. This segment overlaps with the first so that microorganisms from the first segment are deposited on a fresh area of the medium. The process is repeated several times so that each newly streaked segment has fewer and fewer microorganisms deposited upon it (Figure 16.7).

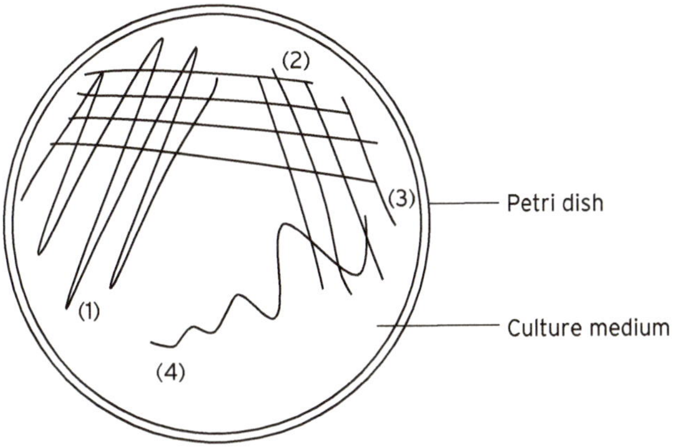

Figure 16.7
Growing bacteria on a Petri dish.
(1) Small amount of material (e.g. pus) is streaked over solid culture medium (e.g. agar). (2), (3), (4) Wire loop is sterilised in a flame and streaked on to uninoculated areas before incubation.

What happens next?

Petri dishes are loaded into an incubator, which maintains the warm conditions ideal for bacterial growth. The result is that bacteria grow and form colonies. These are recognised as clumps on the surface of the medium. The size, shape and colour of the colonies vary according to the species of bacteria that has grown; for example, colonies of *Pseudomonas aeruginosa* are green. If growth on the first segment to be streaked is very heavy, then it will be possible to distinguish individual colonies from other segments. Each colony represents the offspring of a small number of microorganisms deposited there. Once this crop of microorganisms has been obtained, a pure culture of each type can be grown.

Can you think how this might be done?

We start with a fresh batch of Petri dishes and our wire loop once again. The loop is sterilised and material from a single colony is picked up and streaked across the medium in one of the dishes. Just as before, the dish is streaked in segments. The same is done for each different type of colony. The dishes are incubated and the result is a number of dishes, each containing colonies of a single species.

What is the medium on which the bacteria are grown?

The medium is called **agar** – a jelly obtained from seaweed. (Agar was used by the Victorians to make desserts.) Agar consists of polysaccharides (complex sugars), which bacteria cannot use as a nutrient. Thus, the agar is simply a medium on which the bacteria grow. Of course, if microorganisms are to be cultured, they need nutrients, and these are added, mostly in the form of meat extract. The exact makeup of the medium can be adjusted so that different types of bacteria can be grown.

Cultivation of other microorganisms

In the above description, only the cultivation of bacteria has been described. Other types of organism require different cultural techniques that are beyond the scope of this book. It is worth asking one important question, however.

- ***What are the particular problems in cultivating viruses?***

Do you remember that viruses are obligates parasites? That is, they require living cells in which to complete their 'lifecycle'. Consequently, viruses are grown in special preparations of living cells, called **tissue cultures**.

Identifying bacteria

- ***Thus far, we have described how a pure culture is obtained, but how are bacteria identified?***

There are a number of techniques, including microscopy, staining techniques and biochemical tests.

Microscopy

We have previously described that bacteria are initially identified by their shape and consequently examination using the light microscope is performed. When material containing bacteria is smeared on to a glass slide and covered with a thin glass cover slip before examination, the term '**wet film**' is applied. It is more common, however, to use a **dry film** - that is, the slide is passed through a flame. Using a staining technique facilitates visualisation of bacteria. There are a number of staining techniques, and two are described here:

Gram stain

The dry film is stained purple (crystal violet or methyl violet) before being flooded in turn with iodine and acetone. The film is then washed with water. The film is then stained with red carbol fuchsin, washed with water and blotted dry. Some bacteria take up the purple dye, but in some the dye is successfully washed out. These then take up the red stain and appear pink under the microscope - they are referred to as Gram-negative. Gram-positive bacteria are those that appear purple - it has not been possible to wash out the dye. Differences in the structure of the cell wall account for the different staining properties. The Gram stain can help to identify bacteria. For example, the genus *Neisseria* is one of few Gram-negative cocci.

Ziehl-Neelsson stain

The film is stained with hot carbol fuchsin before being washed with water and then flooded with an acid and alcohol solution. The film is stained with methylene blue or malachite green and then washed with water and blotted dry. In most organisms, the acid and alcohol solution will wash out carbol fuchsin. The genus *Mycobacterium* (e.g. *Mycobacterium tuberculosis* - the organism that causes tuberculosis), however, is acid-fast - that is, the acid does not wash out the carbol fuchsin and the bacteria appear red/yellow. This test is performed because

Mycobacteria have thick cell walls that are difficult to stain using Gram's method. Once stained with hot carbol fuchsin, however, they resist decolouration.

Biochemical tests

Metabolic products of bacteria may be demonstrated by the use of specially prepared media. For example, the medium may undergo a colour change when certain substances are present.

Antibiotic sensitivity

The sensitivity of bacteria can be demonstrated by applying an antibiotic-impregnated paper disc to a pure culture of organisms. Where bacteria are sensitive to a particular antibiotic, growth will be inhibited around the paper disc.

Cleaning, disinfection and sterilisation

Cleaning

Think for a moment about a typical hospital ward.

- ***Identify objects that several patients use in the course of a day.***

Perhaps your list includes furniture, toilets, baths, showers, wheelchairs, trolleys and aids for moving and handling. When we think of hospital hygiene, we often think of specialist procedures such as **autoclaving** (more about this later). It is sobering, however, to contemplate that objects used by the greatest number of people are not subject to specialist cleaning or sterilisation. They do not need to be - they simply need to be physically cleaned. Nonetheless, the process of cleaning makes a significant contribution to preventing cross-infection. It is unfortunate, then, that we often think of cleaning as a rather menial task. Worse still, cleaning is often subject to the severest cost-saving measures in health care.

A clinical colleague of the authors visited a hospital in a developing country and commented on how clean it was compared with a UK hospital. It had to be: The staff had no other way of preventing cross-infection and no antibiotics to treat infection if it occurred. Perhaps in the developed world we have become so confident in our ability to deal with infection that we place inadequate emphasis on simple preventive measures. Of course, cleaners are employed to perform most of the cleaning that takes place in care settings, but nurses and other care workers are also involved, and for this reason some important points about cleaning are included in Practice point 16.8.

Disinfection and sterilisation

Disinfection refers to processes that render an object non-infective. It does not mean that there are no organisms remaining but means that the number of microorganisms has been reduced greatly. Spores remain following disinfection. In contrast, **sterilisation** refers to the destruction of all living organisms, including spores. A number of methods are employed, including dry and moist heat, electromagnetic radiation and chemical methods.

Practice point 16.8

Cleaning

- Objects that are used by more than one patient should be cleaned adequately. An appropriate cleaning agent is required. For example, a table on which food is served simply needs to be cleaned with a detergent in order to remove dried spilt food. In contrast, a toilet requires a toilet-cleaning fluid. Just because an object is located in a hospital does not necessarily mean that it requires specialist cleaning, although some objects require more frequent cleaning - just imagine how many times a ward toilet is used in a 24-hour period.
- Cleaning solutions should be changed regularly. Do not carry on 'cleaning' if the solution has become soiled.
- Keep dedicated items (e.g. bowls) for cleaning purposes.
- Use sinks for dedicated purposes. For example, sinks in patient areas may be used for hand-washing, but the kitchen sink should not be used for this purpose. Soiled cleaning solutions should be disposed of in the sluice sink.
- Although cleaners undertake most of the cleaning in care settings, do not be reluctant to get your hands dirty. For example, if a patient soils a commode seat, the seat needs to be cleaned immediately after use.
- Disposable cloths are used for cleaning. Wet non-disposable items are an ideal environment for microorganisms to grow.
- Items that are not disposable should be stored dry. For example, mops should not be allowed to stand in buckets of water but should be wrung dry. Patient washing bowls should be cleaned after use, rinsed and dried with paper towels. They should be stored upside-down, with airflow around them.
- Clean surfaces should be wiped regularly with a fresh damp disposable cloth in order to remove dust. Dust is composed of a number of different materials, including skin cells - not the kind of thing you want to have floating around and landing in someone's wound. A surface that has been damp-dusted should then be dried.
- Clinical procedures, such as wound dressing, should not be performed during or immediately after cleaning. Cleaning may cause dust to circulate. It is always preferable to have a room set aside for clinical procedures. This room should not double-up as an office or storeroom where dust collects and that is difficult to clean because of the volume of stock.
- Take care to avoid solutions seeping into electrical equipment or being spilled and thus creating a danger to others.

Physical methods

Heat

Dry heat: this is used occasionally, for example in sterilising wire loops in the microbiology laboratory and in the burning of infected waste and Petri dishes. Methods that use moist heat are more common, however.

Pasteurisation: this is the process of heating milk in order to kill common bacterial pathogens. Louis Pasteur developed the process as a way to destroy *Brucella abortus* - the bacteria that causes **brucellosis**. One of a number of regimes is used, e.g. heating at 65 °C for 10 minutes.

Autoclaving: the autoclave is a device that employs steam under pressure and is used to sterilise surgical instruments and operating gowns. Heat-sensitive tape with stripes that darken in the autoclave are used so that it is possible to see which materials have been sterilised.

Electromagnetic radiation

You can read about electromagnetic radiation in Chapter 14. Various forms of radiation are effective, including ultraviolet (UV) light. In a primitive way, when hospital staff in developing countries hang out theatre gowns to dry in the sun, they are making use of UV light. Intense, artificially generated UV light is even more effective on the surface of objects, but penetration is poor and therefore it has limited use. Water from wells or boreholes may be treated with UV light in order to make it safe to drink. In health care, **ionising radiation** (e.g. gamma rays) is used to sterilise heat-sensitive objects such as plastic syringes and latex gloves.

Chemical methods

A large number of chemical solutions are available; some are more suitable for particular purposes than others. Suitability is dependent partly upon the ability of the solution to kill specific organisms and partly on the nature of object to be treated. For example, not all solutions are suitable for application on the skin. Chemical solutions rarely destroy spores, and some microorganisms will survive treatment. Consequently, chemical methods cause disinfection rather than sterilisation, and thus such solutions are referred to as **disinfectants**. If a chemical solution is safe to be applied to the skin, then the term '**antiseptic**' is often used instead of 'disinfectant'. Having noted this, strong solutions of antiseptics can cause damage if applied to the skin. Commonly used disinfectants are listed in Table 16.3.

Table 16.3 Common disinfectants.

Type of solution	Examples	Use
Halogens - hypochlorites	Hypochlorite solutions (e.g. Milton - sodium hypochlorite), bleach	Weak solutions are used to clean baby feeding bottles; strong solutions (bleach) are surface disinfectants
Halogens - iodine	Solution of iodine in water or alcohol and iodophors (combination of iodine and surface active agents)	Skin disinfectants, e.g. before surgery
Alcohol	Ethanol, isopropyl alcohol	Variety of uses, e.g. surface disinfection, skin cleansing, hand rubs
Chlorhexidine	Chlorhexidine gluconate (e.g. Hibitane)	Skin disinfection, e.g. as a solution for cleansing wounds, component of hand rubs
Phenols	Phenolic solutions (e.g. Hycolin)	Surface disinfectants

Treating infections

Even if we take the most careful precautions in order to avoid pathogenic microorganisms, our nature as social beings still results in the contraction of infectious diseases. The question that then arises is how to treat infections. Perhaps the immediate response to this question is 'With antibiotics.'

- ***Name an antibiotic.***

You have probably given **penicillin**, the very first antibiotic, as your answer. If you have already gained experience in practice placements, however, you may be able to name some other antibiotics too. It is a sobering thought that until penicillin became widely available, there were few effective treatments for infections, and many people died as a consequence. Scientists had been searching for antimicrobial drugs for a long time, and one of the earliest successes was a compound of arsenic made by Ehrlich in the first decade of the twentieth century. A long course of this drug was successful in killing *Treponema pallidum* - the organism that causes syphilis. In the 1930s, Dogmagk successfully used the dye prontosil to treat animal infections and subsequently antimicrobial drugs called **sulphonamides** were developed.

- ***We began by referring to antibiotics and then antimicrobials. Is there a difference?***

An **antimicrobial** is a drug that is effective in killing microorganisms or preventing their growth. Strictly speaking, antibiotics are antimicrobials that are produced naturally by microorganisms. Perhaps it helps to think of this as a microscopic example of survival of the fittest - one microorganism reducing competition from another by producing chemicals harmful to its competitor. On the basis of these definitions, arsenical compounds and sulphonamides are antimicrobials, and penicillin is an antibiotic. In this book, however, we follow common practice and use the terms 'antimicrobial' and 'antibiotic' synonymously. In addition, we ought also to clarify the proper use of another term - 'chemotherapy'. You have probably heard this used of the drug treatment of cancers. You need to be aware, however, that the term is also used of drug treatment of infections.

The account of the discovery of penicillin in 1929 is worth repeating. In Alexander Fleming's laboratory at St Mary's Hospital in Paddington, London, the fungus *Penicillium notatum* contaminated a culture of *Staphylococcus aureus*. Fleming noticed that the fungus inhibited the growth of the bacteria, but he was unable to isolate the substance responsible (penicillin). Consequently, although Fleming was the first to observe the effects of penicillin, there was no immediate therapeutic benefit from his observations. In 1940, two scientists, Chain and Florey, finally isolated the first penicillin (there are many closely related compounds), but penicillin was not widely available until after the Second World War. The development of other antibiotics was subsequently rapid - **streptomycin**, **chloramphenicol** and **tetracylines** were all identified before the end of the 1940s.

Action of antibiotics

Antibiotics are sometimes distinguished as **bactericidal** (kill bacteria) or **bacteristatic** (inhibit the growth of bacteria). The distinction is not clear cut, however. A number of different mechanisms account for the action of antibiotics.

Prevention of cell-wall formation

The bacterial cell wall is a unique structure - an animal cell does not possess one. Consequently, a selective drug attack on the cell wall is a good way of causing the bacteria to burst while leaving host cells unharmed. Penicillins, **cephalosporins** and **vancomycin** work in this way.

Inhibition of protein synthesis

Bacteria need to synthesise protein, just as animals do. Certain antibiotics, including tetracyclines and **erythromycin**, inhibit bacterial protein synthesis without harming the host's mechanisms.

Enzyme inhibition

Enzymes control the metabolism of bacteria, just as they do in animals. Drugs that interfere with bacterial but not human enzymes function as antibiotics, such as **sulphonamides** and **trimethoprim**.

Blocking DNA replication

Before bacteria divide, they replicate their genetic material (deoxyribonucleic acid/DNA). **Quinolones**, e.g. ciprofloxacin, are antibiotics that interfere with enzymes involved in this process.

Range of action of antibiotics

Certain antibiotics are effective mainly against Gram-positive bacteria (e.g. penicillins and erythromycin). Others are effective mainly against Gram-negative bacteria (e.g. **nalidixic acid**). The expression '**broad-spectrum**' is used of antibiotics that are effective against both Gram-positive and Gram-negative bacteria (e.g. tetracyclines, chloramphenicol, **cephalosporins** and **ampicillin**).

Adverse effects of antibiotics

Pharmacologists describe different types of adverse drug effect. A number of adverse effects are considered here, including toxicity, side effects and secondary effects.

Toxicity

All drugs produce toxic effects if given in high enough doses. The safe effective dose is determined in an extensive research programme before the drug is marketed. Toxicity is largely a problem of administration - that is, giving too much drug. Needless to say, care must be taken to ensure that the correct dose is prescribed, dispensed and administered. Prescription is normally the role of the doctor, but there are increasing numbers of non-medical prescribers, including nurses. Nurses normally dispense drugs - that is, take out the correct number of tablets or pour the correct volume of liquid. Three aspects are important here: identification of the correct patient, identification of the correct drug and calculation of the correct dose. You may find it helpful to review drug administration procedures in a nursing textbook and check the hospital policy in your next clinical placement.

Side effects

A side effect is an adverse effect of a drug that is unrelated to its primary action. For example, the antibiotic **gentamicin** may damage the eighth cranial nerve. (A cranial nerve is a nerve that arises from the brain rather than the spinal cord. The eighth cranial nerve conveys impulses to the brain from the ear.) This damage may result in deafness or **tinnitus** (ringing in the ears).

- ***When you are next with a patient for whom antibiotics are prescribed, find out what the possible side effects are.***

You can do this by consulting the *British National Formulary* (**BNF**). There should be a copy of the BNF in each clinical placement where drugs are administered. Sometimes it is possible to minimise the risk of side effects. For example, in the case of gentamicin, which has to be given by intravenous injection, the dose should be administered slowly so that it becomes diluted in the bloodstream.

Secondary effects

Secondary effects are adverse effects related to the drug's primary action. For example, antibiotics are given for the purpose of treating infection, but the causative organism may be destroyed only to be replaced by another. The expression '**superinfection**' is sometimes used of this phenomenon.

- ***Has this got anything to do with 'superbugs'?***

The expression '**superbug**' is commonly used in the media in a way that is misleading; we shall return to this point later. In common usage, 'super' refers to strength, but in this case it means 'on top of'.

- ***So superinfection is where an infection is treated successfully but the patient contracts a second infection on top of the first?***

Yes, that is correct. One common example of this is oral **thrush** - infection of the oral mucosa by the fungus *Candida albicans*. Thrush is visible as white plaques that cause soreness of the tongue and mouth. Thrush takes hold once the normal bacterial flora of the mouth has been destroyed by a course of antibiotics. This is not the intended effect of the antibiotics - they are used to treat pathogens. It is simply that chemotherapy does not distinguish between harmful bacteria causing an illness and harmless bacteria inhabiting the mouth. You should always look for signs of thrush in any patient who has taken a long course of antibiotics.

- ***How is thrush treated?***

Normally, *Candida albicans* is eradicated by the antifungal drug **nystatin**, although more serious and widespread infection can occur and the second infection is not necessarily a fungus: It might instead be a different species of bacteria or a resistant form of the same species.

In view of the number and potentially serious nature of adverse effects to antibiotics, their prescription and administration thus needs to be undertaken with care, as described in Practice point 16.9. Following this, the problem of antibiotic resistance is explained in Practice point 16.10.

Practice point 16.9

The use of antibiotics

The aim of antibiotic treatment is to eradicate infection while causing the fewest adverse effects as possible. With this in mind, the following points serve as guidance:

- Antibiotics are not prescribed for viral infections and minor self-limiting infections.
- Antibiotics have a limited role in the prevention of infection, for example following surgery.
- The main means by which transmission of infection is prevented are physical measures (e.g. patient isolation) and good hygiene (e.g. washing hands).
- Antibiotic treatment is based both on the patient's condition and on microbiology laboratory reports. It may be necessary for chemotherapy to commence before a laboratory report is available, but ideally suitable specimens are collected before antibiotic treatment begins.
- Chemotherapy is under the control of suitably qualified practitioners and antibiotics are not normally available over the counter.
- A course of antibiotics should always be completed, but sometimes patients stop taking drugs once symptoms have subsided; if the organisms have not been eradicated, the infection may then return. In addition, resistance may develop in microorganisms exposed to antibiotics but not killed. If the reason for non-compliance is unwanted effects, then an alternative drug may be substituted.

In-text review

- ✔ Since microorganisms are not visible with the unaided eye, laboratory tests are required for their identification.
- ✔ Important general points regarding specimens include identification, container, collection and transport.
- ✔ Common microbiology specimens are urine, stools, sputum, wound swabs and blood cultures.
- ✔ Direct tests are those performed on microorganisms, while indirect tests are those performed on patients with diseases.
- ✔ Microorganisms are cultivated in the microbiology laboratory and subjected to a number of tests, including microscopy, staining techniques and biochemical tests.
- ✔ Disinfection refers to processes that render an object non-infective, while sterilisation refers to the destruction of all living organisms, including spores.
- ✔ A number of methods of sterilisation are employed, including dry and moist heat, electromagnetic radiation and chemical methods.
- ✔ An antimicrobial is a drug that is effective in killing microorganisms or preventing their growth.
- ✔ Antibiotics are antimicrobials that are produced naturally by microorganisms.

Practice point 16.10

Antibiotic resistance

The term '**antibiotic resistance**' is probably self-explanatory - it refers to the condition that exists when a microorganism is not susceptible to an antibiotic.

- ***That is quite straightforward – so a particular antibiotic is effective only against certain bacteria?***

This is certainly true. For example, the complex cell wall of Gram-negative bacteria makes these bacteria more difficult to destroy than Gram-positive bacteria. We refer to this type of resistance as 'innate' - meaning inbuilt. It is acquired resistance, however, that is most often referred to. This is the term used when bacteria that are initially sensitive to an antibiotic subsequently become resistant to that antibiotic. This can be observed in the laboratory when bacteria are cultured in the presence of sublethal doses of antibiotics.

Resistance was recognised as a problem very early in the history of the development of antibiotics. Penicillin-resistant strains of bacteria were reported in the 1950s, but newer drugs temporarily proved effective. Certain strains of *Staphylococcus aureus* became resistant to **methicillin** (a type of penicillin), and the expression '**methicillin-resistant *Staphylococcus aureus***' (MRSA) came into being. Methicillin-resistant strains are also resistant to a variety of other antibiotics, and infection by MRSA is particularly difficult to treat. The expression 'superbug' is misused, however, since the organisms are no more virulent than sensitive strains - they are simply resistant to many antibiotics.

Resistant strains of *Staphylococcus aureus* may be carried as skin commensals, just as sensitive strains are. The carrier experiences no ill effects as a result. If the carrier develops a wound, however, MRSA may opportunistically infect that wound. In addition, MRSA can be transmitted from a healthy carrier to other people.

- ***So what should we learn from this?***

The early successes of antibiotic therapy resulted in a degree of complacency concerning infection-control procedures. The current high incidence of infection by resistant forms means that health-care workers are again emphasising the importance of preventing cross-infection rather than relying upon the ability to treat infection once it has occurred.

Summary

This has been a long chapter, with quite a lot of science, including the classification of microorganisms and how they are identified. At times, however, topics related closely to physical health, such as immunity and immunisation, have been explained, and some of the content, such as the prevention of spread of microorganisms, has been highly practical. Despite massive technological advances in the twentieth century, people in modern society experience significant threats to health from microorganisms, including HIV and MRSA, and new threats such as H15N bird flu emerge all the time. The optimism that followed the development of the first antibiotics has given way to an uneasy suspicion that 'out there somewhere' are further organisms ready to cause infections that we shall find very difficult to treat. At present, the role of the nurse in preventing cross-infection and in the care of patients with infections has again become very important indeed.

Summary points

- Four types of microorganism are important in disease: bacteria, viruses, fungi and protozoa.
- Bacteria are identified on the basis of their appearance, staining reactions, metabolism and ability to form spores.
- Various forms of host-microorganism relationship exist, including commensalism and parasitism.
- Various mechanisms exist to resist infectious disease. Immunity may be described as innate or acquired.
- Microorganisms enter the body by inhalation, ingestion, inoculation and congenital routes.
- The means of transmission of microorganism are airborne, contaminated food and water, contact and by insect vectors.
- Microorganisms are identified largely by tests performed in the microbiology laboratory on specimens taken from the patient. These specimens must be obtained without contamination.
- Cleaning, disinfection and sterilisation are important techniques used to reduce the risk of transmission of infection.
- Proper handwashing is the most important single action performed to reduce cross-infection.
- Antimicrobial drugs kill or inhibit the growth of bacteria, but in view of the possible development of resistance their prescription and administration should be controlled carefully.

Self-test questions

1 Match the term on the left with the most appropriate description on the right:

(a) Saprophyte	(i) A microorganism that can complete its lifecycle only at the expense of another organism, in which it causes disease
(b) Obligate pathogen	(ii) A microorganism that lives on dead or decaying matter
(c) Commensal	(iii) A microorganism that has a close relationship with a host on which it confers no benefit or harm
(d) Heterotroph	(iv) A microorganism that obtains its nutrients from organic matter

2 Match the disease on the left with the most appropriate type of microorganism on the right:

(a) AIDS	(i) Bacteria
(b) Ringworm	(ii) Virus
(c) Malaria	(iii) Fungus
(d) Tuberculosis	(iv) Protozoa

3 Match the term on the left with the most appropriate shape description on the right:

(a) Cocci	(i) Curved
(b) Vibrio	(ii) Round
(c) Bacilli	(iii) Rod-shaped
(d) Spirochaetes	(iv) Spiral-shaped

4 Which one of the following is an example of a zoonotic infection?
(a) Cystitis.
(b) Salmonellosis.
(c) Glandular fever.
(d) Chickenpox.

5 Match the type of microorganism on the left with the most appropriate description on the right:

(a) Bacteria	(i) Microorganisms that consists of nucleic acid surrounded by a protein coat (capsid)
(b) Protozoa	(ii) Microorganisms characterised by hyphae
(c) Viruses	(iii) Microorganisms with a prokaryotic cell structure, some forms of which produce resistant spores
(d) Fungi	(iv) Animal-like protists

6 Which one of the following diseases do insect vectors **not** spread?
(a) African sleeping sickness.
(b) Bacillary dysentery.
(c) Malaria.
(d) Tuberculosis.

7 Which one of the following terms best describes the situation characterised by the presence of microorganisms but that produces no response from the host and that does not benefit or harm the host?
(a) Colonisation.
(b) Parasitism.
(c) Mutualism.
(d) Infection.

8 Which one of the following are cells of the immune system that are responsible for antibody production?
(a) Neutrophils.
(b) Macrophages.
(c) Monocytes.
(d) B lymphocytes.

9 Match the organism on the left with the most appropriate description on the right:

(a) *Clostridium tetani*
(b) *Mycobacterium tuberculosis*
(c) *Staphylococcus aureus*
(d) *Salmonella enteritidis*

(i) A microorganism that is an obligate aerobe that infects the lungs
(ii) A microorganism that produces an exotoxin with powerful effects on muscle
(iii) A microorganism that causes food poisoning
(iv) A microorganism that is a skin commensal capable of opportunistic wound infection

10 Match the items on the left with the most appropriate form of treatment to kill microorganisms on the right:

(a) Milk
(b) Operating theatre gowns
(c) Plastic injection syringes
(d) Microbiology wire loops

(i) Autoclaving
(ii) Pasteurisation
(iii) Dry heat
(iv) Ionising radiation

Further study/exercises

1 How is MRSA prevented and treated?

Bissett L. (2006). Reducing the risk of acquiring antimicrobial resistant bacteria. *British Journal of Nursing*, 15(2), 68-71.

Collins F. and Hampton S. (2005). Handwashing and methicillin resistant *Staphylococcus aureus*. *British Journal of Nursing*, 14(13), 703-7.

Fairclough S. (2005). Hand hygiene: a simple way to stem the tide of MRSA. *Nursing and Residential Care*, 7(12), 554-6.

Fairclough S. (2006). Why tackling MRSA needs a comprehensive approach. *British Journal of Nursing*, 15(2), 72-5.

NHS Direct Online Health Encyclopedia - MRSA: www.nhsdirect.nhs.uk/articles/article.aspx?articleId=252

Department of Health: www.dh.gov.uk/Home/fs/en

A simple guide to MRSA: www.dh.gov.uk/PolicyAndGuidance/HealthAndSocialCareTopics/HealthcareAcquiredInfection/HealthcareAcquiredGeneralInformation/HealthcareAcquiredGeneralArticle/fs/en?CONTENT_ID=4093113&chk=7/XgcQ

2 Identify how, as a student nurse, you can help to reduce cross-infection during placements in clinical practice.

Candlin J. and Stark S. (2005). Plastic apron wear during direct patient care. *Nursing Standard*, 20(2), 41-6.

Chalmers C. and Straub M. (2006). Standard principles for preventing and controlling infection. *Nursing Standard*, 20(23), 57-65.

Jeanes A. (2005). Keeping hospitals clean: how nurses can reduce health care associated infection. *Professional Nurse*, 20(5), 35-7.

Johnson D. (2004). Infection thrives when basic cleanliness is ignored. *Nursing Times*, 100(13), 18.

Patel S. (2005). Minimising cross-infection risks associated with beds and mattresses. *Nursing Times*, 101(8), 52-3.

Patel S., Murray-Leonard J. and Wilson A. (2006). Laundering of hospital staff uniforms at home. *Journal of Hospital Infection*, 62(1), 89-93.

Rickard N. (2004). Hand hygiene: promoting compliance among nurses and health workers. *British Journal of Nursing*, 13(7), 404-10.

Answers to self-test questions

Chapter 3

1 a, b, d

2 a, b, d

3 a, c

4 b, c, d

5 a, d

6 a, b, d

7 (a) (iv)
(b) (iii)
(c) (ii)
(d) (i)

8 (a) (ii)
(b) (i)
(c) (iii)
(d) (iv)

9 (a) (iii)
(b) (iv)
(c) (ii)
(d) (i)

10 (a) (ii)
(b) (iv)
(c) (i)
(d) (iii)

Chapter 4

1 b

2 (a) (i)
(b) (ii)
(c) (iv)
(d) (iii)

3 c

4 b

5 d

6 c

7 a

8 a

9 c

10 a

Chapter 5

1 c

2 d

3 b

4 (a) (ii)
(b) (i)
(c) (iv)
(d) (iii)

5 a

6 c

7 c

8 b

9 c

10 c

Chapter 6

1 b

2 c

3 d

4 b

5 d

6 a, b

7 d

8 d

9 a, c

10 a, c, d

Chapter 7

1 (a) (i)
(b) (iii)
(c) (iv)
(d) (ii)

2 (a) (ii)
(b) (iv)
(c) (i)
(d) (iii)

3 (a) (ii)
(b) (iv)
(c) (iii)
(d) (i)

4 (a) (ii)
(b) (i)
(c) (iv)
(d) (iii)

5 (a) (ii)
(b) (iv)
(c) (i)
(d) (iii)

6 (a) (ii)
(b) (iv)
(c) (iii)
(d) (i)

7 (a) (ii)
(b) (iv)
(c) (iii)
(d) (i)

8 (a) (ii)
(b) (i)
(c) (iv)
(d) (iii)

9 c

10 a

Chapter 8

1 b, d

2 a, c

3 b, c, d

4 (a) (iii)
(b) (iv)
(c) (i)
(d) (ii)

5 b, c

6 a, c, d

7 b, d

8 (a) (ii)
(b) (iii)
(c) (iv)
(d) (i)

9 (a) (iv)
(b) (iii)
(c) (ii)
(d) (i)

10 (a) (iv)
(b) (iii)
(c) (ii)
(d) (i)

Chapter 9

1 (a) (iv)
(b) (iii)
(c) (i)
(d) (ii)

2 c

3 d

4 a

5 b

6 c

7 b

8 a, c

9 a, b, c

10 a, b, d

Chapter 10

1 d

2 a, b, c, d

3 b, c, d

4 b, c, d

5 a, b, c

6 a, b, d

7 c

8 d

9 b

10 c

Chapter 11

1 b

2 a, b

3 a, d

4 a, d

5 a, d

6 c

7 a

8 a, b, d

9 b

10 c

Chapter 12

1 a, c

2 a

3 b, c, d

4 a, c, d

5 b, c, d

6 b, c, d

7 a, b, c, d

8 a, c, d

9 c, d

10 a, b, d

Chapter 13

1 b, c

2 a, b

3 a, b, d

4 a, c

5 a, b, d

6 d

7 (a) (iv)
(b) (iii)
(c) (i)
(d) (ii)

8 (a) (i)
(b) (iv)
(c) (iii)
(d) (ii)

9 d

10 b

Chapter 14

1 d

2 c, d

3 (a) (ii)
(b) (i)
(c) (iv)
(d) (iii)

4 d

5 b

6 c

7 d

8 a

9 (a) (iii)
(b) (i)
(c) (ii)
(d) (iv)

10 d

Chapter 15

1 c

2 b, c, d

3 b, c

4 a, b, d

5 a, b

6 a

7 (a) (ii)
(b) (i)
(c) (iv)
(d) (iii)

8 a

9 b

10 (a) (ii)
(b) (iv)
(c) (i)
(d) (iii)

Chapter 16

1 (a) (ii)
(b) (i)
(c) (iii)
(d) (iv)

2 (a) (ii)
(b) (iii)
(c) (iv)
(d) (i)

3 (a) (ii)
(b) (i)
(c) (iii)
(d) (iv)

4 b

5 (a) (iii)
(b) (iv)
(c) (i)
(d) (ii)

6 d

7 a

8 d

9 (a) (ii)
(b) (i)
(c) (iv)
(d) (iii)

10 (a) (ii)
(b) (i)
(c) (iv)
(d) (iii)

Appendix: The Periodic Table*

Key	
1	Atomic number
Hydrogen	Name
H	Symbol
1.01	Atomic mass

Atomic weights are based on carbon-12. Numbers in parentheses are the mass numbers of the most stable isotopes.

Transition elements: groups between II and III (Sc to Zn and below).

I	II											III	IV	V	VI	VII	VIII or 0
1 Hydrogen H 1.01																	2 Helium He 4.00
3 Lithium Li 6.94	4 Beryllium Be 9.01											5 Boron B 10.81	6 Carbon C 12.01	7 Nitrogen N 14.01	8 Oxygen O 16.00	9 Fluorine F 19.00	10 Neon Ne 20.18
11 Sodium Na 22.99	12 Magnesium Mg 24.305											13 Aluminium Al 26.98	14 Silicon Si 28.09	15 Phosphorus P 30.97	16 Sulphur S 32.06	17 Chlorine Cl 35.45	18 Argon Ar 39.95
19 Potassium K 39.10	20 Calcium Ca 40.08	21 Scandium Sc 44.96	22 Titanium Ti 47.90	23 Vanadium V 50.94	24 Chromium Cr 52.00	25 Manganese Mn 54.94	26 Iron Fe 55.85	27 Cobalt Co 58.93	28 Nickel Ni 58.70	29 Copper Cu 63.546	30 Zinc Zn 65.38	31 Gallium Ga 69.72	32 Germanium Ge 72.59	33 Arsenic As 74.92	34 Selenium Se 78.96	35 Bromine Br 79.90	36 Krypton Kr 83.80
37 Rubidium Rb 85.47	38 Strontium Sr 87.62	39 Yttrium Y 88.91	40 Zirconium Zr 91.22	41 Niobium Nb 92.91	42 Molybdenum Mo 95.94	43 Technetium Tc 98.91	44 Ruthenium Ru 101.07	45 Rhodium Rh 102.91	46 Palladium Pd 106.42	47 Silver Ag 107.87	48 Cadmium Cd 112.41	49 Indium In 114.82	50 Tin Sn 118.69	51 Antimony Sb 121.75	52 Tellurium Te 127.60	53 Iodine I 126.90	54 Xenon Xe 131.30
55 Caesium Cs 132.91	56 Barium Ba 137.33	57 * Lanthanum La 138.91	72 Hafnium Hf 178.49	73 Tantalum Ta 180.95	74 Tungsten W 183.85	75 Rhenium Re 186.2	76 Osmium Os 190.20	77 Iridium Ir 192.22	78 Platinum Pt 195.09	79 Gold Au 196.97	80 Mercury Hg 200.59	81 Thallium Tl 204.37	82 Lead Pb 207.20	83 Bismuth Bi 208.98	84 Polonium Po (209)	85 Astatine At (210)	86 Radon Rn (222)
87 Francium Fr (223)	88 Radium Ra 226.03	89 '''' Actinium Ac (227)															

*	58 Cerium Ce 140.12	59 Praseodymium Pr 140.91	60 Neodymium Nd 144.24	61 Promethium Pm (145)	62 Samarium Sm 150.40	63 Europium Eu 151.96	64 Gadolinium Gd 157.25	65 Terbium Tb 158.93	66 Dysprosium Dy 162.50	67 Holmium Ho 164.93	68 Erbium Er 167.26	69 Thulium Tm 168.93	70 Ytterbium Yb 173.04	71 Lutetium Lu 174.97
''''	90 Thorium Th 232.04	91 Protactinium Pa 231.04	92 Uranium U 238.03	93 Neptunium Np 237.05	94 Plutonium Pu (244)	95 Americium Am (243)	96 Curium Cm (247)	97 Berkelium Bk (247)	98 Californium Cf (251)	99 Einsteinium Es (252)	100 Fermium Fm (257)	101 Mendelevium Md (258)	102 Nobelium No (259)	103 Lawrencium Lr (260)

Metals

Non-metals

Noble gases

* Sackheim G. I. (1996). *An Introduction to Chemistry for Biology Students*, 5th edn. California: Benjamin/Cummings

Glossary

A

absolute zero The temperature at which the kinetic energy of matter is at minimum, that is, 0 K or –273 °C.

acceleration The rate of change of velocity in metres per second per second (m/s^2 or ms^{-2}).

accommodation The process of changing the shape of the lens of the eye from relatively flat to more rounded in order to focus light rays on the retina. By this means, parallel rays from a distant object and divergent rays from a near object can be focused.

acetic acid *See* ethanoic acid.

acetone *See* propanone.

acetyl co-enzyme A (acetyl-CoA) A substance that is formed when an acetyl group combines with a co-enzyme molecule. Acetyl-CoA then enters the Krebs cycle.

acetyl salicylic acid The chemical name of the drug aspirin, which is used to reduce temperature in fever and to alleviate pain.

acid A substance that donates hydrogen ions (H^+) during a chemical reaction.

acidity The state of an excess of free hydrogen ions (H^+).

acidosis The state that exists when blood is more acidic than normal (that is, pH is less than 7.35).

actin A protein important in muscle contraction.

action potential A wave of current in nerve and muscle cells that results from the movement of ions across the plasma membrane.

activation energy The energy that must be supplied in order for a chemical reaction to proceed.

acquired immunodeficiency syndrome (AIDS) The disease that results from infection by human immunodeficiency virus (HIV).

Addison's disease The disease caused by under-secretion of steroid hormones produced by the adrenal cortex. Named after Thomas Addison.

adenine An organic compound found in adenosine triphosphate (ATP), adenosine diphosphate (ADP), ribonucleic acid (RNA) and deoxyribonucleic acid (DNA).

adenosine diphosphate (ADP) A substance that consists of the organic base adenine, a five-carbon-atom sugar and two inorganic phosphate groups. The compound that results when a phosphate group is removed from adenosine triphosphate.

adenosine triphosphate (ATP) The body's chemical form of energy. A molecule that consists of the organic base adenine, a five-carbon-atom sugar and three inorganic phosphate groups. ATP is produced when a third phosphate group is added to an adenosine diphosphate (ADP) molecule.

adhesive forces Forces of attraction between unlike particles, for example between water and the vessel in which it is contained.

adipose tissue A type of tissue that is modified to store nutrients. Often referred to as fatty tissue or, simply, fat.

adrenal glands Hormone glands located on top of the kidneys.

adrenal medulla The inner part of the adrenal glands that produces epinephrine (adrenaline) and norepinephrine (noradrenaline).

aerobe A microorganism that requires the presence of oxygen.

aerobic A process that requires the presence of oxygen.

aerosol A colloidal mixture in which a solid or a liquid is dispersed in a gas.

afferent Going to or carrying towards a centre.

afferent nerve A nerve that carries impulses to the brain - that is, a sensory nerve.

after-loading A form of radiotherapy in which empty tubes that will contain the radioisotope are inserted into the body. The radioisotope is then passed to and from the body through the tubing.

agar A gel manufactured from seaweed and used as a medium on which to grow microorganisms.

agranulocyte A leukocyte (white blood cell) that does not contain granules.

albumin A group of water-soluble proteins, some of which are present in blood.

albumin solution A colloidal solution derived from blood that contains 95% albumin and that is used as a plasma volume expander.

alcohols Compounds that contain a hydroxyl group (OH) attached to a carbon atom, the simplest of which conform to the general formula RCH_2OH.

aldehydes Compounds that contain a carbonyl group (C═O) at the end of a carbon-atom chain and conform to the general formula RCHO.

aldosterone A steroid hormone (mineralocorticoid) of the adrenal cortex that regulates sodium ion resorption in the kidney.

aldosteronism The condition of excessive aldosterone secretion that leads to elevated blood sodium levels and reduced blood potassium levels.

algae Plant-like microorganisms belonging to the kingdom protista.

aliphatic Organic compounds in which the ends of the carbon-atom chain are not joined together - that is, a ring is not formed.

alkalosis The state that exists when blood is more alkaline than normal (that is, pH is greater than 7.45).

alkalotic The term used to describe a person who is in a state of alkalosis.

alkanes A group of saturated aliphatic hydrocarbons that conform to the general formula C_nH_{2n+2}.

alkenes A group of unsaturated aliphatic hydrocarbons that contain one double bond and conform to the general formula C_nH_{2n}.

alkynes A group of unsaturated aliphatic hydrocarbons that contain one triple bond and conform to the general formula C_nH_{2n-2}.

alleles Genes that occupy identical loci on homologous chromosomes.

alpha particle A helium nucleus (^4_2He) consisting of two protons and two neutrons.

alveoli Literally, 'little hollows', but referring to air sacs that are the end units of lung tissue across which gas exchange takes place.

amines A group of compounds that are related to ammonia (NH_3), in which one of the hydrogen atoms is replaced by a hydrocarbon chain. Amines contain an amino group (NH_2) and conform to the general formula RCH_2NH_2.

amino acids The component molecules of proteins - organic acids that contain a basic amino group (NH_2) and a carboxyl group (COOH). *Essential* amino acids are those that are required in the diet since they cannot be synthesised in the body. *Non-essential* amino acids are those that are not essential in the diet, since they can be synthesised in the body, provided the essential amino acids are present.

ammonia A gaseous compound that has the molecular formula NH_3.

amniotic cavity The space between the developing embryo/foetus and the amnion (innermost foetal membrane).

amniotic fluid The fluid contained in the amniotic cavity.

amoeba A group of protozoans (animal-like microorganisms belonging to the kingdom protista). Amoebas are shapeless and move by forming pseudopodia ('false feet').

ampere (amp/A) The SI unit of electric current, equivalent to the flow of one coulomb of charge per second.

amphetamines A group of amines that act as nervous-system stimulants and that are abused due to their ability to produce euphoria.

ampicillin An antibiotic; a form of penicillin.

amplitude The maximum displacement of a particle of a wave from its rest position.

amylase A starch-digesting enzyme. *Pancreatic amylase* is produced by the pancreas and secreted into the duodenum through the pancreatic duct. *Salivary amylase* is produced by the salivary glands.

anabolism The synthesis reactions of the body.

anaemia The condition of reduced oxygen-carrying capacity of erythrocytes (red blood cells) due to a reduced number of erythrocytes or a reduction in their haemoglobin content. *Iron deficiency anaemia* results from a deficiency of iron. *Pernicious anaemia* results from a dietary deficiency of vitamin B_{12}, inability of the stomach to secrete intrinsic factor or following surgical removal of the stomach or ileum (the part of the small intestine where B_{12} is absorbed).

anaerobe A microorganism that requires the absence of oxygen.

anaerobic 1. A process that proceeds in the absence of oxygen. 2. See anaerobe.

anaesthesia Loss of feeling or insensibility. *General anaesthesia* is the induction of unconsciousness and loss of feeling. *Local anaesthesia* is the induction of loss of sensation in a part of the body.

anaesthetic A drug that induces anaesthesia.

analgesia The relief of pain.

analgesic A pain-relieving drug.

anaphase The third stage of mitosis, in which the separated chromatids move to the poles of the cell.

anaphylactic shock A type of circulatory shock that results from an allergic reaction and that is characterised by vasodilation (blood-vessel dilation) and low blood pressure.

angina Cardiac (heart) pain that results when the demand for oxygen by the heart muscle exceeds supply. It usually occurs during exercise and is central in the chest, is crushing in nature and may radiate to the neck or left arm.

angiography An X-ray technique in which a radiopaque dye (substance opaque to X-rays) is injected into a blood vessel in order to enable it to be seen as an X-ray image. *Coronary angiography* is angiography of the coronary arteries (arteries of the heart).

anion A negatively charged ion.

annulus fibrosus The strong outer ring of cartilage of an intervertebral disc.

anode A positively charged electrode.

anopheles mosquito The species of mosquito responsible for the transmission of malaria.

anorexia nervosa Literally 'nervous loss of appetite', but used to mean the condition in which appetite is drastically controlled. In its most serious form, the patient may starve to death.

antagonistic Having opposite effects.

antecubital fossa The region of the arm corresponding to the front of the elbow - the brachial pulse can be felt here.

anthrax The condition caused by the bacteria *Bacillus anthracis*. Found in cattle in some parts of the world and can be contracted by humans through inhalation, ingestion and direct contact with infected animals.

antibiotic An antimicrobial drug derived from substances produced naturally by microorganisms.

antibody (immunoglobulin) A globular protein produced by plasma cells of the immune system and that binds to an antigen in order to facilitate phagocytosis.

anticoagulant A drug that acts to delay blood clotting.

anticodon A triplet of nucleotides in tRNA that acts as a code for a particular amino acid.

antidiuretic hormone Literally 'against urine-output hormone'. The hormone produced by the posterior lobe of the pituitary gland and that is responsible for the production of more concentrated urine.

antigen A substance that triggers the production of antibodies.

antihypertensive A drug used to treat high blood pressure.

antimicrobial Any drug that is effective against microorganisms.

antisense strand The stand of DNA that is not used in transcription (synthesis of mRNA).

antiseptic A chemical substance with antimicrobial properties that can be applied to the skin.

antitussive A drug that suppresses cough.

anus The last segment of the large intestine.

aorta The principal artery of the body into which blood flows from the left ventricle.

apoenzyme The protein part of an enzyme; the non-protein part is referred to as a co-factor.

aqueous humour The watery fluid that fills the anterior chamber (the space behind the cornea but in front of the lens) of the eye.

aqueous mixture A mixture of a substance in water.

aqueous solution A solution in which water is the solvent.

archaebacteria A distinctive group of bacteria capable of surviving in extremely hostile environments, such as sulphur springs.

aromatic Literally 'having an aroma'. Used to refer to cyclic organic compounds.

arrhythmia An abnormal heart rhythm.

arteriole A small blood vessel that is formed from a division of an artery.

artery A blood vessel that carries blood away from the heart. All arteries except the pulmonary arteries carry oxygenated blood. The *axillary artery* supplies the upper arm. When a thermometer is placed in the axilla (armpit) for the purpose of measuring body temperature, it rests adjacent to this artery. The *brachial artery* runs down the medial aspect of the humerus bone of the upper arm (the body side of the upper arm). A pulse in the brachial artery can be felt in the antecubital fossa. The *coronary artery* supplies the heart. There are two main coronary arteries, and each has a number of divisions. There is a *carotid artery* on each side of the neck and a common carotid artery in which a pulse can be felt. Each carotid artery divides into an internal carotid artery and an external carotid artery, which supply different structures in the head. The *femoral artery* is a principal artery of the leg that passes down the inside of the thigh. The *pulmonary artery* conveys deoxygenated blood to the lungs from the right ventricle of the heart. The left and right pulmonary arteries supply the left and right lungs, respectively. The *sublingual artery* is literally the 'below-the-tongue' artery. When a thermometer is placed in the pocket between the tongue and the teeth, it rests adjacent to this artery.

aspirin A drug used to reduce temperature in fever and to alleviate pain.

atelectasis The collapse of an alveolus, such that gases can no longer be exchanged across the alveolus.

atherosclerosis Literally 'gruel-like hardening' - used to describe the accumulation of fats and other molecules in artery walls that leads to obstruction.

atom The smallest particle of an element.

atomic mass The average mass of all stable isotopes of an element expressed in atomic mass units and reflecting the relative proportions of the different isotopes.

atomic mass unit (amu/u) A unit equal to one-twelfth of the mass of the most abundant isotope of carbon (^{12}C).

atomic number The number of protons in the nucleus of an atom.

atria The two upper chambers of the heart.

atrioventricular block The condition that exists when an action potential in the conduction system of the heart is delayed or not transmitted by the atrioventricular node.

atrioventricular node (AV node) A part of the conduction system of the heart - a mass (node) of conducting cells in the right atrial wall through which action potentials pass towards the ventricles.

audiometric test A test of a person's hearing by exposing the person to sounds of different intensities.

autoclave A pressurised steam-heated device used for sterilisation.

autosome A chromosome that does not carry information about sex.

axilla The armpit - a site at which body temperature is sometimes measured.

axoplasm The cytoplasm (substance that makes up the cell contents) of a nerve cell.

B

bacillus A rod-shaped bacterium (plural = bacilli).

bacteraemia The presence of bacteria within the bloodstream.

bacteria Microorganisms that belong to the kingdom monera.

bactericidal Used to describe a drug that kills bacteria.

bacteristatic Used to describe a drug that prevents bacteria from reproducing.

barometer A device that measures atmospheric pressure.

basal metabolic rate (BMR) The metabolic rate measured in a subject who is fasted, rested and inactive but awake.

base A substance that accepts hydrogen ions (H^+) during a chemical reaction.

base excess A measure of the amount of acid that would need to be added to the sample of patient's blood in order to restore acid-base balance to normal. The normal value of base excess is, therefore, zero; in metabolic alkalosis it is positive in and metabolic acidosis it is negative.

basilar membrane The membrane that forms the floor of the scala media and the roof of the scala tympani.

basophil A granulocyte (type of leukocyte/white blood cell) that is stained with basic dyes.

becquerel A unit of measurement of radiation in terms of the number of disintegrations per unit of time.

beri beri A condition characterised by fatigue and muscle weakness that results from deficiency of thiamine (vitamin B_1).

beta oxidation The process of forming acetyl-CoA by removing acetyl groups from a carboxylic acid chain.

beta particle The name given to an electron emitted from an unstable nucleus as a consequence of the breakup of a neutron.

bile An alkaline fluid produced by the liver and stored and concentrated in the gall bladder. Bile is important in digestion, especially in the emulsification of fats.

bile salts Substances present in bile that are responsible for the emulsification of fat.

biliary tree The system of ducts that carry bile from the liver to the gall bladder and duodenum.

binary fission The asexual process by which some microorganisms, e.g. bacteria, reproduce. Growth is followed by division into two equal cells, which then proceed to grow and divide.

biopsy Any procedure in which a sample of tissue is obtained from the body for examination and diagnosis.

blood pressure The pressure exerted by blood upon the walls of the vessel in which it is circulating. *Arterial blood pressure* is the pressure that exists in the major arteries. Two values can be measured - systolic and diastolic pressures. *Diastolic blood pressure* occurs during ventricular diastole (relaxation). *Systolic blood pressure* occurs during ventricular systole (contraction). *Central venous pressure* is the pressure that exists in the central (great or major) veins, e.g. the vena cava.

body mass index (BMI) A numerical value without units that is calculated by dividing the weight (in kilograms) by the square of the height (in metres). Used to determine whether a person is underweight or overweight.

Bowman's capsule The capsule that surrounds the glomerulus (capillary network) of the nephron of the kidney.

Boyle's law A law that states that provided the temperature of a gas does not change, then the pressure of a fixed amount of gas will increase as the volume decreases, and vice versa.

bradycardia The condition of an abnormally slow pulse rate.

brachial artery See artery.

brain stem The lowest part of the brain that connects the brain to the spinal cord and that contains important vital centres, e.g. control centres for breathing and heart rate.

bronchitis Inflammation of the bronchi (a division of the airway) of the lung. *Chronic bronchitis* is a long-term condition that results from the inhalation of particles, e.g. in cigarette smoke or industrial dust such as coal dust.

bronchodilation Dilation (widening) of the bronchi of the lungs.

bronchodilator A drug that causes bronchdilation.

Brownian motion The random movement of particles of a gas or liquid.

brucellosis An infectious disease of humans caused by the bacterium *Brucella abortus* and transmitted by contact with infected animals.

buffer An aqueous solution that resists a change in pH upon the addition of an acid or a base.

bulimia nervosa A psychological condition characterised by alternating overeating and self-induced vomiting.

bundle of His (atrioventricular bundle) A part of the conduction system of the heart immediately below the atrioventricular node that conveys impulses from the atria to the ventricles.

Burkitt's lymphoma A malignant neoplasm (cancer) associated with the Epstein-Barr virus, which causes glandular fever.

C

calamine lotion A mechanical suspension of zinc oxide (ZnO) in water used to relieve sunburn.

calcitonin A hormone produced by the thyroid gland that reduces blood calcium levels and stimulates bone mineralisation.

calculi Stone-like masses that form within the body (single calculus). *Gall stones* are calculi that form within the gall bladder. *Renal calculi* form within the kidney.

calorie The calorie (without a capital letter and abbreviated cal) is the amount of energy required to raise the temperature of 1 g of water by one degree Celsius (1 °C). It is a rather small unit of energy, and so the unit of the kilocalorie (kcal - 1000 calories) is more convenient. The kcal is the same as the nutritional Calorie (with a capital letter).

canula A narrow tube inserted into the body, particularly into the bloodstream, e.g. intravenous canula (plural = cannulae).

capacitor A device used to store electric charge.

capillary The smallest type of blood vessel, with a wall only one cell thick.

capillary endothelium *See* endothelium.

capsid The protein coat of a virus.

carbohydrate An organic compound containing only carbon, hydrogen and oxygen.

carbonic acid The compound that has the molecular formula H_2CO_3 and that is formed from a reaction between carbon dioxide and water.

carbonic anhydrase The enzyme responsible for catalysing the reaction between carbon dioxide and water to produce carbonic acid.

carboxyhaemoglobin *See* haemoglobin.

carboxylic acids Organic compounds that contain a carboxyl (COOH) group and conform to the general formula RCOOH; also known as fatty acids, since they react with the alcohol glycerol to form neutral fats.

cardiac Pertaining to the heart. *Cardiac arrest* is the condition that exists when the heart ceases to pump blood effectively.

carotenes Yellow pigments found in a number of plants, including carrots, and from which the liver can make vitamin A.

carpopedal spasm Sustained contraction of the muscles of the wrist and ankle.

catabolism The chemical reactions of the body that involve the breaking down of substances.

catalyst A substance that increases the speed of a chemical reaction but remains unchanged by the reaction.

cataract Opacity of the lens of the eye. It is associated with the ageing process and exposure to ultraviolet light.

catecholamines A group of amines that includes epinephrine (adrenaline), norepinephrine (noradrenaline) and dopamine.

catheter A tube inserted into the body for the purpose of draining fluid or the administration of drugs.

catheterisation The act of inserting a catheter into the body. See also intubation.

cathode A negatively charged electrode.

cathode ray A stream of electrons produced in a cathode ray tube.

cation A positively charged ion.

caustic soda A common name for sodium hydroxide (NaOH). Compounds of sodium are often given the name soda; the description 'caustic' is applied here because of the ability to cause chemical burns.

cell The smallest unit of living matter.

cell membrane *See* plasma membrane.

cellulose A plant polysaccharide that cannot be digested by humans - often referred to as roughage or fibre.

cell wall The structure that encloses the cytoplasm of a bacterial cell, the composition of which determines the staining reactions of the cell.

Celsius scale A scale used to measure temperature in which there are 100 divisions between the melting point of ice and the boiling point of water. Each division is referred to as one degree Celsius (°C).

central venous pressure (CVP) The pressure of blood in the central (great) veins, such as the vena cava.

centre of gravity The point at which the entire weight of an object can be thought of as acting for the purpose of considering torque.

centrioles Cylindrical structures in the cytoplasm of cells that migrate to opposite poles of the cell during cell division and between which spindle fibres form.

centromere The constricted part of chromosomes at which the two chromatids are joined and that attaches to spindle fibres during cell division.

centrosome The area adjacent to the nucleus in which centrioles are normally found.

cephalosporin A type of antibiotic.

cerebrospinal fluid (CSF) The protective fluid contained in the ventricles of the brain, sub-arachnoid space and spinal canal.

cerebrovascular accident (CVA) The condition that results from death of cells in a region of the brain due to ischaemia (lack of blood supply) and most commonly caused by thrombosis (blood-clot formation) of a cerebral artery. May result in paralysis and speech difficulties.

cerumen Earwax.

ceruminous glands *See* gland.

Charles' law A law that states that if the pressure of a gas is constant, then its volume is directly proportional to its absolute temperature.

cheilosis Cracks in the lips caused by a deficiency of vitamin B_2 (riboflavin).

chemoautotrophs Literally 'chemical self-feeders'; used in reference to bacteria that derive energy from inorganic substances.

chemoreceptor A sensory nerve ending that is activated by a chemical stimulus, e.g. CO_2.

chemotaxis The movement of phagocytes to chemicals released at the site of tissue damage.

chief cells *See* zymogenic cells.

chloramphenicol A type of antibiotic.

cholera An acute bacterial intestinal infection caused by *Vibrio cholerae* and characterised by severe diarrhoea and dehydration.

cholesterol A member of a group of lipids called sterols.

chromatid One of two identical structures joined at the centromere that form a chromosome and that appear during interphase.

chromatin Literally, 'coloured material'. The thread-like mass of DNA and its associated proteins found within the nucleus of a cell.

chromosome Literally, 'coloured body'. The structures that are formed within the nucleus of a cell by the super-coiling of DNA and its associated proteins. A *sex chromosome* is a chromosome that carries information that determines sex.

chronic obstructive pulmonary disease (COPD) An umbrella term for long-term lung disease that results in narrowing of the airways. Chronic bronchitis and asthma are included.

chyle The milky contents of the small intestine that results from the emulsification of fat.

chylomicrons Water-soluble lipoprotein droplets present in blood.

chymotrypsin A protein-digesting enzyme produced by the action of trypsin on chymotrypsinogen.

chymotrypsinogen The precursor of chymotrypsin produced by the pancreas and converted to chymotrypsin by trypsin.

cilia Microscopic hair-like projections on the outer surfaces of some cells.

ciliary muscle Literally 'hair-like muscle' - referring to the ring of muscles of the eye that is attached to the lens and that changes the shape of the lens in accommodation.

ciliates Members of a group of protozoa characterised by hair-like cilia that cover the organism. Cilia beat in a coordinated way that enables movement.

ciprofloxacin A type of antibiotic.

circadian rhythm Pertaining to any physiological cycle, e.g. menstruation. A *diurnal rhythm* is a physiological cycle that is repeated every 24 hours, e.g. daily changes in body temperature and the sleep-wake cycle.

citric acid An acid found widely in fruits and important in the energy-producing reactions of cells.

cobalamin A form of vitamin B_{12}.

codon A triplet of nucleotides in DNA or mRNA that acts as a code for a specific amino acid.

coccus A round-shaped bacterium (plural = cocci).

cochlear nerve *See* nerve.

co-enzyme A type of cofactor. A non-protein organic molecule that forms a component of an enzyme and that is essential for its activity.

co-enzyme A A co-enzyme that is derived from the B group vitamin pantothenic acid and that combines with an acetyl group to form acetyl co-enzyme A.

cofactor A non-protein component of an enzyme such as a co-enzyme or an inorganic ion that is essential for the activity of the enzyme.

cohesive forces The forces of attraction that exist between like molecules.

collagen A flexible but inelastic protein that gives strength to soft tissues.

colloid Also referred to as a colloidal suspension or colloidal mixture. An aqueous mixture in which the particles that are dispersed in the fluid are smaller than those of a mechanical suspension but too large to form a true solution.

colonisation A term derived from 'colony' and used in reference to the presence of microorganisms without a response from the body or damage to the body.

combination reaction A type of chemical reaction in which two or more reactants combine to form a new substance.

commensalism A form of symbiosis (association between two species) in which one species benefits from the association while the other neither benefits nor is harmed.

compound A substance that is comprised of atoms of more than one element linked by chemical bonds.

concave Curved inwards.

concave lens *See* lens.

concentration An expression of the relative proportions of solute to solvent in an aqueous mixture commonly given as a percentage or in terms of a number of moles or millimoles of solute per litre of solvent (mol/l or mmol/l).

concentration gradient A difference in concentration between two regions.

condensation reaction A type of chemical reaction in which water is produced.

conduction The property of transmitting - used of heat or electricity, including electrical currents in the body, e.g. the conduction system of the heart (structures that transmit electrical impulses through the heart).

conductive deafness See deafness.

conductor A substance through which electrical current flows or through which heat passes readily.

cone A type of cell of the retina of the eye responsible for black-and-white vision.

control centre A component of a homeostatic control mechanism; a part of the body that regulates a controlled condition.

controlled condition A variable, such as body temperature, that is regulated by a homeostatic control mechanism.

convection A process involved in heat loss whereby air that has been warmed rises and is replaced by cooler, denser air.

convex Curved outwards.

convex lens *See* lens.

cornea The transparent membrane that forms the outer coat of the eye.

cortisone A steroid hormone of the adrenal cortex with anti-inflammatory properties.

coulomb The SI unit of charge (named after Charles Coulomb) equal to the charge of 1.6×10^{19} electrons.

covalent bond The chemical linking of atoms through the sharing of electrons.

covalent compound A compound that is formed when atoms are joined by covalent bonds.

creatinine A waste substance that is the end product of the metabolism of muscle protein.

crenation The shrinking of a cell so that it develops a scalloped surface due to the outward movement of water by osmosis.

crystal A solid that has a geometric form.

crystalloid solution Solution in which the solute has a crystalline structure in the solid phase.

current An expression used to describe the flow of electrons in dynamic electricity. *Alternating current* is current flow in an electrical circuit in alternate directions. *Direct current* is current flow in an electrical circuit flowing in one direction only.

cyclic compound An organic compound in which the ends of the carbon-atom chain are joined together to form a ring structure.

cystic fibrosis An autosomal recessive genetic disorder that leads to the production of excessively thick mucus.

cystitis Inflammation of the urinary bladder as a result of infection.

cytochrome chain *See* electron transport chain.

cytokinesis The division of a cell into two daughter cells.

cytoplasm Literally, 'cell substance'. The living material of the cell, including the cellular organelles but excluding the nucleus.

cytosine A base common to DNA and RNA.

D

Dalton's law A law that states that in a mixture of gases, the total pressure is a sum of the pressures exerted by each of the gases alone.

deafness Loss of hearing. *Conductive deafness* is loss of hearing due to impaired conduction of sound to the cochlea and resulting from a problem affecting the outer ear or middle ear. *Sensorineural deafness* is loss of hearing due to damage to the cochlea or its associated nervous pathways.

deamination The removal of an amino group (NH_2) from a molecule.

decibel (dB) A unit of measurement of the relative loudness of sound.

decomposition A chemical reaction in which a single reactant is broken down to produce one or more products.

defibrillation The application of an electric current to the heart for the purpose of converting ventricular fibrillation to sinus rhythm.

defibrillator The electrical device used to administer an electric current for the purpose of defibrillation.

dehydration The condition that results from a negative water balance.

denaturation A change in the three-dimensional structure of an enzyme that results in its inactivity.

density An expression of the mass of a substance per unit volume.

deoxyribose A pentose (five-carbon-atom sugar) found in deoxyribonucleic acid (DNA).

deoxyribonucleic acid (DNA) The nucleic acid that consists of nucleotides made up of the sugar deoxyribose, a phosphate group and one of four nitrogenous bases (adenine, thymine, guanine or cytosine). Genetic information is encoded in the sequence of these bases.

depolarisation The loss of the resting membrane potential that accompanies the influx of sodium ions during an action potential.

dermatitis Inflammation of the skin.

dermis The layer of skin below the epidermis and consisting of connective tissue.

dextrins Polymers of glucose that are intermediates between starch and glucose and formed during the digestion of starch.

diabetes mellitus An endocrine disorder characterised by a high blood sugar level and caused by a lack of insulin or insulin resistance.

dialysate A solution used in dialysis.

dialysis The exchange of solutes and water between blood and a dialysate across a synthetic or biological membrane. In *haemodialysis*, an extracorporeal circulation is established through a dialyser (artificial kidney) and dialysis occurs across an artificial membrane. In *peritoneal dialysis*, the dialysate is infused into the peritoneal cavity and dialysis occurs across the peritoneum.

diaphragm The principal muscle of breathing that separates the chest from the abdomen.

diastole Relaxation of the heart. The term may be applied to the atria or the ventricles.

diathermy The use of high-frequency alternating current for the purpose of cutting tissue (electrosurgery) or coagulating blood in order to seal blood vessels (electocautery).

diatomic Literally, 'consisting of two atoms'. Used of the gases oxygen (O_2), nitrogen (N_2) and hydrogen (H_2) - the so-called diatomic gases.

diglyceride *See* glyceride.

diffusion The movement of solute particles from an area of high solute concentration, through a semi-permeable membrane, to an area of low solute concentration until an equilibrium is reached.

dihydrogen phosphate ion The $H_2PO_4^-$ ion that forms part of an important buffer systems in intracellular fluid and renal filtrate.

diplococci A term used in the identification and naming of bacteria in which round forms (cocci) are arranged in pairs.

diploid Possessing the full number of chromosomes that is characteristic of somatic cells - that is, 46 in humans.

dipolar ion *See* zwitterion.

disaccharide A compound that is formed from the joining together of two simple sugars (monosaccharides).

disinfectant A chemical substance that can be used for disinfection.

disinfection A chemical treatment that render an object non-infective. It does not mean that there are no organisms remaining, but means that the number of microorganisms has been greatly reduced. Spores may remain following disinfection.

displacement A type of chemical reaction in which a less reactive element is displaced from a molecule by a more reactive element.

dissociation The breakdown of a substance into ions when dissolved in solution.

dissolving The act of forming a true solution.

diuresis The production of urine.

diuretic A drug that causes diuresis.

diurnal rhythm *See* circadian rhythm.

Doppler effect The apparent change in frequency of sound due to the motion of the source relative to the listener.

Down's syndrome The condition of trisomy 21 (possessing three chromosome 21s) that results in learning disability and a number of characteristic features of appearance, including folds of skin over the inner part of the eyelid.

duodenum The first section of the small intestine into which the stomach empties its contents and that produces a number of digestive enzymes.

dysentery Inflammation of the intestines, especially the colon, leading to frequent diarrhoea and caused by one of a number of different microorganisms.

dyspnoea The subjective experience of difficulty in breathing.

E

earth The conductive connection that forms the route by which current flows to earth.

effector An organ that produces an effect as a result of stimulation by the nervous system or the effect of a hormone. Effectors include muscles and endocrine glands.

efferent Literally, 'to carry out'. Refers to any structure that leaves a centre, e.g. efferent nerves transmit impulses away from the brain.

elastin An elastic protein found within the body.

electric current The flow of electrons from a region of high electron density to a region of low electron density. The SI unit of current is the ampere (amp, A).

electrode A solid conductor through which electric current passes in a variety of electrical devices.

electrolyte A substance that dissociates into ions in solution and that accounts for the ability of the solution to conduct electricity.

electromagnet A magnet in which the electromagnetic force is dependent on the flow of electric current.

electromagnetic radiation Energy in the form of transverse waves that do not require a material medium through which to pass but that result from the oscillation of electrical and magnetic fields.

electromagnetic spectrum A term used to encompass the whole range of electromagnetic radiation.

electron A subatomic particle of negligible mass that carries a single negative charge and orbits the nucleus of the atom.

electron cloud The region around the nucleus of an atom that is occupied by electrons.

electron transport chain A sequence of linked chemical reactions in which electrons are passed from one substance to another and ATP is formed. The reactions take place in the mitochondria.

electrocautery *See* diathermy.

electrosurgery *See* diathermy.

element A substance that is composed of identical atoms - that is, they all have the same atomic number.

elemental particle A subatomic particle such as a proton, neutron or electron.

embolism An abnormal circulatory condition in which an object (embolus - a foreign body, blood clot or air) is mobile within the circulation and that eventually lodges and occludes a blood vessel.

emulsification The act of forming an emulsion.

emulsion A colloidal solution in which one liquid is dispersed in another.

encephalopathy Any abnormality of the brain.

endergonic A chemical reaction in which the products possess more energy than the reactants and in which energy is, therefore, required in order for the reaction to proceed.

endocrine glands *See* glands.

endocrine system Pertaining to the system of ductless, hormone-producing glands.

endolymph The fluid contained within the scala media.

endoscope A rigid or fibre-optic instrument used to examine hollow organs and body cavities.

endoscopy Any procedure that employs the use of an endoscope.

endothelium The name given to the tissue that lines body cavities or blood vessels (plural = endothelia). The *capillary endothelium* forms the wall of a capillary.

endothermic A reaction that requires heat - a reaction in which the energy of the products is greater than that of the reactants.

endotoxin A toxin that is contained within the wall of a microorganism and that is released only when the microorganism dies.

endotracheal tube A tube designed to be inserted into the trachea for the purpose of artificial ventilation, i.e. the patient is not breathing and air is forced into the lungs through the tube.

energy The ability to do work.

energy levels/shells The orbitals in which the electrons of an atom are located.

enterokinase An intestinal enzyme that is responsible for activating the protein-digesting enzyme trypsinogen to trypsin.

environment The conditions in which life exists. The *external environment* is the external conditions in which an organism lives. The *internal environment* is the conditions that exist within the body of an organism, e.g. temperature, concentration of substances dissolved in the blood, etc.

enzymes Protein catalysts.

eosin A red dye that can be used as a laboratory stain to colour cells and make them more visible to microscopy.

eosinophil Literally, 'loves eosin'. A granulocyte (leukocyte/white blood cell possessing granules) that can be stained with the red dye eosin.

epidermis The outer layer of the skin formed from epithelial tissue.

epinephrine (adrenaline) A hormone produced by the medulla of the adrenal glands. It has a number of effects, including raising the heart rate and blood pressure.

epithelium A type of tissue characterised by closely packed cells. Different types of epithelia (= plural) are described on the basis of the shape of cells and the number of layers of cells. Epithelia are lining and covering tisues.

equatorial plate The centre of the mitotic spindle to which chromosomes become attached in metaphase.

erythema Redness of the skin, such as occurs in mild sunburn and inflammation.

erythrocyte Literally 'red cell'. Used to identify red blood cells that contain the red oxygen-carrying pigment haemoglobin.

erythromycin A type of antibiotic.

esters Organic compounds formed by a reaction between a carboxylic acid and an alcohol and that conform to the general formula RCOOR.

ethanoic acid The carboxylic acid with the molecular formula C_2H_3COOH; also known as acetic acid and, in dilute solution, as vinegar.

eubacteria A division of bacteria sometimes called 'true bacteria' that includes all bacteria except archaebacteria.

eukaryotic A complex type of cell structure with a separate nucleus that contains genetic information.

eustachian tube A tube that vents the middle ear to the nasopharynx and allows the middle ear to equalise with atmospheric pressure.

evaporation A change in state from liquid to gas.

exergonic A chemical reaction in which the products possess less energy than the reactants and in which energy is liberated during the reaction.

exocytosis The mechanism by which substances too large to diffuse out of a cell are passed to the outside.

exothermic A reaction that releases heat - the energy of the products is lower than that of the reactants.

exotoxin A toxin released by living microorganisms.

external auditory canal The canal that leads from the pinna (ear lobe) to the tympanic membrane (eardrum) and down which sound waves pass.

external-beam radiotherapy *See* radiotherapy.

extracellular fluid Fluid that is located outside cells. The term includes blood and interstitial fluid.

extracorporeal Literally, 'outside the body'. Often used when blood is circulated through a device outside the body.

F

fats *See* lipids.

fatty acids *See* carboxylic acids.

febrile The condition of having a fever.

feedback mechanism A homeostatic response to a physiological change. In *negative feedback*, change is not reinforced but suppressed - most homeostatic mechanisms are of this type. In *positive feedback*, change is reinforced.

femur The bone of the thigh.

fertilisation The fusion of the nucleus of a spermatozoon (sperm) and an ovum (egg).

fibre Thread-like - used to identify indigestible plant carbohydrate such as cellulose. Fibre is also referred to as roughage or non-starch carbohydrate.

fibrillation A highly disorganised and uncoordinated heart rhythm that may affect the atria or the ventricles. Ventricular fibrillation is a cause of cardiac arrest.

fibronectin A glycoprotein (molecule made up of a sugar and a protein) found on the surface of cells.

fibrinogen A soluble plasma protein important in the clotting of blood. When acted upon by the enzyme thrombin, it forms insoluble fibrin - the basis of a blood clot.

fibrous Resembling a fibre - often used of chemical substances, e.g. fibrous protein, to distinguish them from others that resemble a globe or ball, e.g. globular protein.

filtration The process whereby substances are separated by means of a membrane that has pores of a given size.

flagellates A group of protozoa characterised by the possession of at least one flagellum - a whip-like structure that is used for movement.

flagellum A whip-like structure possessed by some microorganisms that enables them to move due to its back and forth motion (plural = flagellae).

flavine adenine dinucleotide (FAD) A derivative of vitamin B_2 important in the energy-liberating reactions of cells.

fluid *See* liquid.

fluoroscopy The procedure in which a real-time image of the body is produced by means of a detector that fluoresces (glows) when struck by X-rays. Often used to aid the accurate positioning of an object (often a needle or tube) inserted into the body.

foam A colloidal suspension produced when a large volume of air is dispersed through a smaller volume of liquid or solid.

focal length The distance between a lens and the focal point.

focal point The point at which light rays converge, having passed through a lens.

focus The effect of a lens in causing light rays to converge at a point referred to as the focal point. For *principle focus*, see focal point.

folic acid Literally, 'leaf acid'. A vitamin found widely in plant and animal sources.

fomite Any non-living object (e.g. nurse's uniform, instrument such as scissors, a bandage, or even a bar of soap) that acts to cause cross-infection (the transfer of microorganisms from one person or place to another).

force An influence that is responsible for changing the state of rest or uniform motion of an object. The SI unit of force is the newton (N).

formula An expression of the chemical composition of a compound. The *molecular formula* states the number of each of the atoms present. The *structural formula* shows the number of each of the atoms present and their structural arrangement.

frequency An expression of how often an event occurs (e.g. change in direction of an electric current), often measured in number of times (cycles) per second (hertz, Hz). For example, in the UK the domestic electricity supply is delivered at 50 Hz.

friction The force that results from the movement of one object across another.

fructose Literally, 'fruit sugar'. Simple sugar with the formula $C_6H_{12}O_6$ - an isomer of glucose.

fulcrum A point of support about which a turning force acts.

functional group A group of two or more atoms that are present in a number of different molecules and that confer similar properties upon all the molecules in which they are present.

fungi A kingdom of eukaryotic organisms, most of which feed on dead or decaying organic material. Some are responsible for disease in humans.

G

galactose Literally, 'milk sugar'. Simple sugar with the formula $C_6H_{12}O_6$ - an isomer of glucose.

gall bladder A structure located beneath the liver, the purpose of which is to store and concentrate bile.

gall stones *See* calculi.

gamete A sex cell (spermatozoa in males, oocytes in females).

gametocyte A sexual cell in the lifecycle of members of the genus *Plasmodium* that cause malaria.

gamma rays Electromagnetic radiation that has a shorter wavelength than X-rays and is emitted by the nuclei of certain radioisotopes.

gas The state of matter in which particles of matter are able to move independently of each other. Gases fill the container in which they are placed.

gaseous *See* gas.

gastrectomy The surgical removal of the stomach.

gastric Pertaining to the stomach.

gel A colloidal suspension formed by the dispersal of a liquid in a solid. A gel exists on the borderline of solidity.

gene The smallest unit of heredity corresponding to a section of DNA that codes for a specific mRNA - that is, a section of DNA located between a start codon and a stop codon.

genetic code A code for the synthesis of protein in the form of a sequence of bases that form part of a nucleic acid molecule.

genetics The study of genes and heredity.

genome The complete gene complement of an organism.

genotype The genetic composition of an individual.

gentamicin A type of antibiotic.

gingivitis Inflammation of the gums.

gland A secretory organ. *Ceruminous glands* are glands of the external auditory canal that produce cerumen (earwax). *Endocrine glands* are glands that do not possess ducts and that secrete their products (hormones) directly into the bloodstream.

glandular fever An infectious illness caused by the Epstein-Barr virus, which produces flu-like symptoms and in some cases a prolonged period of weakness.

globular Resembling a globe or ball - often used of chemical substances, e.g. globular protein, to distinguish them from others that are elongated and resemble a fibre, e.g. fibrous protein.

glomerulus The capillary network located in the renal corpuscle.

glossitis Inflammation of the tongue.

glottis The opening to the larynx.

glucagon The hormone secreted by the alpha cells of the islets of Langerhans of the pancreas. Glucagon stimulates the conversion of glycogen in the liver to glucose and thus raises the blood glucose level.

gluconeogenesis The manufacture of glucose from non-carbohydrate sources such as amino acids.

glucose A simple sugar with the formula $C_6H_{12}O_6$ - the principal source of energy in the body.

glyceride A type of lipid that is formed from the reaction between the alcohol glycerol and one, two or three carboxylic acids. A *monoglyceride* has one carboxylic acid chain. A *diglyceride* has two carboxylic acid chains. A *triglyceride* has three carboxylic acid chains.

glycerol A three-carbon alcohol that reacts with carboxylic acids to form glycerides.

glyceryl trinitrate (GTN) A drug used to relieve angina (heart pain).

glycogen The body's carbohydrate store of energy (in liver and muscle). A polysaccharide consisting of branched chains of glucose molecules.

glycogenesis The process whereby glycogen is manufactured from glucose.

glycogenolysis The breakdown of glycogen to release glucose.

glycolysis A process that occurs in the cytoplasm. The first step in glucose catabolism, which results in the formation of pyruvic acid.

glycoprotein A protein with a sugar molecule attached.

glycosuria The presence of glucose in the urine.

goitre Enlargement of the thyroid gland.

gonads The organs of reproduction.

gonorrhoea A sexually transmitted disease caused by *Neisseria gonorrhoea* that commonly affects the genitourinary tract.

Gram stain A microorganism-staining technique used to distinguish between different types of bacterium.

granulocyte A group of leukocytes (white blood cells) that contain granules within their cytoplasm (substance of the cell). These granules contain chemical substances that affect their staining properties and that are used as a means of identification.

gravity The force of attraction between objects, especially between an object and the earth.

gray A unit of measurement of radioactivity in terms of the amount of energy absorbed by the body.

group A vertical column in the Periodic Table of elements.

guanine A base found in both deoxyribonucleic acid (DNA) and ribonucleic acid (RNA).

H

haematopoiesis Literally, 'blood production'. Refers to the manufacture of blood cells in the bone marrow.

haemodialysis *See* dialysis.

haemoglobin The molecule found in erythrocytes (red blood cells) and responsible for the transportation of oxygen. *Carboxyhaemoglobin* is the molecule formed when carbon monoxide binds with haemoglobin. *Oxyhaemoglobin* is the molecule formed when oxygen binds with haemoglobin.

haemophilia Literally, 'blood love'. Hereditary diseases in which one of the clotting factors is missing, leading to impaired blood coagulation. The most common form concerns the deficiency of factor VIII (haemophilia A).

haemorrhoids Varicose veins of the rectum and anus.

half-life The *biological half-life* is the time taken for the amount of a specific isotope that has entered the body to be reduced by half as a consequence of natural biological processes. The *effective half-life* is the time taken for the amount of a specific isotope that has entered the body to be reduced by half as a consequence of its radioactive decay and its biological elimination. The *physical half-life* is the time taken for half of a given number of atoms of a radioisotope to decay.

halothane An anaesthetic gas used in surgery.

haploid Possessing half the number of chromosomes that is characteristic of somatic cells - that is, 23 in humans.

Heaf gun A multiple-puncture tuberculin skin test (test for immunity to tuberculosis) device named after the physician Frederick Heaf.

heat Energy possessed by a substance as a consequence of the vibration of its particles.

Henry's law A law that states that the mass of a gas that will dissolve in water at a given temperature is proportional to the partial pressure of the gas and its solubility coefficient.

heparin A naturally occurring polysaccharide that prevents intravascular clotting (clotting within blood vessels). Also manufactured as an anticoagulant (prevents blood clotting) drug.

hepatic portal vein Literally, 'the vein that carries blood to the liver'. Refers to the vein that drains blood from the small intestine and supplies the liver.

hepatocyte Literally, 'liver cell'. Refers to the principal type of cell of the liver that performs the functions ascribed to the liver.

heterotrophs Literally, 'other feeders'. Refers to microorganisms that obtain their nutrients from organic molecules.

heterozygous The presence of different alleles of the same gene on homologous chromosomes.

hilum An indentation on the surface of an organ where structures such as blood vessels and nerves enter.

His *See* bundle of His.

histamine A substance produced by cells that is responsible for the inflammatory response.

histones Proteins around which deoxyribonucleic acid (DNA) is wrapped to form chromatin threads.

homeostasis The concept of a relatively stable internal environment.

homologous chromosomes A pair of morphologically identical chromosomes that carry genes for the same traits.

homozygous The presence of identical alleles on homologous chromosomes.

hormone A chemical substance that is secreted directly into the bloodstream by an endocrine (ductless) gland and that produces an effect in a specific target tissue elsewhere in the body.

human immunodeficiency virus (HIV) The virus that destroys T lymphocytes important in cell-mediated immunity and that causes acquired immunodeficiency syndrome (AIDS).

hydrocarbon A compound composed solely of hydrogen and carbon atoms.

hydrochloric acid ($HCl_{(aq)}$) The acid formed when hydrogen chloride gas (HCl) dissolves in water. The acid is also produced by the stomach, where it turns the inactive enzyme precursor pepsinogen into the active protein-digesting enzyme pepsin.

hydrogen bonds Weak forces of attraction that exist between polar molecules or between different regions of the same molecule in which hydrogen atoms with a partial positive charge are attracted to atoms with a partial negative charge.

hydrogen carbonate ion (bicarbonate ion) The HCO_3^- ion.

hydrogenation A process of adding hydrogen to a molecule.

hydrolysis A type of decomposition reaction that requires a water molecule.

hydrophilic Water-attracting.

hydrophobic Water-repelling.

hydrostatic pressure The pressure that results from the collision of particles of a fluid with the walls of the vessel in which it is contained.

hydroxyl ion The OH^- ion.

hypercalcaemia The condition of high blood calcium.

hyperglycaemia The condition of an elevated blood sugar level.

hyperkalaemia The condition of a high blood potassium level.

hypernatraemia The condition of a high blood sodium level.

hyperopia The condition often referred to as long-sightedness, in which light is focused beyond the retina.

hyperosmotic Describing a solution that has a higher osmotic pressure than another.

hypertension An elevated blood pressure.

hyperthermia An abnormally elevated body temperature.

hyperthyroidism The condition of an excess production of hormones of the thyroid gland, e.g. thyroxine.

hypertonic Describing a solution that is capable of causing crenation of cells.

hyperventilation Fast, deep breathing.

hyphae The slender filaments that characterise fungi.

hypocalcaemia The condition of low blood calcium.

hypochromic Literally, 'low colour', e.g. used to describe erythrocytes (red blood cells) lacking the oxygen-carrying pigment haemoglobin in the condition iron deficiency anaemia.

hypoglycaemia The condition of a low blood sugar level.

hypokalaemia The condition of a low blood potassium level.

hyponatraemia The condition of a low blood sodium level.

hypo-osmotic Describing a solution that has a lower osmotic pressure than another.

hypoproteinaemia The condition of a low blood protein level.

hypoprothrombinaemia The condition of a low blood prothrombin (a protein important in blood clotting) level.

hypotension The condition of abnormally low blood pressure.

hypothalamus Literally, 'below the thalamus'. A structure that is located immediately below the thalamus of the brain. The location of important homeostatic control centres, e.g. for temperature.

hypothermia An abnormally low body temperature.

hypothyroidism The condition of reduced production of the hormones of the thyroid gland, e.g. thyroxine.

hypotonic Describing a solution that is capable of causing the plasmolysis of cells.

hypoventilation Literally, 'low ventilation'. Refers to the condition of slow, shallow breathing.

hypoxaemia A low partial pressure of oxygen in arterial blood (P_aO_2).

hypoxia Decreased availability of oxygen to the tissues.

I

iatrogenic Literally, 'doctor-caused'. Refers to a disease or symptoms caused by medical intervention of any kind.

ileum A part of the small intestine, which is the principal site of absorption.

immune system A system within the body that is concerned with protections and especially with fighting infectious disease. Although there are specific cells of the immune system, the system operates in all tissues.

immunity The ability to resist infectious disease. *Acquired immunity* comprises mechanisms that are responsible for individual members of a species developing immunity against a previously encountered microorganism (also referred to as specific immunity). *Cell-mediated immunity* is a type of acquired immunity that involves the activity of specialist types of T lymphocyte.

Humoral immunity is a type of acquired immunity comprising the production of antibodies (immunoglobulins). *Innate immunity* comprises 'inborn' or 'inbuilt' mechanisms that are the same in each member of a species, such as inflammation and phagocytosis. Innate mechanisms do not adapt to different microorganisms that the body encounters, and for this reason innate immunity is also referred to as non-adaptive.

immunoglobulin Literally, 'globular protein of the immune system'. See antibody.

incus Literally, 'anvil'. The name given to one of the bones of the middle ear involved in hearing.

induced fit A model of enzyme action in which the active site is believed to undergo a change in shape in order to accommodate the substrate.

inertia The tendency of an object to resist a force that is applied to it.

infection The state of disease or damage to the body due to the presence and reproduction of microorganisms. The simple presence of organisms, e.g. on the skin, does not mean infection. In *endogenous infection*, the causative organism originates from the patient's own body, e.g. a wound infection caused by organisms from the patient's own skin. In *exogenous infection*, the causative organism originates from another individual or external source, e.g. a wound infection caused by organisms transferred from the wound of another patient. (Often referred to as cross-infection.) A *nosocomial infection* is a hospital-acquired infection. A *zoonotic infection* is an infection acquired from an animal.

inflammation A protective response of the body to damage, irritation or infection and characterised by redness, warmth, swelling, pain and, sometimes, loss of function.

infrared Electromagnetic radiation that has a wavelength of 10^{-5}–10^{-4} m.

inorganic chemistry The branch of chemistry that deals with compounds that do not contain the element carbon.

insulator A substance through which electric current and heat do not pass readily.

insulin The hormone produced by the beta cells of the islets of Langerhans of the pancreas. Insulin lowers blood sugar levels by promoting the uptake of insulin by most cells of the body.

intercellular fluid *See* interstitial fluid.

intercostal drain Literally, 'a drain between the ribs'. Refers to a drain (tube or catheter) inserted into the plural space (surrounding the lungs) for the purpose of removing air or fluid.

intercostal muscles The muscles located between the ribs and that are important in breathing.

interphase Literally, 'in between phases'. Refers to the stage in the cell cycle when the cell is not dividing.

interstitial fluid Fluid that surrounds cells and that is outside the vascular compartment.

interstitium The space around the cells of the body that contains interstitial fluid.

intestine The part of the alimentary system (gut) extending from (but not including) the stomach to the anus. The *small intestine* is the smaller-diameter section of the intestine, consisting of the duodenum, jejunum and ileum and concerned with digestion and the absorption of nutrients. The *large intestine* is the larger-diameter section of the intestine, consisting of the colon and the rectum and concerned with the absorption of water.

intracellular fluid The fluid content within cells.

intradermal Literally, 'into the skin', e.g. intradermal injection.

intramuscular Literally, 'into muscle', e.g. intramuscular injection.

intravascular fluid Fluid in the vascular compartment – that is, blood.

intravenous Literally, 'into a vein', e.g. intravenous injection. An *intravenous infusion* is the administration of fluid directly into a vein.

intrinsic factor A substance secreted by the stomach that is necessary for the absorption of vitamin B_{12}.

intubation The act of inserting a tube into the body via an orifice or a surgical wound. Small-diameter tubes tend to be referred to as catheters, and the term 'catheterisation' is then applied.

inverse square law The law that states that the intensity of radiation is inversely proportional to the square of the distance from the source.

ion Atoms or groups of atoms that have become charged as a consequence of the loss or gain of electrons.

ionic bond The chemical link between ions that arises as a result of the attraction of ions carrying opposite charges.

ionic compound A compound that results from ionic bonding.

ionisation A type of decomposition reaction in which a compound dissociates into ions.

ionising radiation Radiation in the form of electromagnetic waves or particles that is capable of producing ions.

iris The coloured disc of tissue that surrounds the pupil of the eye. It contains smooth muscle, the contraction and relaxation of which is responsible for dilation and constriction of the pupil in order to control the entry of light into the eye.

islets of Langerhans Literally, 'Langerhans' islands' (named after a nineteenth-century German pathologist Paul Langerhans). Used in reference to small areas of endocrine (hormone-producing) cells within the much larger mass of exocrine (enzyme-producing) cells of the pancreas. Within the islets of Langerhans are two main cell types: alpha cells and beta cells. Alpha cells secrete the hormone glucagon and beta cells secrete the hormone insulin.

isomers Compounds that have the same molecular formula but different structural formulae.

iso-osmotic Describing a fluid that has the same osmotic pressure as another.

isotonic Describing a solution that causes neither crenation nor plasmolysis of cells.

isotopes Atoms with the same atomic number but different mass numbers. Isotopes are, therefore, atoms of the same element, but they possess different numbers of neutrons.

J

joule (J) The SI unit of energy.

K

kaolin A type of clay from which a mechanical suspension may be formed for the treatment of diarrhoea. As a paste, it may be used to form a heated poultice.

karyotype The arrangement of chromosomes based upon their size, shape and position of centromeres.

kelvin (K) The SI unit of temperature.

keratin A fibrous protein that forms an important component of the epidermis of the skin and also of hair and nails.

keratinocytes Literally, 'keratin cells'. Refers to cells of the skin that produce keratin.

ketoacidosis/ketosis Metabolic acidosis that results from the production of excess ketoacids.

ketoacids Ketone molecules that also possess an acidic carboxyl (COOH) group.

ketones Organic compounds that contain the carbonyl functional group (C=O) part way along a carbon atom chain and that conform to the general formula RCOR.

kilogram (kg) The SI unit of mass.

kinetic energy The energy of movement.

Korotkoff sounds The sounds (named after Nikolai Korotkoff) made by blood pulsing through blood pressure that are heard when measuring the blood pressure with a stethoscope and sphygmomanometer.

Krebs cycle A series of biochemical reactions (named after Hans Krebs) that take place in the matrix of mitochondria in which electrons are transferred to co-enzymes and, as a consequence, carbon dioxide and ATP are formed.

Kussmaul's respirations Deep, rapid, sighing respirations (named after Adolf Kussmaul) characteristic of ketoacidosis.

L

lacteals Literally, 'pertaining to milk'. Refers to the lymphatic vessel of the small intestine, so called because the fatty chyle absorbed from the small intestine is milky-white in appearance.

lactase The enzyme responsible for breaking down the disaccharide lactose into one molecule of glucose and one molecule of galactose.

lactose The disaccharide found in milk. *Lactose intolerance* is a condition characterised by nausea, diarrhoea, bloating, flatus and abdominal pain due to an inability to digest lactose and caused by a deficiency in the enzyme lactase.

laryngospasm Spasm causing closure of the larynx.

laryngitis Inflammation of the larynx.

larynx The organ containing the vocal cords and responsible for voice production.

laser An acronym for light amplification by the stimulated emission of radiation. Laser light consists of monochromatic waves of visible or invisible electromagnetic radiation, all of which are in phase.

latent heat The energy required to produce a change in state, e.g. to change a solid into a liquid (latent heat of fusion) or to change a liquid into a gas (latent heat of vaporisation).

lavage Literally, 'washing'. Used in reference to any procedure in which a hollow organ (e.g. stomach, bladder or bowel) is irrigated ('washed out').

lecithin A phospholipid found in plants and animals.

lens A structure in the eye, or an optical device responsible for focusing of light. A *concave lens* is narrower in the middle than at the edges. A *converging lens* causes light passing through it to converge; convex lenses are of this type. A *convex lens* is wider in the middle than at the edges. A *diverging lens* causes light passing through it to diverge; concave lenses are of this type.

leukocyte Literally, 'white blood cell'. Used to distinguish a form of blood cell (white blood cells) from those that contain the red pigment haemoglobin (erythrocytes/red blood cells).

lever A bar that connects a mechanical force to an object.

ligaments Fibrous structures that join bone to bone and that are an important component of joints.

light Electromagnetic radiation with a wavelength range of 400-800 nm.

linear accelerator A device used to produce high-energy X-rays for the purpose of radiotherapy.

lipase The enzyme responsible for the digestion of lipids (fats). Lipase breaks the bonds between fatty acids and glycerol.

lipids A diverse group of organic compounds, commonly referred to as fats. Lipids include glycerides (neutral fats), which share the properties of insolubility in water and solubility in organic solvents.

lipoprotein A molecule that has a lipid and a protein component.

liquid A state of matter in which particles are weakly attracted to each other. Liquids conform to the shape of the container into which they are poured.

lithotripsy Literally, 'to wear away'. Refers to the use of ultrasound to break up calculi, e.g. stones of the urinary bladder.

litmus paper Absorbent paper impregnated with a plant pigment and used to indicate the pH of a solution through the process of colour change (i.e. red when acidic, blue when alkaline).

litre (l) A measure of volume. There are 1000 l in one cubic metre (m^3).

liver The largest organ of the body (by weight). The liver is located in the abdomen and has many functions, including manufacture (e.g. plasma proteins, bile), storage (e.g. iron, glycogen, vitamin B_{12}), metabolism (e.g. most drugs) and heat generation.

locus The specific point on a chromosome at which a gene is located.

lumbar Pertaining to the part of the body between the thorax (chest) and the pelvis - especially of the vertebrae of that region.

lumbar puncture Introduction of a needle into the subarachnoid space in the lumbar region, usually for the purpose of aspirating (collecting by suction) a sample of cerebrospinal fluid.

lymphocytes A form of leukocyte (white blood cell) that develops in the bone marrow. *B lymphocytes* are the cells that produce antibodies in response to an infectious disease. *T lymphocytes* are so called because they have been processed in the thymus gland. Some T cells assist B cells, while other T cells are important in resisting the proliferation of cancer cells.

lysosome A structure located within the cytoplasm of cells that contains digestive enzymes.

lysoszyme A enzyme important in destroying some microorganisms and found in body fluids such as saliva and in lysosomes.

M

macrophage Literally, 'big eater'. The name of an agranular leukocyte (white blood cell) that undertakes phagocytosis, e.g. of bacteria in an infection.

magnet An object that demonstrates the property of magnetism.

magnetic field The region in which a magnetic force can be demonstrated.

magnetic resonance imaging (MRI) A medical imaging technique that makes use of the phenomenon of magnetic resonance. The patient is placed in a strong magnetic field and subjected to radio waves. In response, the atoms of the patient's body emit radio waves, which can be used to produce an image of the body.

magnetism The properties and effects of a magnetic substance.

malaria The name given to the infectious disease characterised by chills, fever and anaemia and caused by members of the protozoan genus *Plasmodium*.

malleus Literally, 'hammer'. Refers to a hammer-shaped bone of the middle ear involved in the transmission of sound in the process of hearing.

maltase The enzyme responsible for breaking down each molecule of the disaccharide maltose into two molecules of glucose.

maltose The disaccharide found in malt (germinated grains).

manometer A device for the measurement of pressure by means of a column of fluid.

mass The amount of matter of a substance.

mass number The sum of the number of protons and the number of neutrons in an atom.

matter Anything that occupies space and has mass.

mechanical suspension A mixture in which particles are dispersed but not dissolved in water.

meiosis Cell division characterised by the formation of four daughter cells, each of which possesses the haploid number of chromosomes. Meiosis takes place in the gonads and leads to the production of gametes (sex cells).

melanin A dark pigment found in the skin and hair. One of the pigments that determine the different skin colours of people of different races. In the skin, melanin protects the body from the harmful effects of the sun's rays. Increased production of melanin in response to exposure to the sun is responsible for tanning.

melanocytes Literally, 'melanin cells'. The cells that produce melanin.

meninges The three membranes that cover the brain.

meningitis Inflammation of the meninges. A serious condition that may be caused by bacteria or viruses.

meniscus The bending of the surface of a liquid due to the relative strength of the forces of cohesion and adhesion.

menstrual cycle The monthly cycle of the endometrium (lining of the womb) in which a layer of cells grows, is shed (menstruation) and then regrows.

merozoites One of the developmental stages in the asexual reproduction of the malarial parasite *Plasmodium*.

metabolic rate An expression of the amount of energy released in the body in a given period of time.

metabolism The sum of all the biochemical reactions of the body.

metaphase The second of the four stages of mitosis in which chromosomes are attached to the spindle fibres along the equatorial plate.

methicillin A type of penicillin now discontinued but developed to treat infections by resistant organisms. *Methicillin-resistant Staphylococcus aureus* (MRSA) are strains of *Staphylococcus aureus* that are resistant to methicillin and other antibiotics.

metre (m) The SI unit of length.

micelles Clusters of the products of fat digestion and bile salts that are small enough to diffuse between microvilli of the small intestine.

microbiology The study of microorganisms.

microcytic Literally, 'small cell'. Refers to small erythrocytes (red blood cells) in iron deficiency anaemia.

microorganisms Organisms that are not visible with the naked eye.

microscope An optical instrument used to magnify small objects, such as cells of the body and bacteria.

microscopy Examination with the aid of a microscope.

microvilli Microscopic finger-like projections of certain cells, e.g. the cells lining the ileum of the small intestine, where they provide a large surface area for the absorption of nutrients.

microwaves Electromagnetic radiation with a wavelength of 1 mm–30 cm.

mid-stream specimen of urine (MSU) A specimen of urine collected after a small amount of urine has already been passed and before the bladder has been emptied.

minerals Inorganic substances required in the diet.

mitochondria Cellular organelles that possess an inner membrane and an outer membrane and that are the site of the Krebs cycle and the electron transport chain.

mitosis Cell division characterised by the formation of two daughter cells, each of which possesses the diploid number of chromosomes.

mixture A substance that contains separate elements or compounds that are not bound together.

molality An expression of concentration in terms of the number of moles or millimoles of solute per kilogram of solvent (mol/kg or millimol/kg).

molarity An expression of concentration in terms of the number of moles or millimoles of solute per litre of solvent (mol/l or millimol/l).

mole The relative atomic mass of an element or the molecular weight of a compound in grams. One mole of a substance contains 6×10^{23} particles.

molecular formula See formula.

molecular mass The sum of the relative atomic masses of the atoms that make up a compound.

molecule Two or more atoms joined by a covalent bond.

momentum The product of the mass and the velocity of an object.

monera Literally, 'alone'. One of five kingdoms in which life on earth is classified. Monera is the kingdom of bacteria.

monocyte A type of leukocyte (white blood cell) that has a single nucleus.

monoglyceride See glyceride.

monohydrogen phosphate ion The HPO_4^{2-} ion that forms part of an important buffer system in intracellular fluid and renal filtrate.

monosaccharide A simple sugar that cannot be broken down into a simpler sugar.

morphine A drug used as an analgesic (pain-relieving agent) derived from the opium poppy and named after the Greek god of sleep, Morpheus.

motor Pertaining to movement, e.g. the motor division of the nervous system, which supplies muscle.

mucilages Soluble non-digestible plant carbohydrates.

muscle relaxant A drug used to produce paralysis during general anaesthesia.

mutualism A close relationship between two species in which both organisms benefit.

myalgia Muscle pain.

mycelium A mass of fungal hyphae.

myocardial infarction (MI) A heart attack in which part of the myocardium (heart muscle) dies as a consequence of obstruction of its blood supply.

myopia The condition in which light is focused in front of the retina and that is commonly referred to as short-sightedness.

myosin A protein important in muscle contraction.

myxoedema The most severe form of hypothyroidism (reduced levels of thyroid hormones) characterised by swelling of the tissues, especially of the hands and face.

N

nalidixic acid A type of antibiotic.

narcotic Literally, 'numbing'. Describes drugs derived from the opium poppy or produced synthetically that alleviate pain and induce euphoria.

nasopharynx The uppermost of the three regions of the throat (pharynx). The nasopharynx extends from behind the nasal cavity to the soft palate.

nebuliser A device in which the Bernoulli effect is used in order to produce an aerosol. Nebulisers are used for dispersing liquid medication in a gas so that the drug may be inhaled.

neoplasm Literally, 'new growth'. A swelling due to abnormal and excessive cell growth.

nephrons The functional units of the kidney, each consisting of a renal corpuscle and a renal tubule.

nerve Structures of the nervous system that consist of bundles of nerve fibres that connect the central nervous system (brain and spinal cord) with the rest of the body. The *cochlear nerve* supplies the cochlea of the inner ear and is a division of the eighth cranial nerve (auditory nerve/vestibulocochlear nerve).

neuron A nerve cell. Also spelled neurone.

neutral Having a pH of 7.

neutral fats Triglycerides.

neutralisation The process of combining acids and bases to produce a neutral solution.

neutron A subatomic particle found in the nucleus that has identical mass to that of a proton but that carries no charge.

neutrophil A type of granular leukocyte (white blood cell).

newton (N) The SI unit of force.

niacin A B group vitamin also known as nicotinic acid.

nicotinamide adenine dinucleotide (NAD) A derivative of the vitamin niacin important in the energy-liberating reactions of cells. *Reduced nicotinamide adenine dinucleotide (NADH)* is the reduced form created by the addition of hydrogen to NAD.

night blindness Poor vision at night due to decreased synthesis of the retinal pigment rhodopsin, which may result from a deficiency of vitamin A.

non-disjunction Failure of sister chromatids to separate during mitosis or failure of homologous pairs to separate during meiosis. The result is an abnormal number of chromosomes in daughter cells.

non-steroidal anti-inflammatory drug (NSAID) A drug that is not a steroid but that reduces inflammation. Ibuprofen is an example.

norepinephrine A hormone (previously known as noradrenaline) synthesised by the adrenal medulla. Norepinephrine is also a neurotransmitter in the sympathetic division of the autonomic nervous system.

nuclear membrane The membrane that surrounds the nucleus of the cell.

nucleoplasm Literally, 'nuclear substance'. A colloidal fluid enclosed by the nuclear membrane in which chromatin is suspended.

nucleosome One of the bead-like structures consisting of deoxyribonucleic acid (DNA) wrapped around a core of proteins that form the structure of chromatin.

nucleotide A molecule formed from a sugar, a nitrogenous base and an inorganic phosphate group. Nucleotides are the component molecules of nucleic acids.

nucleus 1. The central part of an atom that contains protons and neutrons. 2. A cellular organelle that contains genetic material.

nucleus pulposus The central elastic part of each intravertebral disc.

numerical prefix A prefix added to a unit in order to simplify the expression of a number. For example, 1000 m (10^3 m) becomes a kilometre ('kilo' is a prefix meaning 1000).

nystatin An antifungal drug.

O

occiput The back of the skull.

oedema The condition of an excess of interstitial fluid.

oesophagus The muscular tube that connects the pharynx to the stomach. Often referred to as the gullet.

oestrogen A group of female steroidal hormones produced by the adrenal cortex and the ovary and responsible for the development of secondary sexual characteristics in women.

ohm (Ω) The SI unit of electrical resistance (named after Georg Ohm).

oocyte An immature ovum (female sex cell).

oncotic pressure The fraction of the plasma osmotic pressure for which plasma proteins are responsible.

opsin A compound that combines with retinal in the retina to form the visual pigment rhodopsin.

organelles Literally, 'little organs'. Membrane-bound structures found within cells that perform specific functions on behalf of the cell.

organic chemistry The branch of chemistry that deals with compounds that contain carbon.

orthostatic Pertaining to the standing position. *Orthostatic hypotension* is hypotension (low blood pressure) that occurs on standing.

oscilloscope An electrical device in which an electron beam is made to cross a fluorescent screen in order to produce a waveform. It is the basis of the electrocardiograph (ECG) monitor.

osmol A unit that corresponds to the number of moles of a solute multiplied by the number of particles into which the solute dissociates.

osmolality The number of osmols per kilogram of solution. This is a measure of the concentration of particles dissolved in solution.

osmolarity The number of osmols per litre of solution. This is a measure of the concentration of particles dissolved in solution.

osmoreceptor A receptor ('detector') that responds to changes in the osmolarity of the blood.

osmosis The movement of solvent particles across a semi-permeable membrane from an area of high solvent concentration to an area of low solvent concentration.

osmotic pressure The pressure required to prevent osmosis.

ossicles The bones of the middle ear (incus, maleus and stapes) that are important in the transmission of sound and as a consequence in hearing.

osteoarthrosis A mechanical condition of chronic joint damage (wear) without inflammation.

osteoblast Literally, 'bone-germinating'. A bone-forming cell.

osteoclast Literally, 'bone breaking'. A bone-destroying cell.

osteomalacia An abnormal bone condition characterised by loss of calcium and phosphorus, leading to weakness and sometimes fracture. It may be caused by a diet lacking these minerals or inadequate vitamin D.

osteoporosis A disorder characterised by a loss of bone density, occurring especially in postmenopausal women and immobilised patients.

ostium A mouth-like opening (plural ostia). The *coronary ostium* is the opening (beginning) of a coronary (heart) artery.

otitis media Inflammation of the middle ear caused by one of a number of possible bacteria.

ovary One of a pair of female gonads (sex organs).

ovulation Expulsion of an ovum from the ovary.

oxidation A type of chemical reaction in which a substance acquires an oxygen atom, loses a hydrogen atom or loses an electron.

oxytocin A hormone of the posterior pituitary gland that stimulates the smooth muscle of the uterus to contract during birth.

oxyhaemoglobin The compound formed when oxygen binds to the erythrocyte (red blood cell) pigment haemoglobin.

oxyntic cells Cells of the stomach that produce hydrochloric acid.

P

pacemaker The name given to the sino-atrial node of the conduction system of the heart since it has the fastest rate of spontaneous depolarisation and sets the pace at which the heart contracts. The term is also used to describe an electronic device used to regulate the heart rate.

pancreas An abdominal organ that possesses both endocrine and exocrine tissue. The pancreas produces a number of digestive enzymes and the hormone insulin.

pandemic The condition that exists when an infection spreads across a whole country or the whole world.

paracetamol A drug used to alleviate pain (analgesic) and reduce fever (antipyretic).

parasitic The type of relationship that exists between two species when one species benefits but the other is harmed.

parasitism The action of behaving as a parasite.

parasympathetic division A division of the autonomic nervous system that has largely antagonistic action to the sympathetic division. It mediates vegetative functions such as digestion.

parathormone The hormone produced by the parathyroid glands.

parenteral Literally, 'besides the gut'. Refers to the administration of substances to the body by a route that does not involve the digestive tract.

partial pressure The pressure exerted by one of the gases present in a mixture of gases or dissolved in solution.

particle Any unit of matter.

partner-exchange reaction A type of chemical reaction in which there is a substitution of elements between two molecules.

pascal (Pa) The SI unit of pressure. A pressure of 1 kPa exists when a force of one newton (1 N) acts over an area of one square metre (1 m^2).

Pascal's law (principle) A law that states that the pressure exerted upon a static liquid is transmitted uniformly throughout the liquid.

Pasteurisation The process (named after Louis Pasteur) of heating milk in order to kill common bacterial pathogens.

Pathogen A disease-causing organism. An *obligate pathogen* is a microorganism that is 'obliged' to cause disease in the process of completing its lifecycle. For example, viruses cannot reproduce outside host cells and thus are obligate pathogens. An *opportunistic pathogen* is a microorganism that can complete its lifecycle without causing disease but that nonetheless sometimes does cause disease. For example, organisms on the skin may reproduce and cause no harm there, but if a wound occurs the organisms infect the wound.

pectins Soluble, non-digestible, gelatinous carbohydrates found in fruits and succulent vegetables.

pellagra A disease caused by deficiency of the B group vitamin niacin and characterised by dermatitis, diarrhoea and dementia.

penicillin Any one of a group of antibiotics derived from cultures of the fungus *Penicillium*.

pepsin The protein-digesting enzyme found in the stomach.

pepsinogen Literally, 'generation of pepsin'. The inactive substance produced by the stomach and turned into the active enzyme pepsin by the action of hydrochloric acid ($HCl_{(aq)}$).

peptidases A group of enzymes, present in pancreatic and intestinal secretions, that break off amino acids from the ends of peptide chains.

peptide A molecule formed from a chain of two or more amino acids.

peptide bond The bond formed between the amino group of one amino acid and the carboxyl group of a second amino acid.

peptones The peptides that result from the digestion of a protein.

perilymph The fluid that fills the scala vestibuli and the scala tympani of the inner ear.

period A horizontal row of the Periodic Table.

Periodic Table A table in which the chemical elements are placed in groups (vertical columns) and periods (horizontal rows). The order of the elements is such that atomic number increases from left to right along a period, while elements with similar properties are found in the same group.

peristalsis The rhythmic contraction of smooth muscle that propels food through the intestines.

peritoneal dialysis *See* dialysis.

Petri dish A shallow disc with a lid in which microorganisms are grown.

phagocyte A cell capable of phagocytosis.

phagocytosis Literally, 'cell-eating'. The process by which certain cells engulf and destroy microorganisms or cellular fragments.

pharynx The throat - the structure that extends from the back of the nasal cavity to the larynx and oesophagus and serves as a common passageway for both food and air.

phenotype The physical expression of the genotype.

phenylalanine One of the essential amino acids.

phenylketonuria Genetic disorder characterised by inability to metabolise phenylalanine, which is toxic to brain tissue and leads to learning disability.

pholcodine A cough-suppressing drug.

phospholipid A group of lipids that consist of the alcohol glycerol combined with two carboxylic acids and one phosphate group.

phosphorylation A type of combination reaction that involves a phosphate group.

photoautotroph Literally, 'light self-feeders'. Refers to bacteria that contain chlorophyll (the green pigment also found in plants) and use energy in the form of light to produce nutrients.

pH scale A numerical scale (0-14) corresponding to the negative logarithm of the hydrogen ion concentration.

piezoelectric effect The property of certain crystals, such as quartz, that when deformed by a force a small voltage is created.

pili Projections on the surface of certain bacteria, e.g. *Neisseria gonorrhoea*.

pinna The ear lobe.

pitch The subjective perception of the frequency of a sound wave.

pituitary gland An endocrine gland situated at the base of the brain.

plasma The fluid part of blood in which the blood cells are suspended.

plasma expander A colloidal suspension that is administered intravenously and that increases plasma osmotic pressure, thus assisting in the maintenance of plasma volume.

plasma membrane The membrane that separates the contents of a cell from the environment.

plasma protein A protein such as albumin that is normally present in blood plasma.

plasma protein solution A colloidal suspension derived from blood plasma that contains 85% albumin.

plasmolysis The rupture of the plasma membrane that occurs as a consequence of the movement by osmosis of water into the cell.

pleura Either of the two membranes that surround the lungs.

pleurisy Inflammation of the pleura.

pleuritis *See* pleurisy.

plural fluid Fluid contained in the plural space.

plural space The space between the two pleurae that contains plural fluid.

pneumonia Inflammation of the lungs.

pneumothorax The presence of air in the plural space.

polar molecule A covalent molecule in which there is an unequal sharing of electrons, such that part of the molecule has a slight negative charge and part has a slight positive charge.

polarisation Production of light in which the light waves oscillate in only one plane.

pole The end of a bar magnet.

polyatomic ion/polyatomic radical An ion made up of atoms of more than one element but that behaves as though it were an ion of a single element.

polycythaemia The condition of an increased number of erythrocytes (red blood cells).

polydipsia Increased thirst.

polypeptide A chain of many amino acids joined together by peptide bonds.

polysaccharide A carbohydrate that consists of many sugar molecules joined together.

polyunsaturated Pertaining to organic molecules with multiple double or triple bonds. A *polyunsaturated fat* is a lipid in which the carboxylic acid (fatty-acid chain) has multiple double bonds.

polyuria Excessive urine output.

pore A small opening through a membrane.

postural drainage The procedure of periodically repositioning a patient so that secretions may drain from different lobes of the lung.

potential difference The difference in electrical potential, measured in volts, between two points.

potential energy The energy possessed by virtue of the position or chemical composition of matter.

power The rate of doing work measured in watts (W).

presbycusis Hearing loss associated with ageing.

pressure The force exerted per unit surface area over which the force acts.

pressure ulcer An ulcer (wound with tissue loss) that results from low sustained pressure to the soft tissues, particularly over bony prominences, caused by the occlusion of the blood supply.

products The substances that are produced as a consequence of a chemical reaction.

progesterone A female hormone produced by the adrenal cortex and the placenta and that plays an important role in regulation of the menstrual cycle and in pregnancy.

prokaryotic A type of cellular organisation characteristic of bacteria in which the cytoplasm contains no compartments or distinct organelles and genetic material is not membrane-bound in a nucleus.

propanone (acetone) The simplest ketone (CH_3COCH_3); often used as a solvent for sticking plaster.

prophase The first stage of mitosis in which chromosomes become visible and it can be seen that each chromosome is made of two chromatids. At the end of prophase, the nuclear membrane breaks down and spindle fibres form between centrioles at opposite poles of the cell.

prostaglandins Unsaturated fatty acids produced by many body tissues, with hormone-like effects.

prostate gland A conical gland situated at the base of the male bladder and that produces a milky fluid that is mixed with semen at ejaculation.

prosthesis An artificial substitute for a body part, e.g. a replacement joint or artificial leg.

proteins Molecules consisting of long chains of at least 100 amino acids.

protista One of the five kingdoms into which all life is classified and that includes algae (plant-like protests), slime moulds (fungus-like protests) and protozoans (animal-like protests).

proton A subatomic particle found in the nucleus. A proton has the same mass as a neutron but carries a single positive charge.

protoplasm All the living substance of a cell that is contained within the plasma membrane.

protozoa Members of the kingdom protista that have animal-like cells.

pseudoephedrine A nasal decongestant drug.

pseudopodia Literally, 'false foot'. Used in reference to the manner in which amoebas and amoeboid cells move by projecting an area of the cell in the direction of movement.

pulley A grooved wheel on an axle that is used to change the direction of a force or to produce a mechanical advantage.

pupil The circular opening in the centre of the iris of the eye and through which light enters.

Purkinje fibres The network of conduction fibres in the ventricles of the heart (named after Johannes von Purkinje) responsible for the transmission of electrical impulses.

pyrexia An abnormally elevated body temperature that results from the action of a pyrogen.

pyrodoxine Vitamin B_6.

pyrogen A substance capable of producing pyrexia (fever).

Q

quinolones A group of antibiotics that prevent the replication of deoxyribonucleic acid (DNA) in bacteria.

R

radiation Energy in the form of electromagnetic waves or particles that radiate from a source.

radioactivity The emission of electromagnetic radiation. *Radioactive* means showing the property of radioactivity. *Radioactive decay* is the process by which an element is formed from another and in the process ionising radiation is released.

radioisotope An isotope that emits radiation.

radio-opaque Opaque to X-rays. Used of contrast media that enables X-ray examination of soft tissue. For example, in a barium meal, a preparation containing barium is swallowed, which enables the outline of the stomach to be seen on X-ray.

radiosensitivity Susceptibility to damage by radiation - different tissues show different degrees of radiosensitivity, rapidly dividing cells being most sensitive.

radiotherapy The treatment of tumours using ionising radiation. In *external-beam radiotherapy*, ionising radiation is directed at the body from outside. In *internal radiotherapy*, a radioisotope is implanted within the body. *Interstitial radiotherapy* is a form of internal radiotherapy in which a radioisotope in the form of beads or needles is implanted directly into the tissues. *Intracavity radiotherapy* is a form of internal radiotherapy in which a receptacle containing a radioisotope is implanted within a body cavity. *Systemic radiotherapy* is a form of internal radiotherapy in which a radioisotope is administered systemically.

rarefaction A reduction in pressure that follows a compression in a longitudinal wave.

reactants The substances that take part in a chemical reaction.

receptors Sensory nerve endings that are capable of responding to a stimulus.

rectum The lower part of the large intestine between the sigmoid ('S'-shaped) colon and the anal canal.

redox reaction A chemical reaction in which both oxidation and reduction take place.

reducing agent A substance that is capable of reducing another substance.

reduction A type of chemical reaction in which a substance loses an oxygen atom, gains a hydrogen atom or gains an electron.

reflection A term used to describe the manner in which a wave 'bounces off' a surface that it strikes.

refraction The bending of a beam of light as it moves from one transparent medium to another of different density.

Reissner's membrane *See* vestibular membrane.

relative atomic mass The average mass, in atomic mass units, of a single atom of an element that takes into account the relative proportions of the different isotopes of that element.

renal Pertaining to the kidney. The *renal corpuscle* (literally, 'little body of the kidney') is a part of the nephron comprising of the glomerulus and Bowman's capsule. The *renal tubule* (literally, the 'small tube of the kidney') is the tubular part of the nephron, consisting of the proximal convoluted tubule, the loop of Henle and the distal convoluted tubule.

repolarisation The restoration of the resting membrane potential following depolarisation.

resistance The property of a material that opposes the flow of electrons. The SI unit of resistance is the ohm (Ω).

resonance The tendency of two objects with identical resonant frequencies to vibrate in time with each other.

resonant frequency The frequency at which an object vibrates maximally.

respiration The act of breathing. *External respiration* is the act of breathing (ventilation). *Internal respiration* is the energy-liberating reactions of the cell.

retina The light-sensitive membrane at the back of the eye - the innermost of three coats of the eye.

retinal A derivative of vitamin A, which together with opsin forms the visual pigment rhodopsin.

reversible reaction A type of chemical reaction in which the reactants can be reformed from the products.

rhodopsin The visual pigment of the rods (type of light-sensitive cell) of the retina of the eye.

riboflavin Vitamin B_2.

ribonucleic acid Nucleic acid that consists of a singe strand of nuceotides. Each nucleotide consists of the sugar ribose, a phosphate group and one of four nitrogenous bases (adenine, uracil, guanine, cytosine). Three forms exist: messenger RNA (mRNA), ribosomal RNA (rRNA) and transfer RNA (tRNA).

ribose A pentose (five-carbon-atom sugar) found in ribonucleic acid.

ribosomes Organelles that are the sites of protein synthesis.

rickets A disorder of calcium and phosphorus metabolism in children associated with deficiency in vitamin D and characterised by softening and bending of the long bones.

ringworm A skin disease caused by a number of fungal species and so called because of characteristic circular scaly areas.

rods Light-sensitive cells of the retina of the eye responsible for black-and-white vision.

roughage *See* fibre.

S

sacrum The name given to the five fused vertebrae located between the fifth lumbar vertebra and the coccyx.

salivary gland Any one of the three pairs of glands that secrete saliva.

salmonellosis The condition characterised by diarrhoea, vomiting and fever caused by gastrointestinal infection by *Salmonella enteritidis* present in contaminated food.

salt An ionic compound that does not dissociate into hydrogen ions (H^+) or hydroxyl ions (OH^-).

saprophytes Microorganisms that live on dead and decaying organic matter.

saturated fat A lipid in which the carbon atoms are linked by single covalent bonds.

scala media The fluid-filled channel of the cochlea of the inner ear that is located between the scala vestibuli and the scala tympani.

scalar A quantity that has size but no direction.

scala tympani The fluid-filled channel of the cochlea of the inner ear that spirals from the apex of the cochlea down to the round window.

scala vestibuli The fluid-filled channel of the cochlea of the inner ear that spirals from the oval window to the apex of the cochlea.

scientific notation A method of expressing very large or small numbers as powers of ten, e.g. 1000 becomes 10^3 and 0.001 becomes 10^{-3}.

schizonts A developmental stage in the asexual reproduction of the malaria parasite *Plasmodium* that exists in the liver.

sclera The tough, white, outer coat of the eye.

scurvy A disease caused by deficiency of vitamin C and characterised by fatigue and haemorrhage.

sebum The fatty secretion of the sebaceous glands of the skin.

selectively permeable membrane A biological membrane, the permeability of which may change due to the opening and closing of channels through it.

semi-permeable membrane A membrane that has pores of a certain diameter. Particles of a smaller diameter can, therefore diffuse, through it, while particles with a larger diameter cannot.

sense strand The strand of DNA alongside which mRNA is transcribed (copied).

sensory Pertaining to the senses, e.g. the sensory division of the nervous system, which conveys impulses from various receptors to the brain.

septicaemia Literally, 'septic blood'. Refers to the persistence of pathogenic organisms in the blood.

serological Pertaining to serum - a blood test for antibodies to specific antigens.

serum Blood plasma without its clotting proteins. Body fluids that resemble serum are described as 'serous fluids' and the moist membranes that line body cavities as 'serous membranes'.

set point The level or value of a controlled condition, such as body temperature, that the body strives to maintain.

sex chromosome *See* chromosome.

sickle cell A genetic disease resulting in the production of abnormal haemoglobin that causes erythrocytes (red blood cells) to become sickle-shaped. The abnormal gene is dominant. *Sickle cell disease* is the homozygous dominant state and is a severe form of the illness. *Sickle cell trait* is the heterozygous state and is a less severe form of the illness.

sickling crisis An acute episode in sickle cell disease characterised by pain, pyrexia, anaemia and jaundice.

sick sinus syndrome The condition of bradycardia (slow heart rate) that results from disease of the sino-atrial node.

sievert A unit of measurement of radiation that takes into account the biological effects of the different forms of radiation and that is, therefore, useful in clinical practice.

sino-atrial node A mass of conduction fibres located in the right atrium of the heart, the spontaneous depolarisation of which sets the pace at which the heart beats and that is therefore often referred to as the 'pacemaker'.

sinus rhythm The normal rhythm of the heart that results when an impulse arises in the sinoatrial node and passes through the normal route of conduction fibres.

sleeping sickness The disease caused by the flagellates *Trypanosoma gambiense* and *Trypanosoma rhodesiense* and characterised by fever, skin eruptions, lethargy and drowsiness.

slime moulds Fungus-like protists.

small intestine *See* intestine.

smallpox Literally, 'small pustule'. Refers to a serious acute infectious disease of viral origin, officially eradicated in 1979.

sodium pump A transport mechanism that pumps sodium (Na) out of cells in exchange for potassium (K).

sol A colloid composed of a solid dispersed in a liquid.

solenoid An electromagnetic switch.

solid A state of matter in which the particles are not free to move but are held by forces of attraction in relatively fixed positions.

solute The least abundant component of a solution.

solution An homogeneous mixture in which the solute particles exist as single ions, atoms or molecules. These particles do not settle out and cannot be separated by simple filters or semipermeable membranes. The Tyndall effect cannot be demonstrated with true solutions.

solvent The most abundant component of a solution.

somatic cell Any cell of the body that is not a sex cell.

somatomotor Literally, 'body motor'. Refers to the part of the motor (movement) division of the nervous system that is under conscious control. This part of the nervous system innervates skeletal muscle.

space-occupying lesion A lesion in the form of a lump (tumour) rather than an ulcer. *Space-occupying lesion effects* are the effects of a space-occupying lesion, such as the compression of adjacent structures.

specific gravity The ratio of the density of a liquid to that of water. For example, the normal specific gravity of urine is in the range 1.001–1.035.

speed An expression of the distance travelled per unit of time, e.g. metres per second (ms^{-1}).

spermatozoa The mature male gamete; also referred to as a sperm cell (singular = spermatozoon).

sphygmomanometer A manometer used in the non-invasive measurement of arterial blood pressure.

spina bifida A congenital spinal defect in which the meninges and spinal cord protrude between the vertebrae.

spindle fibres The fibres that form between the centrioles of the cell during mitosis (cell division).

spore The dormant structure that results when bacteria develop a protective capsule. Spores are able to tolerate extremes of conditions, such as high temperatures, and are resistant to chemical disinfectants.

sporozoa One of the four phyla of protozoa.

stapes Literally, 'stirrup'. One of the three ossicles (bones of the middle ear).

staphylococci A term used in the identification and naming of bacteria in which round forms (cocci) are arranged in groups.

starch The plant-storage polysaccharide.

sterilisation A term used to describe any process that results in the destruction of all living organisms, including spores.

sterols A group of lipid molecules that includes cholesterol.

stimulus An event that provokes a change in a controlled condition.

Stokes-Adams attack Collapse due to bradycardia that occurs in conduction defects such as sick sinus syndrome.

stomatitis Inflammation of the oral mucosa (lining of the mouth).

streptococci A term used in the identification and naming of bacteria in which round forms (cocci) are arranged in chains.

streptomycin A type of antibiotic.

stridor The sound produced when air is drawn in through a narrowed airway, e.g. after inhaling a foreign object.

structural formula *See* formula.

subatomic particle Any constituent particle of an atom, e.g. protons, neutrons and electrons.

subclavian vein *See* vein.

substituent Any chemical group attached to a carbon atom chain.

substitution reaction *See* displacement.

substrate The substance on which an enzyme acts.

sucrase The enzyme responsible for breaking down each molecule of the disaccharide sucrose to one molecule of glucose and one molecule of fructose.

sucrose The disaccharide obtained from sugar cane and sugar beet.

sulphonamide An antimicrobial drug derived from the red dye sulphanilamide.

surface tension The term used to describe the observation that the surface of a liquid behaves as though tense as a consequence of forces of cohesion. Surface tension is responsible for droplet formation.

surfactant A substance that lowers surface tension.

suspensory ligaments The ligaments that attach the ciliary muscle to the lens.

suxamethonium chloride A muscle relaxant used to produce paralysis in general anaesthesia.

symbiosis A close-living association of two different species of organism. A number of forms exist. The relationship may be beneficial to either or both organisms or damaging to one.

sympathetic division A division of the autonomic nervous system that has largely antagonistic action to the parasympathetic division. It mediates the active functions such as the fight or flight response.

synovial fluid The fluid contained in the synovial cavity of a synovial joint.

synovial joint A type of joint characterised by a wide range of movement and a space (synovial cavity) between the articulating surfaces.

synthesis reaction *See* combination reaction.

syphyllis A sexually transmitted disease caused by the spirochaete *Treponema pallidum*.

systole Contraction of the heart. The term may be used of atrial or ventricular contraction.

T

tachycardia A fast heart rate.

tachypnoea A fast respiratory rate.

telophase The last of four stages of mitosis in which deoxyribonucleic acid (DNA) begins to uncoil and form thread-like chromatin again. The mitotic spindle disappears and a nuclear membrane forms around both sets of chromosomes.

temperature A measurement of the degree of hotness. *Core temperature* is the temperature of the organs of the body cavities – the brain in the cranium, the heart and lungs in the chest and the liver in the abdomen. The *peripheral/shell temperature* is the temperature of the surface of the body.

testosterone A male hormone produced by the testes and responsible for male secondary sexual characteristics and for triggering the development of spermatozoa.

tetanus/tetany Sustained muscular contraction that has a number of possible causes, including acute infection by *Clostridium tetani*.

tetracyclines A group of related antibiotics derived from the bacterium *Streptomyces*.

tetrad Literally, 'four'. Refers to the joining together of pairs of homologous chromosomes, each of which consists of two chromatids, during prophase I of meiosis.

thermometer A device used for the measurement of temperature - traditionally, a device that employs a physical property of a substance that changes with temperature, e.g. volume of a fluid. The *mercury-in-glass thermometer* is a device in which temperature is measured by the expansion of mercury up a fine glass tube. The *tympanic membrane thermometer* is a device that measures temperature by detecting the intensity of the infrared radiation emitted by the tympanic membrane (eardrum). A *thermistor* is an electronic device for measuring temperature.

thermoreceptor Literally, 'heat receptor (detector)'. A structure of the nervous system that responds to temperature.

thoracic duct A duct running from the abdomen through the chest, and that drains lymph from most of the body into the left subclavian vein.

thrombus A solid aggregation of the components of blood such as forms in the clotting process.

thrush Infection by the fungus *Candida albicans*.

thymine A base found in deoxyribonucleic acid (DNA) but not in ribonucleic acid (RNA).

thymus gland A gland located in the thorax in front of the heart and that is the site of maturation of T lymphocytes.

thyroidectomy Surgical removal of the thyroid gland.

thyroid gland The endocrine gland located in the neck that secretes the hormone thyroxine.

thyroid-stimulating hormone (TSH) The hormone of the anterior lobe of the pituitary gland that is responsible for stimulation of the thyroid gland.

thyrotoxicosis The condition that results from the excessive production of thyroxine characterised by excessive heat production and fast pulse.

thyroxine The principal hormone of the thyroid gland responsible for the regulation of metabolism.

tinnitus The sensation of noise (hissing, buzzing, etc.) in the absence of external auditory stimulation.

tocopherols A group of related compounds collectively referred to as vitamin E.

tonicity The tendency of a solution to cause crenation or plasmolysis. When cells are placed in a hypotonic solution, water enters the cells by osmosis and the cells burst (plasmolysis). When cells are placed in a hypertonic solution, water leaves the cells by osmosis and the cells collapse (crenation).

torque Turning force.

toxoid A vaccine consisting of a bacterial exotoxin that has been chemically treated to render it safe but still capable of stimulating antibody production.

tracheotomy The formation of a stoma (opening) into the trachea for the purpose of artificial ventilation or the suctioning of secretions.

transcription Formation of a strand of messenger ribonucleic acid (mRNA) in which the sequence of bases is determined by the sequences of bases in deoxyribonucleic acid (DNA). In effect, the genetic code is transcribed (copied) from DNA to mRNA. Transcription takes place in the nucleus.

transcutaneous electrical nerve stimulation (TENS) A technique in which an electric current is applied to the skin in order to relieve pain.

transducer A device that transforms one form of energy into another.

transformer An electrical device that is used to produce a change in voltage.

translation The synthesis of new protein on a ribosome. The sequence of amino acids in the protein is determined by the sequence of bases in the messenger ribonucleic acid (mRNA) attached to the ribosome. In effect, the genetic code carried by mRNA is translated into the sequence of amino acids in protein.

triglyceride *See* glyceride.

trimethoprim An antimicrobial drug.

triplet Three nucleotides that form part of a nucleic acid molecule and act as a code for a specific amino acid.

trypsin A pancreatic enzyme that breaks down peptide chains into smaller peptide chains.

trypsinogen An inactive enzyme precursor that, when acted upon by the enzyme enterokinase (found in intestinal secretions), is converted into the active enzyme trypsin.

tryptophan An amino acid essential for growth in children and for the manufacture of many substances within adults.

tuberculosis The condition caused by infection with *Mycobacterium tuberculosis*. It is normally transmitted by inhalation and affects the lungs, but other organs can be infected.

tumour *See* neoplasm.

tympanic membrane The eardrum, which vibrates in time with sound waves passing down the external auditory canal.

Tyndall effect The scattering of a beam of light that is produced by mechanical suspensions and colloidal suspension but not by true solutions.

U

ulcer A crater-like lesion affecting the skin or mucous membranes that results from an inflammatory process, infection or cancer.

ultrasound Sound waves of a frequency that is too high to be heard by the human ear.

ultraviolet Electromagnetic radiation that has a wavelength range of 20-390 nm.

unsaturated fat A lipid in which some of the carbon atoms are linked by double bonds. In monounsaturates, there is a single double bond; in polyunsaturates, there is more than one double bond.

uracil A base found in ribonucleic acid (RNA) but not in deoxyribonucleic acid (DNA).

urea The end product of the metabolism of ammonia in the liver that is excreted in the urine by the kidneys. (Ammonia is a toxic waste product of protein metabolism.)

urgency The sensation of needing urgently to pass urine, e.g. when cystitis (infection of the urinary bladder) is present.

urinalysis Testing urine in order to determine the presence of a number of substances, such as glucose and protein. Such testing is commonly undertaken in the practice setting using reagent strips that are dipped into a fresh sample of urine and a colour change observed on the indicator pads.

V

vacuole A fluid-filled cavity within a cell.

valence shell The outermost energy shell of an atom. Only the electrons in this shell take part in chemical bonding.

valency A numerical expression of the number of chemical bonds that an element can form.

vancomycin A type of antibiotic.

vasoconstriction Constriction (narrowing) of a blood vessel.

vasodilation Dilation (widening) of a blood vessel.

vector A quantity that possesses both magnitude and direction.

vein A blood vessel that carries blood towards the heart. All veins except the pulmonary veins carry deoxygenated blood. The *subclavian vein* is the vein located below the clavicle (collar bone). The *vena cava* is one of two veins returning deoxygenated blood to the right atrium of the heart.

velocity Speed in a given direction.

vena cava See vein.

ventricle One of the two lower chambers of the heart.

ventricular fibrillation A chaotic disturbance of the rhythm of the ventricles that results in a cessation of effective pumping.

Venturi barrel A device in which the Bernoulli effect is used in order to entrain one gas into another. Venturi barrels are important components of some oxygen masks.

venule A blood vessel that carries blood away from the heart. All arteries except the pulmonary arteries carry oxygenated blood.

vestibular membrane The floor of the scala vestibul, which also forms the roof of the scala media.

vibrio Curved bacteria - an example is *Vibrio cholerae*.

villi Small projections of the small intestine that increase the surface area in order to facilitate the absorption of nutrients (singular = villus).

virulence The ability of a microorganism to cause disease.

virus A microorganism that is so small that it can be seen only with the aid of an electron microscope. Viruses are pathogens (cause disease) with no independent metabolic activity, consisting of nucleic acid surrounded by a protein coat.

vitamins Organic molecules that are essential for life and that are required in relatively small amounts.

vitreous humour The fluid filling the cavity behind the lens of the eye.

volt (V) The SI unit of potential difference.

W

warfarin A drug used as an anticoagulant (prevents blood clotting).

watt (W) The SI unit of power.

wave A disturbance in a medium, e.g. water, in which energy moves through the medium without permanently altering it. An *electromagnetic wave* does not require a physical medium (e.g. water) through which to pass but consists of oscillations in magnetic and electric fields (e.g. light waves). A *longitudinal wave* is a type of wave in which the medium moves back and forth in the direction of travel of the wave. A *mechanical wave* requires a physical medium (e.g. water) through which to pass (e.g. sound waves). A *transverse wave* is a type of wave in which the medium moves back and forth at right-angles to the direction of travel of the wave.

wavelength The distance between two identical points on adjacent waves.

weight The force exerted on an object by gravity.

X

xeropthalmia A disease of the cornea of the eye associated with night blindness and caused by deficiency of vitamin A.

X-ray A form of electromagnetic radiation.

X-ray tube A device for the production of X-rays.

Z

zwitterion A covalent compound that possesses charged ionic regions.

zymogenic cells (chief cells) Cells of the lining of the stomach that secrete pepsinogen and intrinsic factor.

Index

Note: terms in the glossary are indicated by **emboldened page numbers**, Figures and Tables by *italic numbers*

A

ABO blood group system 362-3
absolute zero 207, **426**
acceleration 233, **426**
  Newton's law 238
accommodation (of eye) 293-4, *294*, **426**
acetic acid *see* ethanoic acid
acetone *see* propanone
acetyl co-enzyme A (acetyl-CoA) *195*, 196, 197, **426**
acetylsalicylic acid *100*, 113, 171, **426**
acid(s) 37, 100, 101-2, **426**
  examples *100*
  properties 103-4
acid-base balance 106-12
  by buffer systems 107-10
  by renal regulation 111-12
  by respiratory regulation 110-11
  regulation by hormones 112
acid-base imbalance 112-17
  management of 115-17
  metabolic 113
  respiratory 112-13
  ways of recognising 113-15
acidity 105, **426**
  measurement of 105
acidosis 106, 112, **426**
  metabolic 113, **446**
  respiratory 112-13
acidotic, meaning of term 106
acquired immunity 390-1, **444**
acquired immunodeficiency syndrome (AIDS) 374, **426**
actin 357, **426**
action potential(s) 177, 267, 270-2, **426**
action/reaction, Newton's law 239
activation energy 42, 158, **426**
Addison's disease 112, 113, **426**
adenine 192, 350, 358, **426**
adenosine diphosphate (ADP) 42, 193, **426**
adenosine triphosphate (ATP) 42, 179, 189, 192-4, 196, 197, **426**
ADH *see* antidiuretic hormone
adhesive forces 61, **426**
adipose tissue 166, 224, **426**
ADP *see* adenosine diphosphate
adrenal glands 112, 169, **427**
  role in thermoregulation *220*
adrenal medulla 11, 221, **427**
adrenaline 11, 50, 160, 221, **438**
aerobe(s) 377, **427**
aerobic process(es) 196, **427**
aerosol 66, **427**
afferent arteriole 110
afferent nerve **427**
after-loading (radiotherapy) 342, **427**
agar 66-7, 409, **427**
agranulocyte(s) 387, **427**
AIDS *see* acquired immunodeficiency syndrome
airborne spread of infection 396-7
albumin 88, 163, 165, **427**
albumin solution 69, **427**
alcohol abuse 175
alcohols 47-8, **427**
aldehydes 48, **427**
aldosterone 112, 171, **427**
aldosteronism 112, 113, **427**
algae 380, **427**
aliphatic compounds 45, **427**
alkalosis 106, 112, **427**
  metabolic 113
  respiratory 113
alkalotic, meaning of term 106, **427**
alkanes 45-6, **427**
alkenes 46, **427**
alkynes 46, **427**
alleles 360, **427**
alpha particles 330, 332, **427**
alternating current (AC) 263, **435**

altitude, effect on atmospheric pressure 125, 144
alveoli 63, 141, **427**
diffusion of gases 145-6
amines 49-50, **427**
amino acids 49, *100*, 108, 160, **427**
codes for 351
deamination of 110, 165
in liver 165
in proteins 108, 161-2, 357
structure *162*
ammonia 103, 104, **428**
formation of 110, 165, 198
ammonia buffer system 109-10
ammonium ions 103, 110
amniotic cavity 130, **428**
amniotic fluid 130-1, **428**
amoeba(s) 381, **428**
amoebic dysentry 381
ampere/amp (SI unit) *4*, 261, **428**
amphetamines 50, **428**
ampicillin 415, **428**
amplitude 315, **428**
amylase 159, **428**
anabolism 37, 194, **428**
anaemia 36, 134, 144, 175, 341, **428**
and blood pressure measurement 129
iron deficiency 179, **428**
in malaria 383
pernicious 176, **428**
in sickle cell disease 367
anaerobe(s) 377, **428**
anaerobic process(es) 196, **428**
anaeroid barometer 126
anaeroid sphygmomanometer 126, *127*
anaesthesia **428**
anaesthetic **428**
analgesia **428**
analgesic(s) 50, 73, 116, 171, 235, 248, 367, 379, **428**, **453**
anaphase 354, **428**
anaphylactic shock 88, **428**
angina 136, 171, **428**
angiography 339, **428**
anion(s) 27, **428**
annulus fibrosus 248, **428**
anode 274, **428**
anopheles mosquito 383, 384, **428**
anorexia (loss of appetite) 176
anorexia nervosa 166, 168, **428**
answers to self-test questions 423-4
antacid medication *100*
effects of excess 117
antagonistic, meaning of term 268, **428**
antecubital fossa 128, **429**
anthrax 5, 375, **429**
antibiotic(s) 374, **429**
action of 414-15
adverse effects 415-17
practical use of 417
resistance 417-18
and viral infections 379
antibodies 357, **429**
production of 387, 390-1
anticoagulant 159, **429**
anticodon 360, **429**
antidiuretic hormone (ADH) 91, **429**
antigen(s) 362-3, 390, **429**
antihistamines 88
antihypertensives **429**
blood pressure affected by 128
anti-inflammatory drugs 235
antimicrobials (drugs) 414, **429**
antipyretics (drugs) 171, 224, **453**
antisense strand (of DNA) 358, **429**
antiseptic(s) 63, 400, **429**
antitussive 379, **429**
antiviral agents 378
anus **429**
aorta 111, 237, 273, 339, **429**
apoenzyme 43, **429**
aqueous humour 292, *293*, **429**
aqueous mixture(s) 65-9, **429**
colloidal suspensions 65-7, *68*, **434**
mechanical suspensions 65, *68*, **448**
aqueous solutions 67-8, **429**
characteristics *68*, 69
archaebacteria 376, **429**
area, SI unit *4*, 125
aromatic compounds 45, 50, **429**
arrhythmia(s) 264, 275, **429**
arterial blood, partial pressure of gases in 114, 145, *146*
arterial blood pressure 134
arteriole(s) 86, 110, **429**
artery **429**
artificial pacemakers *187*, 256, 266, 278, *279*, **452**
ascorbic acid (vitamin C) *100*, 177
aspirin *100*, 113, 171, 224, 379, **426**, **429**
asthma 113, 116
atelectasis 64, 113, **430**
atherosclerosis 61, 136, 171, 278, 324, **430**
atmospheric air, partial pressures of gases in *143*
atmospheric pressure 124
measurement of 124-5

atom 16-17, **430**
orbital model of 23-5
structure of 20-1
atomic mass 18, **430**
atomic mass unit 23, **430**
atomic number 21, **430**
ATP *see* adenosine triphosphate
atria *272*, *273*, **430**
atrioventricular block 278, **430**
atrioventricular bundle (bundle of His) 273, **431**
atrioventricular node (AV node) 273, **430**
attenuated microorganisms 392
audiometric test 321, **430**
auscultation 127
autoclaving 226, 411, 413, **430**
autonomous division of nervous system 268
autosomal dominant inheritance 366
autosomal inheritance 361
autosomal recessive inheritance 165, 364-5
autosomes 349, **430**
avian flu 374
Avogadro's number 33, 80
axilla 212, **430**
axillary artery **429**
temperature 212
axoplasm 270, **430**

B

B lymphocytes 387, 390, **448**
bacilli 376, *377*, **430**
back injury 232, 248
bacteraemia 406, **430**
bacteria 375-8, **430**
antibiotic sensitivity 411
cell structure 375
cultivation in laboratory 408-9
enzymes produced by *394*
identifying 376-7, 410-11
nomenclature 374-5
reproduction of 378
toxins produced by 393
types 375-6
bactericidal (drug) 414, **430**
bacteristatic (drug) 414, **430**
barium meal 336
barometer 124-5, 126, **430**
basal metabolic rate (BMR) 198-9, **430**
base(s) 37, 100, 102-3, **430**
examples *100*
in nucleotides 350
properties 104
base excess 115, **430**
basilar membrane *318*, 319, 320, **430**
basophil(s) 387, 389, **430**
batteries *187*, 262-3
becquerel (SI unit) *4*, 338, **430**
bed rest, side effects 123, 240
benign neoplasms 355
benzene 50
beri beri 174, **430**
Bernoulli effect 147-8, 149, **450**, **463**
beta oxidation 197, **430**
beta particle(s) 330, 332, **431**
see also electrons
bicarbonate ion *see* hydrogen carbonate ion
bile 67, **431**
pH range *105*
bile salts 169-70, **431**
biliary obstruction 170
biliary tree 170, **431**
bilirubin 367
binary fission 378, **431**
binomial nomenclature (for microorganisms) 374-5
biochemical tests 411
biological half-life *333*, 334, **442**
biopsy **431**
bird flu 374
birth of baby 12
birth control, body temperature variation and 214
blindness 297-8
blood
components 134
as intravenous infusion 69
normal glucose concentration range 34, 158
pH range *105*, 106
blood flow 133-7
factors affecting 134-7
resistance to 134-6
blood osmolarity, regulation of 91-2
blood pressure 86, **431**
factors affecting 128, 136-7
measurement of 62, 126-9
blood specimens 406
BMR *see* basal metabolic rate
BNF *see* British National Formulary
body mass index (BMI) 168, **431**
body temperature 209-12
cyclic variations in 214
low 224-6
measurement of 207-9, 212-13
raised 221-4
upper (lethal) limit 222
bone marrow, blood cell production in 387
Bowman's capsule 110, **431**
Boyle's law 138-9, **431**

brachial artery 128, 339, **429**
bradycardia 219, 275, 278, **431**
bradytherapy 341
brain stem 11, **431**
breathing 139-42
British National Formulary (BNF) 416
broad-spectrum antibiotics 415
brochodilation **431**
brochodilator(s) 116, **431**
bronchitis 113, **431**
Brownian motion 75, **431**
brucellosis 412-13, **431**
buffer 107, **431**
buffer systems 107-10
bulimia nervosa 168, **431**
bundle of His 273, **431**
bundles (in heart) 272, 273
Burkitt's lymphoma 380, **431**
butane 46

C

calamine lotion 65, **431**
calcitonin 178, **431**
calcium 178
calcium chloride 27-8
calculi 173, **432**
calorie(s) 189-90, **432**
cancer 355
  treatment of 341, 414
cannulae **432**
  bacteria sticking to 393
capacitor 276, **432**
capillaries 86, **432**
capillary endothelium 65, **438**
capsid 378, **432**
carbohydrates 45, 156-61, 188, **432**
  catabolism of 195-7
carbon-atom chain prefixes *45*
carbon monoxide poisoning 36
carbonic acid 43, *100*, 107, 110, 112, **432**
carbonic anhydrase 43, 108, 111, **432**
carboxyhaemoglobin 36, **442**
carboxylic acids 48-9, 101-2, 166, 197, **432**
cardiac, meaning of term **432**
cardiac arrest 264, **432**
cardiopulmonary resuscitation (CPR) 265
cardiovascular system 9
carotenes 173, **432**
carotid arteries 111, **429**
carpopedal spasm 178, **432**
carriers
  of infections 396, 418
  of recessive genes 365, 368
cartilage 235
catabolism 37, 194, **432**
  of carbohydrates 195-7
  of fats 197-8
  of proteins 198
catalysts 42-3, **432**
cataract 290, 298, 306, **432**
catecholamines 49-50, **432**
catheter 236, 405, **432**
catheterisation 236, **432**
cathode 274, **432**
cathode ray(s) 274, **432**
cation(s) 27, **432**
caustic soda 20, 103, **432**
cell 8, 348, **432**
cell division 353-5
cell-mediated immunity 390, **444**
cell membrane 76, 78, 196, 348, 375, **432**
cell nucleus 348-9, **451**
cell wall 415, **433**
cellulose 159, 180, **432**
Celsius scale 206, **433**
  conversion to other temperature scales 206-7
central nervous system (CNS) 268, *269*
central venous pressure (CVP) **431**, **433**
  measurement of 62, 125, 126
centre of gravity 240-3, **433**
centrioles *348*, 354, **433**
centromere 349, *350*, **433**
centrosome 354, **433**
cephalosporin(s) 415, **433**
cerebrospinal fluid (CSF) 89, 111, 382, 403, **433**
  pH range *105*
cerebrovascular accident (CVA) 171, 219, **433**
cerumen 317, **433**
ceruminous glands 317, **441**
charge, SI unit 261, **435**
Charles' law **433**
cheilosis 175, **433**
chemical bonds 25-32
  covalent bonds 30-2
  ionic bonds 26-9
chemical energy *187*
chemical reactions 35-44
  combination 35-6, 49, **434**
  condensation 49, 158, **434**
  decomposition 36-7
  displacement 38, **437**
  endergonic **438**
  endothermic 42, **438**
  and energy 42
  exergonic **439**
  exothermic 42, **439**

chemical reactions (*continued*)
factors affecting rate of 42-4
partner-exchange 38, **453**
redox (oxidation-reduction) 30-1, **456**
reversible 39-40, **457**
chemistry 15-53
chemoautotrophs 376, **433**
chemoreceptor(s) 111, **433**
chemotaxis 389, **433**
chemotherapy 414
chest drains *see* intercostal drain(s)
chickenpox 390
chief cells *see* zymogenic cells
chloramphenicol 414, 415, **433**
chlorine, electron arrangement *24*, 26
chlorophyll 376
cholera 117, 376, **433**
cholesterol 170, 171, **433**
choroid (in eye) 292, *293*
chromatid(s) 349, *350*, **433**
chromatin 349, **433**
chromosomal abnormalities 368-9
chromosome(s) 349, **433**
homologous 349, **443**
chronic obstructive pulmonary disease (COPD) 113, **433**
chyle 171, **433**
chylomicrons 170, **433**
chymotrypsin 164, 165, **433**
chymotrypsinogen 165, **434**
cilia 319, 320, 382, **434**
ciliary body/muscle 292, *293*, *294*, **434**
ciliates 382, **434**
cine radiography 339
ciprofloxacin 415, **434**
circadian rhythm 214, **434**
circulatory system 9, *89*, 133, *272*
citric acid *100*, 103, **434**
cleaning 411, 412
clotting factors 368
CNS *see* central nervous system
cobalamin 175-6, **434**
cobalt-60 (^{60}Co) 333, *333*, 341
cocci 376, *377*, **434**
cochlea *318*, 319
cochlear nerve 317, **450**
codon(s) 351, 358, **434**
co-enzyme(s) 43, 194, **434**
co-enzyme A **434**
cofactor(s) 43, 172, **434**
coherent light 303
cohesive forces 61, **434**
collagen 164, 177, 357, **434**
colloid **434**
colloidal suspensions 65-7, **434**
characteristics *68*, *69*
colonisation 386, **434**
combination reaction(s) 35-6, 49, **434**
in body 36
commensalism 385, **434**
compass 256, 257
compensated acidosis/alkalosis 115
compound(s) 19-20, **434**
common names 20
computerised tomography (CT) 256, 339-40
concave, meaning of term **434**
concave lens *291*, 295, **447**
concentration 72-4, **434**
concentration gradient 75, 77, **434**
condensation reaction(s) 49, 158, **434**
conduction 214-15, *217*, 218, **434**
conduction defects (of heart) 278
conductive deafness 321, **435**
conductor(s) 215, 260, **435**
cones and rods (in eye) 296-7, **435**
congenital transmission 396
conjunctiva 173, 292, *293*
conservation of energy 188-9
conservation of matter 35
contact, infection spread by 399-400, 402
containers, fluids in 131
contaminated food and water, infection from 397-8
contraception 214
contrast medium (radio-opaque medium) 336, 339
control centre 10, 111, 267, **435**
controlled condition(s) 10, 111, 267, **435**
examples *10*, 12, 111
convection 215, *217*, 218, **435**
converging lens 291, *292*, **447**
convex, meaning of term **435**
convex lens(es) 290-2, **447**
applications 294, 298-301
COPD *see* chronic obstructive pulmonary disease
core temperature 209-10, **460**
clinical signs of lower temperatures *225*
upper (lethal) limit 222
variation with activity levels *210*
cornea 173, 292, *293*, **435**
coronary angiography 339, **428**
coronary arteries 136, 171, 275, 339, **429**
coronary ostium 339, **452**
Corti, organ of 319, *320*
cortisone 171, **435**
coulomb 261, **435**
covalent bond(s) 30-2, *32*, 59, 101, **435**

covalent compound(s) *32*, **435**
dissolving in water 71-2
CPR *see* cardiopulmonary resuscitation
cranial nerves *269*, 416
creatinine 165, **435**
crenation (of cell) 83, **435**, **461**
cross-infection, prevention of 399-402, 411
crossing over (in meiosis) 356
crystal **435**
crystalloid solution(s) 69, 84, **435**
CSF *see* cerebrospinal fluid
CT *see* computerised tomography
current 261, **435**, **437**
alternating 262, **435**
direct 262-3, **435**
and electrocution 266
SI unit *4*, 261, **428**
Cushing's disease 168-9
CVA *see* cerebrovascular accident
CVP *see* central venous pressure
cyclic compounds 45, **435**
cystic fibrosis 165, 348, 364-5, **435**
cystitis 386, 403, **435**
cytochrome chain **435**
cytokinesis 353, 355, **435**
cytoplasm 196, 348, **435**
cytoplasmic organelles 196, 357
cytosine 350, 358, **435**

D

Dalton's law of partial pressures 142-3, **435**
daughter cells 352, 353
deafness 321-2, **435**
deamination 110, 165, 198, **435**
deceleration injuries 237, *238*
decibel scale 315-16, **436**
decomposition reactions 36-7, **436**
decongestants 379
defibrillation 265, 275, **436**
defibrillator 265, 275-6, **436**
safety considerations 277
dehydration 93, **436**
effects 93
denaturation 44, **436**
density 93, **436**
SI unit *4*, 93
deoxyribonucleic acid (DNA) 32, *100*, 175, 179, 193, 348, 349, 350-1, **436**
replication of 352, 415
deoxyribose 350, **436**
depolarisation *271*, 272, **436**
dermatitis 175, **436**
dermis 123, 164, **436**
dextrins 159-60, **436**
diabetes insipidus 92
diabetes mellitus 8, 33, 34, 48, 51, 113, 117, 158, 160-1, 198, **436**
ketoacidosis in 46-7, 48, 113, 198, **446**
dialysate 94, **436**
dialysis 93-4, 117, **436**
haemodialysis 94, **436**
peritoneal 94, **436**
diaphragm 139, *141*, **436**
diarrhoea 117, 177, 178, 381
diastole 126, **436**
diastolic blood pressure 129, 134, **431**
diathermy *187*, 276-8, **436**
diatomic gases 30, *31*, **436**
diffusion 75-8, 145, 271, **436**
definition 77, **436**
distinguished from filtration 85
factors affecting rate of 77-8
of gases in alveoli 145-6
digestion 37, 42
of carbohydrates 159-60
of fats 67, 169-71
of proteins 164-5
digestive system 9
diglyceride 166, **441**
dihydrogen phosphate ion 108, 179, **436**
diplococci 376, **436**
diploid, meaning of term 349, **436**
dipolar ion(s) 108
release of hydrogen ion by 108, *109*
removal of hydrogen ion by 108, *109*
see also zwitterion(s)
direct contact, infection spread by 399-400
direct current (DC) 262-3, **435**
disaccharide(s) 158-9, **437**
discs, intervertebral 248
disinfectant(s) 63, *413*, **437**
disinfection 411, **437**
displacement reactions 38, **437**
in body 38
dissociation **437**
dissolving **437**
diuresis 91, 177, **437**
diuretic drugs 88, 113, 178, **437**
diurnal rhythm 214, **434**
diverging lens 295, **447**
DNA *see* deoxyribonucleic acid
dominant genes 360
dopamine 50
Doppler effect 323-4, **437**
use in body 324
Down's syndrome 368-9, **437**

drips *see* intravenous infusions
drug prescribing and dispensing 415
duodenum 67, 158, **437**
dysentry 381, 382, *393*, 402, **437**
dyspnoea 88, 176, **437**

E

earth **437**
earth-leakage circuit breakers 262, 265
ECG *see* electrocardiography
effective half-life 334, **442**
effector(s) 10, 111, 220, 267, **437**
efferent, meaning of term **437**
efferent arteriole 110
elastin 164, **437**
elderly person, heat loss after fall 218–19
electric current **435**, **437**
  SI unit *4*, **428**, **437**
electric shock, first aid in 265
electrical energy *187*
electrical potential 261
electrical potential difference 261, **455**
  in cells 78
  SI unit *4*, 261, 270, **463**
electrical resistance **457**
  SI unit *4*, 262, **451**, **457**
electrical safety 264
electricity 259–62
  in body 267–79
  dynamic 260–2
  static 259
electrocardiography (ECG) 256, 260, 274–5
electrocautery 276, 278, **436**
electrocution 263–7
electrode 274, **437**
electrolyte(s) 56, 70–2, 262, 263, **437**
electromagnet **437**
electromagnetic energy *187*
electromagnetic radiation 286, 330, 413, **437**
electromagnetic spectrum 285–6, 330, **437**
electromagnetic waves 286, 330, **463**
electromagnets 258
electron(s) 20, 259, 330, **437**
  gain of 41, 194
  loss of 41, 101, 194
electron cloud 21, **437**
electron pair 60
electron sharing 30, 59
electron transport chain *195*, 196, **438**
electronic thermometers 208, 212
electrosurgery 276, 278, **436**
element(s) 17, **438**
  importance in body *17*
elementary particle(s) 17, 20, **438**
elephantiasis 89
embolism 113, **438**
emulsification 67, **438**
emulsion(s) 66, 170, **438**
encephalopathy 175, **438**
endergonic reaction **438**
endocrine glands **441**
  acid-base balance regulated by 112
endocrine system 10–11, **438**
endogenous infection 395, **445**
endolymph (fluid) 319, **438**
endoscope(s) *187*, 302, **438**
endoscopy 302, **438**
endothelium 65, **438**
endothermic reactions 42, **438**
endotoxin(s) 393, **438**
endotracheal tube 117, **438**
energy 185–202
  conservation of 188–9
  conversion between forms 188–9
  definition 185, 190, **438**
  expenditure during exercise *192*
  forms 186–7
  kinetic 57, 188, **446**
  potential 188, **455**
  SI unit *4*, 190, **446**
  units *4*, 189–90, **446**
energy levels/shells 23, 24, **438**
energy-liberating reactions of cells 194–5
energy values of food 191
enterokinase 164, **438**
entrainment 148
environment **438**
  external *9*, **438**
  internal 8–9, **438**
enzymes 43, 158, 163, 357, **438**
  denaturation of 44
  inhibition by antibiotics 415
  naming of 159
  production by bacteria *394*
eosinophil(s) 387, **438**
epicanthal folds 369
epidermis 123, 164, **438**
epinephrine 11, 50, 160, 221, **438**
epithelium/epithelia 173, **439**
Epstein-Barr virus 380
equatorial plate **439**
erythema (redness) 305, 389, **439**
erythrocytes (red blood cells) 82, 108, 134, **439**
  in blood matching 362
  sickle-shaped 366, 367
  size 375

erythromycin 415, **439**
Escherichia coli 386, 397-8
essential amino acids 162, **427**
esterification reaction 49
esters 49, 166, **439**
ethanoic acid (acetic acid) 40, 49, 101-2, 103, 104, **439**
ethanol 47
ethene 46
ethyne 46
eubacteria 376, **439**
eukaryotic, meaning of term 375, **439**
eustachian tube 124, *318*, 319, **439**
evaporation 216, *217*, 218, **439**
exercise
  catabolism during 197
  energy expenditure during *192*
  temperature variation during *210*
exergonic reaction **439**
exocytosis 388, *389*, **439**
exogenous infection 395, **445**
exothermic reactions 42, **439**
exotoxin(s) 393, **439**
expiration (breathing) 140
external auditory canal 213, 317, *318*, **439**
external-beam radiotherapy 341, **456**
external environment *9*, **438**
  relationship with internal environment *9*
external respiration **457**
extracellular fluid 86, **439**
extracorporeal, meaning of term **439**
exudate of wound 392

F

faecal contamination 397, 402
faecal specimens 405
Fahrenheit scale 207
  conversion to Celsius scale 207
fainting, causes 223, 240
fallen elderly, heat loss in 218-19
falls in home, causes and prevention of 219
fat-soluble vitamins 172-4
fat/thin considerations 168-9
fats 45, 166, **447**
  catabolism of 197-8
  digestion and absorption of 169-71
  emulsification of 67, 170
  saturated 46, 166, 191, **457**
  unsaturated 46, 166-7, 191, **462**
  see also lipids
fatty acids 49, *100*, 102, 388, **432**
fatty tissue 166, 224, **426**
febrile, meaning of term 204, **439**
feedback mechanism(s) 10-12, 267, *268*, **439**
femoral artery 339, **429**
femur **439**
  fracture 219
fertilisation 349, **439**
fibre (in diet) 180-1, **439**
fibre-optic endoscopes 302
fibres (in heart) 272, 273
fibrillation 275, **440**, **463**
fibrinogen 163, 165, **440**
fibronectin 393, **440**
fibrous molecules 159, 163, **440**
filtration 85, **440**
  distinguished from diffusion 85
  in kidneys 85, 110, 111
first aid
  acids and bases 104
  electric shock 265
fixed pulleys 249, 250
flagellates 382, **440**
flagellum 382, **440**
flavine adenine dinucleotide (FAD) 194, 195, **440**
fluid *see* liquid
fluid balance, regulation within body 90-3
fluoroscopy 339, **440**
foam(s) 66, **440**
focal length 291, *295*, **440**
focal point 291, 295, **440**
focus 291, **440**
folic acid *100*, 176, 367, **440**
fomite **440**
fomites 402
food
  components 156-81
  energy values 191
food hygiene 398-9
food poisoning 376, 395, 398
force 122, 233, 234-6, **440**
  SI unit *4*, 125, 190, 234, **440**, **451**
forces, balanced/unbalanced 236
formulae, molecular/structural 32, 157, **440**
frequency **440**
  electric (AC) current 266-7, 276
  SI unit *4*
  waves 285, 313-14, 323
frequency (of passing urine) 403
friction 234-6, **440**
  and the body 235-6
fructose 157, **440**
fulcrum 241, 245, **440**
functional groups 47, **440**
fundamental quantity 233
fungi 380, **440**

fuses, electrical 262
fusion, latent heat of 206, **447**

G

galactose 157, **441**
gall bladder 67, 170, **441**
gall stones 170, **432**
gamete(s) 349, **441**
gametocyte(s) 384, **441**
gamma rays 286, 330, 331, 333, **441**
gas/gaseous state 16, **441**
gas laws 138-44
gases, in solution 144-6
gastrectomy 176, **441**
gastric, meaning of term **441**
gastric pits 164
gastric secretions, pH range *105*
gastric ulcers, detection of 336
gastrointestinal tract *157*, 159
gastroscopy 302
gel(s) 66, **441**
gene(s) 348, 351, **441**
general anaesthesia **428**
genetic code 350-1, **441**
genetic diseases 364-9
genetic inheritance 360-4
genetics 347-72
  meaning of term 348, **441**
genome **441**
genotype 360, **441**
gentamicin 416, **441**
germicidal lamps 303
gingivitis 179, **441**
glands 91, 112, 169, 180, 199, 340, 387, **441**
glandular fever 380, **441**
globular molecules 159, 163, **441**
glomerular filtrate 110
  glucose in 161
glomerulus 110, **441**
glossary **426-64**
glossitis 175, 176, 179, **441**
glottis 313, **441**
glucagon 160, **441**
gluconeogenesis 160, **441**
glucose 80, 157, 160, **441**
  concentration in blood 33, 34, 51
'glue ear' 321
glycerides 47, 102, 166-71, **441**
  digestion and absorption of 169-71
glycerol 47-8, 102, 166, 197, **442**
glyceryl trinitrate (GTN) 136, **442**
glycogen 159, 194, **442**
glycogenesis 160, **442**
glycogenolysis 160, **442**
glycolysis 160, *195*, 196, **442**
glycoprotein **442**
glycosuria 161, **442**
goitre 180, **442**
gonads 355, **442**
gonorrhoeae 376, **442**
Gram stain 377, 410, **442**
granulocyte(s) 387, **442**
gravity 233, 239-40, **442**
  centre of 240-3, **433**
gray (SI unit) *4*, 338, **442**
group (in Periodic Table) 19, 425, **442**
guanine 350, 358, **442**

H

haematopoiesis 387, **442**
haemodialysis 94, **436**
haemoglobin 36, 108, 163, **442**
  buffer system 108-9
  reduced 109
  and sickle cell anaemia 366
haemolytic disease of the newborn 174
haemophilia 368, **442**
haemorrhage, blood loss due to 137
haemorrhoids 179, **442**
half-life 333-4, **442**
  biological *333*, 334, **442**
  effective 334, **442**
  physical 333, **442**
halothane 224, **442**
handwashing 399, 400-2
haploid, meaning of term 349, **442**
Heaf gun/test 407, **443**
hearing 317-22
  mechanism of 317-20
hearing protection 316
hearing-impaired person, communicating with 322
heart
  conduction defects 278
  conduction system 272-3
heart attack *see* myocardial infarction
heat *187*, 204, **443**
  transmission of 214-19
  see also latent heat
heat exhaustion 223
heat losses
  from body 217-19
  methods of increasing *222*
  prevention of 216-17
heat stroke 223
helium 26
helium nuclei 330

Henry's law 143, 144, **443**
heparin 159, **443**
hepatic portal vein 160, 165, **443**
hepatocyte(s) 160, **443**
heredity 348
heterotrophs 376, **443**
heterozygous, meaning of term 360, **443**
high-density lipoproteins (HDL) 171
hilium 140, **443**
His, bundle of 273, **431**
histamine 88, 387, 389, **443**
histones 349, **443**
HIV *see* human immunodeficiency virus
homeostasis 10, 106, 111, 220-1, **443**
  and nursing care 12-13
homeostatic control mechanisms 10-12, 111
homologous chromosomes 349, **443**
homozygous, meaning of term 360, **443**
hormone(s) 10, 11, 50, 267, 357, **443**
  acid-base balance affected by 112
host-microorganism relationships 385-6
human immunodeficiency virus (HIV) 378, 396, **443**
humoral immunity 390, **445**
Huntington's disease 366
hydrocarbons 45-7, **443**
hydrochloric acid 37, *100*, 101, 104, **443**
  in stomach 101, 164, 388
hydrocolloids 67
hydrogels 67
hydrogen bonds 32, 162, **443**
hydrogen carbonate buffer system 107
hydrogen carbonate ion 29, 39, 40, 102, 103, 112, **443**
hydrogen carbonate ion concentration 114
hydrogen ion 101
  combined with ammonia 110
  concentration 105
  release by dipolar ion 108, *109*
  removal by dipolar ion 108, *109*
  removal from body 111, 112
hydrogen isotopes 22
hydrogenation of fats 46, 167, **443**
hydrolysis 49, 158, **443**
  of disaccharides 158
  of esters 49
  of fats/lipids 197
hydrophilic, meaning of term 170, **443**
hydrophobic, meaning of term 169-70, **443**
hydrostatic pressure 86-7, **443**
  raised 88-9
hydroxide ion 102, 103
hydroxyl groups 47, 166
hydroxyl ion **443**
hypercalcaemia 173, 178, **443**
hyperglycaemia 158, 160-1, **443**
hyperkalaemia 38, 178, **444**
hypernatraemia 177, **444**
hyperopia 294, **444**
  correction of *294*
hyperosmotic, meaning of term 83, **444**
hypersensitivity tests 407-8
hypertension **444**
hyperthermia 218, 221-4, **444**
  factors affecting 222-4
  interventions 222-3
hyperthyroidism **444**
hypertonic, meaning of term 83, **444**
hyperventilation 111, 113, **444**
hyphae 380, **444**
hypocalcaemia 178, **444**
hypochromic, meaning of term 179, **444**
hypochromic megaloblastic anaemia 176
hypoglycaemia 160, **443**
hypokalaemia 178, **444**
hyponatraemia 177, **444**
hypo-osmotic, meaning of term 83, **444**
hypoproteinaemia 89, **444**
hypoprothrombinaemia 174, **444**
hypotension 219, **444**
hypothalamus 11, 91, 220, **444**
hypothermia 12, 204, 218, 221, 224-6, **444**
  clinical signs *225*
  induced 204, 226
  interventions 224-6
hypothyroidism 168, **444**
hypotonic, meaning of term 83, **444**
hypoventilation 112-13, 116, **444**
hypoxaemia 146, **444**
hypoxia **444**

I

iatrogenic, meaning of term 176, **444**
ice
  melting of 56-7, 205-6
  packs 206
ileum 77, 157, 158, **444**
  surgical removal of 176
immune mechanisms 388-92
immune system 387, **444**
immunisation 391-2
immunity 387, **444**
  acquired 390-1, **444**
  cell-mediated 390, **444**
  humoral 390, **445**
  innate 388-9, **445**

immunoglobulin(s) 387, 390, **429**, **445**
imperfect fungi 380
incomplete dominance 362, 366
incus 318, **445**
indirect contact, infection spread by 402
induced-fit model (for enzyme action) 43, **445**
induced hypothermia 204, 226
inert gases 25-6
inertia **445**
  Newton's law 236-7
infection(s) 386, **445**
  endogenous 395, **445**
  exogenous 395, **445**
  nosocomial 395, **445**
  response to 387-92
  sources 394-402
  treatment of 414-18
  zoonotic 396, **445**
inflammation 388-9, **445**
infrared radiation 209, 286, **445**
ingestion of microorganisms 395-6, 397-8
inhalation of microorganisms 395, 396-7
inheritance 360-4
  multiple allele 362-3
  polygenic 363-4
  sex 364
  simple autosomal 361
innate immunity 388-9, **445**
inoculation 392, 396
inorganic chemistry 44, 156, **445**
insect vectors 402
insensible losses (of fluid) 90, 91
insoluble fibre 180-1
inspiration (breathing) 139
insulator(s) 215, 260, **445**
insulin 113, 160, 198, **445**
intensity 315
intercellular fluid *see* interstitial fluid
intercostal drain(s) 140-2, **445**
intercostal muscles 139, **445**
internal communication 10
internal environment 8-9, **438**
  relationship with external environment *9*
internal radiotherapy 341-2, **456**
internal respiration **457**
interphase 353, **445**
interstitial fluid 9, 56, 86, **445**
  excess of 87-8, 177
  formation of 86-8
interstitial implantation radiotherapy 342, **456**
interstitium **445**
intervertebral discs 248
intestine **445**
  large *157*, **445**
  small *157*, 158, 169, **445**
intra-alveolar pressure 141
intracavity implantation radiotherapy 342, **456**
intracellular fluid 86, **445**
intracellular ion(s) 177
intradermal injection 392, **445**
intramuscular injection 392, **445**
intraplural pressure 141
intravascular fluid 86, **445**
intravenous, meaning of term **445**
intravenous infusions (drips) 56, 69, 84, 287
  flow rate regulation 132-3
  movement restricted by 123
  pressure considerations 132-3
  to replace electrolytes 117
intrinsic factor 176, **445**
intubation 236, **446**
inverse square law 337, **446**
iodine 179-80
iodine-131 (^{131}I) 332-3, *333*, 340, 342
ion 26, **446**
ion channels 270
ionic bond(s) 26-9, *32*, **446**
ionic compound(s) *32*, 104, **446**
ionic lattice, effect of water on 70, *71*
ionisation 36-7, **446**
ionising radiation 330-1, **446**
  effects 336, 413
iris 292, *293*, **446**
iron 178
iron deficiency anaemia 179, **428**
islets of Langerhans 160, **446**
isomers 32, 157, **446**
iso-osmotic, meaning of term 81, 82, **446**
iso-osmotic solutions 84
isopropyl alcohol (IPA) *see* 2-propanol
isotonic, meaning of term 82-3, **446**
isotonic solutions 84
isotopes 22, 331, *333*, **446**
  see also radioisotopes

J

jaundice, in sickle cell disease 367
joule (SI unit) *4*, 190, **446**

K

kaolin 65, **446**
karotype **446**
kelvin (SI unit) *4*, 206, **446**
  conversion to Celsius scale 206
keratin 163-4, 388, **446**

keratinocytes **446**
ketoacidosis/ketosis 46-7, 48, 113, 198, **446**
ketoacids 197, **446**
ketones 46-7, 48, **446**
conversion of acetyl-CoA to 197
production in diabetes 46-7, 48, 113
kidney failure 38
kidneys, buffer system in 109-10
kilocalorie 190
kilogram (SI unit) *4*, 5-6, 233, **446**
kilojoule 190
kilowatt 263
kinetic energy 57, 188, **446**
Korotkoff sounds 129, **446**
Krebs cycle *195*, 196, 197, 198, **447**
Kussmaul's respirations 198, **447**

L

lactase 159, **447**
lacteals 170, **447**
lactic acid 197
lactose 158, **447**
digestion of 159
lactose intolerance 159, **447**
Langerhans, islets of 160, **446**
large intestine *157*, **445**
large numbers, scientific notation 3
laryngitis 313, **447**
laryngospasm 313, **447**
larynx 313, **447**
laser(s) 301, 303, **447**
latent heat 206, **447**
of fusion 206, **447**
of vaporisation 206, **447**
lavage 225, **447**
lecithin 170, **447**
Legionella pneumophila 397
length, SI unit 4-5, 190, 232, **449**
lens(es) 290-6, **447**
concave 295, **447**
converging 291, *292*, **447**
convex 290-2, **447**
diverging 295, **447**
leukocyte(s) 381, 387, **447**
lever(s) 245-8, **447**
examples in body 246-8
types 245-6
lifting 232
levers used in body 247-8
ligament **447**
ligament injury 237
light (radiation) 284-6, **447**
particle/wave duality 284
properties 285, 287-90
light receptors 296-7
lightning 259
linear accelerator 331, 335, 341, **447**
linolenic acid 167
lipase 67, 169, **447**
action on triglycerides 170
lipids 166-71, **447**
formation of 49
hydrolysis (decomposition) of 49
see also fats
lipoprotein(s) 170, 171, **447**
liquid 16, **447**
liquid-crystal thermometers 208
Listeria monocytogenes 398
lithotripsy 323, **447**
litmus paper 103-4, **448**
litre (unit) 6, **448**
liver **448**
amino acids in 165
local anaesthesia/anaesthetics 272, **428**
lock-and-key model (for enzyme action) 43
locus 360, **448**
logarithmic scales 105, 315
longitudinal wave(s) 312-13, **463**
long-sightedness *see* hyperopia
loudness (of sound) 314, 315-16
low-density lipoproteins (LDL) 171
lower-limb oedema 89
lumbar puncture 407, **448**
lymph system 88, 171, 172
lymphatic cancer 380
lymphatic obstruction 89
lymphocytes 387, **448**
lysosome *348*, **448**
lysozyme 388, **448**

M

macrophage(s) 387, 388, **448**
macroshock 266
magnet 256-7, **448**
see also electromagnet
magnetic field(s) 257, 258, **448**
and the body 258
magnetic resonance imaging (MRI) 256, **448**
magnetism **448**
magnifying glass 299-300
malaria 383-5, 396, **448**
prevention of 384-5
maligant hyperpyrexia 224
malignant melanomas 305-6
malignant neoplasms 355
malleus 318, **448**

maltase 159, **448**
maltose 158, **448**
digestion of 159, 160
manometer(s) 62, 126, **448**
mass 233, **448**
SI unit *4*, 5-6, 233, **446**
mass number 21, **448**
matter **448**
states of 16, 56
measles/mumps/rubella (MMR) vaccination 391
mechanical energy *187*
mechanical suspension(s) 65, *68*, **448**
mechanical wave(s) 285, 312, **463**
meiosis 355-6, **448**
melanin 305, **448**
melanocytes 305, **449**
melanosomes 305
memory cells 390, *391*
meninges 398, **449**
meningitis *393*, 398, **449**
meniscus 62, **449**
menstrual cycle 214, **449**
mercury, meniscus *62*
mercury-in-glass barometer 124-5
mercury-in-glass sphygmomanometer 62, 126
mercury-in-glass thermometer 204, 207-8, **461**
merozoites 384, **449**
messenger RNA (mRNA) 357, **457**
metabolic acidosis 113, 114, **446**
management of *116*, 117
metabolic alkalosis 113, 114
management of *116*, 117
metabolic rate 198, **449**
metabolism 8, 194, **449**
metals 19
metaphase 354, **449**
methanal 48
methane 45, *46*
methanoic acid (formic acid) 48, *49*
methanol 47
methicillin 417, **449**
methicillin-resistant *Staphylococcus aureus* (MRSA) 417-18, **449**
methylamine *49*
metre (SI unit) 4-5, 190, 232, **449**
MI *see* myocardial infarction
micelles 170, **449**
microbiological samples 403-7
blood specimens 406
sputum specimens 405-6
stool specimens 405
urine specimens 403-5
wound specimens 406
microbiological tests 407-8
microbiology 373-422, **449**
microbiology laboratory 408-11
microcytic, meaning of term 179, **449**
micrograms (mcg) 5-6
microns 5
microorganisms 374, **449**
cultivation in laboratory 408-10
evasion of defences by 393
hosts damaged by 393-4
methods of transmission 396-8
naming 374-5
routes of entry 395-6
virulence 386, 392-3, **463**
see also bacteria; fungi; protozoa; viruses
microscope 300-1, **449**
microscopy 410-11, **449**
microshock 264, 266
microvilli 77, 170, **449**
microwaves 286, **449**
mid-stream specimen of urine (MSU) 405, **449**
milliequivalents per litre (meq/l) 73-4
milligrams (mg) 5
millilitres (ml) 6
millimoles per litre (mmol/l) 33, 34, 73, **449**
millivolts 270
minerals 177-9, **449**
mitochondria 196, *348*, 375, **449**
mitosis 353-5, **449**
mixture **449**
molality *4*, **449**
molarity *4*, 73, **449**
mole *4*, 33-4, 80, **450**
molecular formula(e) 32, 157, **440**
molecular mass 33, **450**
molecule **450**
momentum 234, **450**
monera 374, 375, **450**
monochromatic light 303
monocyte(s) 387, **450**
monoglyceride 166, **441**
monohydrogen phosphate ion 108, 179, **450**
monosaccharide(s) 156-8, **450**
monosaturated fat 167
morphine 50, 65, **450**
motor division of nervous system 268, **450**
moveable pulleys 249, 250, 251
moving and handling techniques 232
MRI *see* magnetic resonance imaging
MRSA *see* methicillin-resistant *Staphylococcus aureus*
MSU *see* mid-stream specimen of urine
mucilages 180, **450**

multiple allele inheritance 362–3
multiple-field radiotherapy 341
muscle relaxant 224, **450**
mutualism 385, **450**
myalgia **450**
mycelium 380, **450**
myocardial infarction (MI) 171, 222, 275, **450**
oedema caused by 89
myopia 295, **450**
correction of *295*
myosin 357, **450**
myxoedema 340, **450**

N

NAD *see* nicotinamide adenine dinucleotide
nalidixic acid 415, **450**
nanometre(s) 5, 286
narcotic drugs 116, **450**
nasopharynx **450**
temperature 208
'natural' birth control 214
nebuliser(s) 63, 116, 149–50, **450**
negative feedback mechanism(s) 11–12, 91, 111, **439**
neoplasm(s) 355, **450**
detection of 323, 336
nephron(s) 65, 109, *110*, **450**
nerve(s) *269*, **450**
nervous system 10, 267–9
neuron(e) 232, 269, **450**
neutral, meaning of term 106, **451**
neutral fats 102, 166, **451**
neutralisation **451**
neutron 20, **451**
neutrophil(s) 387, 388, **451**
newton (SI unit) *4*, 125, 190, 234, **451**
Newton's laws of motion 236–9
niacin 176, **451**
nicotinamide adenine dinucleotide (NAD) 40–1, 176, 194, **451**
reduced (NADH) 41, 194–5, **451**
nicotinic acid *see* niacin
night blindness 173, 298, **451**
nitrogen balance 166
nodes (in heart) 272, 273
non-disjunction 369, **451**
non-electrolyte(s) 72, 80
non-essential amino acids 162, **427**
non-metals 19
non-polar molecule(s) 32
non-starch polysaccharide(s) 180
non-steroidal anti-inflammatory drugs (NSAIDs) 224, **451**
see also aspirin; paracetamol
norepinephrine/noradrenaline 11, 50, 221, **451**
normal saline 20, 68
nosocomial infection 395, **445**
NSAID *see* non-steroidal anti-inflammatory drug
nuclear energy *187*
nuclear membrane 348, 375, **451**
nucleic acid
in viruses 378
see also deoxyribonucleic acid (DNA); ribonucleic acid (RNA)
nucleoplasm 348, 375, **451**
nucleosome 349, **451**
nucleotide(s) 350, **451**
nucleus
of atom 21, **451**
of cell 348–9, 375, **451**
nucleus pulposus 248, **451**
numbers, expressing 2–3
numerical prefix(es) 3, **451**
nutrients
dietary 156–81
for microorganisms 392
nystatin 416, **451**

O

obesity 168–9
and centre of gravity 243
obligate parasites 378, 410
obligate pathogen(s) 377, 386, **453**
occiput 123, **451**
odours 46
oedema 88–9, **451**
causes 88, 177
oesophagus **451**
cancer 168
temperature 208
oestrogen 178, **451**
ohm (SI unit) *4*, 262, **451**
Ohm's law 262, 266
oncotic pressure **451**
oocyte (egg cell) 214, **451**
opportunistic pathogen 385, 386, **453**
opsin 297, **451**
optical instruments 298–303
oral cavity, temperature 212
organ of Corti 319, *320*
organelles 196, 357, 375, **452**
organic chemistry 44–50, 156, **452**
alcohols 47–8, **427**
aldehydes 48, **427**
amines 49–50, **427**

organic chemistry (*continued*)
aromatic compounds 45, 50, **429**
carboxylic acids 48-9, **432**
esters 49, **439**
hydrocarbons 45-7, **443**
ketones 46-7, 48, **446**
orthopaedic traction 250-1
orthostatic hypotension 223, **452**
oscilloscope 274, **452**
osmolality 82, **452**
osmolarity 81, 84, **452**
osmole (unit) 81, **452**
osmoreceptor(s) 10, 91, **452**
osmosis 78-80
definition 79, **452**
osmotic pressure 79-80, **452**
ossicles 318, **452**
osteoarthrosis 235, **452**
osteoblast(s) 240, **452**
osteoclast(s) 240, **452**
osteomalacia 173, **452**
osteoporosis 178, **452**
ostium/ostia 339, **452**
otitis media 321, **452**
ova (eggs) 349
oval window (in ear) *318*, 320
ovary 214, **452**
ovulation 214, **452**
oxidation reactions 40-1, 194, **452**
oxidative phosphorylation 193
oxygen masks *147*, 148-9
oxygen therapy 146-50
oxygen transport 143-4
oxyhaemoglobin 36, 144, 366, **442**
oxyntic cells (parietal cells) 164, **452**
oxytocin 12, **452**

P

pacemaker
artificial *187*, 256, 266, 278, *279*, **452**
node (in heart) 273, **452**, **458**
pain relief
electrical method 278-9
see also analgesics
pallor 137, 176, 221
palmitic acid 166, *167*
pancreas **452**
pancreatic amylase 160, **428**
pancreatic enzymes 164, 165, 169
pancreatic secretions, pH range *105*
pandemic 374, **453**
paracetamol 224, 379, **453**
parasitic, meaning of term 378, **453**
parasitism 385, **453**
parasympathetic division of nervous system 268, **453**
parathormone 178, **453**
parenteral, meaning of term **453**
parietal pleura 140, *141*
partial pressure(s) **453**
of carbon dioxide in arterial blood 114
Dalton's Law of 142-3, **435**
of gases in air *143*
particle **453**
partner-exchange reactions 39, **453**
pascal (SI unit) *4*, 79, 125, **453**
Pascal's law/principle 130, **453**
pasteurisation 412-13, **453**
pathogen(s) 374, 377, 378, 386, **453**
pectins 180, **453**
pellagra 176, **453**
penicillin 414, 415, **453**
pepsin 39, 101, 164, **453**
pepsinogen 39, 101, 164, **453**
peptidases 165, **453**
peptide 162, **453**
peptide bond(s) 162, 357, **453**
peptones 164, **453**
percentage concentration 72-3
perilymph (fluid) 319, **453**
period (in Periodic Table) 19, 425, **453**
Periodic Table 17, 18-19, 425, **453**
peripheral nervous system 268, *269*
peripheral temperature 210, *211*, **460**
and countercurrent heat transfer of blood 210, *211*, 212
peristalsis 181, **454**
peritoneal dialysis 94, **436**
permanent magnets 256-7
pernicious anaemia 176, **428**
Petri dish 408, *409*, **454**
pH scale 105-6, **454**
and microorganisms 393
for various body fluids *105*
phagocyte(s) 387, 388, 389, **454**
phagocytosis 381, 387, 388, *389*, **454**
pharynx 313, **454**
phenol 50
phenotype 360, **454**
phenylalanine 165, **454**
phenylketonuria 165, **454**
pholcodine 73, 379, **454**
phosphate buffer system 108
phospholipid 64, 171, **454**
phospholipid bilayer 179
phosphorus 179

phosphorylation 193, **454**
photoautotroph(s) 376, **454**
photoblation/photocoagulation 303
photoreceptors 296-7
physical half-life 333, **442**
piezoelectric effect 322, **454**
pili 393, **454**
pinna 213, 317, **454**
pitch 314, **454**
pituitary gland 91, 180, **454**
plankton 8-9
plasma 86, 287, **454**
plasma cells 390, *391*
plasma concentrations 74
plasma expander(s) 69, **454**
plasma membrane 76, *348*, **454**
plasma protein 163, **454**
plasma protein solution 69, **454**
Plasmodium parasites 383-4
plasmolysis 83, **454**, **461**
plating out 408
pleura 140, *141*, **454**
pleurisy/pleuritis 140, **454**
plural drains *see* intercostal drain(s)
plural fluid 89, 140, **454**
plural space 125, *141*, **454**
pneumonia 397, **454**
pneumothorax 142, **454**
polar molecule(s) 31, **454**
  water as 31, 60-1, 70
polarisation of light 289-90, **455**
pole(s) 256, **455**
polyatomic ion(s)/radical(s) 28-9, **455**
polycythaemia 134, **455**
polydipsia 161, **455**
polygenic inheritance 363-4
polypeptide(s) 162, **455**
polysaccharide(s) 159-60, 180, **455**
polyunsaturated fat 167, **455**
polyuria 161, 173, **455**
pore **455**
positive feedback mechanism 12, **439**
postural drainage 116, **455**
potassium 177-8
potential difference 261, **455**
  in cells 78
  and electrocution 266
  SI unit *4*, 261, 270, **463**
potential energy 188, **455**
poultices 65
power **455**
  SI unit *4*, **463**
premature babies 64
presbycusis 321, **455**
pressure
  definition 122, **455**
  measurement of 124-9
  SI unit *4*, 79, 125, **453**
  in static liquids 130-3
  units of measurement 125-6
  see also blood pressure
pressure ulcer(s) 122-3, **455**
principal axis 291, 295
principal focus 291, **440**
products 35, **455**
progesterone 171, **455**
prokaryotic, meaning of term 375, **455**
propane 46
2-propanol (isopropyl alcohol) 47
propanone (acetone) 48, **455**
prophase 353-4, 356, **455**
prophylactic drugs 367, 385
prostaglandins 171, **455**
prostate gland 236, **455**
prosthesis 235, **455**
protein(s) 45, 49, 108, 161-6, **455**
  buffer system 108
  catabolism of 198
  digestion of 164-5
  metabolic disturbances 165
  nitrogen balance 166
  structure 162-4
  synthesis of 165, 357-60, 415
prothrombin 165, 174
protists 374, 380, **455**
proton 20, 101, **455**
proton donors 101
protoplasm 348, 375, **455**
protozoa 380-5, **455**
pseudoephedrine 379, **456**
pseudopodia 381, **456**
psoralen UVA therapy 304
pulley(s) 249, **456**
  use 250-1
pulmonary artery 273, **429**
pulmonary embolism 113
pulmonary oedema 88-9
pulmonary veins **463**
punnet square 361-2
  applications 363, 364, 365, 368
pupil (in eye) 292, **456**
Purkinje fibres 273, **456**
pyrexia 136, 221, 223-4, 367, **456**
  in malaria 383, 384
pyridoxine 175, **456**
pyrogen(s) 222, **456**

pyruvic acid, conversion to acetyl co-enzyme A *195*, 196

Q

quinolones 415, **456**

R

radiation 216, *217*, 330, **456**
measurement of 338
radiation protection 337-8
radioactive, meaning of term 331, **456**
radioactive decay 331-3, **456**
alpha decay 331-2
beta decay 332-3
gamma decay 333
radioactivity 331, **456**
units 338
radioisotope(s) 22, 331, **456**
diagnostic testing with 180, 332, 340
half-lives listed *333*
metabolism in body 334, 342
precautions 334, 338, 342
radiological diagnostic procedures 335-6, 339-40
radio-opaque, meaning of term 180, 336, **456**
radiosensitivity 341, **456**
radiotherapy 341-2, **456**
side effects 341
radio waves 286
rarefaction 313, **456**
RDS *see* respiratory distress syndrome
reactants 35, **456**
reactions *see* chemical reactions
receptors 10, 111, 267, **456**
recessive genes 360, 368
rectum **456**
temperature 208
red blood cells *see* erythrocytes
redox reactions 40-1, **456**
reduced haemoglobin 109
reduced nicotinamide adenine dinucleotide (NADH) 41, **451**
reduction reactions 41, 194, **456**
redundancy (in genetic code) 351
reflection 287, **456**
refraction 287-9, **456**
Reissner's membrane *see* vestibular membrane
relative atomic mass 22-3, 33, **457**
relative weights 18
renal, meaning of term **457**
renal calculi 173, 323, **432**
renal corpuscle 109, *110*, **457**
renal failure 38, 113
renal regulation, acid-base balance by 111-12
renal tubule 109, *110*, **457**
repolarisation *271*, 272, **457**
resistance 261-2, **457**
and electrocution 266
SI unit *4*, 262, **451**, **457**
resonance 316-17, 320, **457**
resonant frequency 316, **457**
respiration 139-40, **457**
respiratory acidosis 112-13, 114
management of 116-17
respiratory alkalosis 112-13, 113, 114-15
management of *116*, 117
respiratory distress syndrome (RDS) 64
respiratory regulation, acid-base balance by 110-11
respiratory system 9
resting membrane potential 270
retina *293*, *294*, 296, **457**
damage due to diabetes 161
detachment 298
retinal **457**
retinol 173
reversible reactions 39-40, **457**
Reye's syndrome 224
rhodopsin 297, **457**
riboflavin 175, **457**
ribonucleic acid (RNA) 175, 193, 350, **457**
messenger (mRNA) 357, **457**
ribosomal (rRNA) 357, **457**
transfer (tRNA) 357, **457**
ribose 350, **457**
ribosomal RNA (rRNA) 357, **457**
ribosomes 357, 375, **457**
rickets 173, **457**
ringworm 380, **457**
RNA *see* ribonucleic acid
rods and cones (in eye) 296-7, **457**
dysfunction 298
roughage *see* fibre

S

saccharides *see* disaccharides; monosaccharides; polysaccharides
sacrum 123, **457**
saline manometer 62, 125, 126
saline solution, normal 20, 68
saliva
pH range *105*
in sputum specimen 405
salivary amylase 159, **428**
salivary glands *157*, **457**
salmonellosis 395-6, **457**

salt (common) *see* sodium chloride
salt(s) 37, 104, **457**
as acids and bases 106
saprophytes 374, 380, **457**
saturated fats 46, 166, 191, **457**
saturated hydrocarbons 45-6
saturation (oxygen in blood) 144
scala media *318*, 319, **457**
scala tympani *318*, 319, **458**
scala vestibuli *318*, 319, **458**
scalar quantities 232, **458**
schizonts 384, **458**
scientific notation 2-3, **458**
sclera 292, *293*, **458**
scurvy 172, 177, **458**
sebum 388, **458**
selectively permeable membrane 271, **458**
self-test questions, answers 423-4
semen, pH range *105*
semi-permeable membrane 77, **458**
sense strand (of DNA) 358, **458**
sensorineural deafness 321, **435**
sensory division of nervous system 268, **458**
septicaemia 406, **458**
serological tests 407, **458**
serum **458**
set point 10, **458**
sex cells 349
sex chromosome(s) 349, **433**
sex-linked disorders 368
shell temperature 210, **460**
shivering 10, 221
short-sightedness *see* myopia
SI units 4-6, **428**, **446**, **448**, **449**, **451**, **453**, **463**
base units *4*
derived units *4*
sick sinus syndrome 278, **458**
sickle cell anaemia 366-7, **458**
sickle cell trait 366, **458**
sickling crisis 367, **458**
sievert (unit) 338, **458**
sino-atrial node 273, **452**, **458**
sinus rhythm 275, **458**
skin
role in fighting infection 388
role in thermoregulation *220*, 221
skin cancer 305-6
sleeping sickness 382, 396, **458**
slide projector 298-9
slime moulds 380, **459**
'slipped disc' 248
small intestine *157*, 158, 169, **445**
small numbers, scientific notation 3
smallpox 5, 392, **459**
'soda', confusion of name 20
sodium 177
electron arrangement *24*, 26
sodium balance, factors affecting 90-1
sodium carbonate 20
sodium chloride 19, 27, 34, 35, 36, 37, 68, 70, 80-1, 104, 177
sodium hydrogen carbonate 20, 29, 39, *100*
sodium hydroxide 37, 103, 104
sodium pump 270, **459**
sol 66, **459**
solenoid 258, **459**
solid(s) 16, **459**
soluble fibre 180-1
solute(s) 67, 68, **459**
solution(s) 67-8, **459**
solvent concentration 78
solvent(s) 67, 68, **459**
somatic cell(s) 349, **459**
somatomotor division of nervous system 268, **459**
sonar 322
sound 312-17
space-occupying lesion(s) 355, **459**
specific gravity 93, **459**
specific immunity 390
speech 313
speed, definition 232, **459**
spermatoza 349, **459**
sphygmomanometer 62, 126, **459**
cuff used 126-7, *128*
spina bifida 323, **459**
spinal nerves *269*
spindle fibres 354, **459**
spirochaetes 376, *377*
spoon measure 73
spore 377, **459**
spore-forming organisms 377
sporozoans 382, **459**
sputum
coughing up 379, 395, 406
specimens 405-6
stability 244-5
stable equilibrium 244, 246
stapes 318, **459**
staphylococci 376, *377*, 385, 393, 394, 399, **459**
starch 158, 159, 188, **459**
start codons 351, 358
starvation, biochemical effects 166, 198
states of matter 16, 56, *58*

static electricity 259
static equilibrium 241
static liquids, pressure in 130-3
sterilisation 226, 411-13, **459**
chemical methods 413
physical methods 226, 411-13
sterols 171, **459**
stethoscope 127-8
stimulus 10, **459**
'stitch' 197
Stokes-Adams attack 278, **459**
stomatitis 175, 179, **459**
stool specimens 405
stop codons 351, 358
strength of acids and bases 104-5
streptococci 375, 376, *377*, 393, **460**
streptomycin 414, **460**
stridor 313, **460**
stroke *see* cerebrovascular accident
strong acid(s) 101, 104
strong base(s) 103, 104
structural formula(e) 32, 157, **440**
subatomic particle(s) 17, 20, **460**
subclavian vein 171, **463**
sublingual artery 212, **429**
substituent(s) 45, **460**
substitution reaction *see* displacement reaction
substrate(s) 43, **460**
sucrase 44, 159, **460**
sucrose 44, 158, **460**
digestion of 159
sugar-phosphate backbone (of DNA) 350
sulphonamide(s) 414, 415, **460**
sun, protection from 306
sunburn 305
sunglasses 289-90, 306
super-infection 416
surface tension 61, 62-3, **460**
practical applications 63-4
surfactant 63-4, **460**
surgery
diathermy used 276, 278, **436**
induced hypothermia during 204, 226
lasers used 303
suspensory ligaments 292, *293*, *294*, **460**
suxamethonium chloride 224, **460**
sweat, evaporation of 10, *217*, 218, 221
symbiosis 385, **460**
sympathetic division of nervous system 268, **460**
syncope (fainting) 223, 240
synovial fluid 89, 235, **460**
synovial joint 235, **460**
synthesis reactions *see* combination reactions
syphylis 376, 396, 407, **460**
Système Internationale *see* SI units
systemic radiotherapy **456**
systole 126, **460**
systolic blood pressure 129, 134, **431**

T

T lymphocytes 387, 390, **448**
tachycardia 275, **460**
tachypnoea 88, **460**
tanning 304, 305
tele-radiotherapy 341
telophase 354, **460**
temperature 204, **460**
measurement of 204, 207-9
scales/units 206-7
SI unit *4*, 206, **446**
temperature homeostasis 220-1
temperature regulation 11
abnormalities 221-6
TENS *see* transcutaneous electrical nerve stimulation
testosterone 171, **460**
tetanus/tetany 178, 377, *393*, **461**
tetracyclines 414, 415, **461**
tetrad 356, **461**
thermistor 204, 208, *209*, **461**
see also electronic thermometer
thermometer(s) 207-9, 212-13, **461**
thermoreceptor(s) 10, 220, **461**
thermoregulation abnormalities 221-6
thiamine 174
thoracic duct 171, **461**
thrombus 113, **461**
thrush (candidosis) 416, **461**
thymine 350, 358, **461**
thymus gland 387, **461**
thyroid cancer/disorders, diagnosis and treatment of 180, 332, 340, 342
thyroid gland 199, 340, **461**
role in thermoregulation *220*, 221
thyroid-stimulating hormone (TSH) 180, **461**
thyroidectomy 178, **461**
thyrotoxicosis 175, 222, 340, **461**
thyroxine 168, 175, 180, 199, 221, 340, **461**
tinnitus 321, 416, **461**
tissue cultures 410
tocopherols 174, **461**
tonicity 82-4, **461**
torque 241, **461**
Torricelli's barometer 124-5
toxin-forming bacteria *393*

toxoid(s) 392, **461**
trachea 313
tracheotomy 117, **461**
transcription (in protein synthesis) 357–9, **461**
transcutaneous electrical nerve stimulation (TENS) 278–9, **461**
transducer 323, **462**
transfer RNA (tRNA) 357, **457**
transformer 263, **462**
translation (in protein synthesis) 357, 359–60, **462**
translucent substances 287
transparent substances 287
transverse wave(s) 284–5, 313, **463**
triglyceride(s) 166, *167*, **441**
trimethoprin 415, **462**
triplet **462**
trisomy-21 369
trypsin 164, **462**
trypsinogen 164, **462**
tryptophan 176, **462**
TSH *see* thyroid-stimulating hormone
tuberculosis 374, 395, 407, 410, **462**
tumour *see* neoplasm
tuning fork 312–13
tympanic membrane 124, 209, 317, *318*, **462**
tympanic membrane thermometer 204, 209, *210*, 213, **461**
Tyndall effect 66, **462**

U

ulcer(s) 101, **462**
  blood loss due to 179
  see also gastric ulcers; pressure ulcers
ultrasound 322–3, **462**
  use in body 323
ultraviolet radiation 187, 286, 303–4, **462**
  effects 305, 413
  protection from 306
underwater seal drainage system (intercostal drain) 142
units 4–6
  see also SI units
unsaturated fats 46, 166–7, 191, **462**
unsaturated hydrocarbons 46
unstable equilibrium 244
uracil 350, 358, **462**
uranium-238 (^{238}U) 331–2, *333*
urea 165, 198, **462**
urgency (need to void) 403, **462**
urinalysis 158, 198, 403, **462**
urinary catheter 236, 405
urinary system 9
urine
  pH range *105*
  specific gravity range 93
  specimens 403–5

V

vaccination 391–2
vacuole 388, *389*, **462**
vacuum flask 216–17
valence shell 28, **462**
valency 28, **462**
vancomycin 415, **463**
vaporisation, latent heat of 209, **447**
vaso-active substances 88, 389
vasoconstriction 137, 206, 221, 240, **463**
vasodilation 136, 221, **463**
vasopressin 91
vector(s) 232, 249–50, **463**
vegan/vegetarian diet 162
vein **463**
velocity 232, **463**
  of light 285, 288
vena cava 125, **463**
veneral disease
  serological test for 407
  see also gonorrhoeae; syphilis
venous blood, partial pressure of gases in 145, *146*
ventilators 117, 258
ventricle(s) *272*, *273*, **463**
ventricular fibrillation 275, **463**
  causes 225, 264–5, 266
  treatment 265
Venturi barrel 149, **463**
Venturi nozzle 148
venule(s) 86, **463**
vertebrae, discs between 248
very-low-density lipoproteins (VLDL) 171
vestibular membrane *318*, 319, **463**
vibrio 376, *377*, **463**
villi 77, 165, **463**
vinegar *see* ethanoic acid
viral illnesses 378–9
virulence (of microorganisms) 386, 392–3, **463**
virus(es) 378–80, **463**
  cultivation in laboratory 410
  replication of 379–80
visceral pleura 140, *141*
visible light spectrum 286
vision 284
visual cortex 298
vitamin A 173

vitamin B group 175-6, 367
vitamin C *100*, 172, 177
vitamin D 173
  synthesis in body 305
vitamin E 174
vitamin K 174
vitamins 43, 45, 172-7, **463**
  fat-soluble 172-4
  water-soluble 174-7
vitreous humour 292, *293*, **463**
vocal cords 313
volt (SI unit) *4*, 261, **463**
volume, SI units *4*, 6, **448**

W

warfarin 174, **463**
water 58-61
  chemical bonding in 30, 59-60
  density of 93
  distribution within body 86
  meniscus *62*
  pH 106
  polar nature of 31, 60-1, 70
  states of matter 56-8
water balance, regulation of 10, 91-2, *217*, 218, 221
water loss, factors affecting 92
water-soluble vitamins 174-7
watt (SI unit) *4*, 263, **463**
wave(s) **463**
  longitudinal 312-13, **463**
  transverse 284-5, 313, **463**
wavelength 285, 313, **463**
weak acid(s) 102, 104
weak base(s) 103, 104
weight 233, **463**
Wernicke-Korsakoff syndrome 175
whiplash injury 237, *238*
white light 286
  splitting into separate colours 289
work, definition 186, 190
wound specimens 406

X

X-ray 286, 330, 331, 335-6, **464**
X-ray imaging techniques 339-40
X-ray tube 331, 335, **464**
xerophthalmia 173, **463**

Z

Ziehl-Neelsson stain 410-11
zoonotic infection 396, **445**
zwitterion(s) 108, **464**
zymogenic cells (chief cells) 164, **464**